Sexually Transmitted Diseases
and
AIDS

Sexually Transmitted Diseases
and
AIDS

Editor-in-Chief
Vinod K Sharma, MD, MNAMS
Professor and Head,
Department of Dermatology and Venereology,
All India Institute of Medical Sciences,
New Delhi, India

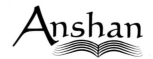

This edition published in 2004

Anshan Limited
6 Newlands Road
Tunbridge Wells
Kent TN4 9AT
UK.
Tel/Fax: +44 (0) 1893557767
E-mail: info@anshan.co.uk
www.anshan.co.uk

Published by arrangement with

Viva Books Private Limited, 4262/3 Ansari Road, New Delhi 110 002, India.

British Library Cataloguing in Publication Data
A catalogue record for this book is available from the British Library

ISBN 1-904798-02-0

Cover Design: Vinod K Sharma and Trilokraj Tejasvi
Cover Photograph (Donovanosis): M Ramam
Printed and bound in India by Replika Press Pvt Ltd, India

Dedicated

to

Late **Dr R V Rajam** and **Dr P N Rangaiah**

Pioneers in the Field of Venereology

Preface

Sexually transmitted diseases (STD) have great impact on health of the individual and community. They can cause genital infection, infertility, abortion, still birth, pneumonia, neonatal deaths, and are associated with cervical cancer; death during and after childbirth, birth defects, impaired vision, blindness; shortened life span and death especially in AIDS. The study and knowledge of STD is essential for improving the health of the community. This book was conceived keeping these aspects in view and an effort was made to address all aspects. STD are more dynamic than other infections and their prevalence and clinical profile varies especially in developing countries like India where syphilis, chancroid and donovanosis are prevalent. However, the picture is undergoing change at fast pace and bacterial STD are becoming less common and viral STD are increasing. The advent of AIDS has caused a sea change in the attitude of all concerned. The STD were a trivial nuisance and now with arrival of AIDS they have become a matter of national concern. We have accorded a high priority to AIDS and STD prevalent in developing countries in this book. STD have a special impact on women and children and this subject has been extensively covered. The prevention of STD especially in viral infections is the only remedy available and special chapters on sexual behaviour, condoms and STD have been included. The NACO is making unprecedented efforts in control of STD and implementing syndromic approach which has been incorporated. The book is meant for postgraduates in dermatology & venereology and general practitioner involved in the care of STD and AIDS. The book has included not only international guidelines of treatment recommended by CDC and WHO but also NACO guidelines for treatment.

The book also includes an Atlas on STD and AIDS along with chapters on clinical approach to a patient with genital ulcer disease, urethral and vaginal discharge. This would help general practitioners and general duty medical officers in the management of STD.

Vinod Kumar Sharma

Acknowledgement

I would like to acknowledge the great opportunity and encouragement provided by Dr C N Sowmini, Patron, Indian Association for the Study of Sexually Transmitted Diseases & AIDS. I am thankful to all the members of the editorial board who gave the constructive suggestions and timely help. I am thankful to all the authors who contributed their best-prepared and revised chapters within the deadline. I must acknowledge the enthusiasm of my young team of resident doctors from the Department of Dermatology and Venereology, All India Institutes of Medical Sciences, New Delhi. I especially acknowledge Dr G Sethuraman and Dr Trilokraj Tejasvi who were involved in many aspects of this endeavour. I also thank Dr Binod K Khaitan and Dr Neena Khanna for the fruitful discussion during the preparation of this book.

I also acknowledge my publisher Viva Books Private Limited and Replika Press Pvt Ltd for following the instruction to last detail.

Vinod Kumar Sharma

Contributors

Veena Acharya, MS, Diploma in STD
Professor
Department of Gynaecology and Obstetrics
Zanana Hospital
S M S Medical College, Jaipur

Praveen Aggarwal, MD
Additional Professor
Department of Medicine
AIIMS, New Delhi 110 029
peekay_124@hotmail.com

P N Arora, MD, SFCP
Former Professor and Head
Department of Dermatovenereology
Armed Forces Medical College, Pune
Visiting consultant
Indraprastha Apollo Hospitals, New Delhi
pranarora18@yahoo.co.in

S Arora, MD
Dermatologist
Base Hospital, New Delhi 110 010
sarora@vsnl.com

Ashok K Bajaj, MD, FICAI
Former Professor and Head
Department of Dermatology
M L N Medical College Allahabad, Uttar Pradesh
bajajak@sancharnet.in

C Balachandran, MD
Professor and Head
Department of Skin and STD
Kasturba Medical College and Hospital
Manipal 576 119
drbalanair@yahoo.com

R Ganesh, MD, DV
Professor and Head
Department of STD
Tirunelveli Medical College and Hospital
Palayamkottai
Tirunelvelli 627 002, Tamil Nadu
ganeshsharma@eth.net

Sarala Gopalan, FRCOG, PhD, FAMS
Professor and Head
Department of Gynaecology and Obstetrics
PGIMER, Chandigarh 160 012
gopalansarala@rediffmail.com

Dinesh C Govil, MD, DVD
Professor and Head
Department of Skin, VD and Leprosy
M L B Medical College
Jhansi 284 128, Uttar Pradesh
drdineshgovil@hotmail.com

Usha Gupta, MD (Skin, VD & Leprosy), PhD in Dermatology, MD (Pathology & Microbiology), DGO
Assistant Professor and Head
Department of Dermatology, STD and Leprosy
NSCB Medical College
Jabalpur, Madhya Pradesh

Rohini Handa, MD
Additional Professor
Department of Medicine, AIIMS, New Delhi 110 029
rohinihanda@hotmail.com

S Handa, MD
Assistant Professor
Department of Dermatology, Venereology and Leprology
PGIMER, Chandigarh 160 012
handa_sanjeev@yahoo.com

H R Jerajani, MD
Professor & Head
Department of Dermatology
L T M Medical College and L T M General Hospital
Sion, Mumbai 400 022
jerajani@rediffmail.com/jerajani@vsnl.com

P L Joshi, MD, MNAMS
Joint Director, Govt. of India
Ministry of Health & Family Welfare
NACO, "Chandra lok", 9th floor, Janpath
New Delhi 110 001

Jaswinder Kalra, MD
Associate Professor
Department of Gynaecology and Obstetrics
PGIMER, Chandigarh 160 012

Sumeet Kane, MBBS
Department of Dermatology
LTM Medical College and LTM General Hospital
Sion, Mumbai

H K Kar, MD, MNAMS
Senior Consultant and Head
Department of Dermatology
Dr Ram Manohar Lohia Hospital, New Delhi
hkkar_2000@yahoo.com

Binod K Khaitan, MD
Assistant Professor
Department of Dermatology and Venereology
AIIMS, New Delhi 110 029
binodkhaitan@hotmail.com

Neena Khanna, MD
Additional Professor
Department of Dermatology and Venereology
AIIMS, New Delhi 110 029
akhanna@mantraonline.com

Sujay Khandpur, MD, DNB, MNAMS
Assistant Professor
Department of Dermatology and Venereology
AIIMS, New Delhi 110 029
shaifalikhandpur@eth.net

Ashok Kumar, MD
Additional Professor and Head
Division of Rheumatology
Department of Medicine, AIIMS, New Delhi 110 029
ashok_145@hotmail.com

Joginder Kumar, MD
Consultant, Department of Dermatology and
Venereology, Safdarjung Hospital, New Delhi

A J Kanwar, MD
Professor
Department of Dermatology, Venereology and
Leprology
PGIMER, Chandigarh 160 012
kd_sandhu@yahoo.co.in

B Loganathan, MD, DV
Former Professor & Head
Kilpak Medical College and Govt. Royapettah
Hospital, Chennai, Tamil Nadu

Sameer Malhotra, MD
Assistant Professor
National Drug Dependence Treatment Centre
Department of Psychiatry
AIIMS, New Delhi 110 029
sameersankalp@hotmail.com

J K Maniar, MD, DVD, DDV
Former Professor of Dermatovenereology and AIDS
Medicine
Grant Medical College, Mumbai.
Consulting AIDS Physician, Jaslok Hospital and
Research Centre, The Bhatia General Hospital and
Masina Hospital, Mumbai.
jkmaniar@vsnl.com

Yogesh S Marfatia, MD
Professor and Head
Department of Skin and VD
Medical College, SSG Hospital, Vadodara 390 001
ym11256@yahoo.com

Dinesh Mathur, MD(Skin), MD (Medicine)
Professor
Department of Skin and STD, Nodal officer AIDS
Control
S M S Medical College and Hospital, Jaipur
drdineshmathur@yahoo.com

R D Mehta, MD
Assistant Professor
Department of Skin and VD
S P Medical College, Bikaner 334 003
mehtard@datainfosys.net

R S Misra, MD
Skin Care Centre
P-I, Prasad Nagar, New Delhi 110 005
drrsm@usa.net

S Mohan, MD, DV
Registrar
Institute of Venereology
Madras Medical College
Chennai 600 003, Tamil Nadu

S Murugan, MD, DV
Former Professor and Head
Department of STD
Govt. Mohan Kumara Mangalam Medical College
Salem, Tamil Nadu
malamurugan@yahoo.com

K P Narendar, MD
Director, Institute of Venereology
Madras Medical College
Chennai 600 002, Tamil Nadu
venereology@helinfinet.com

K Neeladri Raju, MD
Professor of STD
Gandhi Hospital
Secunderabad, Andhra Pradesh
drbenj_anil@rediffmail.com

Sathish Pai B, MD
Associate Professor
Department of Skin and STD
Kasturba Medical College and Hospital
Manipal 576 119

M Ramam, MD
Associate Professor
Department of Dermatology and Venereology
AIIMS, New Delhi 110 029
mramam@hotmail.com

Majumdar Sabyasachi, MBBS
A-13, Vivekanand Apartment
238, NSC Bose Road, Narendrapur, West Bengal

G C Saha, MD
17/13D, Biplabi Barin
Ghosh Sarani
Kolkata 700 067, West Bengal

Pradeep Seth, MD
Professor and Head
Department of Microbiology
AIIMS, New Delhi 110 029
pseth@aiims.aiims.ac.in

Sunil Sethi, MD
Assistant Professor
Department of Medical Microbiology
PGIMER, Chandigarh 160 012

G Sethuraman, MD
Assistant Professor
Department of Dermatology and Venereology
AIIMS, New Delhi 110 029
kgsethu@yahoo.com

Meera Sharma, MD
Professor and Head
Department of Medical Microbiology
PGIMER, Chandigarh 160 012

R K Sharma, MD
Additional Professor
Department of Forensic Medicine
AIIMS, New Delhi 110 029
rksharma1@hotmail.com

Rajeev Sharma, MD
Consultant Dermatologist
Bishen Skin Centre
M-69, Marris Road, Aligarh 202 001
dermdoc@sancharnet.in

Vinod K Sharma, MD, MNAMS
Professor and Head
Department of Dermatology and Venereology
AIIMS, New Delhi 110 029
aiimsvks@yahoo.com

O P Singh, MD
Associate Professor
Department of Dermatology and Venereology
AIIMS, New Delhi 110 029
dsop@rediffmail.com

C S Sirka, MD
Assistant Professor
Department of Dermatology and Venereology
AIIMS, New Delhi 110 029
sirkacs@indiatimes.com

Joseph A Sundharam, MD
Sundharam's Dermatology and Pediatric Centre
Office No.1, KD Market, Pitampura, Delhi 110 034
joseph@mantraonline.com

Gurvinder P Thami, MD
Reader in Dermatology
Govt. Medical College, Chandigarh 160 031
drgurvinder@mantraonline.com

Devinder M Thappa, MD, DHA, MNAMS
Professor and Head
Department of Dermatology and STD
JIPMER, Pondicherry 605 006
dmthappa@satyam.net.in

Trilokraj Tejasvi, MD
Senior Resident
Department of Dermatology and Venereology
AIIMS, New Delhi 110 029
trilokraj_a@yahoo.com

B M Tripathi, MD
Additional Professor
National Drug Dependence Treatment Center
Department of Psychiatry
AIIMS, New Delhi 110 029
bmt_54@yahoo.com

N Usman, MD, DV, PhD
Professor and Head
Department of STD
Kilpak Medical College and Govt. Royapettah
Hospital, Chennai 600 014.
atharusman786@hotmail.com

Madhu Vajpayee, MD
Assistant Professor
Department of Microbiology
AIIMS, New Delhi 110 029
mvajpayee@hotmail.com

K Venkateswaran, MD, DV
Assistant Professor
Institute of Venereology
Madras Medical college
Chennai 600 003, Tamil Nadu

Jyoti Prakash Wali, MD
Professor of Medicine
AIIMS, New Delhi 110 029
jpwali@hotmail.com

Nitin S Walia, MD, DNB
Classified specialist
(Dermatology & STD)
Military Hospital, Secunderabad
Trimulghery, Secunderabad, Andhra Pradesh
slg_nitin@sancharnet.in

Contributors to the Colour Atlas

Vinod K Sharma, MD, MNAMS
Professor and Head
Department of Dermatology and Venereology
AIIMS, New Delhi 110 029
aiimsvks@yahoo.com

J K Maniar, MD, DVD, DDV
Former Professor of Dermatovenereology and
AIDS Medicine, Grant Medical College, Mumbai.
Consulting AIDS Physician, Jaslok Hospital and
Research Centre, The Bhatia General Hospital and
Masina Hospital, Mumbai.
jkmaniar@vsnl.com

R S Misra, MD
Skin Care Centre
P-I, Prasad Nagar
New Delhi 110 005
drrsm@usa.net

P N Arora, MD, SFCP
Former Professor and Head
Department of Dermatovenereology
Armed Forces Medical College, Pune
Visiting consultant
Indraprastha Apollo Hospitals
New Delhi
pranarora18@yahoo.co.in

O P Singh, MD
Associate Professor
Department of Dermatology and Venereology
AIIMS, New Delhi 110 029
dsop@rediffmail.com

M Ramam, MD
Associate Professor
Department of Dermatology and Venereology
AIIMS, New Delhi 110 029
mramam@hotmail.com

Binod K Khaitan, MD
Assistant Professor
Department of Dermatology and Venereology
AIIMS, New Delhi 110 029
binodkhaitan@hotmail.com

G Sethuraman, MD
Assistant Professor
Department of Dermatology and Venereology
AIIMS, New Delhi 110 029
kgsethu@yahoo.com

Manoj K Singh, MD
Additional Professor
Department of Pathology
AIIMS, New Delhi 110 029
makusi@hotmail.com

Devinder M Thappa, MD, DHA, MNAMS
Professor and Head
Department of Dermatology and STD
JIPMER, Pondicherry 605 006
dmthappa@satyam.net.in

S Handa, MD
Assistant Professor
Department of Dermatology, Venereology and
Leprology, PGIMER, Chandigarh 160 012
handa_sanjeev@yahoo.com

Figures Contributed to the Colour Atlas

Vinod K Sharma

Figures 3, 5, 17, 18, 34, 36, 38, 53, 54, 61, 66, 76, 78, 80-83, 87-89, 98, 99, 101, 103

J K Maniar

Figures 1, 2, 4, 5, 7-16, 19-28

O P Singh

Figures 44, 45, 49-51, 55, 58, 64, 65, 67, 68, 70-72, 79, 90, 93, 94, 97

P N Arora

Figures 40, 46, 59, 75, 84, 85, 91, 92, 95

R S Misra

Figures 29, 31, 32, 33, 47, 52, 60, 63

M Ramam

Figures 30, 37, 41, 62, 86, 96, 100, 104

Binod K Khaitan

Figures 35, 39, 42, 44, 45, 56, 58, 102

Sanjeev Handa

Figures 43, 48, 57

G Sethuraman / M K Singh

Figures 69, 77

Devinder M Thappa

Figure 74

Contents

Section 2 : VIRAL AND MISCELLANEOUS SEXUALLY TRANSMITTED DISEASES

Section 3 : SEXUALLY TRANSMITTED PROTOZOAL DISEASES

Section 4 : SEXUALLY TRANSMITTED DISEASES ASSOCIATED SYNDROMES

PART V : SEXUALLY TRANSMITTED DISEASES IN SPECIAL SITUATIONS

PART VI : DRUG RESISTANCE

PART VII : CONTROL OF SEXUALLY TRANSMITTED DISEASES

PART VIII : NON-VENEREAL SKIN DISEASES OF GENITALIA

PART IX : PSYCHOLOGICAL ASPECTS OF SEXUALLY TRANSMITTED DISEASES

PART I
General

Chapter 1

Epidemiology of Sexually Transmitted Diseases

Vinod K Sharma, Sujay Khandpur

Introduction

Sexually transmitted diseases (STD) include diseases that are transmitted by sexual intercourse. Sexual transmission requires the agent to be present in one partner, the other partner to be susceptible to infection with that agent and that the sex partners engage in sexual practices which can transmit the pathogen.

Sexually transmitted infections (STI) differs from sexually transmitted disease (STD) in that STD conventionally includes infections resulting in clinical diseases that may involve the genitalia and other parts of the body participating in sexual interaction eg. syphilis, gonorrhoea, chancroid, donovanosis, non-gonococcal urethritis, genital warts, herpes genitalis etc. STI in addition, includes infections that may not cause clinical disease of genitals, but are transmitted by sexual interaction eg. all STD and hepatitis B, HIV, HTLV-1 etc. Now a days, the term STI is preferred, since it covers all the diseases that can be transmitted by sexual intercourse. **However, for all practical purposes, both STI and STD are used synonymously.**

STD have been known to exist since time immemorial. Medical descriptions date back to the 15th century in Europe where syphilis and gonorrhoea were primarily responsible for the abandonment of public baths. The golden era of microbiology in the late 19th and early 20th centuries identified the microbes responsible for the five traditional venereal diseases- gonorrhoea, syphilis, chancroid, lymphogranuloma venereum and donovanosis. After World War II, new diagnostic techniques and defined clinical and epidemiological studies in North America and Europe established that many 'non-traditional' microbes could also produce infections when transmitted sexually (Table 1).

In the United States, of the top 11 reportable diseases in 1996, five were transmitted sexually (gonorrhoea, chlamydial infection, syphilis, hepatitis B and AIDS). STD rank among the five leading health problems in the developing countries.[1] WHO estimated that during 1995, 400 million cases including 333 million new cases of curable STD occurred in adults globally, of which 150 million were in the South and South-East Asia including 50 million in India.[2] These diseases are endemic in the tropics and the morbidity and mortality caused by them now rivals that by *Plasmodium falciparum* malaria in several African and Asian Nations. STD and HIV may be responsible for up to 17% of productive years lost to disease in certain regions.

STD have a tremendous impact on national health. They are responsible for significant proportion of maternal morbidity, ectopic pregnancy, infant illness and death, malignancies, infertility and increased susceptibility to HIV infection. They are one of the major causes of infertility in both women and men. STD are also one of the significant contributors to foetal death, abortions and low birth weight (Table 2). HIV infection is the most significant STD that has resulted in widespread deaths having considerable impact on the social and economic survival of countries especially in Africa. It is also responsible for renewed interest in the STD and their control.

The epidemiology of STD results from the interaction between STD pathogens, the bahaviours that transmit them and the effectiveness of prevention and control interventions. The epidemiological patterns are very distinct and differ from other diseases since their incubation periods are highly variable, the genetic structure of most of the STD pathogens are so diverse that the researchers have been unable to design a vaccine against them and these diseases are primarily spread by

Table 1.   Sexually Transmitted Agents and Diseases

S. No.	Agents	Disease or Syndrome	Complications
1.	**Bacteria**		
	Neisseria gonorrhoeae	Urethritis, epididymitis, bartholinitis, cervicitis, endometritis, salpingitis, proctitis, pharyngitis	Infertility, ectopic pregnancy, chorioamnionitis, premature rupture of membranes, premature delivery, conjunctivitis, PID, Disseminated gonococcal infection (DGI)
	Chlamydia trachomatis D-K	Urethritis, epididymitis, bartholinitis, cervicitis, endometritis, salpingitis, proctitis, pharyngitis	Same as gonorhoea except DGI, Reiter's syndrome, pneumonia
	Chlamydia trachomatis L1, L2, L3	Lymphogranuloma venereum	Esthiomene, ano-recto-genital syndrome, proctocolitis, skin rashes, pneumonia, hepatitis, meningoencephalitis
	Treponema pallidum	Syphilis- primary, secondary, latent	Benign tertiary syphilis, neurosyphilis, cardiovascular syphilis
	Haemophilus ducreyi	Chancroid	Phimosis, sclerosis, meatal stenosis
	Calymmatobacterium granulomatis	Donovanosis	Phimosis, sclerosis, SCC
	Mycoplasma hominis	Non-gonococcal urethritis, cervicitis, salpingitis	PID, postpartum fever
	Ureaplasma urealyticum	Non-gonococcal urethritis, cervicitis, salpingitis	Chorioamnionitis, low birth weight
	Gardnerella vaginalis and others	Bacterial vaginosis	
	Group B *β-hemolytic streptococcus*		Neonatal sepsis, neonatal meningitis
2.	**Viruses**		
	Herpes simplex virus 1,2	Primary and recurrent genital herpes	Aseptic meningitis, neonatal herpes and associated mortality or neurological sequelae, spontaneous abortion, premature delivery
	Human papilloma virus	Condyloma acuminata	Laryngeal papilloma in infants, squamous epithelial neoplasia of cervix, anus, vagina, vulva and penis
	Hepatitis B virus	Acute, chronic and fulminant hepatitis	Cirrhosis, hepatocellular carcinoma
	Cytomegalovirus	Infectious mononucleosis	Congenital infection, birth defects, infant mortality, cognitive impairment (mental retardation, sensorineural deafness), protean manifestations in immunocompromized hosts
	Molluscum contagiosum virus	Genital molluscum contagiosum	Infection, eczematoid dermatitis, erythema annulare centrifugum
	HIV (Human immunode ficiency virus)	AIDS and related conditions	Opportunistic infections, death
	Human T-lymphotropic virus (HTLV-10)	T-cell leukemia, lymphoma, tropical spastic paraparesis	Death
3.	**Protozoa**		
	Trichomonas vaginalis	Urethritis, balanitis, vaginitis	
4.	**Fungus**		
	Candida albicans	Vulvovaginitis, balanitis, balanoposthitis	
5.	**Ectoparasites**		
	Phthirus pubis	Pubic lice infestation	
	Sarcoptes scabiei	Scabies	Norwegian scabies in immunocompromised host

Table 2. Morbidity Due to Sexually Transmitted Diseases

S.No.	Disease	Morbidity
1.	Gonorrhoea	Reproductive morbidity in men and women (infertility), impaired vision, blindness
2.	Chlamydial infection	Infertility in adults, neonatal death, impaired vision and blindness
3.	Lymphogranuloma venereum	Genital deformity, obstruction during delivery, carcinoma
4.	Syphilis	Involvement of heart and brain, impaired vision and blindness, abortions, foetal and infant deaths
5.	Chancroid	Destruction of genitalia
6.	Donovanosis	Genital destruction, carcinoma, bone involvement (rarely)
7.	Mycoplasma infection	infertility
8.	Ureaplasma infection	Infertility, foetal morbidity, low birth weight
9.	Bacterial vaginosis	Female genital tract infection
10.	Group B *β-hemolytic streptococcus*	Septicaemia, multiorgan failure
11.	Genital herpes	Severe neonatal infection and death, female genital tract cancer (implicated)
12.	Human papillomavirus infection	Respiratory tract obstruction, premalignant and malignant disease of genitalia
13.	Hepatitis B infection	Chronic liver disease, hepatic carcinoma, death
14.	Cytomegalovirus infection	Severe neonatal multiorgan involvement, birth defects
15.	Molluscum contagiosum virus infection	Spread of infection to partner and family members
16.	HIV	Multisystemic involvement, malignancy, death
17.	Trichomoniasis	Reproductive tract infection in men and women
18.	Candida infection	Genital involvement, neonatal complications
19.	Pthriasis	Infection, spread to partner and community
20.	Scabies	Severe skin infection, septicemia, spread to household and community

a class of behaviour which is inherently resistant to change because it is highly motivated and varies considerably within and between social and ethnic groups.

A variety of demographic and medical factors contribute to the high prevalence of STD, especially in the developing countries, where a large percentage of population belongs to the sexually active age-group.[3] Rural to urban migration in these countries has led to family separation and unbalanced sex ratios in both rural and urban areas, loss of traditional values of sexual behaviour and increased sexual promiscuity. In most traditional societies, the stigma associated with STD is still strong and embarrassment may prevent infected persons from seeking medical treatment, thereby increasing the reservoir of infection. The incidence and distribution of these diseases is also influenced by factors such as the lifestyle and susceptibility of the individual, pathogenicity of the microbes, prevailing therapy and disease control measures. A complex set of behavioural factors also determine the risk of acquiring STD (Table 3). Moreover, cure after appropriate antibiotic therapy is no longer certain for some infections such as gonorrhoea and chancroid because of the growing antibiotic resistance.

In the era of HIV infection, there is a resurgence of interest in STD amongst both researchers and health policy makers since their role in facilitating transmission

Table 3. Determinants of Sexually Transmitted Diseases

Behavioural Risk Factors	High risk Groups
Age at first intercourse	CSW
Marital status	Drivers
Frequency of sexual intercourse	Restaurant workers
Number of lifetime partners	Prison inmates
Rate and type of partners recruited	Transsexuals
Age difference between partners	
Addictions- crack cocaine, IV drug-use, alcohol, smoking	

High Risk Sexual Practices	Health Care Behaviour
Receptive and insertive ano-genital intercourse	Contraception: barrier, OCP, IUD
Oro-anal intercourse	Circumcision
Oro-genital intercourse	
Receptive manual-anal intercourse	
Dry sex	
Sex during menstruation	
Vaginal douching	

Demographic and Social correlates
Age
Gender
Education
Socioeconomic status
Ethnicity

of HIV has been well established. Given this situation, the control of STD to prevent the transmission of HIV infection is now considered a public health priority. This recognition has also led to an increased focus on STD cases to be managed at the primary health care level using the syndromic approach in order to reduce their global burden.

The epidemiological profile of STD is more dynamic than many other diseases. Most published data about STD rates is based on surveillance systems that rely heavily on reports from STD, gynecological and family planning clinics. Surveillance data provide valuable information, especially regarding long-term trends, but they represent a biased sample derived from limited subpopulations, which are subject to change over time. Many of the STD rates, especially those obtained from the developing countries are unreliable due to delay in presentation of the disease to a health care facility, lower rate of self-reported STD, lack of recognition of small or asymptomatic lesions as an STD problem and the non-availability of skilled personnel and specific diagnostic tests in most of the Centres. The current trend is to undertake large population-based surveys by experts, supported by necessary diagnostic tests in order to estimate the STD prevalence.

In the developed countries, there has been a steady increase in STD rates, especially the viral STD and genital chlamydia infection, since the development of sophisticated diagnostic tests has helped in the recognition of widespread reservoirs of subclinical infections. In the STD clinics in UK, a 9% increase in the incidence of acute STD was observed between 1996 and 1997.[4] The annual number of genital herpes has almost tripled during the past 15 years in England. This has forced a reappraisal of the importance of sexual and health care behaviour and use of contraceptive devices, since control of the incurable viral STD depends to a great extent on societal efforts at primary prevention through health education and Counselling of the infected carrier rather than early diagnosis and treatment of the disease, which is an effective strategy for the curable bacterial STD. A rapid decline in the incidence of syphilis has been observed in the white communities with however, stable or even increasing rates among the blacks.[5] This rise has occurred especially among the urban, poor and minority populations, particularly among adolescents, with the highest rates recorded among adolescent females. Prostitution has emerged as an STD multiplier and the phenomenon of sex in exchange for drugs has contributed to epidemic spread of syphilis, gonorrhoea

and chancroid in North America. There has been a constant decline in the incidence of gonorrhoea especially among the heterosexual men and all women.[6] However, it has been on the increase in homosexual men.[7,8]

In the developing world, 10-20% of the adult patients attend government health facilities because of STD.[9] In Delhi, between 1954 and 1994, the number of STD cases increased 8 times. However, these figures are most certainly an underestimate, since the infections are rarely treated in the official health sector, patients preferring to visit traditional healers, quacks, pharmacists or private practitioners who are more accessible and less judgemental in their attitudes. In the 1970s and early 1980s, syphilis and chancroid were the main causes of genital ulcer disease (GUD), while the viral GUD such as genital herpes were so rare that they even merited publication as case reports.[10] In India it was recorded under 'other minor STD. The spread of HIV since the late 1980s with subsequent Behavioral change has resulted in significant alterations in STD epidemic patterns, and similar to the developed countries, there is a significant rise in viral STD and a relative fall in the incidence of the traditional infections. In the 1980s, herpes infection accounted for 17% of the genital ulcers in Singapore and 12% in Bangkok. The incidence of gonorrhoea is still very high in African and Asian countries. In the early 90s, the incidence of gonococcal urethritis in Africa was estimated to be approximately 10% annually.[11] Numerous surveys conducted in recent years have shown that gonorrhoea is the commonest cause of male urethritis accounting for approximately 53% - 80% of the cases.[12] In India also, gonorrhoea is a major health problem.

Risk Factors and Risk Behaviours In STD (Table 3)

Determinants of risk of STD including HIV infection and STD distribution patterns include a complex set of ecological and behavioural factors. In industrialized countries, behavioural surveys have provided important insights to help guide public health intervention for preventing STD.

Behavioural Risk Factors

Sexual behaviour is a largely private activity, subject to varying degrees of social, cultural, religious, moral and legal norms and constraints. The behavioural risk factors are related to greater probability of exposure to STD, acquiring the disease and higher risk of developing complications. They play a key role in acquiring the incurable viral STD. The behavioural determinants include age at first intercourse or 'coitarche', marital status of the individual, frequency of sexual intercourse, number of lifetime partners, rate and type of sexual partners recruited, rate of partner change, number of current relationships, age difference between partners, sexual mixing with high risk groups such as commercial sex workers (CSW), truck drivers, mine workers etc., addictions such as drug abuse, alcoholism and smoking and types of sexual practices (vaginal, anal or oral intercourse).

Age at First Intercourse

There is a strong association between the acquisition of STD and young age at first intercourse. Early sexual debut leads to higher rates of partner exchange and greater chance of STD transmission. It also has a bearing on the development of a specific disease. It has been associated with cervical cancer owing to the biological development of the cervix during the teenage period. In a survey conducted in South Africa, the median age at first sex of HIV-positive individuals was 16.6 years for men and 17.2 years for women.[13] The tremendous rise in STD and HIV in this region was possibly due to rise in the proportion of sexually active women aged 15 to 19 years from 57% in 1994 to 67.5% in 1999. In two sub-Saharan urban population groups, women with STD were found to have their sexual debut before age 15.[14] In a survey in Peru, 51% of men with STD had their first intercourse between 15-17 years.[15] Moreover, a greater percentage of women who initiated sexual activity before 18 years of age had antibodies to *Chlamydia trachomatis* than women indulging in sex after 18 years (23% vs 9%). In a study from Sweden, women attaining sexual debut at mean of 15.3 years had greater frequency of genital signs including abnormal vaginal discharge, erythema of the vaginal mucosa, lower genital tract infection as compared to women with sexual debut at mean age of 20.7 years.[16] Similarly, a higher incidence of gonorrhoea, chlamydial infection and genital warts was observed among the teenage population, in a study from Thames, England.[4] A strong correlation has been observed between early age of first intercourse and acquisition of HPV infection, which may be explained by more

visits to prostitutes by husbands of cases with early sexual debut.[17] In several Indian studies, the average age of sexual debut in STD clinic attendees has been observed to be between 15-20 years.[18-21]

Marital Status

Several studies from India and abroad have shown that married individuals especially women are at higher risk of acquiring STD and HIV.[13,14,18-23] This can be explained by the fact that women acquire an additional sex partner after marriage, who is more likely to be infected than casual partners before marriage, since he is older. In addition, a higher frequency of unprotected sex within a marriage results in higher probability of disease transmission compared with casual partnerships where sexual intercourse is less frequent. In two studies from Delhi, majority (54.5% and 62.4% respectively) of the STD patients were married, even though 91.2% of the men had acquired STD outside marriage while 88.1% of the women acquired it from their spouses.[18,24]

Number of Life-time Sexual Partners

Risk of exposure to an STD and the development of cervical and other genital cancers is directly associated with number of lifetime sexual partners, rate of partner recruitment and partner change. However, this correlation is complicated by differences in patterns with respect to choice of partner, partners' own sexual behaviour and the degree of his infectiousness. In the Peruvian study, a direct correlation was noted between STD seropositivity and presence of more than 20 sex partners.[15] In South Africa, HSV-2 seropositivity was also related to the number of partners, the mean number in men being 4.7 and in women, 2.6.[13] In an American study, patients with cervical HPV infection had a mean of 4.8 sex partners as compared to 2.6 for controls.[17] This correlation has been demonstrated in Indian studies as well.[18-24] In 1996, in Delhi/Haryana, the proportion of sexually active persons having atleast one sex partner other than the regular partner in the last 12 months was 2.5, in Maharashtra it was 3.2, in Tamil Nadu 4.2 and in West Bengal, it was 2.7. This has been one of the major cause of rise in STD prevalence in India.[25]

Age Difference Between Sexual Partners

Few studies have shown that a greater age difference

(>11 years) between sexual partners was found to increase the risk of STD and HIV, especially in women.[14]

High-Risk Groups

Commercial Sex Worker (CSW)

CSW or prostitute is defined as a person who provides sexual service for money or other material gains. They include those who work in brothels, night clubs, hotels, massage parlours or bars or are casual freelance sex workers. Contact with CSW has been implicated as an important risk factor for STD transmission, because they experience higher rate of partner change, longer period of exposure to infection, poorer access to health care facilities and efficient transmission from sexual exposure. The role of prostitutes has been assessed by monitoring the incidence of STD in this group and the proportion of male STD patients who acknowledge recent sex with a prostitute. The incidence of STD is directly related to early age of commencement of sexual work, longer duration of prostitution and the current age of the CSW. In Mexico in 1999, significantly high HSV-2 seroprevalence (60.8%) was recorded among the prostitutes.[26] Infection with high-risk and multiple HPV types was also high with the highest rates recorded among younger women. In Japan, CSW showed a greater prevalence of HPV, *C. trachomatis* and gonococcal infection than the control group.[27] In France also, considerably high seroprevalence of anti-HPV type 16, 18, 31 and 58 antibodies was detected in CSW (25%) than the general population (3%), thus indicating that this group is at increased risk of oncogenic infections and that the number of sexual partners is a major determinant in acquisition of oncogenic HPV.[28] Numerous epidemiological studies have shown that in developing countries, GUD are most common among CSW. In a cross-sectional survey undertaken among female CSW in Nigeria, a high sero-prevalence of chancroid and syphilis was observed.[29] Lower class CSW were significantly more likely than upper class CSW to be seropositive for syphilis and *Haemophilus ducreyi*. In women seeking primary care for genital discharge syndrome in Madagascar, highest sero-prevalence of bacterial vaginosis (85%), trichomoniasis (16%), cervical infection (49%) and syphilis (16%) was found in prostitutes, followed by occasional sex traders and the general population, with syphilis being associated with low education, young age at coital debut and more

than one partner in the previous 3 months.[30] An etiological study conducted among the CSW in Dhaka, Bangladesh, revealed 84% of the workers to be positive for STD pathogen, 35.5% for gonorrhoea, 25% for chlamydial infection, 45.5% for trichomoniasis, 32.6% for syphilis and 62.5% for HSV-2 infection.[31]

Several studies conducted in India show that majority of the male patients (74.5% to 89%) give history of contact with CSW.[18-24] In Calcutta, in 1994, a high prevalence of STD (80.6%) was observed among the CSW.[32] Oral infection with HSV-1 and 2 and HPV 16/18 was detected in 24.6%, 11.6% and 29% respectively in the prostitutes and cervical infections in 0%, 44% and 63% of the cases, indicating a high prevalence of oral sex in this group. In a survey of the clients visiting a red-light area in Calcutta, seropositivity of HCV was found in 15.1% cases, while syphilis occurred in 40.9% and HbsAg in 20.4% of the clients.[33] In Pune, 81.5% of the CSW were found to be suffering from STD, thus posing a potential risk of transmitting these diseases to their clients.[34] Syphilis was the commonest STD (36.8%) followed by chancroid (31.3%). CSW differed from women engaged in other works in being of older age group, illiterate, unmarried and staying away from home. 47% of CSW were HIV positive as compared to 14% positivity recorded in the control group. A survey from Tirupati, Tamil Nadu, demonstrated HIV seropositivity in 25% of the CSW, primary chancre in 15%, gonorrhoea in 15%, LGV in 10%, donovanosis in 5%, seropositivity for syphilis in 70% and HbsAg in 50% of the CSW.[35]

Unless prevention strategies are enforced in this high risk group, it is estimated that HIV infection among CSW in India would increase from the 1999 level of 2.49 million to 3.93 million in a favourable scenario and to 6.87 million in a worse scenario by 2005.[36] Hence, their continuous surveillance, early diagnosis, appropriate treatment and rigorous follow-up is of utmost importance in limiting the transmission of STD. Moreover, the focus is on prevention of CSW from acquiring an STD by using barrier contraceptives.

Transport Workers (Drivers)

They have been identified as a male occupational group at high risk of STD and AIDS acquisition, who may play an important role in dissemination of these infections because of their geographical mobility. They often come in contact with various types of sex workers such as homosexuals and prostitutes while they are away from their families for long periods. They also get enough time to visit CSW during the time their trucks are being loaded and unloaded. Poverty, illiteracy and low level of awareness about STD and HIV and lack of healthy recreation facilities are other contributing factors. In a study conducted in Pondicherry between 1997 and 1999, truck drivers were found to have the highest rates of HbsAg (23.8%) and HIV (47.6%) and the second highest rate of hepatitis C positivity (42.8%).[37] In another survey from the same city between 1993 and 1997, 51.4% of the truck drivers reacted seropositive for HIV antibodies.[38] In Nagpur, 43.7% of the long distance truck drivers were found to have one or more STD with HIV infection detected in 15.2% cases, syphilis in 21.9%, gonorrhoea in 6.7% and hepatitis B in 5.1% of the cases.[39] In Delhi, 1% of the truck drivers were found to be HIV positive.[40] The risk behaviours included sex with CSW, homosexuality, illiteracy and non-usage of condoms. In a cross section study conducted among long distance truck drivers in Kenya, seroprevalence for syphilis was 4.6%, 26.5% for chancroid and 18% for HIV.[41] In sub-Saharan Africa, among the truck drivers, rates of HIV infection as high as 26-35% have been reported.[41] The STD detected in Bangladesh's trucking industry were HSV-2 (25.8%), syphilis (5.7%), gonorrhoea (2.1%), and chlamydia (0.8%).[42] The significant risk factors were sex with CSW and lower rates of condom use (in 11.8% drivers only).

Restaurant Workers

They are another high risk group in the transmission of STD. In a survey undertaken among the restaurant workers along a highway in Assam, over one-third had sexual contact with multiple partners or CSW and 2% were engaged in homosexual activity. Majority of them were illiterate, 30% were alcoholic and smokers and 3% were addicted to cannabis.[43] GUD was present in 25.7% of the workers, 11.8% had gonorrhoea, while 5.1% were VDRL reactive.

Transsexuals

In the Indian subcontinent, male sex workers are predominantly transvestites and transsexuals known as 'Hijras'. Their origin dates back many centuries to India where Hijras believed themselves to be the incarnation of Lord Krishna. This community now engages in commercial sex and is at high risk for STD and HIV. It indulges mainly in insertive ano-genital intercourse with men. A survey from Karachi, Pakistan in 1999, documented syphilis in 37%, urethritis in 70%, genital warts in 54% and HbsAg positivity in 3.4% of the transvestite sex workers.[44] 57% of these individuals reported sexual abuse in childhood, the average age of first intercourse with consent was 12 years, condom use by their sexual partners was minimal, almost 50% took drugs while 63% consumed alcohol. Hence, intervention strategies planned for this community can have a great impact on STD and HIV prevention.

Prison Inmates

STD tend to cluster in socially excluded populations and such populations are over-represented in prisons. Consequently numerous studies have found high STD rates among prison inmates. Moreover, the increasing imprisonment rate of drug users is linked to the spread of HIV and hepatitis B and C. A study conducted among female prisoners in Brazil revealed high prevalence of STD including syphilis in 16% cases, gonorrhoea in 7.6%, chlamydial infection in 11%, HPV-infection in 9.3%, trichomoniasis in 30%, and bacterial vaginosis in 15% of the inmates.[45] The fourth Australian National HIV/AIDS Strategy has given priority to prisons as potential environments for the spread of STD. In New South Wales prison in Australia, 2% of the male and 1% of the female inmates had confirmed evidence of syphilis.[46] An outbreak of syphilis was reported in Alabama prisons in 1999 as a result of mixing of prisoners with unscreened jail populations, transfer of infected inmates between prisons and multiple concurrent sexual partnerships.[47] A high risk of urethritis (20.8%) was reported amongst prisoners in Sindh, Pakistan, due to high prevalence of homosexuality and multiple sexual partners.[48] An epidemiologic study conducted among prison inmates in a district jail around Delhi showed that 4.6% of the inmates had primary syphilis, 33.33% were positive for HbsAg positive, 5% were reactive for HCV infection and 1.3% were Western blot confirmed HIV-1 positive cases.[49] 28.8 percent of the inmates were homo/bisexuals, 54.2% had multiple sexual partners, 83% had contact with CSW and 80.6% indulged in unprotected sex. 68 percent of the inmates were alcoholics, 24% consumed smack while 4.8% were IV drug abusers.

Addictions

Populations of drug abusers have been associated with epidemics of STD especially HIV infection.

Crack Cocaine Users

The drug most often associated with STD is smokable freebase (crack) cocaine. Ethnographic research suggests that crack addiction forces young women to sell sex directly for money to buy crack. Also, the sex workers under the influence of the drug may be less careful when choosing sexual practices or partners. Epidemiological data indicate that 'crack for sex' exchange differs from other types of prostitution because of the high proportion of adolescent population involved with drug abuse, oral sex is. the predominant type of sexual activity and the crack users often indulge in unprotected sex.[50] In a study of female drug abusers, use of crack was the most significant predictor of syphilis and more than one-third of the subjects had an STD.[51] In a 1997 survey in Houston, USA, a high prevalence of STD markers was associated with crack smoking-13% positivity for syphilis, 61% for HSV-2, 11% for HIV, 53% for hepatitis B and 42% for hepatitis C infection.[52] The statistics from Atlanta revealed 25% sero- positivity for HIV infection, 37.5% for syphilis and 66.8% for HSV-2 infection among the crack-smoking sex workers.[53] Interestingly, a study from Bahamas showed an outbreak of lymphogranuloma venereum (LGV), associated with the epidemic of crack cocaine use.[54]

Intravenous Drug Abuse

Epidemiological studies in intravenous drug abusers have shown high frequency of blood borne STD including HIV, HBV, HCV infections and syphilis. In Bangladesh, syphilis, HBV and HIV rates were found to be 23%, 66.5% and 1.4% respectively among IV drug abusers.[55] In Manipur, in the year 2000, prevalence of HIV among the IV drug abusers was 80% and vaginal discharge was strongly associated with HIV positivity.[56] A study of the sexual behaviours among drug abusers in Delhi, showed greater number of sex partners, higher rate of anal intercourse (25.7%), greater frequency of visits to CSW and hence a significantly higher prevalence of STD in this group.[57]

Alcoholism and Smoking

Smoking has been shown to be strongly associated with persistence of oncogenic HPV cervical infection. Moreover, adolescent women with alcohol use disorder in the United States appeared to be at substantially high risk of HSV-2 infection, with seroprevalence of 19% as compared to 10% in those without this disorder.[58]

High Risk Sexual Practices

Certain sexual practices are associated with higher risk of acquiring STD. For a specific sexual practice, the number and type of partners and the setting in which the practice occurs, significantly effects the actual risk associated with that practice. The high-risk sexual practices include (a) receptive ano-genital intercourse, which increases the risk of STD such as ano-rectal gonorrhoea, condyloma acuminata, herpes simplex infection, LGV, chancroid etc., (b) oro-anal intercourse, which may lead to oral gonorrhoea, syphilis, chancroid, warts or amoebiasis, (c) insertive ano-genital intercourse, which may cause gonococcal or non-gonococcal urethritis, herpes genitalis, condyloma acuminata, LGV or donovanosis, (d) receptive manual-anal intercourse and (e) rectal douching in association with receptive ano-genital intercourse. The higher risk of STD in these groups is also related to the fact that these individuals also engage in other high risk activities. In San Francisco, both homosexual and bisexual men reporting high prevalence of HSV-2 antibody were associated with increased use of alcohol, ecstasy and heroin and unprotected anal intercourse.[59] A resurgence in syphilis was reported from Washington (increase from 6 cases reported in 1995 to 46 cases in 1999) among men who have sex with men (MSM).[60] A similar outbreak of syphilis in this population was reported in South California, where the number of cases increased from 26% in 1999 to 51% in 2000.[61] Homosexual men are at increased risk of infection with HPV, as manifested by anal warts and anal carcinoma. In 1987, in the United States, the incidence of anal carcinoma among homosexual men was estimated to be 35/100,000. In HIV seropositive men especially those with CD4 counts < 500/ml, there is an increased risk of high-grade anal squamous intraepithelial lesions.[62] In San Francisco, in 1994, anal HPV DNA was detected in 93% of HIV-positive and 61% of HIV-negative homosexual and bisexual men with infection due to multiple HPV types in 73% of

HIV-positive and 23% of HIV-negative men.[63] In Amsterdam, Netherlands, a considerable increase in the incidence of rectal gonorrhoea (from 4% in 1994 to 5.4% in 1999) and syphilis (from 0.5% to 0.8%) was reported in MSM after the introduction of HAART, possibly because of an increase in unprotected anal intercourse due to treatment optimism.[64] In India, STD prevalence among the homosexuals has been shown to vary from 2.2% to 6.16%, confirming that frequent mucosal damage caused by intercourse through the unnatural route in this group poses a high risk for STD transmission.[18,38]

In women having sex with women (WSW), in Australia, a significantly high incidence of bacterial vaginosis, hepatitis C and HIV was reported compared to control group.[65] This group showed higher frequency of IV drug abuse and previous contact with homo/bisexual men. This study corroborated with another report from England in which higher incidence of bacterial vaginosis, cervical HPV infection and trichomoniasis in WSW as compared to heterosexual women was observed.[66] The possibility of sexual transmission via exchange of vaginal secretions or oro-genital contact is suggested. The higher incidence of genital warts in this group may be explained by the fact that the infection can also be transmitted through non-penetrative intercourse from women to women. The transmission of *Trichomonas vaginalis* via fomites or inoculation with infected vaginal secretions may have been responsible for the high incidence in this group. WSW have been reported to have a high incidence of HPV infection. A very high incidence of HPV infection and cervical dysplasia has been reported from USA and UK.[66-68] The sexual practices between female partners that could account for the high rate of HPV transmission include digital-vaginal sex, oral sex and use of insertive sex toys. A recent study demonstrated genital HPV on the fingertips of subjects, substantiating the hypothesis that HPV could be introduced intravaginally with digital vaginal contact between the female partners.[69]

The population groups engaged in high-risk sexual practices should be identified at the earliest, since they require specialized attention including individualized risk-reduction Counselling, assistance with partner notification and follow-up on treatment referrals.

Other Sexual Practices

There are less well characterized health behaviours and sexual practices that may influence the risk of acquiring or transmitting STD. These include dry sex, sex during menses and vaginal douching practices.

'Dry sex' or the practice of removing vaginal secretions with astringent preparations before engaging in vaginal intercourse, has been documented in many sub-Saharan African countries. The most commonly stated reason for engaging in such behaviour is pleasure for the male partner because of the drying effect. This practice is followed by 86% of women in Zambia, 93% women in Zimbabwe and 13% in Malawi.[70,71] The higher risk of STD acquisition is due to the abrasions and ulcers that result from such practice.

Sex during menstruation has been associated with increased risk among women of acquiring gonorrhoea, trichomoniasis and HIV.[72] This practice has been more often found in the educated, white women. According to the National Survey of Women in the United States, 26% of the female population indulge in this practice.[73]

Vaginal douching, a method used to remove vaginal secretions as a preliminary to dry sex or sex during menses, has in the recent National Survey of Family Growth, in United States, been found to be practiced by 55% of the black and 21% of the white women.[74] It is associated with increased risk of pelvic inflammatory disease (PID), cervicitis and endometritis, tubal pregnancy and infertility due to alteration of the vaginal microflora. In Kenya, regular douching was reported by 72% of the women and it was found to be significantly associated with bacterial vaginosis.[75]

Health Care Behaviour

Contraception

The transmission and sequelae of STD is markedly influenced by the pattern of contraception. There has been a recent resurgence in interest in the pattern of contraceptive use as a result of the rising incidence of STD and HIV infection.

Condoms

Barrier methods like condoms offer strong protection against organisms like *Chlamydia trachomatis* and *Neisseria gonorrhoeae* and only partial protection against those which commonly infect the stratified squamous epithelium such as herpes simplex and human papilloma viruses. In the developed countries, rates of condom use range from 3% to 50%.[76] In the developing countries, condom usage has been reported by less than 1% of the couples, the lowest rates being reported from sub-Saharan Africa, which has lead to a high prevalence of HIV infection in these countries. Several STD clinics in India have reported condom use in less than 2% of the attendees.[38] An interesting study undertaken in Ghana, Africa, showed a significant decline in the prevalence of gonorrhoea (from 33% to 11%), genital ulcers (from 21% to 4%), syphilis (from 21% to 2%), trichomoniasis (from 26% to 11%) and HIV infection (from 89% to 32%) between 1992 and 1998, owing mainly to the increase in condom use, through the condom social marketing programs.[77]

Use of diaphragm with spermicide in women offers protection against the organisms transmitted mainly between the columnar or transitional epithelium including *Chlamydia trachomatis* and *Neisseria gonorrhoeae*.

Oral Contraceptives

Oral contraceptives have been associated with a lower risk of PID and higher risk of cervical infections with *Chlamydia trachomatis*, HPV and *Neisseria gonorrhoeae* and candidal vulvovaginitis.[76] High estrogen containing oral contraceptives have shown a strong correlation with risk of hepatitis B and HPV induced cervical cancers.[78]

Intrauterine Devices

There is a strong correlation between the use of intrauterine devices (IUD) and PID. Two reports from the 'Women's Health Study' in United States showed that the use of IUD increased the risk of PID by 60%.[79] Similarly, 'The Oxford Family Planning Association Contraceptive Study' attributed the risk by a factor of 10.[80] However, recent WHO reports have shown the risk of PID in IUD users to be less than 2 episodes per 1000 years of use, which is consistent with the risk in the general population.[81] A meta-analysis of 36 studies has suggested that the risk of PID is related only to the process of inserting the device and that after the first month of use, it is not significantly higher than non-IUD users. In a study from Mumbai, India, prevalence of genital chlamydial infection among the Cu-T users (14%) was found to be significantly lower than among the non-users (20%), with no greater risk of developing PID.[82]

Circumcision

This practice is strongly related to specific religions, ethnicity or culture and socio-economic status. Lack of circumcision has been implicated as a major risk factor for STD including syphilis, chancroid, genital herpes, gonorrhoea, genital warts, candidal and non-specific balanitis and HIV infection.[83] The hypothesis for the higher risk is that the non-keratinized recesses of the preputial sac predispose to physical trauma and microbial infection. The preputial sac serves as a reservoir of STD pathogens acquired during intercourse from where the entire genitalia may get involved.

STD In Special Age-Groups

The sexually active age-group is between 15 to 45 years and the STD are commonly associated with this group. However, other age-groups have also been found to be at high risk for STD.

Adolescence and Teenage Period

Adolescent period, which corresponds to the age-group of 10 to 15 years and teenage period (13 to 19 years) is a stage of psychosocial development when the individuals are intensely aware of their physical changes and are emotionally vulnerable. Their psychosocial maturity does not correspond with their physical maturity. STD are very common in this group and a number of behavioural, social and biological factors have been implicated. In the United States, an estimated 15.3 million new STD cases occur each year, one-quarter of them among teenagers.[84] The higher incidence has been related to greater number of sexual partners, inconsistent and incorrect use of barrier contraceptives, sex with older partners and excessive alcohol and drug use in this population. Moreover, this group shows excessive neglect towards genital hygiene. Individuals in this age-group who suspect an STD are frightened or embarrassed to seek prompt treatment, thus acting as reservoirs of infection. A high frequency of asymptomatic carrier state and the adolescent practice of partial treatment with self-prescribed antibiotics are other risk factors. The biological changes occurring in the genitalia in this age-group make them more susceptible to certain STDs such as gonorrhoea, chlamydial infection and trichomoniasis.

A study conducted in Atlanta, USA, to assess the prevalence of STD in the homeless adolescent population, revealed higher incidence among females (16.7%) than males (9.8%), the prevalence of *C.trachomatis* infection being 10.5%, 18.2% for HSV-2, 3.6% for HBV, 5% for HCV and 0.3% for HIV infection.[85] The HPV infection rates in the sexually active adolescent and teenage girls in the United States have been reported to range from 19% to 30%.[86] In a study from Agra, India, in 1987, syphilis among teenagers was observed in 44% of the cases, chancroid in 18%, genital warts in 14%, gonorrhoea in 10%, herpes simplex infection in 8% and LGV, donovanosis and non-specific urethritis in 2% cases each.[87]

Elderly

The elderly individuals have traditionally not been considered at risk for acquiring STD. However, several factors may put them at risk Older persons are not necessarily monogamous and they use condoms infrequently as they link it with contraception only. The sexual communication skills necessary for adoption of safe sex practices are less well developed in this population. The aging process is also accompanied by biological age-related increase in susceptibility to STD. In older women, the increased friability of the vaginal mucosa can result in tears and microabrasions during sexual intercourse, facilitating disease transmission. The newly available oral medication for erectile dysfunction (Sildenafil citrate) has also precipitated a rise in the incidence of STD, by increasing sexual activity among them. The Washington State STD surveillance data of 1992-1998, reported a prevalence rate of 1.3% in the elderly population.[88] The STD included chlamydial infection (0.4%), gonorrhoea (1.4%), herpes genitalis (3.5%), syphilis (4.1%) and NGU (3.1%). In a retrospective study from Singapore in 1996, 43 cases (41 males and 2 females) of HIV infection in the population aged 50 years and above at first presentation were observed.[89] The proportion of older individuals among HIV-seropositive patients significantly increased from 4.8% in 1991 to 16.7% by mid-1996. They were mainly heterosexuals (93%), majority (79.1%) were previously or currently married and had multiple sexual exposures to commercial sex workers (83.7%). More than half (58%) of the patients had acquired immunodeficiency virus (AIDS) at the time of first presentation, with a low median CD4 count of 17 cells/mm^3.

Demographic and Social Correlates of STD

Demographic and social factors including age-group, gender, educational and socio-economic status also determine the epidemiologic profile of STD in different regions.

Age

The highest proportion of STD clinic attendees are composed of youthful population between 20-30 years. Individuals in this age-group being adventurous and immature with considerable inquisitiveness for sex and lack of healthy recreation may indulge in high-risk sexual practices. In various STD clinics in India, majority of the attendees (42% to 78.6%) were found to belong to this age-group.[18-24,90-102] In other Asian and African developing countries also, the highest incidence of STD has been reported in the 20 to 30 years age-group.[3]

Gender

Several surveys conducted in the developing countries including India have shown significantly high male to female sex ratio among the STD clinic attendees (ranging from 1.3:1 to 11:1).[3,18-24,90-102] This difference may probably be because of the asymptomatic nature of infections in the female sex, lesser degree of freedom given by the society to women to play outdoors, lower awareness amongst women of the need for availing medical facilities or their frequent consultation in gynecological clinics instead of STD clinics, particularly in India.

Educational and Socio-Economic Status

The correlation between the incidence of STD and socioeconomic indicators is epidemiologically very useful, since it helps in predicting the nature of practices which lead to its transmission, informs the policy makers about its effect on the society and helps in the effort to target intervention. In India, illiterates and individuals with primary level of education and lower income groups form a major proportion of the STD clinic attendees.[18-24,90-102] This may be due to lack of general awareness about safe sexual practices such as use of condoms, paucity of healthy recreation facilities and indulgence in high-risk sexual behaviour in this group.

Contrastingly, in sub-Saharan Africa, higher prevalence rates among the richer class have been observed, in view of the relatively greater access of the rich to foreign travel and higher rates of sexual partner change among the high-income adults.[103]

Ethnicity

A strong correlation between ethnicity and STD risk has been observed. Several population-based cross sectional studies in the United States have demonstrated increased rates of gonorrhoea, chlamydial infection and genital herpes in African-Americans populations.[104] In the United Kingdom, gonorrhoea and chlamydial infection rates are substantially higher among the black residents.[105,106] Remote aboriginal communities in northern and central Australia experience high rates of gonorrhoea, chlamydial infection and syphilis. Higher prevalence rates of HPV infection have been reported among the African-American women than in whites or Hispanics.[107] Donovanosis in India is endemic in the south Indian Dravidian population.[108] 30 percent of the tribals of Gadchiroli district in Maharashtra in 1998 were found to be engaged in sex trade, with VDRL positivity recorded in 8% of the individuals during this period.[109]

These ethnic variations may be explained by differences in the educational and socioeconomic status, housing, recreational facilities, rates of drug abuse, geographical variations, genetic predisposition towards greater susceptibility to acquisition and persistence of infection, endogenous hormonal factors or differences in sexual behaviour among the ethnic groups.

Modes of Transmission of STD (Tables 4 and 5)

Table 4. Sexually Transmitted Disease Agents Transmitted Predominantly by Sexual Intercourse

Bacteria	Viruses	Others
Neisseria gonorrhoeae	HIV-1,2	*Trichomonas vaginalis*
Treponema pallidum	HSV-2	*Pthirus pubis*
Haemophilus ducreyi	HPV	
Chlamydia trachomatis	HBV	
Calymmatobacterium		
granulomatis	CMV	
Ureaplasma urealyticum	MCV★	

★ Molluscum contagiosum virus

Table 5. Sexually Transmitted Diseases in Which Fomites are Implicated

- Gonorrhoea
- Syphilis
- Chancroid
- HSV infection-rare
- HPV infection
- Trichomoniasis
- Molluscum contagiosum infection
- Genital scabies

A common biological feature of many microorganisms causing STD is their unique and often exclusive adaptation to humans, the main mode of transmission being genital mucosal contact. i.e. sexual intercourse. However, there is enough evidence to support the non-venereal transmission of these infections via perinatal transmission, parenteral transmission or by fomites, although the relative risk is different for different diseases.

Gonorrhoea

The risk of sexual transmission of gonorrhoea depends on the anatomic site infected and exposed and the frequency of exposures. The risk of acquiring the infection from male-to- female is 50% to 90% as against 20% risk from female-to-male, because of retention of the infected ejaculate within the vagina.[110] Acquisition of rectal gonorrhoea by insertive or receptive anal intercourse or pharyngeal gonorrhoea by fellatio and cunnilingus is also well documented.[111] The possibility of sexual transmission in lesbians through exchange of vaginal secretions has been suggested.[66] Genital infection via contaminated fingers has also been observed.[112]

Non-venereal transmission of gonorrhoea is rare. The organism can survive for upto 24 hours on clothings when periodically rinsed with warm, physiological saline.[112] Since gonococci have been recovered from a variety of materials such as utensils for up to 3 days after contamination, infection through contaminated food or utensils is theoretically possible. There are interesting reports of spread of pharyngeal gonorrhoea via sweets passed by mouth in the absence of direct oral contact between two sisters.[113] Similar transmission from an inflatable doll has also been reported.[114] Moreover, the spread of infection in children by sharing of beds, towels and flannels with infected parents has been documented, but is rare.[112] There are occasional reports of outbreaks of gonococcal infection in children wards by sharing of inadequately sterilized thermometers or toilet articles.[112] Perinatal transmission to neonates causing pharangeal gonorrhoea or urethritis is also documented.

Chlamydia Infection

Chlamydia trachomatis is transmitted sexually, although its transmissibility is less than *Neisseria gonorrhoeae*, since male partners of women with dual infection are found to be more often affected with gonorrhoea than chlamydial infection.[115] Initial studies using less specific diagnostic techniques showed higher infection rates among the female partners of infected males than among male partners of infected women and attributed this to more efficient male-to-female transmission. However, using PCR studies, the frequency of transmission has been found to be equal.[116] Chlamydial proctitis occurs in homosexual men who practice receptive anal intercourse.[117] Pharyngeal infection via oro-genital contact has also been documented.[118] The possibility of sexual transmission in lesbians through exchange of vaginal secretions has been suggested.[66] Perinatal transmission in neonates is reported in 5% of the cases.[119] Chlamydial infection of the pharynx, conjunctiva and middle ear in neonates during perinatal transmission is well documented.

Syphilis

It is acquired via sexual contact by exposure to moist mucosal or cutaneous lesions, through micro or macroscopic breaks in the squamous or columnar epithelium. The rate of acquisition from an infected sexual partner has been estimated to be up to 60%.[120] The incubation period depends upon the size of the treponemal inoculum.

Extragenital syphilitic chancres have been found on lips, tongue, tonsils, fingers, eyelids or nipple as a result of inoculation with contaminated fingers or fomites.[121]

Transplacental transmission of *Treponema pallidum* into the foetal circulation occurs in congenital syphilis, especially in the first four months of gestation. The risk of transmission is higher when the mother is suffering from early syphilis (primary or secondary) than when she has late syphilis.[122] The risk of infecting the foetus declines gradually during the course of untreated syphilis, being inconspicuous after 8 years of untreated infection.

The transmission of syphilis by blood transfusion referred to as 'syphilis d'emblee' is well documented.

Primary stage is usually absent with this mode of transmission. The risk of transmission is greater by fresh blood components rather than transfusion of refrigerated products, although treponema can survive for up to 120 hours in blood stored at 4^0C.[123,124] In both India and other parts of the world, the prevalence of HIV infection and syphilis among blood donors is on the rise.[124–126]

Chancroid

The disease is highly contagious, with the likelihood of male to female spread of 63% during a single act of unprotected exposure.[127] However, studies have shown that the risk of acquiring the disease from a partner with visible lesions is significantly higher than without them. In women, the ulcers may often be subclinical.[128] In such situations, they act as reservoirs of infection, transmitting the disease to their sexually promiscuous clients or spouses. However, in men, the urethra has not been shown to be a reservoir of infection. Extragenital chancroidal ulcers on the hands or breast, transmitted by infected fingers are also documented.[129,130]

Herpes Simplex Infection

The transmission occurs through close contact with individuals who are shedding the virus at a peripheral site, mucosal surface or secretion.[131] Infection occurs via inoculation of virus onto susceptible mucosal surfaces (oropharynx, cervix, conjunctiva) through microabrasions. The transmission is more frequent in women from men than men from women. In one study, the risk of acquisition of HSV-2 infection was found to be 32% in HSV seronegative women while it was 6% in seronegative men.[132] The higher rate of asymptomatic infection in men may be responsible for the greater male-to-female transmission. Since HSV is readily inactivated at room temperature and by drying, transmission via aerosols or fomites is unusual.[133] However, there is some evidence that non-venereal transmission of HSV-2 occurs in humid environment, particularly when children sleep with infected parents or share towel or clothing.[133] Neonatal herpes by perinatal transmission is well documented. However, there are no reports to show transplacental spread of infection.

Donovanosis

The disease is mildly contagious and multiple and

repeated sexual exposures are required for its transmission. Anal intercourse leads to rectal lesions in homosexuals and penile lesions in their partners.[134] The infection can spread from the genitalia by direct contact to the adjoining areas of the thigh, lower abdomen, scrotum or buttocks. Non-venereal transmission to children can occur by sitting on the laps of infected adult patients.[135]

Lymphogranuloma Venereum

Sexual transmission is common, but LGV is not as contagious as gonorrhoea. Perinatal transmission is documented, although transplacental transmission does not occur.[136]

Human Papilloma Virus Infection

Penile or vulvar warts occurring as a result of heterosexual transmission can spread to contiguous sites including the anal canal. Approximately 8% of men and 20% of women with genital warts have concomitant anal warts.[137] Receptive homosexual contact is the commonest cause of anal warts.[138] Sexual transmission amongst lesbians has also been reported, since the transmission of HPV requires mere skin to skin contact rather than penetrative intercourse.[67] The sexual practices that could account for sexual transmission in WSW include digital-vaginal sex, oral sex and use of insertive sex toys. A recent study reported detection of genital HPV on the fingertips of subjects, substantiating the hypothesis that HPV could be introduced intravaginally with digital-vaginal contact.[69] Condyloma acuminata of the lips, tongue or palate can occur by inoculation of the pathogen by contaminated fingers or by oral sex with the infected partner.[139]

In neonates, perinatal transmission of HPV causing infection of the genitalia or buccal and laryngeal mucosa is frequently reported. The detection rate of HPV DNA in oral swabs of newborn babies varies from 4% to 87%.[140] There is evidence that transmission in-utero is possible, either by haematogenous route, by semen at the time of fertilization or as an ascending infection. HPV can also be transmitted non-venereally via fomites.[141] In children, the commonest cause of genital warts is sexual abuse, which has been documented in 30% to 80% of the cases.[142]

Trichomoniasis

Trichomoniasis is most prevalent among sexual partners of patients with documented infection. The organism can be isolated in 70% of men who had sexual contact with infected women within the previous 48 hours and in only 33% cases if their last contact was 2 weeks previously.[143] The infection can be documented in 85% of the female partners of infected men.[144] Asymptomatic men act as reservoirs and are the principle vectors of the disease. Symptomatic infection in men, presenting as urethral irritation and a thin milky white urethral discharge, is responsible for higher risk of transmission. In Zimbabwe, in 1983-1984, 99.4% of men with trichomonal urethritis were symptomatic and were responsible for significantly greater transmission of the infection to their sexual partners than asymptomatic men.[145] Detection of the infection in prepubertal children indicates sexual abuse.[146]

Perinatal transmission in 5% of female babies has been reported.[147] Non-venereal transmission from contaminated lavatory seats, towels or clothings, douche nozzles, rubber gloves or unsterile instruments is possible.[144]

Hepatitis B Infection

The infection is commonly acquired by blood transfusion, needle stick injuries, via body secretions including saliva, vaginal secretions, menstrual blood, semen, sweat, urine and faeces or by homosexual contact. There is a direct correlation between the duration of homosexual activity, number of partners practicing anorectal intercourse and the risk of acquiring the infection.[133] This risk increases with increase in the number of sex-partners engaged in anal intercourse and the duration of homosexuality. There is considerable evidence to support transmission by heterosexual contact as well.[147] In one study, HbsAg was detected in 27% of the spouses of HbsAg carriers and in only 11% of spouses of noncarrier controls. Approximatety 20% of the reported cases of hepatitis B infection in the United States occur by heterosexual contact and 30% cases from India have been contracted through homo/heterosexual route.[149,150] In a study from Mumbai in 1995, HBV prevalence was found to be 8.8%.[151] A quarter of these individuals were seropositive for syphilis and HIV, confirming a definite role of sexual transmission in the spread of of HBV. This was also proved by another study from Pondicherry in 1999, in which HbsAg positivity was found in 10% of the STD clinic attendees, predominantly drivers, bisexuals, patients with infected spouse, sex partners of CSW and those with concomitant presence of another STD.[37]

Regular blood donors and IV drug abusers are also at high risk of acquiring the infection. In Tanzania,

HbsAg and anti HBs antibody were detected in 22% and 11% of the blood donors respectively.[125] In a recent study from Bangladesh, 12% of the IV drug users were positive for HBV infection.[55]

Perinatal transmission in neonates via infected vaginal secretions has also been documented.[152]

Epidemiology of Individual STD

In this chapter, we will discuss the epidemiological aspects of major STD (Tables 6 and 7). The epidemiology of HIV infection is dealt with in a separate chapter.

Table 6. Pattern of Sexually Transmitted Diseases Among STD Clinic Attendees in Major Hospitals in India

S.No	Region	Syphilis	Chancroid	LGV	Donovanosis	HSV	HPV	Gonorrhoea	NGU
1	Chandigarh[98] 1977–1985	10.4	12.2	0.6	6.3	11.4	21.4	16.9	4.1
2	Chandigarh[97] 1985–1992	8.7	8.1	0.9	1.6	19.7	25.2	5.3	4.1
3	Chandigarh[90] 1995–1996	2	3	6	0.5	21	7	3	6
4	Delhi[99] 1955–61	7.3	22.5	0.6	0.25	–	–	15.9	4.9
5	Delhi[24] 1965–1978	54.9	5.9	0.9	1.2	2.5	2	1.9	–
6	Delhi[100] 1989–1995	14.3	23.9	1.6	1.4	11.8	9.2	12.2	3.7
7	Delhi[18] 1995–1999	15.6	11	0.45	0.48	11.8	9.3	11.6	7.4
8	Patiala[94] 1983–1988	29.6	8.8	0.2	0.2	11.6	12	10	5.2
9	Patiala[93] 1990–1998	17.2	1.6	0.15	0.28	9.4	5.1	4.2	10.8
10	Rohtak[96] 1992–1994	30.2	22.1	0.97	1.45	10.6	18.1	12.9	4.7
11	Rohtak[95] 1995–1996	7.4- P 17.5- S	14.5	0.67	0.8	11.1	21.5	12.6	6.7
12	Rohtak[101] 1995–2000	24	10.9	0.2	0.86	16.9	19.4	16.2	4.8
13	Ahmedabad[91] 1993–1994	22.2- P 28.7- S	7.6	0.58	2	8.2	7.2	5.05	–
14	Ahmedabad[21] 1998–1999	28.9	9.6	–	1	27.9	9.1	12.7	1.5
15	Calcutta[92] 1997	23.9	30.8	5.07	0.55	11.3	–	15.3	12.4
16	Kurnool[23] 1992–1996	14.4	2.8	9.7	–	14	11.3	11.7	19.1
17	Pondicherry[102] 1982–1990	18	10.6	8	8.2	14.1	11.9	11.9	0.8

Table 7. Pattern of Sexually Transmitted Diseases Among STD Clinic Attendees in District Hospitals in India

S.No	Region	Syphilis	Chancroid	LGV	Donovanosis	HSV	HPV	Gonorrhoea	NGU
1	Srinagar[20] 1986–1994	20.8	28.8	9.7	0.2	4.1	11.25	11.7	2.6
2	Port Blair[22] 1992–1993	25.4	21.1	–	–	7.7	9.2	19	7.04
3	Port Blair*	12.4	10.7	2.4	–	57.4	4.1	4.1	8.5
4	Tezpur[19] 1986–1990	14.6	35	10	0.013	5	9.2	17.1	3.3

* Data presented in 26th National Conference of IASSTD and AIDS

Syphilis

It is a bacterial STD, caused by the organism *Treponema pallidum*. It is a major cause of GUD and an important risk factor in the transmission of HIV infection. In the developed countries, the prevalence of syphilis has fallen steeply, except for few focal outbreaks, due to improved access to health care, effective control programmes and efficacious treatment. However, in some developing countries, it still remains a major public health problem with an estimated 12 million cases occurring worldwide annually of which 4 million occur in Africa.[2]

In the United States, syphilis is characterized by spontaneous epidemics rather than persistent endemicity. An estimated 70,000 cases of syphilis occur annually.[84] In 1986-1990, an epidemic of syphilis occurred throughout the country .The incidence of primary and secondary syphilis in 1984-1994 ranged from 0 to 87 per 100,000 population, and in 1990 alone, the rate was 20.3 cases per 100,000 persons.[153,154] The rates began to decline in 1991 and have decreased every year since, it being 2.5 per 100,000 population in 1999 and 2.2 per 100,000 in the year 2000.[155-157] (Fig. 1). The rate among the blacks (12.8 per 100,000) was 21 times greater than in whites (0.6 per 100,000), it was 43 times lower than in 1997. Focal outbreaks have

occurred from time to time in different cities including Seattle, Atlanta and Guilford County.[158,159] The factors associated with these outbreaks included missed opportunities for syphilis screening and treatment in high-risk settings, substantial rates of co-infection with HIV virus, sex with multiple partners, exchange of sex for drugs especially crack cocaine and unprotected sex. Syphilis is re-emerging among men who have sex with men (MSM) The focal outbreaks during the periods 1997-1998 and 1999-2000, especially in Chicago, New York, Boston, Miami, Seattle and San Francisco were among this group (comprising 68% of syphilis cases), of which two-thirds were HIV positive.[158] Higher rates occurred among the African-Americans living in poverty in metropolitan areas in the Southeastern United States. The city of Baltimore has the highest number of syphilis cases in the country with an incidence rate of 270 per 100,000 live births for congenital syphilis and 99.3 per 100,000 population for early syphilis, with 96% of the cases occurring in the black population.[160] In the United States, syphilis elimination at the national level has been defined as absence of sustained transmission of the disease within 90 days of the report of an imported case. The national goal of syphilis elimination is to reduce primary and secondary syphilis to < 1000 cases i.e. 0.4 per 100,000 population.[156]

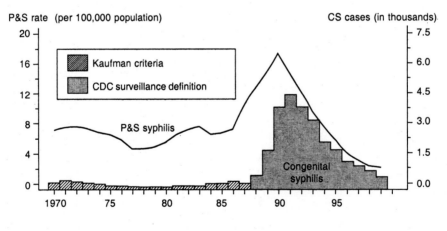

Fig. 1 Congenital syphilis (cs)—reported cases for infants <1 year of age and rates of primary (p) and secondary (s) syphilis among women: United States, 1970–1999

In England and Wales, after almost two decades of consistent decline, infectious syphilis is again on the increase.[161] Since 1997, when the Bristol outbreak heralded the resurgence of the disease, outbreaks have been reported in the North West, South East and London regions of England, such that, by 2000, nearly two-thirds of the nationally reported cases were diagnosed

in these areas. In 1999-2000, the infection rose by 160% in males (from 153 to 248 cases) and 130% in females (from 55 to 73), and in MSM, it rose from 52 to 113 cases. These outbreaks were associated with high rates of partner exchange, travel or migration from endemic areas, predominance of homosexuality and a high proportion of HIV co-infection.

Resurgence of syphilis has also been reported from other European countries. In the STD clinics in Amsterdam, Netherlands, in 1999, 76 new cases of infectious syphilis were reported, an increase of 111% from 1998, with the largest increase seen among MSM (from 9 cases in 1998 to 40 in 1999).[162] This rise was attributed to unsafe sexual practices due to treatment optimism after the introduction of HAART for HIV infection. In Rotterdam, syphilis cases increased dramatically in 1995-1997 with the highest rates reported among CSW.[163] However, with the introduction of prophylactic treatment, the prevalence rate dropped to 1.3% in 1998. A significant increase in the incidence has been noticed in Czech Republic during the past 10 years.[164] From 1992 to 1998, the number of early syphilis cases doubled while the number of stillbirths due to syphilis increased three times. In Belgrade, Yugoslavia, early syphilis incidence rates showed a decreasing trend between 1985-1992 (2.53/100,000 in 1985 to 0.8/100,000 in 1992) as a result of change in sexual behaviour in response to the AIDS epidemic.[165] However from 1993 to 1999, there was a significant rise in the incidence from 1.67/100,000 in 1993 to 3.65/100,000 in 1999. It was highest in men aged 30-39 years and 40-49 years and in women 20-29 years and 30-39 years of age. An alarming increase in the incidence has also been reported in many eastern European countries.[166-168] In Romania, the incidence rose from 7.1/100,000 persons in 1986 to 34.7/100,000 in 1998, in Bulgaria, it increased from 14.4/100,000 in 1994 to 27.3/100,000 in 1996 and in central Russia, it rose from 3.2/100,000 in 1990 to 300/100,000 population in 1997 In all these regions, low education, poor socioeconomic conditions and migration were the main causes of resurgence of infectious syphilis.

Syphilis is an important cause of morbidity in sub-Saharan Africa. In Tanzania, seroprevalence of syphilis in the 90s was unacceptably high, with rates ranging from 5.9% to 12.8%.[169] Higher rates were reported in illiterate individuals with early sexual debut and multiple partners, in individuals with self-perceived high risk of STDs and among uncircumcised males. However in Madagascar, the rates decreased from 56% in 1995 to 29% in 1997 after the introduction of syndromic management for GUD.[170] In Nairobi, Kenya also, a marked decline in the seroprevalence was observed among pregnant women from 1994 to 1997 (7.2% in 1994 to 3.8% in 1997) after the development of a specific syphilis control program.[171]

In many Asian countries especially India, syphilis continues to be a major health problem. However, a constant decline in its prevalence has been observed in recent years. In a retrospective analysis of the data obtained from the STD clinic attendees in a tertiary hospital of Delhi between 1954 and 1994, although the STD cases increased eight times from 1954 to 1984, with prevalence increasing from 5.5% in 1964 to 14.7% in 1994, the syphilis load declined from 61.2% in 1954 to 9.1% in 1994.[172] Males outnumbered females in the ratio of 2.8:1, probably because women report for investigations and treatment much later than their male counterparts, due in part to the asymptomatic nature of the disease in the females. In this analysis it was also observed that the prevalence in adult males increased until 1984 in contrast to children under 14 years in whom it decreased from 12.6% in 1954 to 0.5% in 1994. No case of neurosyphilis was diagnosed during the 40 year study period while 10 cases of cardiovascular syphilis were last reported in 1954. In other Delhi hospitals also, the incidence was shown to decrease from 54.9% in 1965-78 to 15.56% in 1995-99.[18,24] During 1965-1978, two cases each of neuro- and cardiovascular syphilis in the women were reported.[24] In Madurai, in 1992, 17.5% men presenting with neurological manifestations and associated past history of multiple sex partners were diagnosed as neurosyphilis, predominantly meningovascular syphilis.[173] In Himachal Pradesh in the late 1980s, VDRL positivity among the high risk groups was reported in 9% of the cases.[174] Significant decline in syphilis trends have been observed in Chandigarh, with incidence rates reducing from 10.4% in 1977-85 to 2% in 1995-96,[97,98] in Rohtak from 30.2% in 1992-93 to 24% in 1995-2000[95,96,101] and in Patiala from 29.6% in 1983-88 to 17.2% in 1990-98.[93,94] This reduction may be attributed to regular supply and consistent use of effective drugs. A cross-sectional survey of women in the reproductive age group in an urban slum community in Mumbai in 1995, reported VDRL seropositivity of 0.5%, while a study from a similar population in Delhi in 1996-2000, showed seropositivity in 4% of cases.[175,176]

Blood donors are a high-risk group for acquiring and transmitting syphilis (Table 8). In All India Institute of Medical Science, New Delhi, between 1989 and 1995, among the voluntary and replacement blood donors, VDRL reactivity increased from 0.23% to 0.52%.[177] In other parts of India, sero-prevalence of syphilis in this group has been shown to vary from 0% in Lucknow, 2.8% in Delhi, 3.62% in Tirunelvelli to 7% in Bihar.[178-181]

Congenital syphilis (CS) is the most dreaded

Table 8.   VDRL Positivity Among Blood Donors in India

All India Institute of Medical	(1989)	0.23%
Science, New Delhi[177]	(1995)	0.52%
Lucknow[178]	(1996)	0%
Delhi[179]	(1987)	2.8%
Tirunelvelli[180]	(1985)	3.62%
Bihar[181]	(1993)	7%

consequence of untreated syphilis in pregnant women, estimated to occur in 25%-75% of the exposed infants.[103] It has been suggested that approximately 10% to12% of infants born to mothers with positive syphilis serology would die if untreated, yielding a mortality of 1-3% among the under fours. In the United States, chronic drug abuse and inadequate prenatal care has been suggested as the main cause of CS. From 1990 to 1993, in the state of Georgia, 438 deliveries were classified as CS, a prevalence of 0.9%.[182] It was 5 times higher among the black population (9.6 cases per 1000 live births) than among whites (1.7/1000 live births). The CS rates in United States have declined significantly between 1997 and 2000, being 27.8 per 100,000 live births in 1997, 14.5 in 1999 and 13.4 per 100,000 in 2000 (Fig. 1).[183] In Bolivia in 1996, 4.3% of the live-born and 26% of the stillborn infants were found to have syphilis at delivery.[184] In Asian and African countries including India, only sporadic reports of CS have been published. In Delhi, between 1965 to 1978, 82 cases of CS were reported, with a higher female-to-male ratio (1.73:1).[24] In Kurnool, Andhra Pradesh, 7 cases of CS were observed from 1980 to 1990.[185]

The surveys conducted among antenatal women in Africa have shown VDRL seropositivity in 3.6% of cases in Malawi, 9.3% in Gambia and 14% in Zimbabwe, with an average of 10% in Africa.[186-188] In India, it has ranged from 1.8% in Chandigarh to 2.9% in Aligarh and 3.4% in Delhi (1996).[189-191] The seroprevalence of syphilis among pregnant women attending the antenatal clinic in another tertiary level hospital in Delhi in

1998 was found to be 2.5%, with 10% of the cases being HIV-positive.[192] (Table 9)

Table 9.   VDRL Positivity Among Antenatal Women

Africa		
Malawi[186]	(1993)	3.6%
Gambia[187]	(1992)	9.3%
Zimbabwe[188]	(1993)	14%
India		
Chandigarh[189]	(1986)	1.8%
Aligarh[190]	(1987)	2.9%
Delhi[191]	(1996)	3.4%
Delhi[192]	(1998)	2.53%

Chancroid

It is a bacterial GUD, caused by *Haemophilus ducreyi*, and predominantly transmitted through heterosexual contact. The epidemiological data for chancroid may be inaccurate in view of the difficulty in diagnosing the condition on clinical grounds alone since most medical providers do not have the facility to perform laboratory tests. Recently, chancroid has received more attention because of the strong association with HIV transmission. In industrialized countries, it is an uncommon cause of GUD. In United States, 9515 cases were reported in 1947, that steadily declined to fewer than 1000 cases in the late 1970s when the cases reported annually were 646.[193] However, chancroid oubreaks occurred in the 1980s. Between 1981 and 1983, 15% of the GUD cases in California were caused by chancroid. Between 1986 and 1988, in New York city, the number of reported cases increased from 556 to 1140 and in 1987, 4986 cases were reported from USA to the Centre for Disease Control (CDC). Subsequently, from 1993 to 1999, the annual number of cases have constantly declined from 1399 in 1993 to approximately 250 cases in 1999 (Fig. 2). However, in 1997, in New York, chancroid was the third major cause of GUD, observed

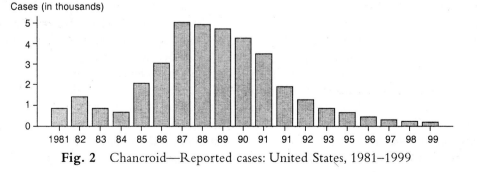

Cases (in thousands)

Fig. 2   Chancroid—Reported cases: United States, 1981–1999

in 33% of the patients.[194] Two outbreaks of chancroid were identified from the inner cities in USA, one in New Orleans (1990-1992), where *H. ducreyi* was isolated by culture in 39% of the GUD patients and the other in Jackson, Mississippi (1994-1995) where it was identified from another 39% of GUD cases by polymerase chain reaction.[195,196] The disease was most prevalent among the urban African-Americans and Hispanics with a high male-to-female ratio. It was significantly associated with alcohol (44%) and cocaine abuse (25%), sex with prostitutes (17%), multiple sex partners, trading drugs for sex (16%) and infrequent use of condoms. Besides the behavioural factors, improvement in diagnostic techniques for isolation and detection of *H. ducreyi* may have been responsible for the higher incidence. In Paris, France, 673 cases were diagnosed between 1973 and 1979.[197] It is a rare disease in Australia and the Scandinavian countries, mainly seen in travelers returning from South-East Asia or in the aborigines population.[103]

Chancroid is the leading cause of GUD in developing countries particularly in sub-Saharan Africa and South-East Asia. In the African countries, the prevalence varies from 9.8% to 68%.[198] The risk factors include early age at first coitus, first coitus before menarche, longer duration of marriage (> 20 years), greater number of lifetime sexual partners, serologic evidence of exposure to another STD and lower socioeconomic status and is highest among divorcees and CSW. In India, the incidence rates have been shown to range from 1.6% in Patiala to as high as 51.9% in Mumbai.[93,199] On comparing the rates from the same region during different periods, a significant decrease in the incidence has been observed. This may be due to the availability of newer antibiotics, their indiscriminate use at the primary care level due to free availability, prophylactic use before or after the sexual exposure, greater awareness regarding early diagnosis and treatment among the masses and the immense success of the syndromic approach and condom promotion campaigns.

Donovanosis

It is a chronic, mildly contagious sexually transmitted disease characterized by granulomatous ulceration of the genitalia and neighbouring sites, caused by *Calymmatobacterium granulomatis*. It has been ignored as a cause of GUD for many years due to the non-availability of specific laboratory diagnostic facilities. However, during the past decade, there has been renewed

interest in the disease, owing to the emergence of HIV infection and consequent increase in the number of donovanosis cases. Although donovanosis has a world-wide distribution, it is endemic in the tropical and sub-tropical countries, especially in India, Papua New Guinea, aborigines of Australia, South Africa and Brazil. Racial and ethnic predispositions have been associated with the disease since it is more common in the local natives than the Europeans staying in Papua New Guinea, in Negroes than the poor whites in United States, in Dravidians in South India and in Pahari dwellers of Himachal Pradesh.[108] In Durban, South Africa, following the introduction of a rapid test (PCR) for its diagnosis, the number of reported cases increased substantially from 312 in 1988 to 2385 in 1995, 2733 in 1996 and 3153 in 1997.[200] 61 women, predominantly pregnant individuals (88.5%) were diagnosed with this condition between 1990-1993.[201] In a Brazilian city, between 1954 and 1990, 259 cases of donovanosis were reported, of which only 56 cases occurred between 1954 and 1974, while 133 cases were found in the last five years.[202] Greater sexual liberty, poor socio-economic conditions and increasing homosexual behaviour were implicated for this augmented disease incidence. In Papua New Guinea, although the disease is endemic for the past 80 years with a prevalence of 54.4%, the incidence has recently increased, particularly in the urban areas and is associated with low socioeconomic status and poor personal hygiene.[203]

The disease is very common in some parts of India, especially in Tamil Nadu, Pondicherry, Andhra Pradesh, Orissa and Himachal Pradesh. It has an uneven geographical distribution with incidence varying from 0.013% in Tezpur[19] to 8.2% in Pondicherry[102] and 10% in Mumbai among STD clinic attendees.[204] It has been speculated that certain climatic factors such as moderate relative humidity and persistent high temperature have influenced the geographical distribution of the disease. A strong association with HLA B57 has also been observed.[205] Two epidemics of donovanosis occurred in Delhi, in 1983, when the reported incidence was 6.38% and another in 1985, when the incidence was 8.33%.[206] The disease mainly affected young unmarried men who contracted the disease during extramarital heterosexual intercourse with prostitutes; illiterate and low socioeconomic groups. In Chandigarh, the incidence declined significantly from 6.3% in 1977-85[98] to 0.5% in 1995-1996.[90] This may be due to the availability of broad-spectrum antibiotics and the changing sexual behaviour in the era of HIV infection. However in Delhi, the incidence increased from 0.25% in 1955-61[99] to 1.4% in 1989-95[100] and then declined to 0.48% in 1995-99.[18] The increase in incidence in Delhi may be attributed to large-scale immigration of high-risk individuals from endemic areas.

Lymphogranuloma Venereum (LGV)

LGV is a less commonly encountered STD in industrialized countries with only sporadic cases reported from North America, Europe and Australia and the cases are mainly seen in immigrants and travelers returning from endemic areas.[207] The rate of reported disease has been declining since 1972 in the United States, with only 113 cases recorded in 1997.[208] In United Kingdom, only 91 cases of chancroid, granuloma inguinale and LGV were reported in 1995 from the genitourinary medicine clinics.[209]

LGV is endemic in several tropical and sub-tropical countries including West, Central and East Africa, India, Malaysia, Korea, Vietnam, South America, Papua New Guinea and the Caribbean Islands.[210-215] The proportion of genital ulcers that can be attributed to LGV in these areas varies from 1-10%.

In India, incidence of 0.15%- 9.74% has been reported from different parts of the country.[18-24,90-102] Perhaps, the lack of specific diagnostic criteria in these studies and the relatively poor degree of clinical suspicion of the condition may have biased these estimates.

In two cross-sectional surveys undertaken in Jamaica in 1982-83 and 1990-91, disease prevalence of 4.1% and 3.9% respectively was reported and in 1996, the incidence decreased to 2.63%.[216] In Madagascar, in 1997, 8% of genital ulcer disease patients were clinically diagnosed as LGV with only 0.5% accounting for confirmed cases by micro-IF test.[217] In Hong Kong, the disease accounted for only 0.001% of all the new STD cases in 1995.[218] An incidence of 1% was recorded in Singapore in 1995.[219] In Nairobi, Kenya, 0.6% of the genital ulcer diseases were attributed to LGV in 1996.[210] A prospective study of inguinal buboes conducted in Thai men between 1987 and 1989 revealed LGV-*C.trachomatis* by immunofluorescent microscopy in 3.9% of the cases.[214]

LGV occurs six times more frequently in men than in women, since it remains undiagnosed because of the asymptomatic nature of the early lesions in females.[220] However, late complications such as ulceration, rectal strictures or esthiomene are more frequently reported in women.

The disease has a peak incidence during the second and third decade of life which corresponds with the peak age of sexual activity. It is more common in urban population, among the sexually promiscuous and lower socio-economic classes.[222] Commercial sex workers play a major role in disease transmission, as was documented during an outbreak in Florida in the late 1980s.[223]

Gonorrhoea

It is a well recognized public health problem. It is still one of the commonest bacterial STD in the world. Approximately 62 million new *Neisseria gonorrhoeae* infections occur annually world wide, making it a major public health problem.[224] The importance of this disease is not only limited to its high incidence and the acute manifestations, but also to the complications and disturbing sequelae it causes besides constituting an important risk factor for the transmission of HIV infection.

In the developed countries, there has been a constant decline in the incidence of gonorrhoea. In Europe, peak incidence of gonorrhoea occurred during World Wars I and II and of late during the 1960s and early 1970s following liberation in sexual values.[225] Thereafter, there has been a sharp decline, initially in North European countries such as Sweden, England, Denmark, Germany etc. In Sweden, the incidence decreased from 487 per 100,000 in 1970 to 3 per 100,000 in 1995. Similarly in England, decline occurred from 210 per 100,000 population in 1970 to approximately 34.1 per 100,000 in 1995. In the United States, the peak incidence occurred around 1975 when it was approximately 473 per 100,000. This was followed by a plateau till 1982, a decrease until 1984 and a slight increase till 1986. Thereafter, the incidence is declining steadily. It was approximately 149.5 per 100,000 in 1995 and gradually declined to 133.2 per 100,000 in 1999.[226-228] (Fig. 3) This decline may be related largely to behavioural changes resulting from the fear of AIDS and treatment of asymptomatic infected persons and their sexual partners thereby interrupting the disease transmission. The incidence of gonorrhoea in the United States is seasonal with the highest rates observed in late summer and the lowest incidence in late winters and early spring.[229] In Canada also, a similar trend in the epidemiology has been observed. The incidence of gonorrhoea declined from 223 per 100,000 in 1980 to 18.6 per 100,000 in 1995.[227]

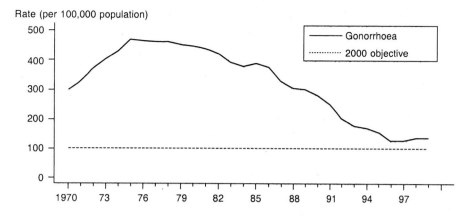

Fig. 3 Gonorrhoea—Reported Rates: United States, 1970-1999 and the Healthy People Year 2000 Objective

In the developed countries, a declining trend in the incidence has been observed among heterosexual men and all women. However, it has been on the increase in homosexual men. In 1996 in England, the incidence in homosexual men was much higher (812 per 100,000 population) compared to heterosexual men (27 per 100,000 population).[230] In 1999 in U.S.A., 13.1% of the Gonococcal Isolate Surveillance Project (GISP) participants were homosexuals as compared to 4% homosexuals in 1988.[227] The male to female ratio of the disease is also decreasing steadily. In England and USA, the ratio of male to female cases has fallen from 3:1 in 1965 to 1.5:1 in the 90s with fewer than 1% men infected with gonorrhoea naming prostitutes as the source of infection. From 1985 to 1995 and 1999, the peak incidence in men was observed in the 20-24 years age group. However, a shift in the age structure was found in women from 20-24 years age group in 1985 to 15-19 years in 1995 and 1999.[231]

In the developing countries, the incidence of gonorrhoea is very high. In Africa, in the early 90s, the incidence of gonococcal urethritis was estimated to be approximately 10% annually.[232] Numerous surveys conducted in recent years have shown that gonorrhoea is the commonest cause of male urethritis accounting for approximately 53-80% of the cases. The prevalence of gonococcal infection in African women is also very high ranging from 20-40% among prostitutes and 3-10% among pregnant women. A study from Bangladesh has shown disease positivity in 35.5% of the female sex workers.[233] In India also, gonorrhoea is a major health problem with incidence rates varying from 3% to 19% among the STD clinic attendees from different regions.[18-24,90-102] Majority of the reported cases are in the 20-24 years age group. However, over the years, there has

been a steady decline in its incidence which may be attributed to the availability of medical facilities at the primary health level, indiscriminate use of over the counter available potent drugs for unrelated illnesses, prophylactic use of antibiotics after sexual exposure and growing awareness about AIDS in the Indian population. A steady decline in the incidence was observed in Chandigarh, Delhi and Patiala, while a marginal increase was reported from Rohtak and Ahmedabad (Table 3). In a survey of women attending an STD clinic in Mumbai in 1996, 9.7% were positive for gonorrhoea.[234] This prevalence rate was much higher than that reported from gynaecological OPD in Amritsar (1995) and Chandigarh (1986) i.e. 0.8% and 1.8% respectively.[235,236] The apparent ratio of male to female cases is 10:1, with 80-90% men acquiring infection from commercial sex workers.[237]

Chlamydial Infection

Genital *chlamydia trachomatis* infection is an STD of epidemic proportions. It causes upto half of all acute non-gonococcal urethritis (NGU) and atleast one-third of acute epididymitis in men. In women, it is responsible for up to half of all mucopurulent cervicitis cases and 20% to 40% cases of pelvic inflammatory disease (PID) with risk of subsequent infertility or ectopic pregnancy.[103] Epidemiologic studies suggest that these sequelae are more closely linked to second or subsequent infection than to the initial infection. 85% of women with chlamydial infection are asymtomatic while 40% of infected men report no symptoms. Perinatal transmission may cause neonatal conjunctivitis and pneumonia.[238]

WHO estimates that the global frequency of infection

has risen to 50 million cases per year and in 1997, 89 million new chlamydial infections were detected.[2,238] In the developed countries, including United States, it is the most commonly reported STD and the commonest nationally notifiable infectious disease, with 3 million cases occurring annually.[84] The prevalence of this infection among women screened in family planning and prenatal clinics, where most of the cases are not seeking care for genital symptoms has been reported to be over 5%. In men seeking health care for reasons other than STD symptoms, prevalence is generally more than 5%.[239] From 1984 to 1994, the disease rates increased dramatically from 3.2 cases per 100,000 population to 188.4 cases.[240] These rates were higher for women (265.3 per 100,000 population) than for men (46.2 per 100,000) (Fig. 4). In 1995 alone, state-specific rates for women were six times higher than for men (46.4 – 622 per 100,000 versus 52.1).[241] This difference was mainly due to increased detection of asymptomatic women through regular screening. The lower rates in men suggest that they are either not diagnosed or are frequently treated but not tested. In 1994, 448,984 cases were reported to CDC from USA, in 1995, this increased to 477,638 cases while in 1997, it was 526,653. In a study conducted as part of the National Health and Nutrition Survey between 1989-1994 to determine the prevalence of chlamydial infection using the ligase chain reaction assay on urine samples, prevalence of 7% was found among non-Hispanic black population, 3% in Mexican Americans and 2% in non-Hispanic whites.[239] The prevalence rate was greater among women than men, with the highest rates in 15-19 years age group. In another study conducted in Washington between 1994-1996 using the same method among the adolescent population, prevalence among female participants was 8.6%, that declined with increasing age, while among the male attendees, it was 5.4%, which increased with age.[242] Disease positivity among women screened at family-planning clinics in 1995 ranged from 2.8% to 9.4%.[241] In HIV-infected women, a prevalence rate of 4% was found. Approximately 1 million cases of PID occur annually in the United States and 15% of the infertility cases are secondary to tubal damage resulting from PID.[8]

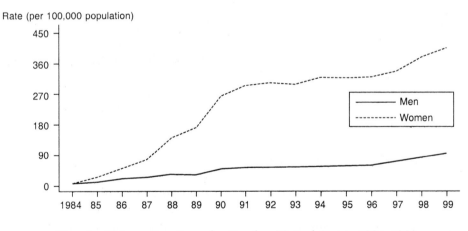

Fig. 4 Chlamydia—Rates by Gender: United States, 1984-1999

In Europe, chlamydial infection is a major bacterial STD with prevalence rates varying from 2.6% to 51.5% among women attending a variety of health Centres including STD, family planning, antenatal and abortion clinics.[243] It has been shown to be higher among the abortion and STD clinic attendees than family planning (prevalence rates of 3% to 4% in UK) and general practice clinic attendees (3% to 7% in UK).[244] The prevalence rates also depend upon the modality used for *C. trachomatis* isolation. In men, prevalence rates of 4.1% to 11.3% have been reported from different parts of Europe.[245] The attendance is highest among women aged 16 to 19, while in men it peaks in the 20-24 years age group.

In Australia, notification for chlamydial infection has been reported to be the highest among the STD and the third highest for all notifiable diseases, predominantly among the female gender and heterosexual adolescent population.[246] In a survey of the heterosexual patients attending an urban sexual health service in Sydney between 1994 and 2000, prevalence rate doubled from 1.8% to 3,5% among women and tripled from 2.1% to 6.6% among men.[247] Among the non-trachoma acute conjunctivitis cases seen in Melbourne in 1991, 2% were due to chlamydial infection of which 83% had concomitant genital infection.[248]

In sub-Saharan Africa, the prevalence is very high ranging from 47% to 52%, predominantly in women in the age group of 21 to 25 years.[249,250] The estimated incidence is 0.4 to 1.5% for PID, 0.3 to 1.5% for bilateral tubal occlusion, 0.01 to 0.04% for ectopic pregnancy and 0.04 to 0.2% for maternal mortality cases resulting from postpartum chlamydial infection complications.[103] In China, the reported prevalence ranges from 9% to 37.6%, with the highest rates recorded among women with high abortion rates, low education, multiple sex partners and non-use of condoms.[251] Seroprevalence of chlamydial infection in China in 1993 was shown to be 20.8% in CSW, 10% in STD clinic attendees, 3% among the antenatal clinic visitors and 1.3% among sexually active men (Fig. 5). In Manila, Philippines, in 1994, chlamydial antibodies were detected in 17.3% of female sex workers and 5.6% of the antenatal attenders (Fig. 6). In rural Thai women attending antenatal, postpartum and family planning clinics, prevalences of *C. trachomatis* infection were 6.8%, 5.2% and 6.7% respectively.[252] In Bangladesh, a lower prevalence of 1.9% has been reported.[253]

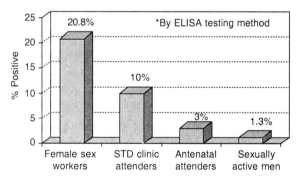

Fig. 5 Prevalence of Chlamydial Infection in High and Low Risk Groups, Nanjing, China, 1993

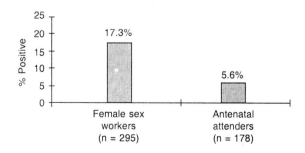

Fig. 6 Prevalence of Chlamydial Infection in High and Low Risk Groups, Manila, Philippines, 1994

Majority of the epidemiological studies conducted in India have used the criteria of demonstration of > 5 neutrophils in urethral smears or 30 neutrophils in endocervical specimens to establish the diagnosis of NGU, without isolating the causative organism. The incidence rates using this criteria have been reported to vary from 1.5% to 19% among the STD clinic attendees from different parts of the country.[18-24,90-102] There are only few studies in which prevalence rates have been established by utilizing specific diagnostic modalities for genital chlamydial infection. Among the STD clinic attendees in Delhi in 1998-99, 50% positivity for *C. trachomatis* was found using the plasmid-based PCR assay, 26% positivity using enzyme immunoassay for antigen detection and 52% positivity using ELISA for antibody detection.[254]

Among the antenatal clinic attendees in Delhi in 1999, 21.3% were found to be infected with *C. trachomatis* with significantly higher incidence of still-births, prematurity and low birth-weight in this group.[255] Another study from the same city published in 1999 showed prevalence of 17% and 18.6% during mid-pregnancy and labour with however, no difference in neonatal complications except for purulent conjunctivitis as compared to the control group.[256] (Table 10)

Table 10. Prevalence of *Chlamydia trachomatis* Infection in Antenatal Clinics

U.S.A.[239]	1990s	5%
U.K.[244]	1990s	3%–4%
China[251]	1993	3%
Phillipines (Fig.6)	1994	5.6%
Thailand[252]	1999	6.8%
India		
Delhi[255]	1999	21.3%
Delhi[256]	1999	17% –18.6%

In women attending gynae OPD in a Delhi hospital between 1990-1992 with symptoms of lower genital tract infection and infertility, prevalence of 41% and 36% respectively was found.[257] In young women undergoing routine gynaecological check-up in Mumbai in 1994, genital chlamydial infection was diagnosed in 15% cases with 53% cases showing clinical signs suggestive of cervicitis and only 2% cases suffering from PID.[258] The contribution of *C. trachomatis* in the Aetiology of PID in this study was much lower than that from Nagpur, in which it was found to be responsible for 33% cases of PID.[259] This infection was detected in 23.3% of gynae OPD attendees of Delhi in 1994.[260]

Among women seeking medical service for reproductive health complications, chlamydial infection rates varying from 0.3%-3.2% to 23.3%-33% have been reported from different parts of the country.[261,262] High risk factors for chlamydial infection identified in India include low socioeconomic factors, multiple sexual partners and use of intrauterine devices, while the protective factors are higher age-group and use of oral and barrier contraceptives (Table 11).

Table 11. Prevalence of *Chlamydia trachomatis* Infection in Gynaecologic Clinic Attendees in India

Delhi[257]	1990-92	36%-41%
Delhi[260]	1994	23.3%
Mumbai[258]	1994	15%
Mumbai[261]	2000	14.3%-20%
Chandigarh[262]	1989	33%

Genital Herpes Infection

Genital herpes is the second most prevalent STD worldwide and the commonest cause of GUD in the developed world.[263] This infection has important public health implications since undiagnosed cases contribute to the population reservoir and transmission of the virus, perinatal transmission to the neonate may result in disseminated disease, neurologic damage and high mortality and the herpetic ulcers facilitate HIV transmission. Approximately 60% of the seropositive persons are able to identify symptoms of genital herpes after receiving symptom-recognition Counselling while more than 80% of asymptomatic seropositive women shed HSV intermittantly from the genital tract.

The spread of HIV since the 1980s and subsequent behaviour change has resulted in considerable alteration in STD pattern in which the relative importance of genital herpes has increased significantly. In 1990s, HSV-2 seroprevalence from different parts of the world in population-based studies has been found to be 3.4% to 23.4%. Among specific target-groups such as STD clinic attendees, CSW, factory workers, army recruits and blood donors, it has ranged from 12% to 80%.[264]

Genital herpes is one of the 3 most prevalent STD in the United States (with chlamydial and HPV infections) and probably of greatest concern to sexually active people, apart from HIV infection.[265] In USA, about one in five persons over age 12 i.e. approximately 45 million people are infected with, HSV-2 infection with up to one million new HSV-2 infections transmitted annually. There has been a constant increase, both in the incidence and prevalence of genital herpes From 1970 to 1985, the annual incidence of HSV-2 infection increased by 82% from 4.6 per 1000 to 8.4 per 1000. Incidence in 1985 was higher in women, black population and in the age-group of 20-29 years. The age-adjusted seroprevalence of HSV-2 has also increased by 30% from the National Health and Nutrition Examination Survey II (NHANES II) 1976-1980 figures of 16.7% to NHANES III (1988-1994) rates of 21.9%.[265,266] (Fig. 7). In the third survey, seroprevalence was higher among women (25.6%) than men (17.8%) and greater among black population (45.9%) than whites (17.6%).[265] These surveys have also shown increased HSV-2 seroprevalence in Hispanic (25%) and black women (55%) as compared to white women of child-bearing age (21%). It quintupled among the white teenagers and doubled among the white population in their twenties. The other risk factors included older age, illiteracy, poverty, cocaine use and greater number of lifetime sexual partners. Among the STD clinic attendees in USA, the seroprevalence is even higher, varying from 30% to 70%.[267] In California, among young women in the low-income group, HSV-2 seropositivity was detected in 34.8% individuals in 1999-2000.[268]

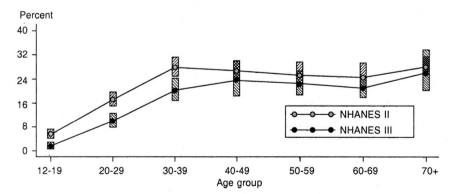

Fig. 7 Genital Herpes Simplex Virus Type 2—Percent Seroprevalence According to Age in NHANES II (1976–1980) AND NHANES III (1988–1994)

In Australia, HSV-2 infection is a major cause of STD, although its prevalence in pregnant women is less than in USA. Between 1995 and 1998, 12.5% of the antenatal clinic attendees were found to be positive for HSV-2, while 79.3% were positive for HSV-1 antibodies.[269]

In Europe, HSV-2 prevalence has been reported to range from 8% in pregnant women to 50% in homosexual men, while that for HSV-1 ranges from 60% to 90%.[270,271] In 1999-2000, seroprevalence of HSV-1 and 2 among HIV-infected women in Europe was found to be 76% and 42% respectively.[271] Majority of the genital herpes cases are caused by HSV-2, HSV-1 has been reported in an increasing number of genital ulcer cases in UK. In UK among the STD clinic attendees from 1995-1999, 62% of males and 77% of females were found to have HSV-1 isolate in their genital lesions. Among the general population groups in UK, HSV-2 seroprevalence was found to be low (3.3% in men and 5.1% in women) as compared to HSV-1 positivity observed in 24%-54% individuals, during 1994-95.[272]

In Rotterdam, Netherlands, seroprevalence of both HSV-1 and 2 was found to decrease from 68% and 59% to 30% and 22% respectively between 1993 and 1998 among the STD clinic attendees.[273] In Amsterdam also, HSV-2 seroprevalence was found to decrease from 32% in 1986 to 22% in 1998.[274] The decreasing trend in Netherlands could be an effect of the ongoing national public health campaigns promoting safer sexual practices.

In Scandinavia, the seroprevalence of HSV-2 infection among pregnant women has nearly doubled over the past two decades from 19% to 33%.[275] Studies from Scandinavia also indicate that HSV-1 is also responsible for significant proportion of genital herpes in women. This was identified in a study from Norway in 1990s, in which HSV-1 was identified in 70%-90% of suspected female genital herpes infection cases.[276] In 1992-94, in Norway, seroprevalence of HSV-2 among pregnant women was 27%, that increased with age, since 17% of the 20-24 year olds and 34% of the 35-year-olds and above were infected with this disease.[277] 25% of the STD clinic attendees in UK, 14% to 90% of the STD population in Sweden and 5% to 40% in other European populations are infected with HSV-2.[278]

Genital herpes is a significant problem in central and South America. In the 1990s, HSV-2 type-specific antibodies were detected in 61% of the CSW in Mexico city, 53% of STD patients in Brazil and 39% of women in Costa Rica.[279,280,264] In a seroepidemiologic survey undertaken in Brazil in 1994 among the voluntary blood donors, HIV-positive homo/heterosexual men and CSW, HSV-2 seropositivity was detected in 72% of the cases.[281]

In sub-Saharan Africa, the proportion of herpes-culture positive GUD have increased from 3%-11% in the 1980s to 21%-48% in the 1990s.[282] In rural populations, HSV-2 antibodies were detected in 75% of women > 25 years and 60% of men > 30 years. According to the data published in 2001, in four urban African populations, HSV-2 seroprevalence was 50% among women and 25% among men.[283] The significant increase in HSV-2 as a cause of GUD may be explained by the fact that in the era of HIV infection, immunosuppression during advanced HIV disease can increase the duration, severity and incidence of herpetic recurrences, leading to an increased herpes ulcer load. Decrease in the prevalence of bacterial STD especially chancroid, may induce a relative increase in HSV-2 as a cause of GUD. The apparent increase in genital herpes may also reflect changes in detection rates rather than a true shift in the GUD Aetiology. The improved HSV-2 detection could result from increased awareness among clinicians and patients as well as improved diagnostic choices including viral culture, specific serologic tests and PCR.

In Asia, a considerable shift in the pattern of GUD has occurred since the early 1980s when syphilis and chancroid were the primary cause of genital ulcers. In Singapore, seroprevalence of herpes infection has changed from 17% in 1980 to 72% in 1993.[284] In Kuala Lumpur, Malaysia in the 1990s, HSV-2 was identified by culture and immunofluorescence in 19% of the GUD cases.[285] Similarly, in Papua New Guinea, genital herpes was identified as the commonest cause of GUD.[286] In Dhaka, Bangladesh, seroprevalence among married women was found to be 12%.[253] In young men recruited in the armed forces in Thailand, HSV-2 seroprevalence was 41%. Among the STD clinic attendees with GUD, using the multiplex-PCR technique, prevalence of HSV-2 was found to be 82%.[287] In another study among female STD clinic attendees with clinical symptoms of genital herpes between 1994 and 1996, HSV-1 was isolated by culture in 18.7% and HSV-2 in 81.3% of the cases in Thailand.[288]

In India, there has been a significant increase in the proportion of viral STD especially HSV infection, with the incidence rates varying from 4.11% to 27.9% among STD clinic attendees in different regions of the country.[18-24,90-102] In Pune, in 1994, 26% of GUD patients were diagnosed with herpes Aetiology using the multiplex-PCR technique.[289] In a study published from Nagpur in 1998, seroprevalence of HSV-2 was shown to be 40.22% among the GUD.[290] It was higher among the sexually active, unmarried men. During 1983-86, genital herpes was diagnosed in 19% of STD clinic attendees in south India, with culture positivity in 38.7% cases with primary infection and 38.2% patients with recurrent disease.[291] The wide variation in the incidence rates may be attributed to differences in the pattern of sexual behaviour, frequency of contact, abstinence during the period of viral replication or variations in the use of barrier contraceptives. The exact prevalence is difficult to ascertain because of the large percentage of subclinical cases and limitations of serologic assays for HSV-2 antibody detection. In Chandigarh, a fourfold increase in genital herpes was observed among the STD clinic attendees from 1977 to late 1990. The incidence rose from 11.4% in 1977-85 to 21% in 1995-96.[97,98] In Ahmedabad, the incidence increased from 8.23% in 1993-94 to 27.9% in 1998-99.[21,91] In Delhi also, significant increase in the proportion of herpes genitalis was observed with the incidence rising from 2.5% in 1965-78 to 11.8% in 1995-99.[18,24] In a cross-sectional study of gynaecological clinic attendees in a Delhi hospital in 1994, IgA antibodies to HSV were detected in 20.6% of women.[260] The increasing incidence of genital herpes infection may be attributed to a decrease in the incidence of bacterial STD owing to their treatment at the primary level with large number of over-the-counter available newer antibiotics and changes in the pattern of sexual behaviour.

Seroepidemiologic studies have established that HSV is among the most common viral coinfection in AIDS patients, with 95% of MSM and 40.5% to 60% of IV drug users demonstrating serum antibodies to HSV-1, 2 or both.[292] In 1998, in the United States, anogenital HSV-2 cultures were found to be positive in 9.7% of HIV-positive men as compared to 3.1% in HIV-negative individuals.[293] Risk factors for increased viral shedding included low CD4 counts and antibodies to both HSV-1 and 2. Similarly in an Indian study, herpes genitalis was diagnosed in 7.7% of the HIV-positive individuals.[294]

The prevalence of HSV-1 varies between 50% and 90% across various study populations.[271-273] Although HSV-I is associated with orolabial disease, upto 50% of new genital ulcers in some developed countries are caused by this virus.

The most serious consequence of genital HSV infection is neonatal herpes which results from perinatal transmission from mother to infant. The transmission is greatly influenced by the mother's serologic status. If the infection is recently acquired and the mother is seronegative, 15% to 50% of the vaginally delivered infants acquire infection. However, the risk is lower among women with long–standing infection.[295]

The incidence of culture proven cases of neonatal herpes in Netherlands from 1992-1998 was 2.4 per 100,000 live-births and HSV-1 was the primary cause (73%) of neonatal herpes infection.[296] In British Isles, during 1986-1991, 76 infants with neonatal herpes were reported, an incidence of 1.65 per 100,000 live births.[297] In majority of the cases, the infection was caused by HSV-1 with 25% fatalities occurring in the neonatal period and further 33% showing long-term sequelae. The reported incidence of neonatal HSV infection in the United States is approximately 11-33 cases per 100,000 live births. During 1985, 1990 and 1995, 11.7, 11.3 and 11.4 infants per 100,000 live births were diagnosed to have HSV infection.[298] British Columbia in Canada records 1-3 cases of neonatal herpes per 45000 live births.[299]

Human Papilloma Virus (HPV) Infection

Genital HPV infect the epithelial lining of the anogenital tract. Of the 100 HPV types identified today, approximately 30 have affinity for the anogenital tract. The low risk HPVs (6 and 11) are the causative agents of genital warts and the high risk types (16, 18, 31, 33, 45), which exhibit oncogenicity, have been implicated in penile, vulval, vaginal and cervical cancers. Recent advances in laboratory techniques have made large-scale epidemiological investigations of HPV more feasible.

Genital HPV infection is the commonest viral STD in the developed world, with an estimated 30 million new cases diagnosed annually worldwide.[300] Approximately 15% of the general population harbour subclinical infection.[301]

In the United States, genital HPV infection is the third most commonly diagnosed STD, behind chlamydial infection and trichomoniasis, and the most frequently reported viral STD.[302] 99 percent of all cervical cancers and over 50% of other anogenital cancers are due to oncogenic HPV infection.[303] CDC estimates that 24 million Americans are infected with HPV and 7,50,000 new cases are diagnosed annually.[302] The incidence of genital warts has increased over the past four decades (increased from 13/100,000 population in 1950 to 106/100,000 in 1978 in Minnesota) with a 5-fold increase in the number of visits to physicians for its diagnosis and treatment.[304] The number of visits increased significantly from 60,000 in 1966 to 3,40,000 in 1988, after which they declined marginally to 2,00,000 visits in 1996 and then increased to 2,40,000 in 1999 (Fig. 8).[302] In a seroepidemiologic study of HPV infection in a male cohort of STD clinic attendees in Louisiana between 1993 and 1995, seroprevalence of HPV-6/11 and HPV-16 were 31.6% and 36.1% respectively.[305] The significant predictors for HPV-6/11 antibodies included history of syphilis, NGU and genital warts, presence of concomitant HSV-2 antibodies and increased

number of partners in the previous one year. History of trichomoniasis, syphilis and presence of HSV-2 antibodies, more than 10 years of sexual activity, older age, exchanging drugs or money for sex and cocaine or IV drug abuse were strongly associated with oncogenic HPV infection. Condoms were shown to have no protective effect against HPV-6/11 acquisition and only marginally protective against HPV-16 infection, since they do not prevent exposure to the external genital warts which are predisposed to infect keratinized epithelium and can be present outside the coverage range of condoms.

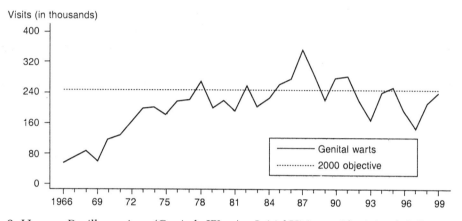

Fig. 8 Human Papillomavirus (Genital Warts)—Initial Visits to Physicians' Offices: United States, 1966-1999 and the Healthy People Year 2000 Objective

At the United States-Mexico border, in 1997-1998, the overall HPV prevalence among women attending gynecological care Centres was 14.4%, with HPV-16 being the commonest type detected.[306] The prevalence declined linearly with age from 25% among the 15-19 years old to 5.3% among 56-65 years age-group. Other risk factors included multiple sex partners, concurrent chlamydial infection and current use of injectable contraceptives.

Mexico and central America have the highest cervical cancer incidence rates with age-adjusted incidence of 44.4 cases per 100,000 women.[307] In a study conducted during 1996-1999 among Mexican women with normal cervical cytology, an overall prevalence of cervical HPV DNA was found to be 14.5%, with the highest rate of 16.7% observed under 25 years of age, which declined to 3.7% in the age-group of 35-44 years and then increased progressively among women 65 years and older. Low education was associated with high risk HPV, while low socioeconomic status correlated with low risk HPV. In Brazilian women with abnormal cervical cytology, HPV prevalence ranged from 85.6%

in low-grade squamous intraepithelial lesions to 55.2% in frank squamous cell carcinoma.[308] History of another STD mainly syphilis, but not oral contraceptive use or smoking were associated with progression to malignancy. Among women prison inmates in Sao Paulo, in 1997-1998, prevalence of 16.3% for high risk HPV and 4.8% for low risk HPV was reported.[309]

In United Kingdom, the incidence of HPV infection is on the rise. It increased 2.5-fold in both the sexes between 1971-1982.[310] Among asymptomatic women in Hungary, HPV prevalence was 17%.[311] The risk factors included young age, unmarried marital status, unemployment and smoking. The lowest prevalence rates in cytologically normal women have been reported among Spanish (4.7%) and Colombian (10.5%) women.[312] The prevalence of HPV infection among the indigenous women in Australia attending various health Centres in 1996 was low (0.42%).[313] The rates decreased with increasing age.

In sub-Saharan Africa, cervical cancer is the commonest malignancy in women, with incidence rates being fourfold higher than in United States or Europe.[314]

In Tanzania, in 1994, among the antenatal clinic attendees, HPV prevalence was found to be 34%, with high risk HPV DNA detected in 83% of women.[315] The infection was strongly associated with short duration of relationship, single marital status, non-usage of condoms and gonorrhoea.

In India, incidence of genital warts range from 2% to 25.2% in STD clinic attendees.[18-24,90-102] The data collected from the STD clinics show contradictory trends in different regions. In Delhi, in 1955-61, no case was reported,[99] the incidence in 1965-78 was 2%,[24] which increased to 9.3% in 1995-99.[18] In women attending gynae OPD in Delhi in 1994, HPV was found to be the leading infection, affecting 49.4% of women.[260] In Rohtak, during the 90s, it marginally increased from 18.1% to 21.54% and then declined to 19.35%.[95,96,101] Similarly in Ahmedabad, a slight increase in the incidence of HPV infection was observed from 7.17% in 1993-94 to 9.1% in 1998-99.[21,91] However, in Chandigarh and Patiala, the incidence of genital warts has been declining (Table 3). These studies are based on clinical diagnosis only, rather than detection of HPV DNA or serologic diagnosis. The subclinical and asymptomatic nature of HPV infection, especially in women may have been responsible for the wide disparity in the incidence rates.

Infection with oncogenic HPV is the leading cause of cervical cancer in India (Table 12). In a study from Delhi during the late 90s among women STD clinic attendees, HPV-16 DNA was detected in 30% of cases, which increased to 52% and 72% among women with precancerous and cancerous cervical lesions.[254] In Mumbai, using the method of Southern hybridization of the HPV PCR product using HPV 16/18 probes, HPV 16/18 was detected in 77% of cervical cancer patients, 38% of low-grade squamous intraepithelial squamous neoplasia lesions (LSIL), 80% of high-grade intraepithelial squamous neoplasia lesions (HSIL) and 15.2% of healthy women.[316] In the same city, using the non isotopic in-situ hybridization technique, HPV DNA was detected in 76.4% of the cervical cancer lesions, with HPV 16/18 found in 29.4% cases with squamous cell carcinoma, HPV 18 only in all cases with adenocarcinoma and neuroendocrine carcinoma of the cervix.[317] HPV 16 was isolated in 29.1% and HPV 18 in 8.3% of SIL lesions. In Calcutta, HPV DNA was detected in 50% of the biopsy specimens and none of the exfoliative cervical cell specimens of carcinoma cervix patients, with HPV 16/18 isolated in 56% of the positive biopsy material.[318]

Table 12. Prevalence of Oncogenic HPV Types in Cervical Disease in India

Delhi[254]	HPV-16	Healthy women-	30%
		SIL*-	52%
		Carcinoma cervix-	72%
Mumbai[316]	HPV-16/18	Healthywomen-	15.2%
		LSIL**-	38%
		HSIL***-	80%
		Carcinoma cervix-	77%
Mumbai[317]	HPV-16/18	SIL-	37.4%
		Carcinoma cervix-	76.4%
Calcutta[318]	HPV-16/18	Carcinoma cervix-	37%

*squamous intraepithelial neoplastic lesion
**low-grade squamous intraepithelial neoplastic lesion
***high-grade squamous intraepithelial neoplastic lesion

In majority of the studies cited above, it has been observed that the risk of acquiring HPV infection, especially among cytologically normal women is inversely associated with age and directly with the number of sexual partners, poor socioeconomic status, low education, use of oral contraceptives, reproductive characteristics, concomitant presence of other STD, smoking and dietary factors. Some of the highest prevalence rates have been found among the adolescent population, ranging from 15.6% to 46% in the early 1990s.[319] The inverse association with age may be explained by the fact that immunologic or hormonal changes occurring in old age may clear or suppress the existing infection. Moreover, lesser number of sexual partners in older women, may reduce the rate of infection. In a study from Japan, it was observed that the risk of acquiring premalignant and malignant cervical lesions with HPV-16 was 8 times higher in women 44 years of age or younger than women, 45 years of age or older.[320] Use of oral contraceptives may influence the transcription and translation of the HPV genome, hence they play an important role in the causation of cervical neoplasia. Ethnographic variations have also been observed in the epidemiology of HPV infection.[321] Higher prevalence rates have been reported among African-American women than in whites or Hispanics. This may be due to differences in the probability of encountering HPV-positive partner, genetic predisposition towards greater susceptibility to acquisition and persistence of infection, endogenous hormonal factors or differences in sexual behaviour among the ethnic groups.

Several studies have also demonstrated higher risk of cervical cancer in HIV-positive women especially with lower CD4 counts as compared to HIV-negative women or HIV-positive cases with higher CD4 counts. This may be due to persistence of greater HPV load in this group of women. The prevalence of oncogenic HPV types in HIV-positive patients varies from 14.4% to 93%, depending upon the circulating CD4 levels.[322,323] Combinations of several HPV types have been found simultaneously in most of the studied groups. In a study from Atlanta, it was shown that HIV-positive women with CD4 counts less than 200/mm³ were 1.8, 2.1 and 2.7 times more likely to have high-, intermediate- and low-risk HPV infection respectively compared with HIV-negative women.[324] Also, the cumulative prevalence of HPV infection after 3 years of follow-up was 90.2% in the former group as compared to 54.6% in the latter group. In Mexico, HPV DNA was detected by PCR in 69% of HIV-positive women and only 29% of the healthy controls.[325] In a survey conducted in 12 European countries between 1993-1998 among HIV-infected women, individuals with CD4 counts < 200/mm³ had a twofold increase in prevalence of squamous intraepithelial lesions (SIL) and non-regression from low-grade SIL as compared to women with CD4 count > 500/mm³.[326]

A strong causal association exists between HPV infection and anal and vulvar carcinoma. The incidence of anal cancer is increasing in the United States among both men and women, being twice more common in women.[327] Since 1960, the incidence of anal cancer in Connecticut increased 2-fold among men and 2.3-fold among women, being the highest among African-American women (0.74/100,000 between 1973-89) and lowest among white men (0.41/100,000).[328] In men, anal cancer is common among those indulging in receptive anal intercourse, with an incidence of 36/100,000 population.[329] The incidence of anal cancer in this group of men is 5 times higher than the incidence of cervical cancer among women in the United States. With the advent of HIV infection, the incidence has increased 2-fold from the pre-AIDS era. In a study conducted in San Francisco during 1995-1997, 76% of HIV-positive and 42% of HIV-negative women were found to have anal HPV DNA.[323] In HIV-positive women, lower CD4 counts and concomitant cervical HPV infection were strongly associated with anal infection. Younger white women were at increased risk as compared to older African-American women. Al-Ghamdi et al[330] detected HPV DNA in 85% cases of vulvar carcinoma reported between 1970-1998 in Canada

The epidemiology of STD depends upon several distdnct and complex yet interrelated behavioural, socio-

Table 13. Community Prevalence of Sexually Transmitted Diseases in Tamil Nadu[331]

Genital Symptoms (47.3%)	
Genital discharge	52.5% women
	1.7% men
Vaginal discharge, abdominal pain, dyspaerunia	60% women
Asymptomatic infection	32% women
	72% men

STD Syndromes	
GUD (men)	0.1%
GUD (women)	2.7%
Vaginal discharge	41.5%
Urethral discharge (men)	0.2%
Bubo (men)	0.02%
Scrotal swelling	2.5%
PID	0.6%

Pattern of STD	
Any STD	15.8%
Classical STD	9.7%
Gonorrhoea	3.7%
Syphilis	0.3%
Chlamydia infection	3.9%
Trichomoniasis	5.1%
HbsAg	5.3%
HIV	1.8%

demographic, economic, geographical and ethnic factors. A comprehensive knowledge of the various epidemiological parameters is extremely essential in order to design preventive and control strategies against these infections, which are responsible for significant morbidity and mortality throughout the world.

References

1. Centres for Disease Control and prevention. Summary of notifiable diseases in the United States, 1996. MMWR 1997; 45: 1-103.
2. World Health Organization. World Health Report 1998. Geneva: WHO, 1998.
3. Mabey D. Sexually transmitted diseases in developing countries. Trans R Soc Trop Med Hyg 1996; 90: 97-99.
4. Hughes G, Simms I, Rogers PA, et al. New cases seen at genitourinary medicine clinics: England 1997. Commun Dis Rep CDR (Suppl) 1998; 8: S1-11.
5. Panchaud C, Singh S, Fievelson D, et al. Sexually transmitted diseases among adolescents in developed countries. Fam Plann Perspect 2000; 32: 24-32.
6. Fox KK. Gonorrhoea in the United States, 1981-1996. Sex Transm Infect 2000; 76: 18-24.
7. Hughes G. Investigation of the increased incidence of gonorrhoea diagnosed in genitourinary medicine clinics

in England, 1994-1996. Sex Transm Infect 2000; 76: 18-24.

8. Eng TR, Butler WT. Reported rates of gonorrhoea in selected developed countries. In: The hidden epidemic: Confronting sexually transmitted diseaes. Washington DC, National Academy Press, 1997, p 29.

9. Arya OP, Lawson JB. Sexually transmitted diseases in the tropics. Epidemiological, diagnostic, therapeutic and control aspects. Tropical Doctor 1977; 7: 51-56.

10. O'Farrell N. Increasing prevalence of genital herpes in developing countries: implications for heterosexual HIV transmission and STD control programme. Sex Transm Infect 1999; 75: 377-384.

11. Perine PL. Sexually transmitted diseases in the tropics. Med J Australia 1994; 160: 360-364.

12. De Schryver A, Meheus A. Epidemiology of sexually transmitted diseases: The global picture. Bull World Health Org 1990; 68: 639-654.

13. Auvert B, Ballard R, Campbell C, et al. HIV infection among youth in a South African mining town is associated with herpes simplex virus-2 seropositivity and sexual behaviour. AIDS 2001; 15: 885-898.

14. Auvert B, Buve A, Ferry B, et al. Ecological and individual level analysis of risk factors for HIV infection in four urban populations in sub-Saharan Africa with different levels of HIV infection. AIDS 2001; 15(Suppl 4): S15-30.

15. Sanchez J, Gotuzzo E, Escamilla J, et al. Gender differences in sexual practices and sexually transmitted infections among adults in Lima, Peru. Am J Public Health 1996; 86: 1098-1107.

16. Mardh PA, Creatsas G, Guaschino S, et al. Correlation between an early sexual debut and reproductive health and Behavioural factors: a multinational European study. Eur J Contracept Reprod Health Care 2000; 5: 177-182.

17. Melissa S, Becker TM, Masuk M, et al. Risk factors for cervical intraepithelial neoplasia in Southwestern American Indian women. Am J Epidemiol 2000; 152: 716-726.

18. Khandpur S, Agarwal S, Kumar S, et al. Clinico-epidemiological profile and HIV seropositivity of STD patients. Indian J Sex Transm Dis 2001; 22: 62-65.

19. Jaiswal AK, Bhushan B. Pattern of sexually transmitted diseases in North-Eastern India. Indian J Sex Transm Dis 1994; 15: 19-20.

20. Jaiswal AK, Singh G. Pattern of sexually transmitted diseases in Jammu & Kashmir region of India. Indian J Sex Transm Dis 1998; 19: 113-115.

21. Parmar J, Raval RC, Bilimoria FE. Clinical profile of STDs at Civil Hospital Ahmedabad. Indian J Sex Transm Dis 2001; 22: 14-16.

22. Sharma PK. A profile of sexually transmitted diseases at Port Blair. Indian J Sex Transm Dis 1994; 15: 21-22.

23. Ranganayakulu B, RaviKumar GP, Bhaskar GV. Pattern of STDs at Kurnool. Indian J Sex Transm Dis 1998; 19: 117-121.

24. Reddy BSN, Jaitley V. Profile of sexually transmitted diseases: A 14-year-study. Indian J Sex Transm Dis 1985; 6: 37-40.

25. UNAIDS/WHO Epidemiological fact sheet (India) on HIV/AIDS and sexually transmitted infections. 2000 Update (revised).

26. Conde-Glez CJ, Juarez- Figueroa L, Uribe-Salas F, et al. Analysis of herpes simplex virus 1 and 2 infection in women with high risk sexual behaviour in Mexico. Int J Epidemiol 1999; 28: 571-576.

27. Ishi K, Suzuki F, Saito A, et al. Prevalence of human papilloma virus, *chlamydia trachomatis* and *Neisseria gonorrhoeae* in commercial sex workers in Japan. Infect Dis Obstet Gynecol 2000; 8(5-6): 235-239.

28. Touze A, de Sanjose S, Coursaget P, et al. Prevalence of anti-human papilloma virus types 16, 18, 31 and 58 virus-like particles in women in the general population and in proSTDtutes. J Clin Microbiol 2001; 39: 4344-4348.

29. Dada AJ, Ajayi AO, Diamond stone L, et al. A serosurvey of *Haemophilus ducreyi*, syphilis and herpes simplex virus type 2 and their association with human immunodeficiency virus among female sex workers in Lagos, Nigeria. Sex Transm Dis 1998; 25: 237-242.

30. Behets F, Andriamiadana J, Rasamilalao D, et al. Sexually transmitted infections and associated socio-demographic and Behavioural factors in women seeking primary care suggest Madagascar's vulnerability to rapid HIV spread. Trop Med Int Health 2001; 6: 202-211.

31. Rahman M, Alam A, Nessa K, et al. Aetiology of sexually transmitted infections among street-based female sex workers in Dhaka, Bangladesh. J Clin Microbiol 2000; 38: 1244-1246.

32. Chatterjee R, Mukhopadhyay D, Murmu N, et al. Prevalence of human papilloma virus infection among prostitutes in Calcutta. J Environ Pathol Toxicol Oncol 2001; 20: 113-117.

33. Thawani G, Singh US, Jana S. Prevalence of antibodies to hepatitis-C virus among visitors of red light areas in Calcutta. Indian J Sex Transm Dis 1998; 19: 105-108.

34. Urmil AC, Dutta PK, Basappa K, et al. A study of morbidity pattern among proSTDtutes attending a municipal clinic in Pune. J Indian Med Assoc 1989; 87: 29-31.

35. Lakshmi N, Kumar AG. HIV infection among commercial sex workers. Indian J Sex Transm Dis 1994; 15: 11-12.

36. Venketaramana CB, Sarada PV. Extent and speed of spread of HIV infection in India through the commercial sex network: a perspective. Trop Med Int Health 2001; 6: 1040-1061.

37. Singh S, Thappa DM, Jaisankar TJ, et al. Risk factors in transmission of HIV, hepatitis B, C in STD clinic attenders. Indian J Sex Transm Dis 2001; 22: 17-23.

38. Singh S, Jaisankar TJ, Thappa DM, et al. Risk factors for transmission of HIV infection among STD clinic attenders at Pondicherry. Indian J Sex Transm Dis 2001; 22: 27-30.

39. Gawande AV, Vasudeo ND, Zodpey SP, et al. Sexually

transmitted infections in long distance truck drivers. J Commun Dis 2000; 32: 212-215.

40. Singh YN, Malviya AN. Long distance truck drivers in India: HIV infection and their possible role in disseminating HIV into rural areas. Int J STD AIDS 1994; 5: 137-138.

41. Bwayo JJ, Omari AM, Mutere AN, et al. Long distance truck-drivers: 1. Prevalence of sexually transmitted diseases (STDs). East Afr Med J 1991; 68: 425-429.

42. Gibney L, Saquib N, Macaluso M, et al. STD in Bangladesh's trucking industry: prevalence and risk factors. Sex Transm Infect 2002; 78: 31-36.

43. Biswas D, Hazarika NC, Hazarika D, et al. Prevalence of communicable disease among restaurant workers along a highway in Assam, India. Southeast Asian J Trop Med Public Health 1999; 30: 539-541.

44. Baqi S, Shah SA, Baig MA, et al. Seroprevalence of HIV, HBV and syphilis and associated risk behaviours in male transvestites (Hijras) in Karachi, Pakistan. Int J STD AIDS 1999; 10: 300-304.

45. Miranda AE, Vargas PM, St Louis ME, et al. Sexually transmitted diseases among female prisoners in Brazil: prevalence and risk factors. Sex Transm Dis 2000; 27: 491-495.

46. Butler T, Robertson P, Kaldor J, et al. Syphilis in New South Wales (Australia) prisons. Int J STD AIDS 2001; 12: 376-379.

47. Wolfe MI, Xu F, Patel P, et al. An outbreak of syphilis in Alabama prisons: correctional health policy and communicable disease control. Am J Public Health 2001; 91: 1220-1225.

48. Akhtar S, Luby SP, Rahbar MH. Risk behaviours associated with urethritis in prison inmates, Sindh. J Pak Med Assoc 1999; 49: 268-273.

49. Singh S, Prasad R, Mohanty A. High-prevalence of sexually-transmitted and blood-borne infections among the inmates of a district jail in Northern India. Int J STD AIDS 1999; 10: 475-478.

50. Ratner M, ed. Crack pipe as pimp: An ethnographic investigation of sex for crack exchanges. New York: Lexington Books, 1993; p. 1-35.

51. De Hovitz JA, Kelly P, Feldman J, et al. Sexually transmitted diseases, sexual behaviour and cocaine use in inner city women. Am J Epidemiol 1994; 140: 1125-1134.

52. Ross MW, Hwang LY, Leonard L, et al. Sexual behaviour, STDs and drug use in a cocaine house population. Int J STD AIDS 2000; 10: 224-230.

53. Jones DL, Irwin KL, Inciardi J, et al. The high-risk sexual practices of crack-smoking in sex workers recruited from the streets of three American cities. Sex Transm Dis 1998; 25: 187-193.

54. Baumens JE, Orlanders H, Gomez MP, et al. Epidemic lymphogranuloma venereum during epidemics of crack cocaine use and HIV infection in the Bahamas. Sex Transm Dis 2002; 29: 253-258.

55. Azim T, Bogaerts J, Yirrell DL, et al. Injecting drug users in Bangladesh: prevalence of syphilis, hepatitis, HIV and HIV subtypes. AIDS 2002; 16: 121-125.

56. Agarwal AK, Singh GB, Khundom KC, et al. The prevalence of HIV in female sex workers in Manipur, India. J Commun Dis 1999; 31: 23-28.

57. Sharma AK, Aggarwal OP, Dubey KK. Sexual behaviour of drug-users: Is it different? Prev Med 2002; 34: 512-515.

58. Cook RL, Pollock NK, Rao AK, et al. Increased prevalence of herpes simplex virus type 2 among adolescent women with alcohol use disorders. J Adolesc Health 2002; 30: 169-174.

59. Waldo CR, McFarland W, Katz MH, et al. Very young gay and bisexual men are at risk for HIV infection: The San Francisco Bay Area Young Men's Survey II. J Acquir Immune Defic Syndr 2000; 24: 168-174.

60. Resurgent bacterial sexually transmitted diseases among men who have sex with men- King county, Washington, 1997-1999. MMWR 1999; 48: 773-777.

61. Outbreak of syphilis among men who have sex with men- Southern California, 2000. MMWR 2001; 50: 117-120.

62. Daling JR, Weiss NS, Hislop TG, et al. Sexual practices, sexually transmitted diseases and the incidence of anal cancer. N Engl J Med 1987; 317: 973-977.

63. Palefsky JM, Holly EA, Ralston ML, et al. High incidence of anal high-grade squamous intraepithelial lesions among HIV-positive and HIV-negative homosexual and bisexual men. AIDS 1998; 12: 495-503.

64. Stolte IG, Dukers NHTM, de Wit JBF, et al. Increase in sexually transmitted infections among homosexual men in Amsterdam in relation to HAART. Sex Transm Infect 2001; 77: 184-186.

65. Fethers K, Marks C, Minder A, et al. Sexually transmitted infections and risk behaviours in women who have sex with women. Sex Transm Infect 2000; 76: 345-349.

66. Skinner CJ, Stokes J, Kirlew Y, et al. A case-controlled study of the sexual health needs of lesbians. Genitourin Med 1996; 72: 272-280.

67. Edwards A, Thin RN. Sexually transmitted diseases in lesbians. Int J STD AIDS 1990; 1: 178-181.

68. Robertson P, Schachter J. Failure to identify venereal disease in a lesbian population. Sex Transm Dis 1981; 8: 75-76.

69. Sonnex C, Strauss S, Gray JJ. Detection of human papilloma virus DNA on the fingers of patients with genital warts. Sex Transm Infect 1999; 75: 317-319.

70. Nyirenda MJ. A study of the Behavioural aspects of dry sex practice in urban Lusaka. Int Conf AIDS 1992; 8: D101.

71. Runganga A, Pitts M, McMaster J. The use of herbal and other agents to enhance sexual experience. Soc Sci Med 1992; 35: 1037-1042.

72. Tanfer K, Aral SO. Sexual intercourse during menstruation and self-reported sexually transmitted disease history among women. Sex Transm Dis 1996; 23: 395-401.

73. Foxman B, Aral SO, Holmes KK. Interrelationships among

douching practices, risky sexual practices and history of self-reported sexually transmitted diseases in an urban population. Sex Transm Dis 1998; 25: 90-99.

74. National Survey of Family Growth. From Vital and Health Statistics. Data from the National Survey of Family Growth. Hyattsville, MD: U.S. Department of Health and human Services, Public Health Service, National Centre for Health Statistics, 1995.

75. Fonck K, Kaul R, Keli F, et al. Sexually transmitted infections and vaginal douching in a population of female sex workers in Nairobi, Kenya. Sex Transm Infect 2001; 77: 271-275.

76. Aral SO, Holmes KK. Epidemiology of sexual behaviour and sexually transmitted diseases. In; Holmes KK, Mardh PA, Sparling PF, eds, Sexually Transmitted Diseases. 2nd ed. New York: McGraw-Hill; 1990. p. 19-36.

77. Ghys PD, Diallo MO, Ettiegne-Traore V, et al. Increase in condom use and decline in HIV and sexually transmitted diseases among female sex workers in Abidjan, Cote d' Ivoire, 1991-1998. AIDS 2002; 16: 251-258.

78. Daling JR, Madeleine MM, McKnight B, et al. The relationship of human papillomavirus-related cervical tumours to cigarette smoking, oral contraceptives use and prior herpes simplex virus type 2 infection. Cancer Epidemiol Biomarkers Prev 1996; 5: 541-548.

79. Kramer RL. The intrauterine device and pelvic inflammatory disease revisited: new results from The Women's Health Study. Obstet Gynecol 1989; 73: 300-301.

80. Vessey M, Doll R, Peto R, et al. A long-term follow-up study of women using different methods of contraception-an interim report. J Biosoc Sci 1976; 8: 373-427.

81. Farley TM, Rosenberg MJ, Rowe PJ, et al. Intrauterine devices and pelvic inflammatory disease: an international perspective. Lancet 1992; 339: 785-788.

82. Palayekar V, Joshi JV, Hazari KT, et al. *Chlamydia trachomatis* detected in cervical smears from Copper-T users by DFA test. Adv Contracept 1996; 12: 145-152.

83. Fink AJ. Circumcision: A parent's decision for life. Mountain view, CA, Kavanah Publishing Co., 1988.

84. American Social Health Association. Sexually transmitted diseases in America: How many cases and at what cost? Menlo Park, CA: Kaiser Family foundation, 1998.

85. Noell J, Rohde P, Ochs L, et al. Incidence and prevalence of chlamydia, herpes and viral hepatitis in a homeless adolescent population. Sex Transm Dis 2001; 28: 4-10.

86. Moscicki AB, Palefsky J, Gonzales J, et al. Human papillomavirus infection in sexually active females: prevalence and risk factors. Pediatr Res 1990; 28: 507-513.

87. Sharma RP, Dhir GG. Sexually transmitted diseases in teenagers. Indian J Sex Transm Dis 1987; 8: 51-52.

88. Xu F, Schillinger JA, Aubin MR, et al. Sexually transmitted diseases of older persons in Washington state. Sex Transm Dis 2001; 28: 287-291.

89. Lee CC, Leo YS, Snodgrass L, et al. The demography, clinical manifestations and natural history of HIV infection in an older population in Singapore. Ann Acad Med Singapore 1997; 26: 731-735.

90. Mehta Swami D, Jaswal R, Bedi GK, et al. Pattern of sexually transmitted diseases in a new Northern Indian Hospital. Indian J Sex Transm Dis 1998; 19: 109-112.

91. Raval RC, Desai N, Bilimoria FE. Clinical profile of STDs at BJ Medical college and Civil Hospital, Ahmedabad. Indian J Sex Transm Dis 1995; 16: 54-55.

92. Majumdar S, Saha SS. Epidemiological survey of chancroid in Calcutta area. Indian J Sex Transm Dis 1997; 18: 9-11.

93. Chopra A, Dhaliwal RS, Chopra D. Pattern of changing trends of STDs at Patiala. Indian J Sex Transm Dis 1999; 20: 22-25.

94. Chopra A, Mittal RR, Singh P, et al. Pattern of sexually transmitted diseases in Patiala. Indian J Sex Transm Dis 1990; 11: 43-45.

95. Gupta SK, Jain VK, Aggarwal K. Trends of sexually transmitted diseases at Rohtak. Indian J Sex Transm Dis 1997; 18: 2-3.

96. Gupta SK, Jain VK. Pattern of sexually transmitted diseases in Rohtak. Indian J Sex Transm Dis 1995; 16: 28-29.

97. Kumar B, Handa S, Malhotra S. Changing trends in sexually transmitted diseases. Indian J Sex Transm Dis 1995; 16: 24-27.

98. Kumar B, Sharma VK, Malhotra S. et al. Pattern of sexually transmitted diseases in Chandigarh. Indian J Sex Transm Dis 1987; 53: 286-291.

99. Singh R. Pattern of VDs as seen at VD training demonstration Centre, Safdarjung Hospital, New Delhi. Ind J Dermatol Venereol leprol 1962; 28: 62-67.

100. Narayan R, Kar HK. Pattern of STDs in a Delhi Hospital. Indian J Sex Transm Dis 1996; 17: 14-16.

101. Aggarwal K, Jain VK, Brahma D. Trend of STDs at Rohtak. Indian J Sex Transm Dis 2002; 23: 19-21.

102. Reddy BSN, Garg BR, Rao MV. An appraisal of trends in sexually transmitted diseases. Indian J Sex Transm Dis 1993; 14: 1-4.

103. Over M, Piot P. HIV infection and other sexually transmitted diseases importance and priorties for resource allocation. J Infect Dis 1996; 174 (Suppl 2). 162-75

104. Laumann EO, Youm Y. Racial/ethnic group differences in the prevalence of sexually transmitted diseases in the United States: a network explanation. Sex Transm Dis 1999; 26: 250-261.

105. Shahmanesh M, Gayed S, Ashcroft M, et al. Geomapping of chlamydia and gonorrhoea in Birmingham. Sex Transm Infect 2000; 76: 268-272.

106. Miller PJ, Law M, Torzillo PJ, et al. Incident sexually transmitted infections and their risk factors in an Aboriginal community in Australia: a population based cohort study. Sex Transm Infect 2001; 77: 21-25.

107. Ley C, Bauer HM, Reingold A, et al. Determinants of genital human papilloma virus infection in young women. J Natl Cancer Inst 1991; 83: 997-1003.

108. Reddy BSN, Rao MV, Gharami RC, et al. Clinico-epidemiological study of donovanosis in Pondicherry. JIPMER Bulletin 1994; 13: 14-17.

109. Aswar NR, Wahab SN, Kale KM. Prevalence and some epidemiologic factors of syphilis in Madia tribes of Gadchiroli district. Indian J Sex Transm Dis 1998; 19: 53-58.

110. Holmes KK. An estimate of the risk of men acquiring gonorrhoea by sexual contact with infected females. Am J Epidemiol 1970; 91: 170.

111. Tice RW, Rodriguez VL. Pharyngeal gonorrhoea. JAMA 1981; 246: 2717-2719

112. King A, Nicol C, Rodin P, eds. Gonorrhoea: Mode of infection; Diagnostic methods; Pathology; The Incubation period. In: Venereal Diseases. 4ᵗʰ ed. London: ELBS; 1980. p. 189-199.

113. David IM. Acquisition of pharyngeal gonorrhoea via sweets passed by mouth. Genitourin Med 1997; 73: 146.

114. Kleist E, Mei H. Transmission of gonorrhoea through an inflatable doll. Genitourin Med 1993; 69: 321-325.

115. Lycke E, Lowhagen GB, Halhagon G. The risk of genital *chlamydia trachomatis* infection is less than that of *Neisseria gonorrhoeae* infection. Sex Transm Dis 1980; 7: 6-10

116. Quinn TC, Gaydos C, Shepherd M, et al. Epidemiologic and microbiologic correlates of *Chlamydia trachomatis* infection in sexual partnerships. JAMA 1996; 276: 1737-1742.

117. Goldmeier D, Darougar S. Isolation of *Chlamydia trachomatis* from the throat and rectum of homosexual men. Br J Vener Dis 1977; 53: 184-185.

118. Jones RB, Rabinovitch RA, Kats BP, et al. *Chlamydia trachomatis* in the pharynx and rectum of heterosexual patients at risk of genital infection. Ann Intern Med 1985; 102: 757-762.

119. Hammerschlag MR, Andenka M, Semine DZ, *et al.* Prospective study of maternal and infantile infection with chlamydia trachomatis. Paediatrics 1979; 64: 142-148.

120. Schroeter AL. Therapy for incubating syphilis.: Effectiveness of gonorrhoea treatment. JAMA 1971; 218: 711.

121. King A, Nicol C, Rodin P, eds. Early acquired syphilis. In: Venereal Diseases, 4ᵗʰ ed, 1980, ELBS, Great Britain, p.15-43.

122. Harter CA, Benirschke K. Foetal syphilis in the first trimester. Am J Obstet Gynecol 1976; 124: 705-711.

123. Chambers RW, Foley HT, Schmidt PJ. Transmission of syphilis by fresh blood components. Transfusion 1969; 9: 32-34.

124. Harris VK, Nair SC, Das PK, et al. Prevalence of syphilis and parasitic infection among blood donors in a tertiary-care centre in southern India. Ann Trop Med Parasitol 1999; 93: 763-765.

125. Matee MI, Lyamuya EF, Mbena EC, et al. Prevalence of transfusion associated viral infections and syphilis among blood donors in Muhimbili Medical Centre, Dar-es-Salaam, Tanzania. East Afr Med J 1999; 76: 167-171.

126. Azim T, Islam MN, Bogaerts J, et al. Prevalence of HIV and syphilis among high-risk groups in Bangladesh. AIDS 2000; 14: 210-211.

127. Plummer FA, D'Costa LJ, Nsanze H, et al. Epidemiology of chancroid and *Haemophilus ducreyi* in Nairobi, Kenya. Lancet 1983; 2: 1293-1295.

128. Plummer FA, D'Costa LJ, Nsanze H, et al. Clinical and microbiological studies of genital ulcers in Kenyan women. Sex Transm Dis 1985; 12: 193-197.

129. Diaz-Mitoma F. Aetiology of non-vesicular genital ulcers in Winnipeg. Sex Transm Dis 1987; 14: 33.

130. King A, Nicol C, Rodin P, eds. Chancroid. In: Venereal Diseases. 4ᵗʰ ed. London: ELBS; 1980, p251-257.

131. Cesario TC, Poland JD, Wulff H, et al. Six years' experience with herpes simplex virus in a chidren's home. Am J Epidemiol 1969; 90: 416-422.

132. Stanberry L, Cunningham A, Mertz G, et al. New developments in the epidemiology, natural history and management of genital herpes. Antiviral Res 1999; 42: 1-14.

133. King A, Nicol C, Rodin P, eds. Herpes genitalis and Hepatitis B infection. In: Venereal Diseases. 4ᵗʰ ed. 1980, ELBS; London: 1980, p 325-332.

134. Marmell M. Donovanosis of the anus in the male: An epidemiologic consideration. Br J Vener Dis 1958; 34: 213.

135. King A, Nicol C, Rodin P, eds. Granuloma inguinale. In: Venereal Diseases. 4ᵗʰ ed. London: ELBS; 1980, p. 268-273.

136. Perine PL, Osoba AO. Lymphogranuloma venereum. In: Holmes KK, Mardh PA, Sparling PF, et al, eds. Sexually Transmitted Diseases. 2ⁿᵈ ed. New York: McGraw-Hill, 1990, p. 195-204.

137. Oriel JD. Natural history of genital warts. Br J Vener Dis 1971; 47:1-13.

138. Oriel JD. Anal warts and anal coitus. Br J Vener Dis 1971; 47: 373-376.

139. Judson FN. Condyloma acuminatum of the oral cavity: A case report. Sex Transm Dis 1981; 8: 218-19.

140. Puranen M, Yliskoski M, Saarikoski S, et al. Vertical transmission of human papillomavirus from infected mothers to their newborn babies and persistence of the virus in childhood. Am J Obstet Gynecol 1996; 174: 694-699.

141. Tang CK, Shermeta DW, Wood C. Congenital condylomata acuminata. Am J Obstet Gynecol 1978; 131: 912-913.

142. De Jong AR, Weiss JC, Raent RL Condylomata acuminata in children. Am J Dis Child 1982; 136: 704-706.

143. Weston TET, Nicol CS. Natural history of trichomonal infection in males. Br J Vener Dis 1963; 39: 251.

144. Honigberg B. Trichomonads of importance in human medicine. In: Kreier JP ed., Parasitic protozoa, New York: Academic; 1978, p. 275.

145. Latif AS, Mason PR, Marowa E. Urethral trichomoniasis in men. Sex Transm Dis 1987; 14: 9-11.

146. Jones JG, Lamauchi T, Lambert B. *Trichomonas vaginalis* infestation in sexually abused girls. Am J Dis Child 1985; 139: 846-848.

147. Al-Sahili FL, Curran JP, Wang J. Neonatal *Trichomonas*

vaginalis: Report of 3 cases and review of literature. Paediatrics 1974; 53: 196-200.

148. Szmuness W, Much I, Prince AM, et al. On the role of sexual behaviour in the spread of hepatitis B infection. Ann Intern Med 1975; 83: 489-495.

149. Centre for Disease Control. Changing patterns of groups at high risk for hepatitis B in the United States. MMWR 1988; 37: 429.

150. Mehendale SM, Shepherd ME, Divekar AD, et al. Evidence of high prevalence and rapid transmission of HIV among individuals attending STD clinics in Pune. Indian J Med Res 1996; 104: 327-335.

151. Kura KM, Hira S, Kohli M, et al. High occurrence of HBV among STD clinic attenders in Bombay, India. Int J STD AIDS 1998; 9: 231-233.

152. Villarejos V, M, Visona KA, Gutierrez A, et al. Role of saliva, urine and faeces in transmission of type B hepatitis. N Engl J Med 1974; 291: 1375-1378.

153. Koumans EH, Sternberg M, Gwinn M, et al. Geographic variation of HIV infection in childbearing women with syphilis in the United States. AIDS 2000; 14: 279-287.

154. Cook RL, Royce RA, Thomas JC, et al. What's driving an epidemic? The spread of syphilis along an interstate highway in rural North Carolina. Am J Public Health. 1999; 89: 369-373.

155. Finelli L, Levine WC, Valentine J, et al. Syphilis outbreak assessment. Sex Transm Dis 2001; 28: 131-135.

156. Primary and secondary syphilis- United States, 1999. MMWR 2001; 50(7): 113-117.

157. Division of STD Prevention. Sexually Transmitted Disease Prevention, 2000. Atlanta, Centres for Disease Control and Prevention, US Department of Health and Human Services, Public Health Service, 2001.

158. Kahn RH, Heffelfinger JD, Berman SM. Syphilis outbreaks among men who have sex with men. A public health trend of concern. Sex Transm Dis 2002; 29: 285-287.

159. Outbreak of primary and secondary syphilis- Guilford County, North Carolina, 1996-1997. MMWR 1998; 47: 1070-1073.

160. Williams PB, Ekundayo O. Study of distribution and factors affecting syphilis epidemic among inner-city minorities of Baltimore. Public Health 2001; 115: 387-393.

161. Fenton KA, Nicoll A, Kinghorn G. Resurgence of syphilis in England: time for more radical and nationally coordinated approaches. Sex Transm Infect 2001; 77: 309-310.

162. Fennema JS, Cairo I, Coutinho RA. Substantial increase in gonorrhoea and syphilis among clients of Amsterdam sexually transmitted diseases clinic. Ned Tijdschr Geneeskd 2000; 144: 602-603.

163. Bosman A, de Zwart O, Schop WA, et al. Increase of early syphilis in a red light district of Rotterdam (1995-1997) and preventive treatment. Ned Tijdschr Geneeskd 1999; 143: 2324-2328.

164. Machovcova A, Konkolova R, Schmiedbergerova R, et

al. Syphilis in the third millenium. Cas Lek Cesk 2002; 141: 96-100.

165. Bjekic M, Vlajinac H, Sipetic S, et al. Trends of gonorrhoea and early syphilis in Belgrade, 1985-99. Sex Transm Infect 2001; 77: 387-389.

166. Diaconu JD, Benea V, Muresian D, et al. Incidence of sexually transmitted disease in Romania in the transition period. JEADV 1999; 12 (Suppl 2): 342.

167. Dencheva R, Spirov G, Gilina K, et al. Syphilis in Bulgaria-epidemiological survey 1990-1999. CEEDVA, Bulletin 2000; 2: 10-13.

168. Karieva MT, Umanov TM. Incidence of syphilis in the Republic of Uzbekistan: epidemiological aspects. JEADV 1997; 9 (Suppl 1): 228.

169. Todd J, Munguti K, Grosskurth H, et al. Risk factors for active syphilis and TPHA seroconversion in a rural African population. Sex Transm Infect 2001; 77: 37-45.

170. Behets F M-T, Andriamiadana J, Randrianasolo D, et al. Chancroid, primary syphilis, genital herpes and lymphogranuloma venereum in Antananarivo, Madagascar. J Infect Dis 1999; 180: 1382-1285.

171. Temmerman M, Fonck K, Bashir F, et al. Declining syphilis prevalence in pregnant women in Nairobi since 1995: another success story in the STD field? Int J STD AIDS 1999; 10: 405-408.

172. Rathore AS, Ray K, Ramesh V, et al. Periodic syphilis profile in a New Delhi hospital. J Commun Dis 1999; 30: 153-157.

173. Ganesh R, Stanley A, Ganesh N, et al. Prevalence of neurosyphilis at Government Rajaji Hospital, Madurai, India. Int J STD AIDS 1994; 5: 290-292.

174. Thakur TS, Sharma V, Goyal A, et al. Seroprevalence of HIV antibodies, Australia antigen and VDRL reactivity in Himachal Pradesh. Indian J Med Sci 1991; 45: 332-335.

175. Pandit DD, Angadi SA, Chavan MK, et al. Prevalence of VDRL sero-positivity in women in reproductive age group in an urban slum community in Bombay. Indian J Public Health 1995; 39: 4-7.

176. Garg S, Sharma N, Bhalla P, et al. Reproductive morbidity in an Indian urban slum: need for health action. Sex Transm Infect 2002; 78: 68-69.

177. Nanu A, Sharma SP, Chatterjee K, et al. Markers of transfusion-transmissible infections in north Indian voluntary and replacement blood donors: prevalence and trends 1989-1996. Vox Sang 1997; 73: 70-75.

178. Choudhary N, Ramesh V, Saraswat S, et al. Effectiveness of mandatory transmissible diseases screening in Indian blood donors. Indian J Med Res 1995; 101: 229-232.

179. Bhargava NC, Ray K, Kumari S, et al. Incidence of HIV versus VDRL antibody positivity in a major STD clinic in Delhi. Indian J Sex Transm Dis 1987; 8: 44-46.

180. Murugan S, Srinivasan G, Kaleellulah MCA. Screening of blood donors for syphilis. Indian J Sex Transm Dis 1991; 12: 45-46.

181. Gupta AK, Saran R. Detection of antibodies to HIV-

infection among high risk group in Bihar, India. Indian J Public Health 1993; 37: 54-56.

182. Warner L, Rochat RW, Fichtner RR, et al. Missed opportunities for congenital syphilis prevention in an urban Southeastern Hospital. Sex Transm Dis 2001; 28: 92-98.

183. Congenital syphilis- United States, 2000. MMWR 2001; 50: 573-577.

184. Southwick KL, Blanco S, Santander A, et al. Maternal and congenital syphilis in Bolivia, 1996: prevalence and risk factors. Bull World Health Organization 2001; 79: 33-42.

185. Anandam K, Seethamma R. Variegated presentation of congenital syphilis. Indian J Sex Transm Dis 1999; 20: 57-59.

186. McDermott J, Steketee R, Larsen S, et al. Syphilis associated perinatal and infant mortality in rural Malawi. Bull World Health Organization 1993; 71: 773-780.

187. Greenwood AM, D'Alessandro U, Sisay F, et al. Treponemal infection and the outcome of pregnancy in a rural area of the Gambia, West Africa. J Infect Dis 1992; 166: 842.

188. Rutger S. Syphilis in pregnancy: a medical audit in a rural district. Cent Afr J Med 1993; 39: 248-253.

189. Sharma M, Kumar B, Sharma SK, et al. Blood VDRL reactivity in STD and antenatal clinics in Chandigarh. Indian J Sex Transm Dis 1986; 7: 14-15.

190. Rattan A, Maheshwari N, Sharma R, et al. Significance of low titre VDRL reactions. Indian J Sex Transm Dis 1987; 8: 5-6.

191. Nair D, Bhalla P, Mathur MD. A study of antenatal screening for syphilis. Indian J Sex Transm Dis 1996; 17: 54-56.

192. Vajpayee M, Seth P, Malhotra N. HIV and syphilis in pregnant women at a tertiary care hospital. Tropical Doctor 2001; 31: 56.

193. Schmid GP, Sanders Jr LL, Blount JH, et al. Chancroid in the United States- Reestablishment of an old disease. JAMA 1987; 258: 3265-3268.

194. Dillon SM, Cummings M, Rajagopalan M, et al. Prospective analysis of genital ulcer disease in Brooklyn, New York. Clin Infect Dis 1997; 24: 945-950.

195. DiCarlo RP, Armentor BS, Martin DH. Chancroid epidemiology in New Orleans men. J Infect Dis 1995; 172: 446-452.

196. Mertz KJ, Weiss JB, Webb RM, et al. An inveSTDgation of genital ulcers in Jackson, Mississippi, with use of multiplex polymerase chain reaction assay: High prevalence of chancroid and human immunodeficiency virus infection. J Infect Dis 1998; 178: 1060-1066.

197. Morel P, Casin I, Gandiol C, et al. An epidemic of chancroid. 587 cases. Nouv Presse Med 1982; 11: 655-656.

198. Kamali A, Nunn AJ, Mulder DW, et al. Seroprevalence and incidence of genital ulcer infections in a rural Ugandan population. Sex Transm Infect 1999; 75: 98-102.

199. Hira SK. Sexually transmitted diseases in the era of AIDS. AIDS Watch. WHO South-East Asia Region Newsletter 1997; 2: 1-2.

200. Annual Reports of the Medical Officer of Health for Durban 1996, 1997.

201. Bassa AG, Hoosen AA, Moodley J, et al. Granuloma inguinale (Donovanosis) in women. An analysis of 61 cases from Durban, South Africa. Sex Transm Dis 1993; 20: 164-167.

202. Siva D, Salgado U, Macedo C, et al. Donovanosis in Peru. Rev Soc Bras Med Trop 1991; 24: 251-252.

203. Kuberski T, Philips P, Tabua TW. Status of granuloma inguinale in Papua New Guinea. P N G Med J 1979; 22: 5-12.

204. Jamkhedkar PP, Hira SK, Shroff HJ, et al. Clinico-epidemiologic features of granuloma inguinale in the era of acquired immune deficiency syndrome. Sex Transm Dis 1998; 25: 196-200.

205. O'Farrell N, Hammond M. HLA antigens in donovanosis (granuloma inguinale). Genitourin Med 1991; 67: 400-402.

206. Sehgal VN, Jain MK. Pattern of epidemics of Donovanosis in the nonendemic region. Int J Dermatol 1988; 27: 396-399.

207. Abrams AJ. Lymphogranuloma venereum. JAMA 1968; 205: 199-202.

208. Division of STD Prevention. Sexually Transmitted Disease Surveillance, 1997. U.S. Department of Health and Human Services, Public Health Service. Atlanta, Centre for Disease Control, September 1998.

209. Department of Health. New cases of genitourinary medicine clinics in England. Annual figures 1995, Summary information from KC 60. London, 1996.

210. Ndinya-Achola JO. Presumptive specific clinical diagnosis of genital ulcer disease in a primary health care setting in Nairobi. Int J STD AIDS 1996; 7: 201-205.

211. Mabey DCW. Aetiology of genital ulceration in the Gambia. Genitourin Med 1987; 63: 312-315.

212. O'Farrel. Genital ulcer disease: accuracy of clinical diagnosis and strategies to improve control in Durban, South Africa. Genitourin Med 1994; 70: 7-11.

213. Ray K. Usefulness of immunoperoxidase for serodiagnosis of genital chlamydial infections. Ind J Med Res 1993; 97: 67-71.

214. Viravan C. A prospective clinical and bacteriological study of inguinal buboes in Thai men. Clin Infect Dis 1996; 22: 233-239.

215. Piot P. Sexually Transmitted Disease. In: Warren KS, Mahmoud AAF, eds. Tropical and Geographical Medicine. 2nd ed. New York: McGraw-Hill; 1990. p. 894-910.

216. Brathwaite AR. A comparison of prevalence rates of genital ulcers among persons attending a sexually transmitted disease clinic in Jamaica. West Indian Med J 1997; 46: 67-71.

217. Frieda MT. Chancroid, primary syphilis, genital herpes and lymphogranuloma venereum in Antananarivo, Madagascar. J Infect Dis 1999; 180: 1382-1385.

218. Luk NM. Lymphogranuloma venereum. In: Social Hygiene Handbook, Handbook of Dermatology and Venereology. 2nd ed. 1996. p. 1-14.

219. Chua SH. Genital ulcer disease in patients attending a public sexually transmitted disease clinic in Singapore: an epidemiological study. Ann Acad Med Singapore 1995; 24: 510-514.

220. Schachter J. Lymphogranuloma venereum and other non-ocular *Chlamydia trachomatis* infections. In: Manual of Clinical Microbiology. Hobson D, Holmes KK, eds. Washington, American Society of Microbiology, 1977: 91-97.

221. Koteen H. Lymphogranuloma venereum. Medicine 1945; 24: 1.

222. Annamuthoda H. Rectal Lymphogranuloma venereum in Jamaica. Ann R Coll Surg Engl 1961; 29: 141.

223. Chamber S, Henry F. Infectious Diseases: Bacterial and Chlamydial. In: Lawrence M, Tierney Jr, eds. Current Medical Diagnosis and Treatment, 1998, Stamford, CT: Appleton and Lange, 1997.

224. Tapsall JW. Surveillance of antibiotic susceptibility of *Neisseria gonorrhoeae* in the WHO western pacific region 1992-1994. Genitourin Med 1997; 73: 355-361

225. Cates W Jr. Sexually transmitted diseases, pelvic inflammatory disease and infertility - an epidemiologic update. Epidemiol Rev 1990; 12: 199-220.

226. Low N. Success and failure in gonorrhoea control. Dermatol Clin 1998; 16: 713-720.

227. Eng TR. Butler WT. Reported rates of gonorrhoea in selected developed countries. In: The hidden epidemic: Confronting sexually transmitted diseases. Washington DC: National Academy Press; 1997. p. 29.

228. Division of STD Prevention. Sexually transmitted disease surveillance, 1999. US Department of Health and Human Services, Public Health Service. Atlanta: Centres for Disease Control and Prevention, October 2000: 1-112.

229. Wright RA, Judson FN Relative and seasonal incidences of the sexually transmitted diseases: A two-year statiSTDcal review. Br J Vener Dis 1978; 54: 433-440.

230. Hughes G. Investigation of the increased incidence of gonorrhoea diagnosed in genitourinary medicine clinics in England, 1994-1996. Sex Transm Infect 2000; 76: 18-24.

231. Fox KK. Gonorrhoea in the United States, 1981-1996: Demographic and Geographic trends. Sex Transm Dis 1998; 25: 386-393.

232. Cates W Jr. Sexually transmitted diseases, pelvic inflammatory disease and infertility - an epidemiologic update. Epidemiol Rev 1990; 12: 199-220.

233. Rahman M. Aetiology of sexually transmitted infections among street-based female sex workers in Dhaka, Bangladesh. J Clin Microbiol 2000; 38: 1244-1246.

234. Divekar AA, Gogate AS, Shivkar LK, et al. Disease prevalence in women attending the STD clinic in Mumbai, India. Int J STD AIDS 2000; 11: 45-48.

235. Kaur H, Saini JS, Jasmeen. Prevalence of gonorrhoea in Punjabi women. J Obstet Gynecol India 1995; 45: 100-105.

236. Kaur S, Kumar B, Malhotra S, et al. Screening for gonococal infection in patients attending gynaecological clinics. Indian J Sex Transm Dis 1986; 7: 44-46.

237. Hook EW. Gonococcal Infections. Ann Int Med 1985; 102: 229-243.

238. Tchoudomirova K, Nuhov Ph, Tchapanova A. Prevalence, epidemiological and clinical correlates of genital *chlamydia trachomatis* infection. JEADV 1998; 11: 214-220.

239. Mertz KJ, McQuillan GM, Levine WC, et al. A pilot study of the prevalence of chlamydial infection in a national household survey. Sex Transm Dis 1998; 225-228.

240. Centre for Disease Control. Ten leading nationally notifiable infectious diseases- United States, 1995. MMWR 1996; 45: 883-884.

241. *Chlamydia trachomatis* genital infections- United States, 1995. JAMA 1997; 277: 952-953.

242. Marrazzo JM, White CL, Krekeler B, et al. Community-based urine screening for *chlamydia trachomatis* with a ligase chain reaction assay. Ann Intern Med 1997; 127: 796-803.

243. Oakeshott P, Hay P. General practice update: chlamydia infection in women Br J Gen Pract 1995; 45: 615-620.

244. Stokes T. Screening for chlamydia in general practice: a literature review and summary of the evidence. J Public Health Med 1997; 19: 222-232.

245. Shafer MA, Schachter J, Moncada J, et al. Evaluation of urine-based screening strategies to detect *chlamydia trachomatis* among sexually active asymptomatic young males. JAMA 1993; 270: 2065-2070.

246. Thompson J, Lin M, Halliday L. Australia's notifiable disease status, 1998. Annual report of the National Notifiable Diseases Surveillance System. Commun Dis Intell 1999; 23: 277-305.

247. Donova B. Rising prevalence of genital *chlamydia trachomatis* infection in heterosexual patients at the Sydney Sexual Health Centre, 1994 to 2000. Commun Dis Intell 2002; 26: 51-55.

248. Garland SM, Malatt A, Tabrizi S, et al. *Chlamydia trachomatis* conjunctivitis. Prevalence and association with genital tract infection. Med J Aust 1995; 162: 363-366.

249. Harms G, Matull R, Randrianasolo D, et al. Pattern of sexually transmitted diseases in a Malagasy population. Sex Transm Dis 1994; 21: 315-320.

250. Azenabor AA, Eghafona NO. Association of *chlamydia trachomatis* antibodies with genital contact disease in Benin City, Nigeria. Trop Med Int Health 1997; 2: 389-392.

251. Bai H, Bo N, Huan Li, et al. Prevalence of genital *Chlamydia trachomatis* infection in selected populations in China. Sex Transm Dis 1995; 383-384.

252. Thongkrajai P, Thongkrajai E, Pengsaa P, et al. The prevalence of *Chlamydia trachomatis* infection in rural Thai women. Southeast Asian J Trop Med Public Health 1999; 30: 52-57.

253. Bogaerts J, Ahmed J, Akhter N, et al. Sexually transmitted infections among married women in Dhaka, Bangladesh: unexpected high prevalence of herpes simplex type 2 infection. Sex Transm Infect 2001; 77: 114-119.

254. Gopalkrishna V, Aggarwal N, Malhotra VL, et al. *Chlamydia trachomatis* and human papillomavirus infection in Indian women with sexually transmitted diseases and cervical precancerous and cancerous lesions. Clin Microbiol Infect 2000; 6: 88-93.

255. Rastogi S, Kapur S, Salhan S, et al. *Chlamydia trachomatis* infection in pregnancy: risk factors for an adverse outcome. Br J Biomed Sci 1999; 56: 94-98.

256. Paul VK, Singh M, Gupta U, et al. *Chlamydia trachomatis* infection among pregnant women: prevalence and prenatal importance. Natl Med J India 1999; 12: 11-14.

257. Mittal A, Kapur S, Gupta S. Screening for genital chlamydial infection in symptomatic women. Indian J Med Res 1993; 98: 119-123.

258. Joshi JV, Palayekar S, Hazari KT, et al. The prevalence of *Chlamydia trachomatis* in young women. Natl Med J India 1994; 7: 57-59.

259. Shrikhande SN, Joshi SG, Zodpey SP, et al. *Chlamydia trachomatis* in pelvic inflammatory disease. Indian J Pathol Microbiol 1995; 38: 181-184.

260. Singh V, Sehgal A, Satyanarayana L, et al. Clinical presentation of gynaecologic infections among Indian women. Obstet Gynecol 1995; 85: 215-219.

261. Brabin L, Gogate A, Gogate S, et al. Reproductive tract infections, gynaecological morbidity and HIV seroprevalence among women in Mumbai, India. Bull World Health Organization 1998; 76: 277-287.

262. Sharma M, Nayak N, Malhotra S, et al. Chlamydiazyme test for rapid detection of *Chlamydia trachomatis*. Indian J Med Res 1989; 89: 87-91.

263. Brugha R, Keersmaeker K, Renton A, et al. Genital herpes infection: a review. Int J Epidemiol 1997; 26: 698-709.

264. Corey L, Hansfield HH. Genital herpes and public health. Addressing a global problem. JAMA 2000; 283: 791-794.

265. Fleming DT, Mcquillan GM, Johnson RE, et al. Herpes simplex virus type 2 in the United States, 1976 to 1994. N Engl J Med 1997; 337: 1105-1111.

266. Johnson RE, Nahmias AJ, Magder LS, et al. A seroepidemiologic survey of the prevalence of herpes simplex virus type 2 infection in the United States. N Engl J Med 1990; 321: 8-12.

267. Koutsky L, Stevens CE, Holmes KK, et al. Underdiagnosis of genital herpes by current clinical and viral isolation procedures. N Engl J Med 1992; 326: 1533-1539.

268. Buchacz K, McFarland W, Hernandez M, et al. Prevalence and correlates of herpes simplex virus type 2 infection in a population-based survey of young women in low-income neighbourhoods of North California. The young women's survey team. Sex Transm Dis 2000; 27: 393-400.

269. Mindel A, Taylor J, Tideman RL, et al. Neonatal herpes prevention: a minor public health problem in some communities. Sex Transm Infect 2000; 76: 287-291.

270. Nahmias AJ, Lee FK, Beckman-Nahmias S. Seroepidemiological and sociological patterns of herpes simplex virus infection in the world. Scand J Infect Dis Suppl 1990; 69: 19-36.

271. Van Benthem BHB, Spaargaren J, van den Hoek JAR, et al. Prevalence and risk factors of HSV-1 and HSV-2 antibodies in European HIV infected women. Sex Transm Infect 2001; 77: 120-124.

272. Vyse AJ, Gay NJ, Slomka MJ, et al. The burden of infection with HSV-1 and HSV-2 in England and Wales: implications for the changing epidemiology of genital herpes. Sex Transm Infect 2000; 76: 183-187.

273. Roest RW, van der Meijden WI, van Dijk G, et al. Prevalence and association between herpes simplex virus types 1 and 2-specific antibodies in attendees at a sexually transmitted disease clinic. Int J Epidemiol 2001; 30: 580-588.

274. Van der Laar MJW, Termorshuizen F, Slomka MJ, et al. Prevalence and correlates of herpes simplex virus type 2 infection: evaluation of Behavioural risk factors. Int J Epidemiol 1998; 27: 127-134.

275. Forsgren M. Genital herpes simplex virus infections and incidence of neonatal disease in Sweden. Scand J Infect Dis 1990; 69(Suppl 1): 37-41.

276. Nilsen A, Myrmel H. Changing trends in genital herpes simplex virus infection in Bergen, Norway. Acta Obstet Gynecol Scand 2000; 79: 693-696.

277. Eskild A, Jeansson S, Jenum PA. Antibodies against herpes simplex virus type 2 among pregnant women in Norway. Tidsskr Nor Laegeforen 1999; 119: 2323-2326.

278. International Herpes Management forum. Report from the sixth Annual meeting of the IHMF. Herpes 1999; 6: 1-27.

279. Uribe-Salas F, Hernandez-Avila M, Juarez-Figueroa L, et al. Risk factors for herpes simplex virus type 2 among female commercial sex workers in Mexico city. Int J STD AIDS 1999; 10: 105-111.

280. Carvalho M, de Carvalho S, Pannuti CS, et al. Prevalence of herpes simplex type 2 antibodies and a clinical history of herpes in three different populations in Campinas city, Brazil. Int J Infect Dis 1998-99; 3: 94-98.

281. Da Rosa-Santos OL, Goncalves Da Silva A, Pereira AC Jr. Herpes simplex virus type 2 in Brazil: seroepidemiologic survey. Int J Dermatol 1996; 35: 794-796.

282. Korenromp EL, Bakker R, De Vlas SJ, et al. Can behaviour change explain increase in the proportion of genital ulcers attributable to herpes in sub-Saharan Africa. A simulation modeling study. Sex Transm Dis 2001; 29: 228-230.

283. Weiss HA, Buve A, Robinson NJ, et al. The epidemiology of HSV-2 infection and its association with HIV infection in four urban African populations. AIDS 2001; 15(Suppl 4): S 97-108.

284. Chua SH, Cheong WK. Genital ulcer disease in patients

attending a public sexually transmitted disease clinic in Singapore: an epidemiologic study. Ann Acad Med Singapore 1995; 24: 510-514.

285.   Zainah S, Sinniah M, Cheong YM, et al. A microbiological study of genital ulcers in Kuala Lumpur. Med J Malaysia 1991; 46: 274-182.

286.   Hudson BJ, van der Mehden W, Lupiwa T, et al. A survey of sexually transmitted diseases in five STD clinics in Papua New Guinea. PNG Med J 1994; 37: 152-160.

287.   Beyrer C, Jitwatcharanan K, Natpratan C, et al. Molecular methods for the diagnosis of genital ulcer disease in a sexually transmitted disease clinic population in Northern Thailand: predominance of herpes simplex virus infection. J Infect Dis 1998; 178: 243-146.

288.   Puthavathana P, Kanyok R, Horthongkham N, et al. Prevalence of herpes simplex virus infection in patients suspected of genital herpes; a virus typing by type specific fluorescent monoclonal antibodies. J Med Assoc Thai 1998; 81: 260-264.

289.   Risbud A, Chan-Tack K, Gadkari D, et al. The Aetiology of genital ulcer disease by multiplex polymerase chain reaction and relationship to HIV infection among patients attending sexually transmitted disease clinics in Pune, India. Sex Transm Dis 1999; 26: 55-61.

290.   Ambhore NA, Thakar YS, Gaval SR, et al. Seroprevalence of herpes simplex virus type-2 in STD patients with genital ulcers. Indian J Sex Transm Dis 1998; 19: 81-84.

291.   Jacob M, Rao PS, Sridharan G, et al. Epidemiology and clinical profile of genital herpes. Indian J Med Res 1989; 89: 4-11.

292.   Enzensberger R, Braun W, July C, et al. Prevalence of antibodies to human herpesviruses and hepatitis B virus in patients at different stages of HIV infection. Infection 1991; 19: 140-145.

293.   Schacker T, Zeh J, Hu HL, et al. Frequency of symptomatic and asymptomatic herpes simplex virus type 2 reactivations among human immunodeficiency virus infected men. J Infect Dis 1998; 178: 1616-1622.

294.   Kumarasamy N, Soloman S, Madhivanan P, et al. Dermatologic manifestations among human immunodeficiency virus patients in south India. Int J Dermatol 2000; 39: 192-195.

295.   Whitley RJ. Neonatal herpes simplex virus infections. J Med Virol 1993; Suppl 1: 13-21.

296.   Gaytant MA, Steegers EA, van Cromvoirt PL, et al. Incidence of herpes neonatorum in Netherlands. Ned Tijdschr Geneeskd 2000; 144: 1832-1836.

297.   Tookey P, Peckham CS. Neonatal herpes simplex virus infection in the British Isles. Pediatr Perinat Epidemiol 1996; 10: 432-442.

298.   Gutierrez KM, Meira S, Halpern F, et al. The epidemiology of neonatal herpes simplex virus infections in California from 1895 to 1995. J Infect Dis 1999; 180: 199-202.

299.   Patrick DM, Dawar M, Cook DA, et al. Antenatal seroprevalence of Herpes simplex virus type 2 (HSV-2) in Canadian women. Sex Transm Dis 2001; 28: 424-428.

300.   Khanna J, Van Look PFA, Griffin PD. Reproductive health: a key to a brighter future. Biennial report 1990-91, Geneva, World Health Organization, 1992.

301.   Koutsky L. Epidemiology of genital human papillomavirus infection. Am J Med 1997; 102: 3-8.

302.   Centres for Disease Control and Prevention: The challenge of STD prevention in the United States. Atlanta, Centres for Disease Control and Prevention, Division of STD Prevention, 1996.

303.   Severson J, Evans TY, Lee P, et al. Human papillomavirus infections: epidemiology, pathogenesis and therapy. J Cutan Med Surg 2001; 5: 43-60.

304.   Chuang TY, HO P, Kurland LT, et al. Condyloma acuminatum in Rochester, Minnesota, 1950-1978. I. Epidemiology and clinical features. Arch Dermatol 1984; 120: 469-475.

305.   Slavinsky J, Kissinger P, Burger L, et al. Seroepidemiology of low and high oncogenic risk types of human papillomavirus in a predominantly male cohort of STD clinic patients. Int J STD AIDS 2001; 12: 516-523.

306.   Giuliano AR, Papenfuss M, Abrahamsen M, et al. Human papillomavirus infection at the United States- Mexico border: implications for cervical cancer prevention and control. Cancer Epidemiol Biomarkers Prev 2001; 10: 129-136.

307.   Lazcano-Ponce E, Herrero R, Musoz N, et al. Epidemiology of HPV infection among Mexican women with normal cervical cytology. Int J Cancer 2001; 91: 412-420.

308.   Cavalcanti SM, Zardo LG, Passos MR, et al. Epidemiological aspects of human papillomavirus infection and cervical cancer in Brazil. J Infect 2000; 40: 80-87.

309.   Lopes F, Latorre MR, Campos Pignatari AC, et al. HIV, HPV and syphilis prevalence in a women's penitentiary in the city of Sao Paulo, 1997-1998. Cad Saude Publica 2001; 17: 1473-1480.

310.   Koutsky LA, Galloway DA, Holmes KK. Epidemiology of genital human papillomavirus infection. Epidemiol Rev 1988; 10: 122-163.

311.   Nyari T, Cseh I, Woodwart M, et al. Screening for human papillomavirus infection in asymptomatic women in Hungary. Human Reprod 2001; 16: 2235-2237.

312.   Bosch FX, Munoz N, de Sanjose S, et al. Human papillomavirus and cervical intraepithelial neoplasia grade III/ carcinoma in situ: A case-control study in Spain and Columbia. Cancer Epidemiol Biomarkers Prev 1993; 2: 415-422.

313.   Bowden FJ, Paterson BA, Mein J, et al. ESTDmating the prevalence of *Trichomonas vaginalis, Chlamydia trachomatis, Neisseria gonorrhoeae* and human papillomavirus infection in indigenous women in northern Australia. Sex Transm Infect 1999; 75: 431-434.

314.   Parkin DM, Pisani P, Ferlay J. Estimates of the worldwide incidence of 25 major cancers in 1990. Int J Cancer 1999; 80: 827-841.

315. Mayaud P, Gill DK, Weiss HA, et al. The interrelation of HIV, cervical human papillomavirus and neoplasia among antenatal clinic attenders in Tanzania. Sex Transm Infect 2001; 77: 248-254.

316. Saranath D, Khan Z, Tandle AT, et al. HPV 16/18 prevalence in cervical lesions/cancers and p53 genotypes in cervical cancer patients from India. Gynecol Oncol 2002; 86: 157-162.

317. Menon MM, Sinha MR, Doctor VM. Detection of human papillomavirus types in precancerous and cancerous lesions of cervix in Indian women: a preliminary report. Indian J Cancer 1995; 32: 154-159.

318. Chatterjee R, Roy A, Basu S, et al. Detection of type specific human papillomavirus DNA in cervical cancers of Indian women. Indian J Pathol Microbiol 1995; 38: 33-42.

319. Jamison JH, Kaplan DW, Hamman R, et al. Spectrum of genital human papillomavirus infection in a female adolescent population. Sex Transm Dis 1995; 22: 236-243.

320. Tanaka H, Karube A, Tanaka T, et al. Much higher risk of premalignant and malignant cervical diseases in younger women positive for HPV 16 than in older women positive for HPV 16. Microbiol Immunol 2001; 45: 323-326.

321. Portolero-Luna G. Epidemiology of genital human papillomavirus. Haematol Oncol Clin North Am 1999; 13: 245-256.

322. Palefsky JM, Holly EA, Ralston ML, et al. Prevalence and risk factors for anal human papillomavirus infection in human immunodeficiency virus-positive and high-risk HIV-negative women. J Infect Dis 2001; 183: 383-391.

323. Palefsky JM, Holly EA, Ralston ML, et al. Prevalence and risk factors for human papillomavirus infection in human immunodeficiency virus-positive and HIV-negative homosexual men. J Infect Dis 1998; 177: 361-367.

324. Ahdieh L, Klein RS, Burk R, et al. Prevalence, incidence and type-specific persistence of human papillomavirus in human immunodeficiency virus-positive and HIV-negative women. J. Infect Dis 2001; 184: 682-690.

325. Volkow P, Rubi S, Lizano M, et al. High prevalence of oncogenic human papillomavirus in the genital tract of women with human immunodeficiency virus. Gynecol Oncol 2001; 82: 27-31.

326. Delmas MC, Larsen C, van Benthem B, et al. Cervical squamous intraepithelial lesions in HIV-infected women: prevalence, incidence and regression. AIDS 2000; 14: 1775-1784.

327. Holmes F, Borek D, Owen-Kummer M, et al. Anal cancer in women. Gastroenterology 1988; 95: 107-111.

328. Melbye M, Rabkin C, Frisch M, et al. Changing patterns of anal cancer incidence in the United States, 1940-1989. Am J Epidemiol 1994; 139: 772-780.

329. Daling JR, Weiss NS, Hislop TG, et al. Sexual practices, sexually transmitted diseases and the incidence of anal cancer. N Engl J Med 1987; 317: 973-977.

330. Al-Ghamdi A, Freedman D, Miller D, et al. Vulvar squamous cell carcinoma in young women: a clinicopathologic study of 21 cases. Gynecol Oncol 2002; 84: 94-101.

331. Thomas K, Thyagarajan SP, Jeyaseelan I, et al. Community prevalence of sexually transmitted diseases and human immunodeficiency virus infection in Tamil Nadu, India: A probability proportional to size cluster survey. Natl Med J India 2002; 15: 135-140.

Chapter 2

Sexually Transmitted Diseases and Reproductive Health

H R Jerajani, Sumeet Kane

Introduction

The sexually transmitted infections (STI) or sexually transmitted diseases (STD) are a group of communicable diseases that are transmitted predominantly by sexual contact and are caused by a variety of bacterial, viral, protozoal, fungal agents and ectoparasites[1-3]. Many of these conditions also have non-sexual routes such as scabies, molluscum contagiosum, cytomegalovirus infection and hepatitis B virus infection. The term reproductive tract infections (RTI) includes bacterial vaginosis in addition to the conditions listed under STD. Bacterial vaginosis is a debatable issue in reference to its inclusion as a STD[1] as some of the organisms may not be pathogenic and their presence may be due to mere colonization.

The true incidence of STD will probably never be known, not only because of inadequate reporting but also because of the taboo and secrecy that surrounds them. Most of the diseases are not even notifiable. All available data however indicates a very high prevalence of STD ranging from 1% to 14% in the vulnerable population worldwide. For viral STD, the true incidence can only be roughly estimated due to the presence of asymptomatic infections. WHO estimates that in 1999, 340 million new cases of STD have occurred worldwide (Table 1).[2] The largest number of new infections occurred in the region of South and South-East Asia, followed by Sub-Saharan Africa, Latin America and the Caribbean. However, the highest rate of new cases per 1000 population has occurred in Sub-Saharan Africa. The worldwide estimates of annual incidence of the four major bacterial STD for the year 1999 are gonorrhoea: 62.35 million, genital chlamydia: 91.98 million, syphilis: 23.59 million and trichomonas infection: 87.68 million respectively.

Table 1. Estimated Prevalence and Annual Incidence of Curable STD by Region

Region	Population (15-49 years) in millions	Prevalence in millions	Prevalence per 100	Annual incidence in millions
North America	156	3	19	14
Western Europe	203	4	20	17
North Africa and Middle East	165	3.5	21	10
Eastern Europe and Central Asia	205	6	29	22
Sub Saharan Africa	269	32	119	69
South and South East Asia	955	48	50	151
East Asia and Pacific	815	6	7	18
Australia and New Zealand	11	0.3	27	1
Latin America and Caribbean	260	18.5	71	38
Total	3040	116.5		340

Reproductive Health[4]

The International Conference on Population and Development held in Cairo in 1994 defined reproductive health as a state of complete physical, mental and social well being and not merely the absence of disease or infirmity. It goes on to add that the reproductive health care should enhance the right to decide freely and responsibly the number and spacing of one's children and the right to a satisfying and safe sex life. Implicit in this last condition is the right of men and women to be informed of and to have access to safe, effective, affordable and acceptable methods of fertility regulation of their choice and the right of access to appropriate health care services that will enable women to go safely through pregnancy and childbirth and provide couples with the best chance of having a healthy infant.

As a result of above understanding from April 1996 India has moved to a "target free" dispensation of reproductive health services through a demand driven, decentralized, client centered, participatory planning approach. There has been a paradigm shift whereby the hitherto segregated programmes are to be converged under the common Reproductive and Child Health (RCH) Programme.[4]

The RCH programme incorporates the components covered under the Child Survival & Safe Motherhood Programme and includes two additional components; one relating to STD and the other related to RTI. The reproductive health component of the RCH programme rests on effective intervention of STD and RTI. The impact of STD on reproductive health is paramount and checking them is critical to the successful implementation of the RCH programme.[4]

As shown in Table 2, untreated STD have profound impact on the reproductive health especially of females. Children are vulnerable to acquire diseases from the infected mothers. Thus an asymptomatic STD could have far reaching consequences if not detected and treated effectively. This chapter attempts to discuss complications of the STD that are categorized on the basis of their impact on the reproductive health.

Chlamydial Infection[5]

Chlamydia infection is a STD that is caused by the *Chlamydia trachomatis*. Approximately 75% of infected women and 50% of men have no symptoms, and therefore may not seek health care. Untreated chlamydia

infection can result in both short and long term consequences related to the reproductive tract which include pelvic inflammatory disease (PID), which is strongly linked to infertility and tubal pregnancy.[5] Chlamydia is known to cause conjugal infection. When female partners of *C. trachomatis* positive and *C. trachomatis* negative men with non gonoccocal urethritis were examined, 60-70% of the former and 0-10% of the latter group were found to have *C. trachomatis* induced cervicitis.[6]

When the infection remains undetected and therefore untreated, 40% will develop PID, 20% will become infertile, 18% will experience debilitating, chronic pelvic pain, and 9% will have a life threatening tubal pregnancy. Tubal pregnancy is the leading cause of first trimester, pregnancy related deaths in American women.[5]

Chlamydia infection may also result in adverse outcomes of pregnancy, neonatal conjunctivitis and pneumonia. In addition, recent research has shown that women infected with chlamydia have a 3–5 fold increased risk of acquiring HIV. Chlamydia is also common among young men, who are seldom offered screening. Untreated chlamydia in men typically causes urethral infection, but may also result in complications such as epididymitis. Based on reports to CDC provided by states that collect age-specific data, teenage girls have the highest rates of chlamydia infection. In these states, 15 to 19-year-old girls represent 46% of infections and 20 to 24-year-old women represent another 33%. These high percentages are consistent with high rates of other STD among teenagers.[5]

Strong evidence is now available that chlamydia screening and treatment not only reduces the prevalence of lower genital tract infection, but also decreases the incidence of dreaded complications like PID. CDC has developed recommendations for the prevention and management of chlamydia infection for all providers of health care.[5] These recommendations call for screening of all sexually active females under 20 years of age at least annually, and annual screening of women ages 20 years and older with one or more risk factors for chlamydia (i.e., young age, use of oral contraceptives, new or multiple sex partners and lack of barrier contraception). All women with infection of the cervix and all pregnant women should also be tested for chlamydia.[5]

Lymphogranuloma venereum (LGV) caused by *Chlamydia trachomatis* serovar L1, L2, and L3 has many acute and chronic complications, which affect the reproductive health of untreated cases. Acute LGV is

Table 2.   Complications of STD and the Associated Pathogens

Complications	Pathogens
In males:	
1 Urethritis	*N. gonorrhoeae*, *C. trachomatis*, HSV
	U. urealyticum, *M. genitalium*, *T. vaginalis*
2 Epididymitis	*N. gonorrhoeae*, *C. trachomatis*
3 Intestinal infections	
Proctitis	*N. gonorrhoeae*, *C. trachomatis*, HSV
Proctocolitis	*Campylobacter* sp, *Shigella* sp,
	E. histolytica, Helicobacter sp.
Enteritis	*Giardia lamblia*
In females:	
1. Lower genitourinary infections	
Vulvitis	*C. albicans*, HSV
Vaginitis	*T. vaginalis*, *C. albicans*
Vaginosis	*G. vaginalis*, Mobiluncus sp and other
	Anaerobes, *M. hominis*
Cervicitis	*N. gonorrhoeae*, *C. trachomatis*, HSV
2. Pelvic inflammatory disease (PID)	*N. gonorrhoeae*, *C. trachomatis*, *M. hominis*
	Anaerobes, Group B streptococcus
3. Infertility	*N. gonorrhoeae*, *C. trachomatis*, *M. hominis*
4. Pregnancy morbidity	Several STD
In males and females	
1. Neoplasia	
Cervical, vulvar, vaginal, anal, penile, intraepithelial neoplasia & cancer	Human papillomavirus (HPV)
Hepatocellular carcinoma	Hepatitis B virus, Hepatitis C virus
Kaposi's sarcoma, body cavity lymphoma, multiple myeloma? Multicentric Castleman's disease	Human herpes virus type 8
T-cell lymphoma/leukaemia	HTLV 1
2. Genital ulceration	HSV, *T. pallidum*, *H. ducreyi*, *C. granulomatis*, *C. trachomatis* (LGV strains)
3. Acute arthritis with urogenital or intestinal infection	*N. gonorrhoeae*, *C. trachomatis*, Campylobacter sp, Shigella sp.
4. Hepatitis	Hepatitis A, B & C viruses, cytomegalovirus *T. pallidum*
5. Genital warts	Human papilloma virus
6. Molluscum contagiosum	Molluscum contagiosum virus
7. Ectoparasitic infestations	*Sarcoptes scabiei*, Phthirus pubis
8. Heterophil-negative mononucleosis	Cytomegalovirus, EB virus
9. Tropical spastic paraparesis	HTLV type 1 virus
In neonates:	
1. Systemic infection, deafness, death	Cytomegalovirus, HSV, T. pallidum, HIV
2. Conjunctivitis	*N. gonorrhoeae*, *C. trachomatis*
3. Pneumonia	*C. trachomatis*, *U. urealyticum*
4. Otitis media	*C. trachomatis*
5. Sepsis, meningitis	Group B streptococcus infection
6. Laryngeal papillomatosis	HPV

more common in males while the late complications such as hypertrophy of genitalia called as esthiomene (Greek: eating away) and rectal strictures are more common in women.[7]

The inguinal syndrome results in genital elephantiasis due to primary infection affecting the lymphatics of the area involved. Chronic progressive lymphangitis, chronic oedema and sclerosing fibrosis of the subcutaneous tissues are the chronic sequelae leading to esthiomene formation. Accompanying ulcers are superficial and later deep and give rise to severe pain. The ulcers are commonly situated on labia majora, at the genitocrural folds and perineum in the later stages. About one third women with abdominal pain could have deep pelvic and lumbar lymph nodes. Periadenitis results in adhesions, which eventually give rise to adhesions of many pelvic organs together, causing marked morbidity in reference to female reproductive health.[8]

Urethral and vaginal fistulae and vaginal stenosis are added complications.[9] All these changes interfere with normal sexual functions and also would pose obstruction to normal vaginal delivery.

Penoscrotal elephantiasis (saxophone penis), which appears after 1 to 20 years of infection, causes severe oedema and induration of the area involved.[10] These changes are of long standing in nature and interfere with sexual function due to deformities and erectile dysfunction.

Gonorrhoea

In males, fibrous strictures both diaphragmatic and tubular found in the bulbar area, persistent urinary fistulae, and scarring at the site of opening of periurethral abscesses on the surface are the known sequelae but are rare now due to availability of effective antimicrobial therapy.[11] Painful erections suggest seminal vesiculitis and on microscopic examination of the seminal fluid, besides polymorphonuclear cells, granular debris and mucinous material, spermatozoa are found to be few in number and show degenerative changes and sometimes may be absent.[12] Penile lymphangitis associated with inguinal lymphadenopathy is an uncommon complication. Acute epididymitis and/or epididymo-orchitis due to *N. gonorrhoeae* present as unilateral painful testicular swelling and are always associated with active urethritis.[13] Sterility ensues if the fine tubules of epididymis get permanantly blocked following chronic infection.[12]

In females, acute salpingitis and PID are the expected complications in 10 to 20% of cases with acute gonoccocal infection and may be bilateral.[13] It has varied presentations such as dysparaeunia, lower abdominal pain and abnormal menstrual cycles. The affected female appears grossly ill with fever and severe malaise. The physical examination reveals marked tenderness of lower abdominal, uterine and adnexal regions. The cervix shows active discharge and cervical pain on manouvering could be elicited. Tubo-ovarian abscesses often present as tender adnexal mass. Leucocytosis, elevated ESR and adnexal mass on ultrasonography support the diagnosis. The younger females (15%) are particularly at risk of developing salpingitis following vaginitis (prepubertal age) and are also prone to develop PID.[15] Younger age of acquisition of gonorrhoea, multiple sex partners and use of intrauterine device for contraception are the major risk factors for PID.[15] Puerperal infection and infection following dilatation and curettage of the infected cervix, douching, sexual intercourse and menstruation are the added risk factors.[13] The risk for ectopic pregnancy is increased by ten folds following an attack of acute salpingitis. The incidence of gonoccocal infection in pregnant women has remained high even when the men from the same setting have shown declining trend. In America, young unwed mothers, nonwhite and from low socioeconomic background are particularly vulnerable. Newborns who have not received ocular prophylaxis and are exposed to maternal gonoccocal infection are at higher risk for ophthalmia neonatorum especially after prolonged rupture of membranes and gonoccocal amniotic fluid infection syndrome may be the eventual event.[14]

Syphilis

In USA, 80% of women with infectious syphilis are within the age group of 15-34 years and the prevalence rate of syphilis in pregnant women receiving antenatal care is 2.2 to 3.9% and those who do not have access to antenatal care, the rate is higher up to 11 percent.[16] The morbid reproductive health sequelae of syphilis are found in pregnant women. Syphilis is a common cause of stillbirth especially in the developing countries. In a study of pregnant women in Zambia, serological tests were reactive in 43% of women delivering stillborn babies, 19% in women who aborted and 13% in normal first time antenatal care clinic attendees.[14] It has been observed that syphilis has benign effect on the mother due to the prevalent immunosuppressive state during pregnancy however it has disastrous effect on the foetus.

In males, gummatous syphilis may cause localized or generalized infiltration of the testis, usually unilaterally, however the epididymis remains unaffected. If left untreated, interstitial fibrosis ensues. There are no reports suggesting sterility following gummatous syphilis of testis.

Granuloma Inguinale (Donovanosis)[17]

Granuloma inguinale (GI) has a long insidious course with ulceration if left untreated and involves genitals, genitocrural folds, perineum and anal area and, rarely extending to cervix uteri. Occasionally, phagaedena supervenes causing severe destruction of the genitals. The eventual scarring could be keloidal in some cases. Scarring results in elephantine enlargement of the genitals in both genders with resultant impact on the reproductive health. Malignant transformation is known to occur in the long standing cases. Rajam and Rangiah found 0.25% of 2000 cases of GI developing squamous cell carcinoma.[18] It is often difficult to differentiate the carcinomatous changes from the pseudoepitheliomatous changes. The general health too deteriorates due to accompanying anaemia, anorexia and cachexia. Urethral, vaginal and anal orifices develop sclerosis and stenosis with resultant complications such as dysparaeunia and difficulty in defaecation.

Bacterial Vaginosis (BV)[2]

Bacterial vaginosis (nonspecific vaginitis) is the most common disease affecting the females and often coexists with trichomoniasis and candidiasis. *Gardernella vaginalis*, mycoplasmas, Bacteroid species, anaerobic organisms such as peptostreptococci, mobiluncus and prevotella are the main causative organisms of BV. Multiple sex partners, douching and presence of intrauterine devices are the risk factors promoting BV. It is seldom found in women who have never had intercourse.[19]

BV in pregnancy raises incidence of intraamniotic infections, chorioamnionitis and post partum endometriosis and resultant premature or low birth weight babies following ascension of the organisms from the vagina.[14] In a study, it was reported that the women with BV in second trimester had 50% more chances to develop fever during labour as compared to women with lactobacillus predominant flora. In the United States, as many as 16% of pregnant women have BV.[20] This varies by race and ethnicity from 6% in Asians and 9% in whites to 16% in Hispanics and 23% in African Americans.[20] BV is generally more commonly seen in women attending STD clinics than in those attending family planning or prenatal clinics.[21] Vaginal cuff cellulitis occurs when vaginal bacteria contaminate the operative field during hysterectomy. It is known to occur four times more commonly in patients with BV

than the ones with normal flora. BV also has a strong association with PID especially in post abortal phase.[21] In a study, 174 women with BV underwent double-blind randomization to a placebo or metronidazole prior to abortion.[14] Placebo treated women had higher rates of postabortal PID. Spontaneous PID is also strongly linked with BV. Abnormal bleeding in the intermenstrual period and heavy bleeding during menstrual period are some of the subtle signs of silent endometriosis.[14] A study by Paavonen et al reported 29% of 31 patients who had histologic evidence of endometriosis also had BV, while none of the 14 controls without endometriosis had BV.[21] PID can cause infertility or damage the fallopian tubes enough to increase the future risk of ectopic pregnancy and infertility. BV can increase a woman's susceptibility to HIV infection if she is exposed to the virus. Having BV increases the chances that an HIV infected woman can pass HIV to her sex partner and also increases a woman's susceptibility to other STD, such as chlamydia and gonorrhoea[14]

Trichomonas Vaginalis (TV) Infection[22]

Trichomonas vaginalis infection accounts for 200 million males suffering from nonspecific urethritis and females with vaginitis. In males, besides urethritis, TV is known to be the causative organism detected in cases of prostatitis (9-100%) especially in long standing cases not responding to antimicrobials.[22] Balanoposthitis with phimosis, chronic sinus formation along the median raphe,[23,24] urethral stricture formation, epididymitis and infertility are some of the sequelae in males. *T. vaginalis* has adverse effect on the sperm motility and is considered to contribute to male infertility. Gopalkrishnan et al have found *T. vaginalis* in 4% of 1,131 semen specimens of infertile males.[22] Further, abnormality of sperm morphology and motility along with abnormal seminal fluid viscosity and increased particulate debris were reported in the group with *T. vaginalis* infection than the non-infected group. There are some reports linking *T. vaginalis* infection with erectile dysfunction and premature ejaculation.

T. vaginalis infection in women can have postcoital bleeding due to cervicitis and 12% of women are reported to have abdominal pain perhaps due to salpingitis or endometriosis. Pregnant women with *T. vaginalis* infections are reported to have reproductive complications such as post caesarian infection, premature rupture of membranes and pre-term birth. Approximately

2-17% female infants of mothers infected with TV are reported to have developed vaginal infection.[25] This infection may not be overt in all the cases. Within 3 to 4 weeks, by which time the maternal oestrogens, which cause the neonatal vaginal epithelium to predispose to the TV infection, are now in low levels and thus the neonatal vagina reverts to the prepubertal stage and resists the TV infection.

Mycoplasma[19]

Mycoplasma hominis has a role in the development of nonspecific vaginosis and usually coexists with *T. vaginalis* and anaerobic gram-negative rods in the vagina. *M. hominis* was recovered from 63% of bacterial vaginitis and 10% of the normal controls.[26] The role of *Ureaplasma urealyticum* in bacterial vaginosis is not well defined. The mycoplasmas are the copathogens to *N. gonorrhoeae* and *C. trachomatis* in causing PID. Mardh and Westrom in their study reported isolation of *M. hominis* from 8% of 50 women with salpingitis but not from women without salpingitis.[27] The direct yield of mycoplasma by laparoscopy has been achieved in 11% of women with salpingitis.[19,27] *Mycoplasma genitalium* has been implicated in PID especially in women without the infection with *N. gonorrhoeae* and *C. trachomatis.*

There exists an association with colonization of vagina with mycoplasma and postabortal and postpartum fever due to endometriosis especially where there is evidence of early rupture of membranes and prolonged labour.[28] The mycoplasma associates with virulent bacteria and have symbiotic relation with these bacteria to cause endometriosis. In one study, *M. hominis* was isolated from blood of nine out of 125 febrile postpartum women, compared to none of 60 afebrile postpartum women ($p < 0.005$).[29]

Ureaplasmas have profound effect on the motility of sperms and can cause oligospermia (low sperm count).[30] Elimination of these offending agents has improved sperm motility, quantity and appearance. Ureaplasmas have been recovered more frequently from the infertile couples than the fertile ones.[30] Conception rate ranging from 23 to 84 percent have been recorded among ureaplasma colonised infertile couples. But later studies have not substantiated these claims. Thus, to date role of mycoplasma in infertility remains doubtful. Similarly despite their isolation from lower genital tract in women with habitual abortions and still birth, mycoplasma is not the predominant organism in these cases. Low birth weight is associated with isolation of *U. urealyticum* in the infants. Mycoplasma colonization of vagina in women with bacterial vaginosis and the resultant effect on the pregnancy in terms of pre term delivery or low birth weight of the foetus have to be taken with due consideration that these effects may be due to organisms coexisting with mycoplasma.

Genital Herpes Simplex Virus 2 (HSV 2) Infections

There is tremendous increase in genital HSV 2 infections world wide. HSV 2 infections predisposes the infected to acquisition of HIV infection. The frequency of HSV 2 antibody is higher in STD clinic attendees and homosexual men.[31] It is linked to age of initiation of sexual activities, multiple sexual partners in lifetime, history of present and past STD, advancing age and low socioeconomic status. The conjugal infection transmission rate is about 12% per year.[32] Women and seronegative individuals have more chances for acquisition of HSV.

Many times the primary and the secondary episodes remain asymptomatic. Subclinical shedding from various mucosal surfaces such as oral, genital and anorectal canal is an important issue. It has been observed that candidial vaginitis is frequently encountered with active HSV infection. A study recorded 14% of women with primary genital HSV infection also had candial vaginitis.[31] Bacterial superinfection may add to severe discomfort and pain of the primary infection. HSV cervicitis can be found without the infection on the external genitals and often could be asymptomatic. HSV infection of pregnant women is linked to age, past sexual activities and poor socioeconomic status. The clinical course of infection, both primary and recurrent, does not change during pregnancy. The frequency and severity of episodes may increase during pregnancy.

Cytomegalovirus (CMV) Infections[33]

CMV infection in the developing countries takes place in early age group than the developed countries especially in low socioeconomic group. Recently there are many indications that have emerged which point to CMV infection as a STD. A significant correlation was found with seropositivity to CMV and increased number of sex partners and past or current infection with chlamydia and history of STD. Increased seroprevalence of CMV and shedding of virus is observed in women attending STD clinic and young group of homosexuals. Virus shedding is noted in semen, cervical secretions and saliva and these sites form a potential source of infection and sexual transmission of CMV. The viral shedding takes place from multiple sites following primary or recurrent secondary infection. Pregnancy has marginal impact on viral shedding however the rate of shedding is lowest in the first trimester. Maternal infection and perinatal infections often are subclinical.

As CMV is secreted in breast milk, perinatal infection could be attributed due to breast feeding practices. Maternal primary CMV infection could be acquired during pregnancy with resultant congenital perinatal CMV infections and variable outcomes.

Juvenile Onset Recurrent Respiratory Papillomatosis (JO-RRP)[34]

JO-RRP is a benign condition caused by human papilloma virus (HPV), usually subtypes 6 and 11 and presents as papilloma in the respiratory tract from nasal vestibule to the lung tissue in infants and children. Hoarseness of voice and symptoms of obstruction of upper airway tract are the presenting features. Maternal condyloma is the usual source of infection and is found in 50% mothers giving birth to JO-RRP babies. Young motherhood, first pregnancy and vaginal delivery form a triad of high risk-profile for JO-RRP. Subclinical infection with HPV in mother could give rise to JO-RRP.

Infertility due to STD

Infertility is defined as the lack of conception after one year of regular sexual (penovaginal) intercourse without the use of any contraception.[35]

Exceptionally, STD in male result in infertility. Bilateral epididymitis and blocking of vas deferens due to *N. gonorrhoeae* and *C. trachomatis* could result in obstruction to the passage of sperms. *T. vaginalis* and mycoplasma are known to affect motility, quantity and morphology of spermatozoa. However, these changes are reversible following antimicrobial therapy. *T. pallidum* infection of testis result in orchitis, which is usually unilateral and therefore less likely to cause infertility.

The greater impact of STD is seen in women. The common causes of STD related infertility are given in Table 3. Salpingitis is the most common preceding event. It is an inflammation of the epithelial surfaces of the fallopian tubes due to one or more active organisms, which have ascended from the lower genital tract. The local peritonitis, tuboovarian adnexal masses and PID are the recognized complications. Many women remain asymptomatic or minimally symptomatic despite having PID. These are called as atypical PID and are significant unrecognizable causes of salpingitis and eventually infertility.[35]

Table 3.   Common Causes of Female Infertility

1.   Bilateral tubal adhesions
2.   Pelvic adhesions
3.   Acquired tubal abnormalities
4.   Anovulatory normal menstrual cycles
5.   Anovulatory oligomenorrhoea
6.   Hyperprolactinaemia
7.   Endometriosis

N. gonorrhoeae and *C. trachomatis* are the two most important causative agents of PID and infertility. In Uganda, 15 districts recorded a significant inverse correlation between annual reported incidence of gonoccocal urethritis in men and the general fertility rate.[36] A WHO multicentric study was undertaken to compare STD related infertility in five different regions of the world.[37] Out of the 8000 infertile couples, 71% completed evaluation of the fallopian tubes. In Africa, approximately, 66% infertility was due to infection. Bilateral tubal occlusion accounted for 49% and pelvic adhesions for 24% of infertility.[35] Developed countries had far less prevalence of tubal occlusion (11%) as the cause of infertility. The non-African developing countries had higher rates of tubal occlusion than the developed countries but certainly less than the African countries. The risk factors for tubal infertility are shown in Table 4

Table 4.   Risk Factors for Tubal Infertility

1.   Number of episodes of pelvic inflammatory disease
2.   Severity of pelvic inflammation
3.   Delay in access to treatment
4.   Type of contraceptives used
5.   Smoking

Acute salpingitis due to both *N. gonorrhoeae* and *C. trachomatis* results in varying degree of inflammation. The proportion of women who become infertile after the fist episode of inflammation are 0.6% after mild,

Table 5.   Prevalence of Clinically Detectable Gynecological Morbidity

Study	Total women	Vaginal discharge (%)	Lower backache (%)	Lower abdominal pain (%)
Bombay (urban slum)	1001	30.8	39.3	21.5
Baroda (urban slum)	840	22.4	24.1	9.3
West Bengal (rural)	875	50.1	5.3	17.5
South Gujarat (rural)	835	57.0	29.7	—
Ambala (Urban slum)	2325	45.1	47.9	—
Chandigarh (urban slum)	576	42.4	30.4	39.3

Source: Kumar B, Sharma NM. Ind J Sex Transm Dis 2000: 21; 4-7

Table 6.   Correlation of Gynaecologic Conditions with Aetiological Agents

Total %	Clinical condition	Candida	T. vaginalis	G. vaginalis	N. gon	C. trachom	M. hom	U. urealyt
43.18	Vaginitis	27.97	23.31	20.98	1.29	1.81	10.88	32.53
32.21	Cervicitis	15.28	10.42	9.37	2.08	7.29	5.21	24.31
15.21	Infertility	11.02	3.67	6.62	2.94	15.44	9.55	19.83
5.26	PID	6.38	2.12	4.25	6.38	21.27	12.76	31.91
4.14	Miscellaneous	13.51	10.81	5.40	8.10	8.10	18.91	4.14
100	Total	19.57	14.54	13.42	2.24	6.94	8.84	27.18
100	Control	9.06	5.14	4.9	0.0	1.22	1.47	12.5

Aetiological agents in %

N. gon-*N. gonorrhoeae*, C. trachom-*C. trachomatis*, M. hom-*M. hominis*, U. urealyt-*U. urealyticum*

Source: Gogate A. Reproductive tract infections (RTI) in women of childbearing age from Dharavi slums of Mumbai. Ind J Sex Transm Dis 1999: 20; 11-15

6.2% after moderate and 21% after severe inflammation of the fallopian tubes.[38]

Morbidity and risk of infertility increases with each episode of PID. A single episode of PID would be responsible for 8%, two episodes for 19% and three or more for 40% of infertility.[35] The necrosis of the ciliated epithelium gives rise to permanent damage and therefore, despite surgical correction of adhesions and assuring tubal patency, conception does not take place. Women taking steroidal contraceptives have milder impact and suffer from less severe type of PID.[39] As compared to gonoccocal infection, chlamydial infection has more chances to cause PID and tubal infertility. In large studies, 70% women with tubal infertility had chlamydia antibodies as compared to 26% of control women.[40] A special antigen called as chlamydial heat shock protein 60 (hsp 60), which is now available in the recombinant form, has facilitated many studies related to PID and infertility.[41] It is possible to detect antibodies to hsp 60 by microimmunofluorescence. It is observed that 16-25% of normal fertile women have these antibodies as compared to 44% cases of cervicitis, 48-60% of PID and 81-90% cases of fallopian tube obstruction caused by *C. trachomatis*.[41] The women with hsp 60 antibodies have more damaging inflammation than those without, suggesting the role of hsp 60 in inciting inflammation. The atypical PID is largely asymptomatic but can cause infertility and is mainly caused by *C. trachomatis* induced silent damage.[41] Type of contraceptives choice has definite impact on the degree of inflammation of PID. Intrauterine devices (IUCD) are associated with increased risk of tubal infertility.[42] Condoms and spermicides, the barrier contraceptives provide significant protection against tubal infertility. Oral contraceptives mask the degree of inflammation and therefore reduce the signs and symptoms of PID but do not reduce the potential of tubal obstruction.[43] Smoking has direct suppressive effect on the immune mechanisms, which prevent the upward, ascent of organisms from the lower genital tract.[44,45] Women who smoke and also use an IUCD have greater risk to develop tubal infertility.

Infertility is not only a medical but also a social problem. The sterile woman has to face wrath of family members and the society at large. It is prudent to say that early and prompt treatment of these STD causing infertility would prevent stigma and ostracization faced by many unfortunate women. The health-seeking behaviour of most women especially in the rural setting is dismal and along with to poor access to family planning, antenatal and gynaecology clinics, results in chronic debilitating PID and related conditions. These undiagnosed STD have direct effect on the general health and the reproductive health of women.

STD and Pregnancy[14]

STD have many untoward influences on the outcome of pregnancy. They are spontaneous abortions, stillbirths, ectopic pregnancy, prematurity, intrauterine growth retardation of the foetus, congenital and perinatal infections and post abortal and post puerperal maternal infections. Primary infections are usually severe due to lack of host defense and therefore, pregnant adolescents and younger women have more morbidity following STD contracted during pregnancy as compared to older women. Chlamydia and cytomegalovirus infection is observed to be more frequent in the pregnant adolescents. Gonorrhoea, syphilis, HSV infection and HIV are now considered the diseases with pronounced effect on outcome of pregnancy. There is also increased incidence and severity of viral hepatitis in pregnancy. The different factors as shown below are operative during pregnancy and have great impact on the outcome of pregnancy.

1. Immunosuppresive State During Pregnancy[46]

Due to prevalent immunosuppression following reduction in T-helper subset of lymphocytes due to pregnant state, the STD have different morphological features and also different response to therapy. This immunosuppression is more marked in the third trimester. Venereal warts are the prime example wherein there is increased virulence of HPV during pregnancy.

2. Anatomical Changes

Anatomical changes such as increased blood flow in the pelvis also aggravate venereal warts becoming enlarged and more vascular. The vagina becomes hypertrophic and has increased content of glycogen, which in turn alters the vaginal pH. The cervical os becomes dilated and larger area of columnar epithelium of exocervix is exposed to the microbial flora of the vagina. There could be reactivation of infections of exocervix.

3. Alteration in Microbial Flora

Alteration in vaginal pH due to increased glycogen content result in increased colonization of *C. albicans*. The bacterial flora diminishes during pregnancy especially the anaerobes. The lactobacilli increase in number while the facultative bacteria remain unchanged.

4. Cervical Mucous Plug

The cervix has a protective mechanism in the form of a mucous plug. This plug becomes more viscid during pregnancy and offers protection against the ascent of pathogenic organisms to the upper genital tract.

5. Alteration of Uterus

As the uterine cavity obliterates due to juxtaposition of chorioamnion on decidua vera, the risk of infection to uterus and fallopian tubes diminishes greatly. Risk of chorioamnionitis increases after 16 weeks of gestation as it lies on the cervical os.

6. Placental Factor

The trophoblastic layer, which lies in close proximity of the maternal blood vessels, has a challenging task of uptake of nutrient for the growing foetus. The placenta has many macrophages, which are the first line of defence for the foetus.

Ectopic Pregnancy

Ectopic pregnancy is the dreaded complication of salpingitis and with each episode of salpingitis there is an increased risk of development of ectopic pregnancy. 50% of surgically removed ectopic mass had evidence of prior salpingitis thus confirming the role of salpingitis in inducing tubal pregnancy.[47] There is a worldwide increase in ectopic pregnancy, which also reflect the rising incidence of tubal infection with *N. gonorrhoeae* and *C. trachomatis*. It is reported that *C. trachomatis* is responsible for at least 30% of tubal pregnancies.[14]

Intrauterine Infections and Congenital Infections[14]

The STD could infect the intrauterine cavity by the direct ascent of organisms from the lower genital tract. Chorioamnionitis is associated with infections due to *N. gonorrhoeae, C. trachomatis,* and Mycoplasmas. Syphilis causes infection via the haematogenous spread. CMV infection spreads by continuity to the adjacent areas therefore maternal infection is also transmitted via placenta with resultant disastrous effects on the foetus such as the intrauterine death, stillbirths, intrauterine growth retardation and congenital anomalies. HSV, CMV, *T. pallidum* and HIV infections are the prime examples giving rise to congenital anomalies of the foetus. Many studies give credence to antibiotic therapy in pregnancy with fewer incidences of preterm deliveries, perinatal infections and postpuerperal sepsis.[48] *N. gonorrhoeae, C. trachomatis* and *T. vaginalis* infection and bacterial vaginosis are linked with preterm birth. Recent studies have shown that TNF-α, IL-1 and IL-6 are associated with preterm deliveries and presence of chorioamnionitis.[49,50,51] Prostaglandins E2 and F2α levels are also increased in women with chorioamnionitis and resultant preterm births.[52] These cytokines also have damaging effect on the foetus in the form of respiratory distress syndrome and intraventricular haemorrhages.[14] The organisms causing bacterial vaginosis secrete proteases which weaken the foetal membranes causing early rupture of the membranes thereby exposing the amniotic fluid to the organisms from the lower genital tract.[53]

Puerperal sepsis due to preceding STD is more common in the developing countries than the developed ones. Endometriosis is the main manifestation of puerperal sepsis. *N. gonorrhoeae* and *C. trachomatis* are the main organisms causing puerperal sepsis in about 35% of cases reported from an African study.[54] Chances of puerperal sepsis are higher following caesarean section in the developed countries. Mycoplasmas are often implicated in puerperal fever and the women may not show any signs of puerperal infection. *M. hominis* and anaerobes from the vaginal tract often cause sepsis following vaginal delivery especially if there are additional factors of early rupture of membranes and prolonged labour.[14] Late postpartum endometriosis (occurring between 3 days to 6 weeks after delivery) is associated with *C. trachomatis* infection and is considerably milder than the early onset endometriosis but could give rise to secondary infertility due to salpingitis.[55]

There are three routes of transmission of HSV from mother to child; they are (1) in-utero infection (2) intrapartum infection and, (3) postnatal infection. Intrapartum route accounts for the majority of neonatal infections (90%).[14]

From 70-90% of women with primary episode HSV-2 infection have cervicitis in compared to 15-20% of women with recurrent secondary genital herpes.[56]

Genital HSV infection is associated with increased frequency of spontaneous abortion and premature delivery especially with women having primary infection during pregnancy.[31] Primary cervicitis in women has more complications during pregnancy than other forms. The acquisition of HSV and occurrence of primary HSV disease during pregnancy is associated with serious complications such as visceral dissemination, hepatitis, pneumonitis, and coagulopathy.[14,57] Mortality rate of pregnant women with disseminated disease is about 50 percent. Neonatal morbidity is very high with pregnant women having primary episode, which promotes chorioamnionitis via direct and haematogenous routes. Women having recurrent mild episodes during pregnancy do not have great pregnancy related morbidity. The risk of foetal transmission is 50% when the primary infection takes place during pregnancy, 20% in mother with past HSV-1 but new HSV-2 infection before pregnancy and 1% in women with recurrent episodes during pregnancy.[57] These findings support the hypothesis that the maternal antibodies have a protective role and prevent acquisition of the disease by the foetus. Maternal infection prior to 20 weeks gestation is associated with spontaneous abortions. The gestation period does not have any impact on neonatal infection, however early rupture of membranes is a risk factor for foetal transmission. Intrauterine infection can lead to an infant with congenital herpes simplex infection presenting with blistering disease with or without neurological abnormalities. If the mother has active lesions on the genitals during delivery, it is advisable to deliver by caesarean section especially if the membranes are ruptured for less than 6 hours. Intrauterine infection is apparent at the time of birth in the form of skin vesicles, eye disease in the form of keratoconjunctivitis and chorioretinitis and microcephaly or hydranencephaly. In homosexual men, HSV proctitis is associated with fever, severe rectal pain, tenesmus and sacral autonomic nervous dysfunction that may present as impotence.

Intrauterine infection with CMV could be following a primary maternal infection or reactivation of a secondary infection (mother infected before pregnancy). A particular phenomenon is observed in CMV infection during pregnancy that the infected mother who is highly immune i.e. mother having high humoral antibodies has more chances to transmit infection in utero.[57,58] Thus the countries, which have higher rates of CMV seropositivity, also have higher rates of CMV congenital infections. When primary infection of CMV occurs during pregnancy, there are 30% chances to transmit the infection to the foetus as compared to the secondary reactivation of previous infection taking place in pregnancy wherein the mother could infect the foetus in only 2% cases.

CMV transmission from mother to child is effective if there are lower levels of neutralizing antibodies. The congenital infection with CMV may remain asymptomatic in about 90% of cases.[57] Failure to thrive, neonatal jaundice and mild splenomegaly are some of the features of these mild manifestations. As many as 5-15% cases of congenital CMV infection are at risk to develop serious sequelae. The psychomotor retardation, neurological complication and hearing loss could remain undetected for many years. The other long-term complications include microcephaly, seizures, paraparesis, diplegia, learning disabilities, chorioretinitis and optic atrophy.

Syphilis is transmitted to the foetus from mother via placental route or through direct access to foetal circulation by traversing the foetal membranes and reaching amniotic fluid.

The rate of active syphilis is about 6% in Africa; in some areas it is as high as 10%.[59,60] The infected untreated mother to her foetus can transmit syphilis in first 9 weeks of gestation however the manifestation in the foetus is more obvious after 18 weeks. An explanation for this phenomenon rests on the hypothesis that the effect of *T. pallidum* on the foetus is not due to cytopathic effects but due to immune response. The foetus develops immunocompetence after 16 weeks. Syphilis causes placentitis and due to endartertis obliterans, extensive infarcts and increased fibrosis take place. The placenta is bulky, pale and greasy and *T. pallidum* could be demonstrated with silver stains. The umbilical cord also could be infected with *T. pallidum* causing funisitis,

which may have deep necrotizing inflammation in the matrix of the cord. There are varied outcome of pregnancy in syphilis depending upon the time of infection during pregnancy.[59] If the mother is infected in early pregnancy and has primary or secondary syphilis, the chances of foetus aborting at the 4th month of gestation are 100% (abortion before 3rd month of gestation are less likely due to syphilis). The foetus may die in utero (macerated foetus) or there would be a stillbirth. There are 50% chances of premature delivery or perinatal death. The child may be born with early syphilis or the child would appear normal at time of birth but manifest symptoms and signs of syphilis within few weeks or months. The child may not manifest early signs of congenital syphilis but directly presents with late sequalae. The child may escape infection if the duration of infection is longer or the mother is infected in the advanced stage of pregnancy. Intrauterine infection with *T. pallidum* is associated with prematurity, low birth weight and small for age babies. In Ethiopia 5% of pregnancies are lost due to syphilis[57] while in Zambia the rate is 19%.[59] The spontaneous abortion rate among syphilitic pregnant women in Africa is estimated to be 50%. Another study from Zambia reported 42% stillbirths due to syphilis during pregnancy and congenital syphilis was attributed for 20 to 30% of perinatal death.[61] About 2.9% positivity rate of serological tests of syphilis was observed in children below six months of age in Zambia. Half of these babies had signs and symptoms of congenital syphilis and 60% of them required hospitalization.[61] CDC defines syphilitic stillbirth as death of foetus weighing > 500 gms or having gestational age > 20 weeks and the mother is untreated or inadequately treated for syphilis. Long bone radiography showing classical changes of congenital syphilis and confirmation of presence of *T. pallidum* in foetal tissues on autopsy are other corroborative features. Ultrasonography during pregnancy has certain characteristic findings which point towards foetal syphilis. They are skin thickening, placental thickening, serous cavity effusions, hepatosplenomegaly and hydramnios.

The risk of congenital syphilis is directly related to duration of diseases in the mother, and is highest in the first four years of acquiring the infection. A study by Ingraham reported 41% of babies being born with congenital syphilis, 25% with stillbirths, 14% perinatal death, 2% with prematurity and only 18% being born healthy in mothers who acquired syphilis in less than 4 years of duration. In contrast, only 2% infants had congenital syphilis when the duration of infection was more than 4 years.[62] With advancing time the risk of infection from mother to child decreases but does not disappear.

Perinatal Infection

Perinatal infection is strongly linked with chorioamnionitis, early rupture of membranes and prolonged labour. Perinatal infection occurs within the first 48 hours of birth is usually caused by the ascent of bacterial infection from the vagina and cervix. Mycoplasmas are the prime organisms causing chorioamnionitis. The perinatal infection is often polymicrobial in nature and the organisms involved are, anaerobes, Group B streptococci (GBS), gram negative rods etc. These organisms cause neonatal sepsis, pneumonia and meningitis, which may prove fatal. Viruses such as HSV and cytomegalovirus and protozoal infection also cause perinatal infection.[31]

GBS was reported to cause fatal perinatal infection in as high as 50% infants affected in 1980 in USA. Administering antibiotics during labour to women at risk of transmitting GBS to their newborns could prevent invasive disease in the first week of life (i.e., early-onset disease). Penicillin remains the first line agent for intrapartum antibiotic prophylaxis, with ampicillin an acceptable alternative. The women with obstetric risk factors such as delivery at <37 weeks gestation, duration of membrane rupture ≥18 hours, or temperature ≥100.4°F [≥38.0°C].[63]

During pregnancy or the postpartum period, women can contract amnionitis, endometriosis, sepsis, or rarely, meningitis caused by GBS. Women with prenatal GBS colonization are 25 times more likely than women with negative prenatal cultures to deliver infants with early onset GBS disease.

Virtually most neonatal herpes infection occurs in the perinatal stage during the passage through infected birth canal. More than 70% of infants with neonatal disease have mothers having asymptomatic disease suggest the pivotal role of silent shedding in causing neonatal infection. Neonatal HSV infection is always symptomatic and has great morbidity and mortality. Many of them have disease localized to skin, some have predominant neurological disease such as encephalitis and fatal visceral disease (80%). The most likely causes of death are pneumonitis and disseminated intravascular coagulopathy.[57] The infection manifests between 9-11 days. About 75% babies present with signs of encephalitis. Presence of skin vesicles provides a diagnostic clue to

neonatal HSV infection however 20% of disseminated HSV do not have skin vesicles.

The long-term sequelae of neonatal infection are grave. About 50% surviving children manifest neurological deficit such as microcephaly, spasticity, chorioretinitis, blindness, psychomotor retardation and learning disabilities. The neonatal HSV infection localized to skin and mucosa has lower mortality rates but can have neurological impairment in about 30% cases.

The perinatal transmission of CMV is considered when there is no evidence of viral shedding in the first 15 days after birth. The incubation of CMV in the perinatal period is about 4 to 12 weeks. Perinatal transmission of CMV is linked to maternal shedding of the virus in the genital tracts (57% transmission rate) and in the breast milk (61% transmission rate).[57] Young mothers from low socio-economic strata who breastfeed their infants are more likely to transmit the disease. Most healthy infants remain asymptomatic and the infection has no effect on the physical and mental growth of the infant. Pneumonitis due to CMV could occur in the infants less than 4 months of age. The preterm and premature babies have the worst prognosis. Infants weighing less than 1500 g at birth have more chances to develop haematological abnormalities such as neutropenia, thrombocytopenia and lymphocytosis. Hepatosplenomegaly, and neuromuscular impairments are the other major complications.

The infant could be infected by the transfusion of infected blood during perinatal period and the worst outcome is in the infant weighing less than 1500 g at time of birth. Deterioration of respiratory function, septicaemia, hepatosplenomegaly and haematological abnormalities comprise the post-transfusion CMV syndrome. In 20% of infants, it may prove fatal.

Perinatal mortality rates of infants are two to four folds higher in women who continued coitus during pregnancy than those who maintained abstinence from sex. The frequent coitus is associated with amniotic fluid infection and abruptio placentae. However current data do not show any harmful effect of coitus in pregnancy especially in healthy women with normal vaginal flora.

The changing face of epidemiology of STD in view of emerging resistance of antimicrobials particularly in gonococcal infection, emergence and rapid spread of HIV worldwide and changing sexual practices will have greater impact on reproductive health. It is imperative at part of policy makers and health care providers to take cognizance of these facts for future planning of national policy on detection and treatment of STD.

References

1. Holmes KK, Sparling PF, Mardh PA, et al. Introduction. In: Homes KK, Sparling PF, Mardh PA, eds Sexually Transmitted Diseases. 3rd edition. New York: McGraw-Hill; 1999. p. xxi – xxiii

2. Global estimates In: WHO/HIV-AIDS/2001.02, 2001 http://www.who.int/HIV_AIDS/STIGlobalReport/index.htm

3. Park K, Epidemiology of communicable diseases. In: Park K, edr. Textbook of Preventive and Social medicine. 16th edition. Jabalpur: Banarasidas Bhanot; 2001. p. 251-255.

4. Training Module of medical health personnel on RCH, Study fellowship on reproductive and child health, 1999-2000, Family Welfare training and research Centre, Mumbai. Sponsored by Department of Family Welfare, Government of India and World Health Organization (WHO).

5. Chlamydial infections In: WHO/HIV-AIDS/2001.02, 2001 http://www.who.int/HIV_AIDS/STDGlobalReport/index.htm

6. Stamm W. *Chlamydia trachomatis* infections of the adults. In: Holmes KK, Sparling PF, Mardh PA, eds. Sexually Transmitted Diseases. 3rd edition. New York: McGraw-Hill; 1999. p. 407-422.

7. Perine P, Stamm WE. Lymphogranuloma venereum. In: Holmes KK, Sparling PF, Mardh PA, eds. Sexually Transmitted Diseases. 3rd edition. New York: McGraw-Hill; 1999. p. 423-432.

8. von Haam EV, D'Aunoy R: Is Lymphogranuloma a systemic disease? Am J Trop Med Hyg 1936; 16: 527.

9. Hopsu-Havu VB, Sonck CE. Infiltrative, ulcerative and fistular lesions of the penis due to Lymphogranuloma venereum. Br J Vener Dis 1973; 49: 49-193.

10. Willcox RR, Willcox JR. Lymphogranuloma venereum. In: Willcox RR, Willcox JR, eds. Pocket consultant of venereological Medicine. 1st edition. Bombay: Oxford University Press; 1992. p. 248-255.

11. Willcox RR, Willcox JR. Gonorrhoea. In: Willcox RR, Willcox JR, eds. Pocket consultant of venereological Medicine. 1st edition. Bombay: Oxford University Press; 1992. p. 41-86.

12. King A, Nicol C, Rodin P. Gonorrhoea in the male. In King A, Nicol C, Rodin P, eds. Venereal Diseases. 4th edition. London: ELBS; 1986. p. 200-213.

13. Hook III EW, Handsfield HH. Gonococcal infections in the adult. In: Holmes KK, Sparling PF, Mardh PA, eds. Sexually Transmitted Diseases. 3rd edition. New York: McGraw-Hill; 1999. p. 451-472.

14. Watts DH, Brunham RC. Sexually transmitted diseases, including HIV infection in pregnancy. In: Holmes KK, Sparling PF, Mardh PA, eds Sexually Transmitted Diseases. 3rd edition. New York: McGraw-Hill; 1999. p. 1089-1132.

15. Berman SM, Hein Karen. Adolescents and STDs. In: Holmes KK, Sparling PF, Mardh PA, eds. Sexually Transmitted Diseases. 3rd edition. New York: McGraw-Hill; 1999. p. 129-142.

16. Syphilis. In: WHO/HIV-AIDS/2001.02, 2001 http://www.who.int/HIV_AIDS/STDGlobalReport/index.htm

17. Farrell N. Donovanosis. In: Holmes KK, Sparling PF, Mardh PA, eds. Sexually Transmitted Diseases. 3rd edition. New York: McGraw-Hill; 1999. p. 525-531.

18. Rajam RV, Rangiah PN. Donovanosis (Granuloma Inguinale, Granuloma Venereum). Geneva, World Health Organization, WHO Monograph Series No 24, 1954: 1-72.

19. Hillier S, Holmes KK. Bacterial vaginosis. In: Holmes KK, Sparling PF, Mardh PA, eds. Sexually Transmitted Diseases. 3rd edition. New York: McGraw-Hill; 1999. p. 563-586.

20. Bacterial Vaginosis In: WHO/HIV-AIDS/2001.02, 2001 http://www.who.int/HIV_AIDS/STDGlobalReport/index.htm

21. Westrom L, Eschenbach D. Pelvic inflammatory disease. In: Holmes KK, Sparling PF, Mardh PA, eds. Sexually Transmitted Diseases. 3rd edition. New York: McGraw-Hill; 1999. p. 783-803.

22. Kriegar JN, Alderete JF. *Trichomonas vaginalis* and Trichomoniasis. In: Holmes KK, Sparling PF, Mardh PA, eds. Sexually Transmitted Diseases. 3rd edition. New York: McGraw-Hill; 1999. p. 587-604.

23. Sowmini CN, Vijayalakshmi K, Chellamuthiah C, Sundaram SM. Infection of the median raphe of the penis: report of three cases. Br J Vener Dis 1973; 49: 469-474.

24. Pavithran K. Trichomonal abscess of the median raphe of the penis. Int J Dermatol 1993; 32: 820-821.

25. Salihi FL et al. Neonatal *Trichomonas vaginalis*: Report of three cases and review of the literature. Paediatrics 1980; 53: 196-199.

26. Pheifer TA. Nonspecific vaginitis. Role of *Haemophilus vaginalis* and treatment with metronidazole. N Eng J Med 1978; 298: 1429-1433.

27. Mardh PA, Westrom L. Tubal and cervical cultures in acute salpingitis with special reference to *Mycoplasma hominis* and T-strain mycoplasmas Brit J Vener Dis 1970; 46: 179-185.

28. Harwik HJ. *Mycoplasma hominis* and abortion. J Infect Dis 1970; 121: 260-266.

29. Wallace RJ. Isolation of mycoplasma hominis from blood cultures in patients with post partum fever. Obstet Gynecol 1989; 73: 181.

30. Toth A. Light microscopy as an aid in predicting ureaplasma infection in human semen. Fertil Steril 1978; 42: 586-593.

31. Corey L, Wald A. Genital herpes. In: Holmes KK, Sparling PF, Mardh PA, eds. Sexually Transmitted Diseases. 3rd edition. New York: McGraw-Hill; 1999. p. 285-312.

32. Bryson Y. Risks of acquisition of genital herpes simplex virus type 2 in sex partners of persons with genital herpes: a prospective couple study. J infect Dis 1993; 167: 942-946.

33. Drew WL, Bates MP. Cytomegalovirus.In: Holmes KK, Sparling PF, Mardh PA, eds. Sexually Transmitted Diseases. 3rd edition. New York: McGraw-Hill; 1999. p. 313-326.

34. Kashima H, Shah K, Mounts P. Recurrent respiratory papillomatosis. In: Holmes KK, Sparling PF, Mardh PA, eds. Sexually Transmitted Diseases. 3rd edition. New York: McGraw-Hill; 1999. p. 1213-1218.

35. Cates W Jr, Brunham RC. Sexually transmitted diseases and infertility. In: Holmes KK, Sparling PF, Mardh PA, eds. Sexually Transmitted Diseases. 3rd edition. New York: McGraw-Hill; 1999. p. 1079-1087.

36. Griffith HB. Gonorrhoea and fertility in Uganda. Eugen Rev 1963; 55: 103-108.

37. World Health Organization Task Force on the prevention and management of infertility: Tubal infertility: serological relationship to past chlamydial and gonococcal infection. Sex Transm Dis 1995; 22: 71.

38. Westrom L. Pelvic inflammatory disease and fertility. A cohort study of 1,844 women with laparoscopically verified diseases and 657 control women with normal laparoscopic results. Sex Transm Dis 1992; 19: 185-192.

39. Svensson L Mardh PA, Westrom L. Infertility after acute salpingitis with special reference to *Chlamydia trachomatis*. Fertil Steril 1983; 40: 322-329.

40. Cates W Jr. Genital chlamydia infections: Epidemiology and reproductive Sequalae. Am J Obstet Gynecol 1991; 164: 1777-1781.

41. Cerrone MC. Cloning and sequence of the gene for heat shock protein 60 from *Chlamydia trachomatis* and immunological reactivation of protein. Infect immun 1991; 59; 79.

42. Darling JR. Primary tubal infertility in relation to the use of an intrauterine device. N Eng J Med 1985; 312: 937.

43. Cramer DW. The relationship of tubal infertility to barrier method and oral contraceptive use. JAMA 1987; 257: 2446-2450.

44. Phipps WR Cramer DW, Schiff Z, et al. The association between smoking and female infertility as influenced by cause of the infertility. Fertil Steril 1987; 48: 377-382.

45. Hershey P. Effects of cigarette smoking on the immune system. Follow-up studies in normal subjects after cessation of smoking. Med J Aust 1983; 2: 425.

46. Sridama V. Decrease levels of helper T cells: A possible cause of immunodeficiency in pregnancy. N Eng J Med 1982; 307: 352.

47. Bone NC, Greene RR. Histologic study of uterine tubes with tubal pregnancy. Am J Obstet Gynecol 1961; 82: 1166.

48. Temmerman M. Mass antimicrobial treatment in pregnancy: A randomised placebo-controlled trial in a population with high rates of sexually transmitted diseases. J Reprod Med 1995; 40: 176-180.

49. Romero R. Tumour necrosis factor in preterm and term labour. Am J Obstet Gynecol 1992; 166: 1576-1587.

50. Romero R, Brody DT, Oyarzum E, et al. Infection and labour: III. Interleukin-1: A signal for the onset of parturition. Am J Obstet Gynecol 1989; 160: 1117-1123.

51. Coultrip LL. The value of amniotic fluid interleukin-6 determination in patients with pre-term labour and intact membranes in the detection of microbial invasion of the amniotic cavity. Am J Obstet Gynecol 1994; 171: 901-911.

52. Romero R. Prostaglandin concentrations in amniotic fluid of women with intra-amniotic infection and preterm labour. Am J Obstet Gynecol 1987; 157: 1461-1467.

53. McGregor JA. Bacterial protease-induced reduction of chorioamniotic membrane strength and elasticity. Obstet Gynecol 1987; 69: 167-174.

54. Plummer FA. Postpartum upper genital tract infections in Nairobi, Kenya: Epidemiology, aetiology and risk factors. J Infect Dis 1987; 156: 92.

55. Wager GP, Martin OH, Koutsky L, et al. Puerperal infectious morbidity: relationship to route of delivery and to antepartum *Chlamydia trachomatis* infection. Am J Obstet Gynecol 1980; 138: 1028-1033.

56. Corey L. Holmes KK. Genital herpes simplex virus infections: current concepts in diagnosis, therapy, and prevention. Ann Intern Med 1983; 98: 973-983.

57. Stagno S, Whitley RJ. Herpesvirus infections in neonates and children: cytomegalovirus and herpes simplex virus. In: Holmes KK, Sparling PF, Mardh PA, eds. Sexually Transmitted Diseases. 3rd edition. New York: McGraw-Hill; 1999. p. 1191-1212

58. Stagno S, Pass RF, Dworsky ME, Alford CA Sr. Maternal cytomegalovirus infection and perinatal transmission. Clin Obstet Gynecol 1982; 25: 563-576.

59. Radolf JD, Sanchez PJ, Schulz KF, Murphy FK. Congenital syphilis. In: Holmes KK, Sparling PF, Mardh PA, eds. Sexually Transmitted Diseases. 3rd edition. New York: McGraw-Hill; 1999. p. 1165-1185.

60. Ratnam AV, Din SN, Hira SH, et al. Syphilis in pregnant women in Zambia. Br J Vener Dis 1982; 58: 355-358.

61. Manning B, Moodley T, Ross SM. Syphilis in pregnant black women. S Afr Med J 1985; 67: 966-967.

62. Ingraham NR. The value of penicillin alone in the prevention and treatment of congenital syphilis. Acta Derm Venereol (Stockh) 1951; 31 (suppl 24): 60.

63. Hughes JM, Cohen ML. Prevention of Group B Streptococcal Infection. Revised Guidelines from CDC. www.cdc.gov.

PART II
HIV/AIDS

Chapter 3

Global and National Overview of HIV/AIDS Epidemic

P L Joshi

Introduction

AIDS (Acquired Immuno Deficiency Syndrome) represents the late clinical stage of infection with human immunodeficiency virus (HIV). The syndrome was first recognized in 1981, but probably existed at a low endemic level in Central Africa before the HIV epidemic spread to several areas of the World during 1980s.[1]

Two decades into the epidemic and there is still no vaccine and no "cure" for AIDS. There is considerably more information now available on how the HIV leads to AIDS, its spread, and a wealth of "lessons learned" in implementing prevention strategies and increased understanding about what constitutes effective management of HIV/AIDS patients. The social and economic conditions that facilitate the spread of HIV are also well understood. Despite all that we know, risk behaviour and risk environments persist and HIV continues to spread among individuals and across national and regional borders, the latest frontier being Asia.

AIDS has crossed geographic borders around the world, within Asia and nations, the epidemic has also challenged traditional cultural boundaries. Effective prevention involves addressing traditional "taboos" in many cultures. Discussing sensitive issues around sexuality, critical to effective AIDS education, requires a change of traditional "culture of silence" so people can more openly talk about safe sex.

Due to the association of HIV/AIDS with commercial sex, drugs and men having sex with men, the disease has also acquired a stigma that has been difficult to overcome. Those infected and affected by HIV and AIDS have faced discrimination and alienation. The early uncertainty about the mode of HIV spread and knowledge that it is a fatal illness with no currently available cure, created considerable fear and consequent alienation of people living with HIV and AIDS as well as their close family members. Stigma is one of the most crucial impediments in breaking the chain of transmission of HIV in the community. It is a time to cross the boundaries laid by misinformation, fear and stigma and break the barriers in taking proactive, sensible and effective measures to contain the spread of HIV/AIDS in the country.

Historical Milestones

The first indication, that the disease is caused by a retrovirus, came in 1983 from French scientists, when Prof. Montagnier and his co-workers isolated the causative viral agent, which was later named as HIV.[2] Enzyme Linked Immunosorbent Assay (ELISA) technique to detect the presence of antibodies in blood against HIV was developed in 1984. The CD4 molecule was identified as the major receptor for HIV. HIV was isolated from semen[3] and central nervous system[4]. Thus, by 1984, it became apparent that the virus is lymphocytotrophic and also has neurotropism. The viral isolation in the semen explained the reason behind the epidemic being observed in gay groups. In 1986, Montagnier's group discovered a new type of HIV in West Africa and labeled it as HIV 2.[5] In 1987, zidovudine was reported to be useful in managing the patients with HIV infection for the first time.[6] Later combination therapy came in vogue which became more popular after the discovery of protease inhibitors.

An Overview of the Epidemic

The HIV/AIDS Pandemic

WHO and UNAIDS estimates that at the end of 2001, 40 million people around the World were living with HIV, 4 million more than at the end of the previous year. During 2001, it is estimated that there were 5 million new HIV infections and 3 million deaths due to AIDS. Among the new infections, 8,00,000 occurred among children under 15 years and more than 2 million were among women. Since the first clinical evidence of AIDS was reported in June 1981, some 22 million people have died of AIDS, including 3.6 million children. Nearly 14 million children have become orphaned due to AIDS.[7]

Adult and children estimated to be living with HIV/AIDS as of end of 2001[7] are shown in Fig. 1.

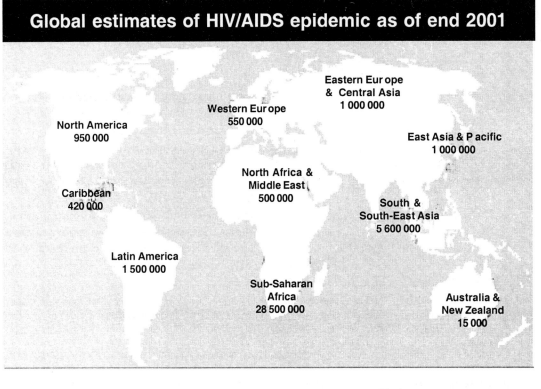

Global estimates of HIV/AIDS epidemic as of end 2001

North America
950 000

Western Europe
550 000

Eastern Europe
& Central Asia
1 000 000

East Asia & Pacific
1 000 000

Caribbean
420 000

North Africa &
Middle East
500 000

South &
South-East Asia
5 600 000

Latin America
1 500 000

Sub-Saharan
Africa
28 500 000

Australia &
New Zealand
15 000

People newly infected with HIV in 2001	Total	5 million
	Adults	4.2 million
	Women	2 million
	Children <15 years	800 000
Number of people living with HIV/AIDS	Total	40 million
	Adults	37.1 million
	Women	18.5 million
	Children < 15 years	3 million
AIDS deaths in 2001	Total	3 million
	Adults	2.4 million
	Women	1.1 million
	Children < 15 years	580 000
Total number of children orphaned** by AIDs, and living, end 2001		14 million

**Defined as children aged 0–14, as of end 2001, who have lost one or both parents to AIDS.

Fig. 1   Adults and Children Living with HIV/AIDS: 40 million

The diversity of HIV spread throughout population is striking: 16 countries (all in sub-Saharan Africa) report an overall adult HIV prevalence over 10%; 8 countries between 5% and 8% (all in sub-Saharan Africa); 28 countries between 1% and 5% and the remaining 119 countries of the World have less than 1% of HIV prevalence among adults. Several countries currently have concentrated epidemics whereby overall population prevalence remain low, but high risk groups such as commercial female sex workers (FSW), injecting drug users (IDU) and men have sex with men (MSM) have rising rates.[8]

As of mid 2001, the HIV/AIDS epidemic comprises many separate and basically independent epidemics, each involving different modes of HIV transmission and each developing at separate times and in different countries. Even within the countries, HIV epidemics have primarily been localized and diverse. What appeared about two decades ago to be focal epidemics in industrialized countries that mainly involved MSM and IDU, has evolved into a more complex pandemic. HIV/AIDS is currently endemic at varying but usually high prevalence levels among MSM in most regions of the world. Explosive spread of HIV still occurs within pockets of susceptible IDU populations worldwide and sexual transmission occurs throughout the world among both males and females who have unprotected sex with multiple partners. However, extensive heterosexual spread of HIV has occurred predominantly, only in sub-saharan African countries, a few countries in the Caribbean and in Central America, and a few countries in South and South-east Asia.

Sub-Saharan Africa

Sub-Saharan Africa remains by far the worst affected – but most poorly resourced region in the World. More than 28.5 million Africans are living with HIV and a further 17 million have already died of AIDS. By the end of 1999, 12.1 million children in the region have been orphaned by AIDS. Across the continent, an estimated 1.1 million children under 15 years were living with HIV/AIDS at the end of 2000. In this region, the virus spreads mainly through heterosexual intercourse, in all social groups. Women's physiological, social and economic vulnerability, however, contribute to their higher rates of infection in this region. Mother to child transmission of HIV is also claiming increasing number of lives. Indeed, the region is home for 90% of all children in the World who became infected through mother to child transmission in 2000.

In southern Africa, the epidemic is still spinning out of control, despite belated efforts to contain it. In several countries like Lesotho, Namibia, South Africa, Swaziland, Zambia and Zimbabwe etc, at least one in five adults is HIV positive. In Botswana, the adult prevalence is approaching 36%. In 2000, the HIV prevalence among pregnant women in South Africa rose to its highest level ever: 24.5%. Uganda is the only African country to have turned around a major epidemic. Its extra-ordinary efforts pushed down the adult prevalence to 5% at the end of 2001, however, new infections continue to occur in Uganda.[7]

Latin America and the Caribbean

The spread of HIV is driven by a variety of factors, including unsafe sex between men and women, MSM and injecting drug abuse. At 5%, Haiti has the highest HIV adult prevalence rate in the World outside sub-Saharan Africa.

Asia and the Middle East

Asia is seeing alarming increase in the number of infections, 6 million people are living with HIV/AIDS. In 2000, an estimated 7,80,000 people became infected in South and South-East Asia, with adult HIV prevalence rate exceeding 2% in Cambodia, Myanmar and Thailand. Unsafe sex and drug injecting practices largely account for the rising prevalence rates. While East Asia and the Pacific region still appear to be holding HIV at bay, the recent steep rise in sexually transmitted diseases (STD) in China and vast transmigration of people could unleash an epidemic. In North Africa and the Middle East, infections are rising from a low base.

Central and Eastern Europe

Infection rates are climbing unabated in Eastern Europe and Central Asia, where overlapping epidemics of HIV of injecting drugs use and STD are swelling the ranks of people living with HIV/AIDS. New epidemics have emerged in Estonia, Uzbekistan, while, in Ukraine, 2,40,000 people were living with HIV/AIDS in 1999. In year 1996, only a few cities in the Russian Federation reported HIV cases; today, 82 of its 89 regions harbour the virus. The epidemic is still concentrated among injecting drug users and their sexual partners.[7]

Industrialized Countries

Almost 1.5 million people live with HIV in those regions, many of them productively and on antiretroviral therapy. In some countries, a new pattern is emerging, with the epidemic shifting towards poorer people especially ethnic minorities who face disproportionate risks of infection and are more likely to be missed by a prevention campaign and deprived of access to treatment. The HIV prevalence rates among IDU give cause for alarm: 18% in Chicago and as high as 30% in parts of New York. By contrast, needle exchange schemes in Australia have kept prevalence rates low among IDU. There are reports that in some American cities HIV infection rates are rising and also reported a sharp increase in STD among MSM in Amsterdam, an indication that unsafe sex threatens to become the norm again. The prospect of larger HIV/AIDS epidemic cannot be ruled out if wide spread public complacency is not addressed and if inappropriate or stalled prevention efforts are not adapted to reflect changes in the epidemic.

The HIV epidemic in western Europe is the result of multitude of epidemics that differ in terms of their timing, their scale and population they affect. In Spain, a significant share of HIV infections (24%) is occurring via heterosexual transmission. But injecting drug use is the main mode of transmission, reported HIV prevalence among drug users in 2000 was 20-30% nationwide, while in France, prevalence rates ranged between 10% and 23%. Portugal, meanwhile faces a serious epidemic among IDU of the 3680 new HIV infections reported, there in 2000, more than half were caused by injecting drug use and just under a third occurred via hetrosexual intercourse. At 37.3 per 1,00,000 persons, Portugal's rate of reported new infections is the highest among all reporting countries in western Europe.

There are signs that the sexual behaviour of young people in Japan could be changing significantly and put this group at greater risk of HIV infection. Higher rates of chlamydia among female and gonorrhoea among males, as well as doubling of the number of induced abortion among teen age women in the past five year, indicated increased rates of unprotected sexual intercourse. Sex between men remains an important transmission route in several countries, while recently becoming a more prominent mode of HIV transmission

in others, such as Japan. There, the number of HIV infections detected in MSM has risen in recent years.

In Australia, Canada, the United States of America and countries of Western Europe, an apparent increase in unsafe sex is triggering higher rates of STD and, in some cases, higher HIV incidence among MSM. A syphilis outbreak in Los Angles among MSM, reported in 2001, confirmed warnings that safe sex was on the decline in the city. In a French Study, in year 2000, 38% of surveyed HIV positive MSM said they had recently practiced unsafe sex, compared to 26% in 1997.[10]

The reasons for this are debatable. Part of the explanation could lie in the perceived life saving effects of antiretroviral therapy, introduced in high income countries in 1996.

HIV Epidemic: Indian Scenario

Based on nationwide sentinel surveillance, the National AIDS Control Organization estimated that atleast 3.97 million persons have been infected by HIV (2001). Estimations of 2001 indicated that atleast 0.8% adults between the age group of 15-49 years were infected. The predominant mode of transmission of HIV infection is sexual in India (Fig. 2). The HIV epidemic has become generalized in six Indian states–Maharashtra, Tamilnadu, Karnataka, Andhra Pradesh, Manipur and Nagaland. (Fig. 3).

Surveillance for HIV infection was initiated in India by the Indian Council of Medical Research (ICMR) in late 1985 as a part of AIDS Task Force. Anti-HIV antibodies were first detected among sex workers from Chennai in south India in 1986 and soon thereafter, the first AIDS case in India was reported from Mumbai in 1986. Realizing the high HIV prevalence rates amongst the professional blood donors, anti- HIV screening of all the blood units to be used for transfusional purposes was made mandatory in July 1989 in four metropolitan cities of India. Presence of HIV 2 infection in India was reported for the first time from Bombay in 1991. Two different types of HIV epidemic are seen in India. In the north-eastern India, the epidemic is mainly among IDU whereas it is mainly spread through heterosexual route in rest of the country.

India-an Evolving HIV Epidemic

Based on the results of sentinel surveillance, States/ Union Territories (UT) can be categorized into: (i)

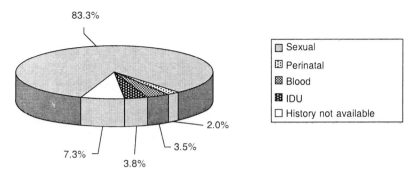

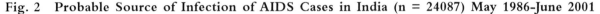

Fig. 2 Probable Source of Infection of AIDS Cases in India (n = 24087) May 1986-June 2001

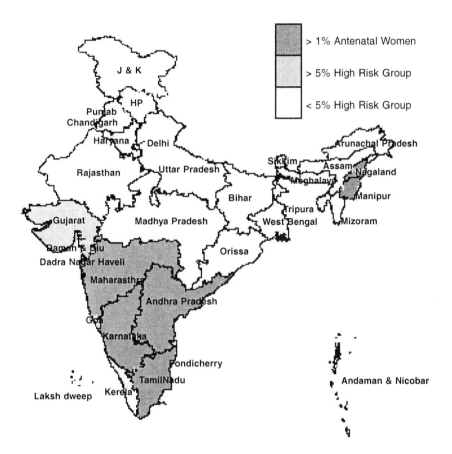

Fig. 3 Prevalence of HIV Infection in India.

High prevalence States- where HIV prevalence among antenatal mothers is 1% or more. These States are Maharashtra, Tamil Nadu, Andhra Pradesh, Karnataka, Manipur, and Nagaland; (ii) Moderate prevalence States, where HIV prevalence rate in antenatal women is less than 1% but the prevalence among high risk group is 5% or more. The States/UT like Gujarat, Pondicherry and Goa fall in this category; and (iii) Low prevalence states: where HIV prevalence among high risk group is less than 5% and among antenatal women is less than 1%. All other States belong to this category. The national estimate of HIV infections is about 4 million. Most of them do not know their HIV status, making prevention of spread of HIV infection more complex.

India's epidemic is not a single epidemic but is made up of a number of distinct epidemics, often co-existing in the same state. Primarily driven by heterosexual transmission, HIV infection is steadily moving beyond its initial focus among commercial sex workers into the wider population. At the same time sub-epidemics have evolved with potentially explosive spread among groups of IDU. There has been a broadening of the epidemic in the Southern, Western and a few Northeast States of India. In other parts of the country overall levels of HIV are still low.

High levels of STD, the evident presence of sexual networks and presence of migration all indicate to a significant vulnerability. The epidemic continues to shift towards women and young people with an expected accompanying increase in the vertical transmission and pediatric HIV. Migration both within and between states is a source of transmission of HIV between urban and rural populations but remains poorly studied. Gender bias, unequal power in decision making, between men and women and the latter's inability to negotiate safer sex remain major obstacles. In the case of drug users indications are that there is a shift from inhaling to over the counter injecting drugs. Harm minimization approach is followed in areas having high drug use, like the North Eastern State of Manipur and the metropolises of Mumbai, Chennai and Delhi.

Pattern of Spread

India's epidemic seems to be following the so called Type 4 pattern, first described in Thailand. The epidemic shifts from the highest risk groups (commercial sex workers, drug users) to bridge populations (clients of sex workers, STD patients, partners of drug users) and then to the general population. The shift usually occurs where the prevalence in the first group reaches 5%. There is a time lag of 2-3 years between shift from one group to the next. Forecasting the future of an epidemic is as complex as HIV, will always be problematic. Important new elements are entering into the picture. The burden of AIDS cases will soon begin to be felt in states affected early in the epidemic, like Tamil Nadu, Maharashtra and Manipur.

Basic Epidemiology

Human Immunodeficiency Virus

HIV is a retrovirus belonging to the subfamily of lentiviruses. It contains a genome comprising of two single-stranded RNA molecules. HIV gets integrated into the chromosomal DNA of the host cell by using reverse transcriptase enzyme to produce a double-stranded proviral DNA. Majority of the proviral particles may go into latency for a variable period of time. Upon activation, it reproduces RNA transcripts and proteins which are used to synthesize new HIV virions. There are two main types of HIV: HIV 1 and HIV 2. HIV 1 and -2 have originated from the simian immunodeficiency virus (SIV) probably from the ones found in chimpanzees (SIVcpz) and in sooty mangabey monkeys (SIVsm). HIV is a lymphocytotropic and neurotropic virus. Therefore it is found in almost all the body fluids and organs. It is present in infective dosages in semen, vaginal & cervical secretions and blood. Exchange of these body fluids from an HIV infected individuals can lead to transmission of HIV infection to another person. Semen contains about fifty times higher concentration of the virus as compared to vaginal and cervical secretions and blood. The central nervous system, testis, lymphnodes, etc act as reservoirs of HIV. The highest concentration of HIV among the body fluids is found in cerebrospinal fluid.[5]

Molecular Epidemiology

There are two types of HIV, HIV 1 & HIV 2. The transmission efficiency of HIV 2 infection through sexual route is lower than HIV 1. The efficiency of mother to child transmission (MTCT) of HIV 2 is reported to be 1.2% when compared to 24.7% of HIV 1[11]. Moreover, the incubation period of HIV 2 infection is reported to be longer than that of HIV 1. Of the persons infected with HIV in India, 1.7-4.6% have been reported to be due to HIV 2 alone and 3.3-20.1% due to HIV 1 and 2. Presence of dual infection of HIV 1 and 2 and not of HIV 2 alone has been also reported among IDU from Manipur.

Genetic mutations are very frequent in most of the RNA viruses especially so in HIV. Therefore every patient is likely to have a swarm virus variants (quasi-species). Development of recombinant HIV has also been well reported. Such mutations can, theoretically, confer some selective advantage to HIV. It can theoretically lead to evolution of species that may have a higher sexual transmission efficiency and slower disease progression, advantageous to the virus. Identification of mutations and subtypes are likely to be important in HIV vaccine development.

The strains of HIV 1 are divided into two groups as Major and Outlier, which are designated as M and O groups, respectively. Recently, a new HIV 1 group N has been discovered in Cameroon. The viruses belonging to the M group are more closely related to one another which is not the case with the viruses belonging to the O group. The M group is further classified into ten different subtypes, named alphabetically from A to K.[9]

The predominant HIV 1 subtype in United States and Europe is subtype B. In Thailand HIV 1 subtype E and subtype B are commonly seen. However, with increasing international travel and migration, more and more subtypes are being seen in a specified geographic area. A distribution profile of the subtypes of HIV 1 viruses prevalent in India has emerged as a result of a few studies. These strains are closely related to those isolated from South Africa. According to phylogenetic analysis, most of the the Indian HIV-1 strains belong to the subtype C.

Reports from the National AIDS Research Institute reveal that of the 46 samples studied, 44 were identified as subtype C and one each of subtype A and B. Of the samples belonging to subtype C, 15 were most homologous to the C2 reference strain from Zambia and others to Indian reference strain C3. Predominance of HIV 1 subtype C was also shown in samples collected from Punjab, Delhi and Vellore. Surprisingly a study has shown that all the four isolates from Hyderabad belonged to subtype B. Additionally, a recombinant HIV between subtype C and A has been reported from Pune.[10]

Waves of HIV Epidemic

Predominant route of transmission of HIV is sexual. Hence this epidemic spreads as one would envisage in a classical epidemic of STD. HIV epidemic spreads classically in three waves. In the first wave, HIV infection is seen amongst sex workers or IDU which are also called as *core transmitters* or *core groups*. In its second wave, HIV infection reaches the clients of sex workers or partners of IDU. When evidences suggest affection of spouses and children of the clients of sex workers, the HIV epidemic is understood to have reached its third wave. HIV infection is brought into the low risk population from the *core transmitters* through the *bridge population*, a term used to connote mobile population such as truck drivers, single male member migrants etc. (Fig. 4) Some scientists, consider that IDU constitute the first wave which is followed by the sex workers

and so on. Recently, a fourth wave comprising of adolescents has also been proposed to indicate the severity of epidemic.

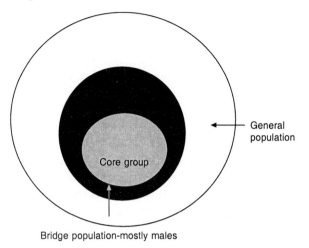

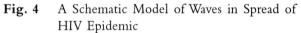

Fig. 4 A Schematic Model of Waves in Spread of HIV Epidemic

Estimating the Magnitude

It is essential to know the number of cases of any disease or disorder for undertaking advocacy, planning extension of health care services and control strategies including budgetary allocation, and evolving research priorities. Such estimations can be made by initiating surveillance among the most vulnerable population groups. The proportion of people found to be infected at any given time of point is called as prevalence rate. However, such a rate may not be very useful in chronic diseases. In these circumstances, one needs to estimate the rate of occurrence of new cases in the community every year. This rate is called as the incidence. However, estimation of incidence requires establishment of a cohort of susceptible population group (s). It is a costly and time consuming activity. Hence a rough estimate is made through use of surveillance at periodic intervals in various vulnerable groups. Most often such studies are carried out from the clinics or hospital settings. This limits the generalizability of the findings. However, using certain assumptions and using data from various geographical areas and risk groups, the estimates of cases can be made using different statistical models.

HIV Incidence and Prevalence, and AIDS Mortality

The rate of spread of HIV and current levels of infection

are measured by incidence and prevalence. The incidence of HIV is the number of new cases, that is, the number of people who become infected during a specified period of time, usually over a twelve month interval.

The prevalence of HIV is the number of people currently infected with HIV at a given point of time. Because there is no cure for HIV/AIDS, HIV prevalence reflects the cumulative number of infections from the past and mortality rate of those infected.

Incidence and prevalence of HIV/AIDS are often expressed as a rate e.g. in terms of the number of infections per 1000 adults. At the beginning of the epidemic, HIV prevalence grows rapidly and AIDS mortality is not evident because of the long asymptomatic period of most of those infected. Years later, when the first few cases of AIDS appear, large numbers of people are already infected with HIV. Incidence may still be climbing but growth in prevalence may slow because of rising HIV/AIDS mortality or saturation of the population. As long as incidence exceeds mortality, the prevalence of HIV will continue to rise. Prevalence will peak in the year in which incidence exactly equals the rising mortality rate. Whether prevalence then levels off, declines or resume climbing toward new peak will depend on whether the number of new infections—incidence is equal to, less than, or greater than the number of deaths of people with HIV/AIDS. In the absence of a cure, the key to reducing future HIV prevalence is by preventing new cases i.e. is lowering incidence.

Stable or declining prevalence does not necessarily signal the end of the epidemic. Eventually, HIV prevalence will level off in all populations, in some it will stabilize at a high level, and in others at a low level. However, a plateau simply indicates that there is an equilibrium in which the number of new infections exactly offsets AIDS mortality. In populations where prevalence is declining, mortality is occurring at a faster rate than new infections. The number of new infections may still be quite high, coexisting with high mortality.

The relationship between HIV incidence and prevalence and the lag in the appearance of AIDS cases have important implications for public policy:

- Early intervention is critical to prevent an AIDS epidemic that can persist for decades. Only a fraction of those infected with HIV are showing symptoms of AIDS at any given point of time. By the time the AIDS morbidity becomes a significant health issue, HIV may have spread widely in the population, making prevention efforts very difficult. Countries with few reported AIDS cases should not be complacent about launching prevention campaign.

- The full impact of infection levels on mortality is delayed. Even if all HIV infections could be prevented, in absence of cure, AIDS deaths would continue for years because of the population already infected and the long asymptomatic period between HIV infection and AIDS. Countries where HIV prevalence is high are only beginning to experience the profound mortality impact of the epidemic, which will last for decades even with the best prevention efforts.

- Biology and behaviour affect the spread of HIV. Not all infectious agents introduced into a population will be self sustaining. If each infected person transmits the infection, on an average, to less than one other person over his or her life time, then the infection disappears, if to more than one other person, then the infection will expand. The reproductive rate of a sexually transmitted disease is the average number of susceptible people infected by an infected person over his or her life time. If each person infected with a disease transmits it to exactly one other person, then the reproduction rate is one[1].

In population in which HIV has a reproductive rate of less than 1, the epidemic will not be self sustained. Thus, greater the reproductive rate of HIV, the more rapidly the epidemic will spread. Three main factors have a large influence on the reproductive rate of all STD, including HIV

- The amount of time a person remain infectious
- The risk of transmission per sexual contact
- The rate of acquisition of new partners

These factors are similar for transmission through contaminated injecting equipment, except that the risk per injection and the number of partners refer to number of people with whom injecting equipment is shared.

Each of these three factors in turn influenced by the biology of the virus and by individual behaviour.

Duration of Infectiousness

The lack of cure and the long duration of infectiousness are the main characteristics that distinguish HIV from most other STD. The long duration of HIV infectiousness increases the likelihood that an infected individual will pass the infection to others. Further, because a person with HIV typically remains asymptomatic for years, an infected individual or his or her sexual (or injecting) partners are often unaware of the risk of transmission. Thus the long duration of asymptomatic HIV infection potentially puts many more partners at risk than is the case for other STD.

Risk of Infection per Contact

The average risk of infection per sexual exposure is much smaller than that for other STD, however, because of long period of infectious-ness and numerous cofactors that enhance HIV transmission, the chance that an HIV positive person who does not take precautions will eventually infect others can be quite high.

The most extensive studies of the risk of HIV transmission have been conducted in industrial countries. Because of generally superior health levels and the ready availability of treatment for other STD, the average risk of HIV infection per sexual contact in industrial countries is quite small. For example, the average chance that an infected male will transmit HIV to an uninfected female partner by unprotected vaginal sex is estimated at between 1 and 2 per 1000 exposure. The risk of transmission from an infected female to an uninfected male partner through unprotected vaginal sex is one-third to one half.[11]

Anal sex carries the highest risk, especially for the receptive partner. However, all these figures very likely underestimate the average transmission probability of HIV infection per exposure.

Probability of HIV–I Infection per exposure is shown in Table 1.

Probability of HIV infection per sexual act are generally based on studies of transmission within discordant couples-couples in which one partner is HIV-positive and other is HIV negative. The "per contact" risk of HIV transmission with a commercial or casual partner is likely to be substantially less than that for other STD. In the case of gonorrhoea, for example, the probability that an infected woman will transmit the disease to an uninfected male partner during intercourse is 20-30% per exposure, while the probability that an infected male will transmit the disease to his female partner is 50-70%.

The risk of infection per contact is not constant; it can be influenced by a variety of factors, some of

Table 1. Probability of HIV 1 infection per exposure

Mode of transmission	Infection per 100 exposure
Male to Female, unprotected vaginal sex	0.1 to 0.2
Female to male, unprotected vaginal sex	0.033 to 0.1
Male to male, unprotected anal sex	0.5 to 3.0
Needle stick	0.3
Mother to child transmission	13 to 48
Exposure to contaminated blood products	90 to 100

which may exacerbate the epidemic. Some of these are: stage of HIV infection, untreated STD, use of latex condoms, male circumcision, etc.

Role of Partner Change

Both the average rate of partner change in a population and the variation of the rate across individuals have an impact on the spread of HIV in populations. Other factors being constant, the higher the average rate of partner change is, the higher the reproductive rate of HIV. However, in a population in which a few people have very high rates of partner change, and many people have very low rates, HIV and other STD will spread more quickly than if the same average number of partners were distributed more equally across the entire population.

Mixing Patterns

The path of the epidemic within the overall population depends on the degree of pattern of mixing among people with the high risk behaviour and the mixing between people with high risk behaviour and people with low risk behaviour. By "high risk behaviour, we mean unprotected sexual intercourse with multiple partners or sharing of unsterilized infecting equipment. People with high risk behaviour, who have few partners, who consistently use condoms, who do not inject drugs, or (if they do) do not share injecting equipment, are less likely to pass HIV to others.

In sexually transmitted HIV epidemic, the speed at which HIV spreads from people with large number of partners to those with very few partners depends on the extent of mixing between people with different levels of sexual activity. If people with large numbers of partners have intercourse only with other who are similarly active (known as assortative sexual mixing), then HIV will tend to rise rapidly within those groups but only very slowly and to a limited extent to the rest of the population. As a result, the epidemic will achieve lower peak levels of infection in the entire population than if those with large number of partners also have sex with those who have fewer partners (known as random or disassortative mixing).

Mixing patterns explain why HIV does not spread through a population at a uniform rate. Rather, it spreads in a series of smaller epidemics that race through overlapping subpopulations whose behaviours puts them at various degree of risk than those with less risky behaviour with whom they mix.

HIV Prevalence in Risk Groups in India

Core Groups

HIV infections have been reported from all the states in India and heterosexual contact is the predominant mode of transmission. However, intravenous drug use was recognized as important risk behaviour among youth for the first time in the North-eastern Indian state of Manipur. High HIV prevalence rate among the IDU was observed along the National Highway linking India and Myanmar. The HIV seroprevalence of almost 50% in IDU in 1991 has increased to about 87% in 1996, highlighting the explosive HIV epidemic faced in the North-eastern states. However, the HIV prevalence rate among IDU in Calcutta is reported to be about 1%.[12]

In Vellore, the prevalence of HIV 1 antibody among commercial sex workers (CSW) increased from 1.8% in 1986 to 28.6% in 1990, while in the western cities of Pune and Bombay, the HIV sero-prevalence among female sex workers has also greatly increased to 47% and 70%, respectively. Alarmingly high HIV incidence of 20.2 per 100 person years among CSW was observed in HIV incidence study in Pune. Surprisingly, a slow rise in HIV prevalence rates among sex workers in Calcutta from 0.53% (1991) to 5.5% (1998) has been observed.[13]

STD Patients

The prevalence of HIV infection in STD patients increased from 0.19 per cent in 1986 to 3.9 per cent in 1992 in south India[14]. However, reported HIV sero-prevalence in Bombay was as high 14-26% in 1992-93 and that in Pune was 19.9% in 1998. HIV incidence of

9.7 per 100 person years and 5.6 per 100 person years was observed among males who had recent exposure to sex workers and those who did not have, respectively, in Pune.[15] Factors like number of sex partners, lack of condom use and history of previous or present STD were found to be important predictors of prevalent and incident HIV infection. Recent use of condoms reduced the risk of acquiring HIV infection by almost half. A high HIV prevalence of about 14 % was found amongst women attending STD clinic who denied history of sex work[16]. Surprisingly, the small difference in HIV prevalence rates between male STD patients who reported multi-partner sex and those married monogamous women, suggests that the epidemic has established its roots in the low risk population.

'Bridge' Population

A high HIV point prevalence of 5.2% was found amongst 500 truck drivers and helpers in West Bengal in 1994[17] provides epidemiological support to the findings of other studies that have shown little or no awareness about AIDS and higher practice of risk behaviour among the *bridge* population groups.

Blood Donors and Recipients

HIV prevalence among voluntary blood donors in the metropolitan cities of India during the period of 1990-93 was reported to be 0.3 to 0.9%. HIV prevalence rate amongst blood donors at Vellore showed a statistically significant increasing trend from 1.5 per 1000 in 1988-89 to 3.1 per 1000 in 1992-93[18] and similar rates have been observed in Bombay and Pune cities.

Mandatory testing of blood and blood products for HIV antibodies was initiated in July 1989. Consequent to reports of high HIV prevalence in commercial blood donors and HIV reactivity among some commercially available blood products[19], a ban on manufacture of blood products in India was enforced. It was subsequently lifted following improvement in the manufacturing process and quality control procedures. However, no HIV seroconversions were observed among women receiving Anti-D immunoglobulins during pregnancy.

Different studies among thalassemic and other children who received multiple transfusions reported a high HIV sero-prevalence between 8.9% and 30.4%[20], mostly due to transfusions of commercially available cryoprecipitate. Multi-transfused thalassemic children showed no evidence of HIV 2 infection in New Delhi.

Pregnant Women

The HIV sero-prevalence among the pregnant women primarily attending the public hospitals has been reported to be between 0.5-3.3% in various parts of the country. The HIV sentinel surveillance data amongst pregnant women shows that six states in India; Maharashtra, Tamilnadu, Andhra Pradesh, Karnataka, Manipur, and Nagaland have a HIV prevalence of more than 1%[21]. Most of these states are highly industrialized or are affected due to internal strife.

Mother to Child Transmission (MTCT)

The risk of transmission from a pregnant mother to her baby is reported to be between 21-43% in developing countries.[22] A prospective study involving 143 tribal pregnant women and their infants followed until 18 months of age reported an overall mother to child transmission efficiency of 48%.[23] Almost 30-50% of the neonates acquire HIV infection during antenatal period and about 50-70% during delivery. The risk of acquiring HIV infection through breast milk is 14-29%, according to a study based on meta-analysis of other studies.[24] The only observation study being conducted in Malawi has reported that the HIV incidence amongst infants who are breastfed between 1-5 months is higher (0.7% per month) when compared to that between 6-11 months (0.6% per month) and between 12-17 months (0.3% per month).[25] However, exclusive breastfeeding has now been shown to be better than mixed feeding.[26]

The Interplay of Factors Driving Sexual Transmission

There is evidence from around the world that many factors play a role in kick-starting a sexually transmitted HIV epidemic or driving it to higher levels.

Behavioural and Social Factors

- Little or no condom use
- Large proportion of the adult population with multiple sexual partners
- Overlapping (as opposed to serial monogamy)

sexual partnerships- individuals are highly infectious when they first acquire HIV and thus more likely to infect any concurrent partners
- Large sexual networks (often seen in individuals who move back and forth between home and a distant workplace)
- "Age mixing", typically between older men and young women or girls
- Women's economic dependence on marriage or prostitution, robbing them of control over the circumstances or safe sex.

Biological Factors

- High rates of STD, especially those causing genital ulcers, low rates of male circumcision
- High viral load-HIV levels in the bloodstream are typically high when a person is first infected and again in the late stages of illness.

Men Who Have Sex with Men

In many countries around the world, openly "gay communities are rare or non existent". Male homosexual behaviour, on the other hand, exists in every country. It often involves penetrative anal sex between men, an act that carries a high risk of HIV infection. Sex between men is one of the major factors behind the spread of the HIV epidemic in many high-income countries and in some parts of Latin America. In Asia, the contribution of male homosexuality to the HIV epidemic has been recorded regularly but has rarely been quantified. In India, HIV transmission among men has been reported from Mumbai and Chennai. In most of the developing countries including India, MSM are far more likely to do so secretly, and they are less likely to have access to prevention, information and care services.

Bridging Population—the Key for Further HIV Spread

Bridge population can be defined as those men and women who have sex with both high risk and low risk partners. Bridging risk beahvior involves transmission of HIV across the sub-populations having different risk behaviours. Studies have suggested that men having sex with both commercial and non-commercial sex partners play a significant role in transmission of HIV. Scientists have also highlighted in Ukraine the significant "bridging role of IDU" in spreading HIV from a drug user population to other populations through unprotected heterosexual intercourse. In Ukraine, most injecting drug users were described as unaware of the risks of unsafe sex; more than 50% reported sexual encounters with multiple partners, most of them being non-drug-users. Similar observations have been made in the state of Manipur among IDU. The HIV epidemic may or may not spread in the region, depending on the extent of expansion from localized IDU epidemic to so called general population through sexual contacts. Widespread HIV transmission among sexual partners of IDU is likely to occur due to their low level of protected sex, according to the behaviour surveillance.

Vulnerability of Women to HIV

Women are biologically more susceptible to HIV infection than men. Male to female transmission of HIV is 2-4 times more efficient than female to male. This is because women have a larger mucosal surface exposed during sexual intercourse. Another reason is that semen contains a much higher concentration of HIV than vaginal fluid. Women are also disproportionately represented among those who receive blood or blood products as a consequence of their childbearing role, which exposes them to the risk of yet another mode of transmission. The fact that it is the norm for young women to have sex with, or marry older men, also increases the risk of infection. This is because age and or delayed marriage in men is associated with a higher likelihood of premarital sex with more than one partner, including with CSW, thereby creating a greater likelihood of infection.

Poverty, lack of education and limited income earning opportunities often propel women to commercial sex, significantly increasing their risk of infection. There is, for example, a sharp increase in HIV prevalence rates among CSW in Mumbai from 1% to 51% between 1987-1993. The risk of HIV transmission is known to increase with the number of male partners a sex worker has intercourse within the course of a day's work. For many women, high risk activity can simply mean being married. Social norms which accept extra-marital and pre-marital sexual relationships in men as normal, and women's inability to negotiate safe sex practices with their partners are factors that make it difficult for women to protect themselves from HIV infection.

Men's unwillingness to use condoms further accentuates women's risk. For example, in a study of the prevalence of and risk factors for HIV infection in Tamil Nadu, India (1994-95) covering a population of about of 97,000, less than 2% of married men were found to be condom users. Negotiating condom use with male partners becomes especially difficult in contexts where the vast majority of women using contraception have undergone sterilization, as is the case in India and Sri Lanka.

The presence of untreated STD, especially if ulcerative, multiplies the risk of HIV infection by 300-400%. Women with STD face a higher risk of HIV infection than men with STD for a number of reasons. To begin with, more women in the developing world have an STD as compared to men. Secondly, many STD in women are asymptomatic and therefore less likely to be recognized. Yet another reason is that the stigma attached to visiting an STD clinic together with other barriers such as lack of time, money and decision making power, discourages women from seeking treatment.

For all the above reasons, the prevalence of HIV infection is increasing among women who have traditionally been considered low risk populations. The perinatal transmission is bound to increase under these conditions, leaving behind more and more infants and children infected with HIV. A holistic approach needs to be taken into consideration in prevention of mother to child transmission of HIV.

Barriers in Access to Reproductive Health Services

Studies from India on gynaecological morbidity mention "shame and guilt" as important reasons why women do not seek medical treatment. A study from Karnataka (1995) found that the proportion of women reporting untreated reproductive morbidity ranged from 44% to 57% across different socio-demographic groups. In a study (1989) of gynecological morbidity in rural Maharashtra, 92% of the women with a self-reported problem had not sought treatment prior to the screening camp conducted as a part of the study.

National Family Health Survey, India 1992-93, asked women for reasons why they did not seek antenatal care. Almost 60% of women, 66% in urban and 58% in rural areas felt that antenatal care was unnecessary. The higher proportion of women in urban areas stating that it was not necessary must be interpreted in the context of a much smaller proportion over all (18%) in urban than in rural areas (43%) who did not receive antenatal services. 13% of the women did not know about the existence of antenatal services, about 7% could not afford the cost involved and little over 5% did not have the time or had not been given permission to go. In India just over 30% of births are attended by a trained person. The proportion of institutional deliveries is approximately one-fourth of the total annual deliveries.

For an effective prevention of perinatal transmission, it is essential that there should be over all improvement in coverage, maternity and child health services and STD/RTI and HIV/AIDS prevention, screening and management should be incorporated in MCH package.

Survival Time After Diagnosis of AIDS and Advent of Anti-HIV Treatment

The survival time after onset of severe AIDS characteristic illness is also variable, but prior to the development of effective anti-HIV therapy, average survival time was about 2-4 years in most developed countries and about 6 months or less in developing regions was most likely due to diagnosis at a later stage of disease and limited access to good supportive medical care. In the absence of anti-HIV drug treatment, the case fatality rate attributable to HIV is among the highest of any human infectious agent.

The proportion of HIV infected persons who, in the absence of anti-HIV treatment, will ultimately develop AIDS has been estimated to be over 90%. Less than 5% of HIV-infected persons who have been followed with detailed clinical and laboratory studies for 10 years or longer have been classified as possible non-progressors. In the absence of effective anti-HIV treatment, the AIDS cases fatality rate is very high most (80-90%) patients in developed countries die within 2-4 years after the diagnosis of AIDS is made. However, in the United States of America and most developed countries, routine use of prophylactic drugs for the prevention of *P. carinii* pneumonia and other opportunistic infections was able to delay the development of AIDS and death significantly, even prior to the routine available of effective anti-HIV treatment is variable. Access ranges from one extreme, such as in Hong Kong where triple anti-HIV drug therapy is provided to all Hong Kong residents, to the other extreme in the poorer Asian countries, such as Cambodia and Myanmar, where anti-HIV drug treatment is virtually unavailable.

National Response

The Government of India is determined to take all necessary steps to contain the HIV epidemic within manageable limits. Since 1986, Government of India has implemented several HIV/AIDS Control initiatives including: (1) launching the National AIDS Control Programme in 1987, which focused on increasing awareness, blood safety and surveillance; (2) expanding sero-surveillance facilities; (3) implementing a medium term plan to those States and cities considered worse affected by the epidemic, focusing on strengthening programme management capacities, targeted interventions; IEC campaign, surveillance and preventive capacities such as STD control and Condom Promotion, and developing and implementing the five year strategic plan (NACP-I).[27]

The establishment of the National AIDS Committee, the National AIDS Control Board, the National AIDS Control Organization and State AIDS Control Societies considerably strengthened India's management capacity to respond to the epidemic; sentinel surveillance activities have been significantly expanded and steps have been taken to improve the coverage and reliability of the data; the implementation of awareness raising strategy including mass media, advocacy and NGO involvement has resulted in awareness level going up sharply, particularly in urban areas; a comprehensive programme to modernize blood banks has been implemented. NACO has framed and disseminated a National HIV testing policy and campaigns to increase voluntary blood donations have been successfully implemented. The STD control, Condom Promotion activities have been expanded and strengthened.

The lessons learnt during the implementation of NACP-I have been reviewed and applied in preparing NACP-II. In this phase of the programme, the building of ownership and capacity at State and local levels through the de-centralization of planning and implementation of AIDS Control Programme has been a priority. Best practices in interventions targeting the high risk behaviour of populations at highest risk of HIV infection as well as in caring for people living with HIV/AIDS have been scaled up significantly. Technical support and the capacity for research and development have been strengthened through the establishment of technical resource groups. Efforts have been made to mobilize wide spectrum of stakeholders, including the community, private sector and others both within and outside the health sector. A comprehensive monitoring and evaluation system is in place for measuring performance of the programme in quantitative terms.

During the last one and half decade policy decision makers and civil society have realized the threat of an unchecked HIV/AIDS epidemic and its wide spread fall out on socio-economic development. The nature of national response, its urgency, scale and quality has varied critically over time. In the late 1980s and early 1990s, the growing presence of HIV was met largely with denial or indifference from most political quarters. The late 1990s when the new phase of the programme was being prepared saw much openness and realism to emerge in facing the difficult problems posed in developing a strong and broad based national response to the epidemic.

Government of India is currently implementing the second phase of the National AIDS Control Programme (NACP). The main stress of the programme is to adopt a decentralized framework by giving more responsibility to State Governments for the expeditious implementation of the programme in collaboration with other sectors, NGO and civil society. State AIDS Control Societies have been created in all States for this purpose. There is a firm commitment of the Indian Government at the highest political level to do every thing to contain the epidemic. This is sea change from the initial efforts, when the first cases were reported in India during 1986. The national response has gradually evolved and improved over past decade. Strengths and weaknesses were analyzed and the lessons learnt incorporated into the present programme after detailed consultations with all the stakeholders.

1980s The first cases of HIV were reported during 1986. The initial response was aimed at creating mass awareness, carrying out of sero surveillance and ensuring blood safety. As the full impact was not realized the response albeit was a little slow, but once the looming magnitude was appreciated their was an up scaling of the National effort in the control of HIV/AIDS.

1992-1999 The scaled up programme concentrated on the following areas which conform to the global AIDS Prevention and Control strategy:

(a) Programme management
(b) Surveillance and research
(c) Information, education and communication including social mobilization through NGO
(d) Control of STD
(e) Condom programming
(f) Blood safety
(g) Reduction of impact

The Government can look back at the seven years of the first phase of the programme with a measure of satisfaction for its success in important areas like generation of awareness about HIV/AIDS among the urban and rural population of the country. Awareness levels, which were almost insignificant at the beginning of the epidemic, have substantially increased in urban areas even though the level of awareness in rural areas continues to remain low.

Several important actions were taken to ensure blood safety by modernization and strengthening of blood banks, introduction of licensing system of blood banks and phasing out of professional blood donors. Introduction of component separation facilities has also helped in proper clinical use of blood for transfusion. Some very successful intervention programmes among the high risk groups like CSW in the Sonagachi area of Calcutta, men having sex with men in Chennai and IDU in Manipur were carried out through the dedicated involvement of NGO. Emphasis has been laid on control of STD by strengthening STD clinics at the district level by early diagnosis and proper management of STD. Availability of good quality condoms through social marketing has made a significant increase.

1999-2004 The preparation of the new national programme saw a thorough review of the earlier phase I of the programme. It was realized that the programme needed a multi-pronged approach, the targeted interventions needed high coverage and saturation, an enabling environment needed to be created for the marginalized groups, and the blood banking needs improvement for maintaining blood safety. It was further realized that the distribution of the HIV was not uniform, monitoring should be done as a routine function and implementation should be decentralized to States and Municipalities.

As a result all States were mobilized as part of the phase II of the national programme. Thus leading to growing partnerships between government, NGO and the private sector. Participation of NGO in policy making, capacity building was initiated, and guidelines for NGOs developed. Safety of blood and blood products is to be ensured by the National Blood Council and the State Blood Councils. All the Blood banks have to be licensed under the Drugs and Cosmetics Act. Mandatory testing is done for five diseases viz malaria, syphilis, hepatitis B, HIV and hepatitis C. There are still, however formidable challenges ahead, especially in the area of implementation. Discussions between all stakeholders emphasized the value of evolving a collaborative framework in which each agency could participate and yet feel their individual approaches and distinctive contributions find place. Recognizing the importance of encouraging different approaches to meet the diversity of local settings, the framework was deliberately kept broad and flexible as a first step towards harmonizing approaches to the HIV epidemic by external partners. The development of this external partnership framework was based on the global experience that prevention of HIV works, if and only if, (1) effective partnership between government, NGO and civil society are at the heart of the response and continually renewed and refined, and (2) interventions are based on respect for and maintain the dignity of both vulnerable and affected individuals.

The preparation of the new programme has contributed to a growing momentum behind the national response, symbolized by the Prime Minister's strong statement to Parliamentarians in December 1998 calling for renewed efforts to combat HIV, not as a health problem but as a threat to India's development. The country has clearly moved, beyond denial, into a new phase of response.

The Phase II of the National AIDS Control Programme was prepared from the lessons learnt from the first Phase of the programme with five key components: (1) Targeted interventions for communities at highest risk, (2) Prevention of HIV transmission among the general population, (3) Provision of low cost care, (4) Strengthening institutional capacities, and (5) Inter-sectoral collaboration.

This Phase was developed through a participatory process with Government of India, State governments, UNAIDS and bilateral working in partnership with community members, PLWA, industry and labour organizations, NGO and civil society. Each state and Union Territory has registered a State AIDS Control Society [SACS], which will be responsible for implementation of the programme at the state level. The cities of Mumbai, Chennai and Ahmedabad have

formed Municipal AIDS Control societies to effectively implement the AIDS Control programme in these large metropolises. Each SACS developed a Project Implementation Plan (PIP) as part of preparation for Phase II, which allows for addressing the specific needs of the state and the epidemic. Key features of the Phase II are: (1) Special delegation of financial and administrative authority to NACO, (2) A greater ownership of the decentralized programme plans by the states, (3) A major role for NGO in the implementation of intervention programmes with marginalized populations, (4) Involvement of democratic institutions (Panchayati Raj) and youth organizations at the district, block and village level, and (5) Involvement of the community in social mobilization and awareness at grass root levels.

National AIDS Control Programme Phase II: Aims

(a) To shift the focus from raising awareness to changing behaviour through interventions, particularly for groups at high risk of contracting and spreading HIV;

(b) To support decentralization of service delivery to the States and Municipalities and a new facilitating role for National AIDS Control Organization. Program delivery would be flexible, evidence-based, participatory and to rely on local programme implementation plans;

(c) To protect human rights by encouraging voluntary counselling and testing and discouraging mandatory testing;

(d) To support structured and evidence-based annual reviews and ongoing operational research;

(e) To encourage management reforms, such as better-managed State level AIDS Control Societies and improved drug and equipment procurement practices. These reforms are proposed with a view to bring about a sense of 'ownership' of the programme among the States, Municipal Corporations, NGO and other implementing agencies.

Objectives Phase II of National AIDS Control Programme has two key objectives namely:

(a) To reduce the spread of HIV infection in India; and

(b) Strengthen India's capacity to respond to the HIV/AIDS on a long term basis.

Targets   The programme has the following firm targets to be achieved during project period:

(a) To reduce blood-borne transmission of HIV to less than one percent of the total transmissions.

(b) To introduce Hepatitis C as the fifth mandatory test for blood screening.

(c) To attain awareness level of not less than 90% among the youth and those in the reproductive age group.

(d) To train up at least 600 NGO in the country in conducting targeted intervention programmes among high-risk groups and through them promote condom use of not less than 90% among these groups and control of STD.

(e) To conduct annual Family Health Awareness Campaigns among the general population and provide service-delivery in terms of medical advice and provision of drugs for control of STD and Reproductive Tract Infections (RTI). These campaigns are conducted jointly by NACO and RCH programme managers at the State level. Through this it is proposed to reduce the prevalence of STD/RTI in the general community to a significant level.

(f) Promotion of voluntary testing facilities across the country. At the end of the project, it is visualized that every district in the country would have at least one voluntary testing facility.

(g) Awareness campaigns will now be more interactive and use of traditional media such as folk arts and street theatre will be given greater priority in the rural areas. It is proposed to cover all the schools in the country targeting students studying in Class IX and Class XI through school education programmes and all the universities through the "Universities Talk AIDS" programme during the project period.

(h) Promotion of Organizations of people living with HIV/AIDS and giving them financial support to form self-help groups.

Components of Phase II

Priority targeted interventions for populations at high risk. This component of the project aims to reduce the spread of HIV in groups at high risk by identifying target populations and providing peer counselling, condom promotion, treatment of STD etc. This component is delivered largely through NGO, Community based organizations and the Public sector.

Preventive interventions for the general population. The main activities are: (a) IEC and awareness campaigns; (b) provide voluntary testing and counselling; (c) reduction of transmission by blood transfusion; and (d) prevention of occupational exposure.

Low cost care for people living with HIV/AIDS. Under this component financial assistance for home based and community based care, including increasing the availability of cost effective interventions for common opportunistic infections are provided to State Governments and NGO.

Institutional strengthening. This component aims to strengthen effectiveness and technical managerial and financial sustainability at National, State and Municipal levels, strengthening surveillance activities and building strong Research & Development component, including operational research etc.

Inter-sectoral collaboration. This component promotes collaboration amongst the public, private and voluntary sectors. The activities are being co-ordinated with other programmes within the Ministry of Health & Family Welfare and other central ministries and departments. Collaboration focuses on; (I) learning from the innovative HIV/AIDS programmes that exist in other sectors; and (II) sharing in the working, generating awareness, advocacy and delivering interventions.

Achievements

(a) Political commitment has been achieved at the highest level, which is evident by Indian Prime Minister's address to countrymen on the eve of Independence day 2000, emphasising the need for effective control of HIV/AIDS spread in India. This has triggered political commitment and advocacy in the States.

(b) Intensive awareness campaigns through electronic and print media and the field publicity units of the Ministry of Information & Broadcasting in both the urban and rural areas resulted in generation of awareness about the disease both in the high risk groups and the general population. Awareness levels are of the order of

60-65 per cent on an average in urban areas and 35-40 per cent in rural areas. The highest awareness levels are in Tamil Nadu where it is 95% in urban areas and 75% in rural areas.

(c) Awareness programs through school and college education have been taken up on a large scale by State Governments by involving NGO and Department of Education.

(d) To ensure safe blood to the population, blood banks in the Government and voluntary sector modernized in phases and blood component separation facilities have been established in major blood banks throughout the country. Mandatory testing of blood units collected in blood banks for HIV, Syphilis, Malaria and Hepatitis B and C, has been introduced throughout the country. Infection through blood transfusion has been brought down appreciably over the last 2-3 years. There is a complete phasing out of professional blood donation in the country.

(e) For control of STD, which have a direct correlation with HIV/AIDS, STD clinics in district hospitals have been established. Medical and paramedical workers have been trained in Syndromic management of HIV/AIDS.

(f) Voluntary Counselling and Testing Centers [VCTC] facilities have been established in all medical colleges and major hospitals, and the process of providing such facilities in all district hospitals is in progress.

(g) For tracking the epidemic in the country, 384 sentinel sites have been established. These sites include both high-risk groups like Sex Workers, IDU as well as low risk group i.e., pregnant women attending antenatal clinic. One round of sentinel surveillance is carried out each year during the period of August – October.

(h) Over 550 targeted intervention projects have been implemented all over the country for groups practicing risky behaviour. These interventions include outreach activities, IEC and interpersonal communication, condom promotion, and general health and STD service provision. Targeted intervention projects such as that for CWS in Calcutta's Sonagachi area, the MSM project in Chennai, truck drivers in Rajasthan and IDU in Assam, Manipur and Nagaland have increased the use of condoms and reduced STD, yielding lessons in best practice.

(i) Role of NGO: NGO have played a major role in initiating and ensuring effective interventions, defending the human rights of people living with HIV/AIDS and in providing care and support to people living with HIV/AIDS.

(j) Inter-sectoral Collaboration: NACO has promoted inter-sectoral collaboration with other Ministries/Departments such as Human Resource Development, Information and Broadcasting, Railways, Defence, Labour, Steel, Social Justice and Empowerment etc. for the implementation of HIV/AIDS prevention and control programme.

(k) Private Sector Collaborations: Effective collaborations have also been built with the private sector through the Confederation of Indian Industries (CII), the Indian chamber of Commerce and Industries and the Bengal Chamber of Commerce. The Tata Iron and Steel Company has incorporated HIV/AIDS prevention in their ongoing family welfare programme and control activities.

Conclusions

In India, the first case of AIDS was reported in 1986. Currently about 4 million people are estimated living with HIV/AIDS, more than any country in the world except South Africa. With a huge population even low HIV prevalence rate translate into huge number of people living with HIV. India's epidemic is highly diverse but surveillance data indicate that HIV infection is prevalent in all parts of country spreading from urban to rural and from individual with high risk behaviour to general population. The multifaceted national response to contain the epidemic since 1986 has yielded some results in slowing of spread of HIV infection as evident from sentinel surveillance data in year 1998, 1999 and 2000. The estimated number of people living with HIV was 3.5 million in 1998, 3.71 million in 1999, 3.86 million in 2000 and 3.97 million in 2001. The most populous States of India are least affected, e.g. Uttar Pradesh, Bihar, Madhya Pradesh, Rajasthan etc; the present situation offers a window of opportunity to diminish the spread of HIV into these populous States. But the opportunity is closing fast. India's strategy at present should be to prevent small epidemics whenever they occur from becoming larger. Other challenges for the country to tackle the epidemic effectively are to confront discrimination and stigma associated with HIV/AIDS patients and addressing the urgency of care and support to such patients.

References

1. HIV/AIDS in Asia and Pacific Region, World Health Organization, 2001.

2. Barre Sinoussi F, Chermann JC, Rey F, et al. Isolation of a T-lymphotropic retro virus from a patient at risk for acquired immune deficiency syndrome (AIDS). Science 1983; 220: 868-871.

3. Zagury D, Bernard J, Leibowitch J, et al. HTLV III in cells cultured from semen of two patients with AIDS. Science 1984; 226: 449-451.

4. Levy JA, Shimabukuro J, Hollander H, Mills J, Kaminsky L. Isolation of AIDS associated retroviruses from cerebrospinal fluid and brain of patients with neurological symptoms. Lancet 1985; 2: 586-588.

5. Clavel F, Guetard D, Brun-Vezilnet F, et al. Isolation of human retrovirus from west African patients with AIDS. Science 1986; 233: 343-346.

6. Fischi MA, Richman DD, Gricco MH, et al. The efficacy of 3'-azido-3' deoxythymidine (azidothymidine) in the treatment of patients with AIDS and AIDS related complex: a double blind, placebo controlled trial. N Eng J Med 1987; 317: 185-191.

7. Report on the global HIV/AIDS epidemic UNAIDS: 2001 and 2002.

8. Effective Prevention strategies in low HIV prevalence settings: UNAIDS Best Practices key Material: 2001.

9. HIV/AIDS Round Table Conference Series Number-6, April 2000. Ranbaxy Science, Foundation, New Delhi, India.

10. Lole KS, Bollinger RC, Paranjape RS, et al. Full length human immunodeficiency virus type-1 genome from subtype C-infected seroconvertes in India; with evidence of intersub type recombination. J Virol 1999; 73: 152-160.

11. Haverkos HW, Battjes RJ. "Female to male transmission of HIV. JAMA 1992; 268: 1855-1856.

12. Panda S, Chatterjee A, Bhattacharjee S, et al. HIV, hepatitis B and sexual practices in the street-recruited injecting drug users of Calcutta: risks perception versus observed risk. Int J STD AIDS 1998; 9: 214-218.

13. Jana S. Intervention through peer-based approach–A lesson from Sonagachi, AIDS Res Rev 1999; 2: 58-63.

14. Jacob M, John TJ, George S, Rao PS, Babu PG. Increasing prevalence of human immunodeficiency virus infection among patients attending a clinic for sexually transmitted diseases. Indian J Med Res 1995; 101: 6-9.

15. Mehendale SM. HIV infection amongst persons with high risk behaviour in Pune city: Update on findings from a prospective cohort study. AIDS Res Rev 1998; 1: 2-9.

16. Gangakhedkar RR, Bentley ME, Divekar AD, et al. Spread of HIV infection in married monogamous women in India. JAMA 1997; 278: 2090-2092.

17. Mistry S, Misra K, Rao A, Dey A, Verma K, Islam A. An HIV point prevalence study among truck driver at Uluberia, West Bengal. Abstract no. Pub.C. 1111 published in XI International Conference on AIDS, Vancouver, July 7-12, 1996.

18. Bhushan N, Pulimood BR, Babu PG, John TJ. Rising trend in the prevalence of HIV infection among blood donors. Indian J Med Res 1994; 99: 195-197.

19. Banerjee K, Rodrigues J, Israel Z, Kulkarni S, Thakar M. Outbreak of HIV seropositivity among commercial plasma donors in Pune, India. Lancet 1989; 2: 166.

20. Sen S, Mishra NM, Giri T, et al. Acquired immunodeficiency syndrome (AIDS) in multi-transfused children with thalassemia. Indian Pediatr 1993; 30: 455-460.

21. Joshi PL, Prasada Rao. Changing epidemiology of HIV/AIDS in India. AIDS Res Rev 1999; 2: 7-9.

22. Working Group on Mother-to-Child Transmission of HIV. Rates of mother-to-child transmission of HIV 1 in Africa, America and Europe; results from 13 perinatal studies. J Acquir Immune Defic Syndr Retroviral 1995; 8: 506-510.

23. Kumar RM, Uduman SA, Khurranna AK. A prospective study of mother-to-infant HIV transmission in tribal women from India. J Acquir Immune Defic Syndr Hum Retroviral 1995; 19: 238-242.

24. Dunn DT, Newell ML, Ades AE, Peckham C. Risk of human immunodeficiency virus type 1 transmission through breastfeeding. Lancet 1992; 340: 585-588.

25. Miotti PG, Taha ET, Kumwenda NI, et al. HIV transmission through breastfeeding A study in Malawi. JAMA 1999; 282: 744-749.

26. Coutsoudis A, Pillay K, Spooner E, Kuhn L, Coorodia HM. Influence of infant-feeding patterns on early mother-to-child transmission of HIV 1 in Durban, South Africa: a prospective cohort study. Lancet 1999; 354: 471-476.

27. Combating HIV/AIDS in India 1998-1999, 1999-2000 and 2000-01; Ministry of Health & Family Welfare (National AIDS Control Organization), Govt. of India, New Delhi.

Chapter 4

Clinical Presentation of HIV Infection

J K Maniar

Introduction

The clinical presentation of HIV infection in India[1-4] is grossly similar to that of global scenario except for minor variations. HIV 1 is seen worldwide and is responsible for most of the disease globally. HIV 2 was mostly confined to West Africa, but now it is being detected in Asia and India. HIV 1 is categorized into two groups: M and O. The M group is further subdivided into A-J. In India HIV 1 subtypes A, B, C and E have been identified along with HIV 2. There is no consolidated indigenous data on the study of natural history of HIV 1, HIV 2 or dual infection from India.[5] It is important to recognize HIV/AIDS medicine, as a distinct speciality by itself. In this era of matured HIV epidemic in India, vigilant clinical acumen is required to recognize symptoms and signs of HIV/AIDS related diseases in clinical practice. The differential diagnosis of HIV/AIDS as a possible etiological factor should be given consideration while managing common clinical problems like pyrexia of unknown origin (PUO), chronic cough, chronic diarrhoea, weight loss, lymphadenopathy, anaemia and idiopathic thrombocytopenic purpura (ITP). The clinical spectrum of both HIV 1 and HIV 2 diseases are almost similar except that HIV 2 infection has milder and slower progression of the disease with longer incubation period and is poorly transmitted vertically.[6] The spectrum of opportunistic events is similar for both. The infectivity of HIV 2 is much lower than that of HIV 1. The laboratory diagnosis needs careful evaluation using appropriate Western Blot kit specific for HIV 2 detection. Currently HIV 2 viral load measurement kits are not available in India. Even in moderately immunosuppressed HIV 2 infected individuals with absolute CD4 count around 200 cells/

mm^3, the HIV 2 viral load is likely to be undetectable or even in advanced stage of HIV 2 infection the viral load is not so high. The effectiveness of currently available non-nucleoside analogues against HIV 2 infection is unknown.

Natural History of HIV Infection[7]

In short within 2-3 weeks of viral transmission, acute retroviral syndrome develops that lasts for about 2-3 weeks. It is followed by chronic HIV infection and after an average period of 8 years, patient develops asymptomatic infection/AIDS defining complex and in India after a mean period of 1.3 years, death may occur. The course of the disease from the time of initial infection to the development of full blown AIDS is divided into the following stages (Fig. 1):

1. Primary HIV infection
2. Asymptomatic chronic infection with or without PGL
3. Symptomatic HIV infection previously known as AIDS related complex
4. AIDS (AIDS indicator conditions according to 1993 CDC criteria)
5. Advanced HIV disease characterized by CD4 cell count of $50/mm^3$

Acute Retroviral Syndrome/Primary HIV Infection [8-10]

Acute retroviral syndrome is the symptom complex that follows and is experienced by 80-90% of HIV infected patients. Most symptomatic patients seek medical

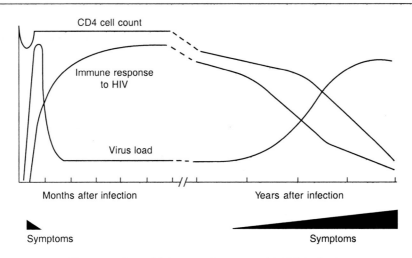

Fig. 1   Natural history of untreated HIV infection.

consultation, but this diagnosis is infrequently recognized.[13] The time from the initial exposure to onset of symptoms is usually 2-4 weeks, but the incubation may be as long as ten months in rare cases. The clinical symptoms include fever, lymphadenopathy, pharyngitis, erythematous maculopapular rash, arthralgia, myalgia, diarrhoea, nausea, vomiting, headache, mucocutaneous ulceration involving mouth, oesophagus or genitals, hepatosplenomegaly, and thrush. The neurological features include meningoencephalitis, peripheral neuropathy, facial palsy, Guillain Barre syndrome, brachial neuritis, radiculopathy, cognitive impairment and psychosis. The laboratory findings include lymphopenia followed by lymphocytosis with depletion of CD4 cells, CD8 lymphocytosis, and often, atypical lymphocytes. The transaminase levels may be elevated. The diagnosis is established by demonstrating quantitative plasma HIV RNA or qualitative HIV DNA and negative or indeterminate HIV serology. The complete clinical recovery with a reduction in plasma levels of HIV RNA follows. The cytotoxic T lymphocyte (CTL) response occurs first and precedes detectable humoral responses. The preliminary studies indicate that aggressive antiretroviral therapy protects activated HIV specific CD4 cells from HIV infection to preserve a response analogous to the response seen in non-progressors. This observation emphasizes the importance of early recognition and aggressive antiretroviral therapy. The seroconversion with positive HIV serology generally takes place at an average of three weeks after transmission with the standard third generation Enzyme Immunoassay (EIA). By using standard serological tests it now appears that more than 95% of patients seroconvert within 5.8 months following transmission.

Asymptomatic Infection With or Without Persistent Generalized Lymphadenopathy[8,11]

During this period the patient is clinically asymptomatic and generally has no findings on physical examination except in some cases for persistent generalized lymphadenopathy (PGL). PGL is defined as enlarged lymph nodes involving at least two noncontiguous sites other than inguinal nodes. Quite often patients living with HIV/AIDS present in asymptomatic phase following screening test either for pre-blood or organ donation, pre-emigration medical check up, or testing done at voluntary testing and counselling centre (VTCT). Post-test counselling needs to be offered as a priority to such individuals. Detailed history taking followed by thorough clinical examination is necessary. Incidental findings could be scars from previous genital ulcer disease or herpes zoster, lymphadenopathy, oral hairy leukoplakia (OHL) and even asymptomatic dermatological manifestations. HIV screening of conjugal partner or relevant children after informed consent is essential. The baseline investigations to be undertaken viz. complete haemogram (including platelets count), ESR, serological tests for syphilis (STS), hepatitis B and C serology, liver function test, urine examination, chest x-ray, sonography of abdomen/pelvis and Mantoux test. The evaluation of CD4/CD8 lymphocytes as well as estimation of HIV 1 viral load is optional in Indian setup in the absence of plan to initiate antiretroviral therapy. It may only help to decide regarding initiation of chemoprophylaxis against opportunistic infections.

It is important to offer counselling emphasizing on maintaining food and water hygiene, life style modification such as practicing safer sex and refraining from organ donation (viz. blood, semen, kidney etc.). The periodical follow up (every three to six months) consisting of history taking, clinical examination, baseline investigations and counselling.

Symptomatic HIV Infection[8,11] (CD 4 count 200-499 cells/mm³, Category B symptoms, CDC Clinical classification, Table 2)

During the symptomatic HIV infection, the skin and mucous membranes are predominantly involved. Widespread seborrhoeic dermatitis is the most common presentation. Other features include multidermatomal herpes zoster, molluscum contagiosum, OHL, pruritic dermatitis, folliculitis, dermatophytic infection, recurrent vulvovaginal candidiasis and oral candidiasis. Upper and lower respiratory tract infections caused by *Streptococcus pneumoniae*, *Haemophilus influenzae* and *Mycoplasma pneumonia* may also occur. Other features during this stage include Kaposi's sarcoma, pulmonary tuberculosis, cervical dysplasia and Idiopathic thrombocytopenic purpura (ITP).

AIDS[8,11] (CD 4 count 50-200 cells/mm³, Category C symptoms, CDC Clinical classification, Table 2)

This stage is characterized by opportunistic infection and malignancy. They are described in detail in later part of the chapter. Other features are persistent and progressive constitutional symptoms, wasting disease and neurological disease.

Advanced HIV Disease[8,11] (CD 4 count < 50 cells/mm³)

As in the previous stage it is also characterized by AIDS defining opportunistic infections and malignancy. Some of the infections are more frequently seen like *M.avium complex*, CMV, cryptococcal meningitis, histoplasmosis, slow virus disease and cervical dysplasia. CNS involvement also is very prominent: AIDS dementia complex, CNS lymphoma and CMV infection. AIDS wasting syndrome with a weight loss of >10% of ideal body weight is common.

Diagnosis of AIDS

Clinical: For the purposes of AIDS surveillance an adult or adolescent (>12 years of age) is considered to have AIDS if at least 2 of the following major signs are present in combination with at least 1 of the minor signs listed in Table 1, and if these signs are not known to be due to a condition unrelated to HIV infection.

Table 1. WHO Case Definition for AIDS Surveillance[13]

Major signs
- Weight loss $\geq$ 10% of body weight
- Chronic diarrhoea for more than 1 month
- Prolonged fever for more than 1 month (intermittent or constant).

Minor signs
- Persistent cough for more than 1 month
- Generalized pruritic dermatitis
- History of herpes zoster
- Oropharyngeal candidiasis
- Chronic progressive or disseminated herpes simplex infection
- Generalized lymphadenopathy
  The presence of either generalized Kaposi's sarcoma or cryptococcal meningitis is suffcient for the diagnosis of AIDS for surveillance purposes.

Expanded WHO case definition for AIDS surveillance
  For the purposes of AIDS surveillance an adults or adolescent (>12 years of age) is considered to have AIDS if a test for HIV antibody gives a positive result and one or more of the following conditions are present.
- > 19% body weight loss or cachexia, with diarrhoea or fever, or both, intermittent or constant for at least 1 month, not known to be due to a condition unrelated to HIV infection.
- Cryptococcal meningitis
- Pulmonary or extra-pulmonary tuberculosis
- Kaposis sarcoma
- Neurological impairment that is sufficient to prevent independent daily activities, not known to be due to a condition unrelated to HIV infection (for example, trauma or cerebrovascular accident)
- Candidiasis of the oesophagus (which may be presumptively diagnosed based on the presence of oral candidiasis accompanied by dysphagia).
- Clinically diagnosed life threatening or recurrent episodes of pneumonia, with or without aetiological confirmation.
- Invasive cervical cancer.

The CDC has proposed the following clinical classification for HIV infection in adults and adolescents. It is based on three ranges of CD4 cell counts and three clinical categories (Table 2).[14]

Dermatological Manifestations of HIV Infection.[8,15–17]

There are wide range of dermatological manifestations

Table 2. 1993 Revised Classification for HIV Infection and Expanded Case Definition for AIDS in Adolescents and Adults

CD4 cell count	A	B	C
>500/mm^3 (>29%)	A1	B1	C1
200 to 499/mm^3 (14% to 28%)	A2	B2	C2
<200/mm^3 (<14%)	A3	B3	C3

CATEGORY A
  Asymptomatic HIV infection
  Persistent generalized lymphadenopathy
  Acute retroviral syndrome

CATEGORY B
  Bacillary angiomatosis
  Oral or recurrent vulvovaginal candidiasis
  Cervical dysplasia
  Constitutional symptoms (fever of 38.5°C, diarrhoea >1 month)
  Oral hairy leukoplakia
  Herpes zoster
  Idiopathic thrombocytopenic purpura
  Listeriosis
  Pelvic inflammatory disease
  Peripheral neuropathy

CATEGORY C (AIDS-Defining Conditions)
  CD4 count <200 cells/mm^3
  Candidiasis of oesophagus, pulmonary
  Cervical cancer[a]
  Coccidioidomycosis
  Cryptococcosis, extrapulmonary
  Cryptosporidosis
  Cytomegalovirus infection
  Herpes simplex with esophageal, pulmonary, or mucocutaneous involvement of >1 month
  Histoplasmosis
  HIV encephalopathy
  Isosporiasis
  Kaposi's sarcoma
  Lymphoma
  Mycobacterium avium complex or *M. kansasii*
  Mycobacterium tuberculosis[a]
  Pneumocystis carinii pneumonia
  Pneumonia, recurrent with more than two episodes in 12 months[a]
  Progressive multifocal encephalopathy
  Salmonellosis
  Toxoplasmosis

[a]Added in the 1993 Centres for Disease Control revised case definition.

which prompts the clinician to screen attending individual patient for HIV. Each of these dermatological markers has different positive predictive value for HIV / AIDS. Those with high positive predictive value are: herpes zoster, herpes simplex infection, seborrhoeic dermatitis, Reiter's syndrome, pruritic papular eruptions, extragenital molluscum contagiosum, Kaposi's sarcoma, Norwegian scabies, ITP, cutaneous histoplasmosis, cutaneous cryptococcosis, cutaneous penicilliosis, pyomyositis, candidiasis (oral, genital or oesophageal), OHL, Stevens Johnson syndrome, eosinophilic follicultis and bacillary angiomatosis (**P I-V, Fig. 1-21**). The remaining dermatological manifestations include; psoriasis, vasculitic leg ulcer, addisonian pigmentation,

tinea incognito including onychomycosis, demodicidosis, melasma, photosensitivity (including porphyria cutanea tarda) hair changes, nail changes, acquired ichthyosis, recalcitrant eczema, erythroderma, orificial cancer, pyoderma, tuberculides and acne conglobata (Table 3). Almost all dermatological manifestations of HIV/AIDS respond to currently recommended highly active antiretroviral therapy (HAART).

STD and HIV/AIDS

It is a well known fact that the presence of sexually transmitted diseases (STD) viz. genital ulcer disease,

Table 3. Dermatological Manifestations of HIV/AIDS

Cutaneous manifestations	Clinical features
Herpes zoster	Ophthalmic division commonly involved, eye complication common, multisegmental or bilateral, necrotic, haemorrhagic, some time generalized, recurrent,
Herpes simplex infection	It is a reactivation of HSV, often aggressive and extensive, recurrent, response to acyclovir is variable
Seborrhoeic dermatitis	Quite often presenting feature of HIV, chronic disease
Reiter' syndrome	Almost AIDS defining illness, persistent, of varied severity, oral retinoid safer and effective drug.
Pruritic papular eruptions	Chronic, recurrent or persistent, intense itching, difficult to treat
Molluscum contagiosum	Severity varies, more often extragenital location, cosmetically disturbing,
Norwegian scabies	Unusual location of skin eruptions on face or scalp besides other usual parts of the body, itching almost absent, recurrent
Cutaneous cryptococcosis	Mimics molluscum contagiosum, invariably systemic involvement, histopathology study of skin biopsy is diagnostic.
Pyomyositis	AIDS defining illness, localized or extensive, besides appropriate antibiotics, surgical intervention may be required.
Candidiasis	Recurrent, quite often oesophageal without oral involvement, varied morphological appearance (erosive, membranous, vegetative)
Oral hairy leukoplakia	Almost specific to clinical presentation of HIV infection, sometimes difficult to distinguish from oral candidiasis, Epstein Barr virus (EBV) infection, asymptomatic
Stevens Johnson syndrome	More often drug induced viz. sulphonamides (cotrimoxazole), nevirapine, abacavir, dilantin, pyrazinamide, rifampicin and carbamazepine. Complication of septicemia not uncommon, death can result if not appropriately managed
Psoriasis	Wide spread lesions, wet or pustular psoriasis
Addisonian pigmentation	Occurs without adrenal dysfunction, progressive disease, cosmetically stigmatizing, reversible pigmentation with HAART,
Erythroderma	Could be presenting feature, mostly it is primary HIV related erythroderma, disturbing condition for patient and others, responds to HAART
Tuberculides	Papulonecrotic or lichen scrofulosorum lesions common, most often associated with detectable tuberculous focus
Idiopathic thrombocytopenic purpura	Chronic, varied severity, difficult to correct
Acquired ichthyosis	Quite often marked and extensive, irritation common, reversible disease on HAART
Acne conglobata	Quite often severe, extensive, only high index of suspicion could prompt clinician to carry out HIV screening, responds to oral retinoids or HAART
Hair changes	Lusterless hair, thin hair, various types of alopecia, discoloration of hair, premature graying, long eye lashes
Nail changes	Leuconychia, pigmentation, half and half nail, clubbing, onychomycosis, paronychia, yellow nail syndrome

urethritis, vaginitis or cervicitis favour transmission of HIV during unprotected sexual intercourse. Therefore syndromic management or management after etiological diagnosis of various STD should help to control HIV transmission. In people infected with HIV / AIDS the serological tests for syphilis (STS) may either be reactive in higher dilutions or may be false negative or false positive. In such circumstances specific tests for syphilis may help to confirm the diagnosis in addition to clinical suspicion. There could be rapid progression in natural history of syphilis, thereby precocious occurrence of tertiary syphilis viz. neurosyphilis or cardiovascular syphilis. Depending upon the severity of immunosuppression, the clinical features of various STD show varying degrees of aggressiveness. The recommended therapy for respective STD may need modification depending upon individual case study. The reactivation of genital / perianal herpes simplex virus infection is fairly common and its presence helps in algorithmic clinical diagnosis of HIV / AIDS. The dosage and duration of oral acyclovir therapy vary with the severity of clinical presentation. The occurrence of more than one STD at a given time carry higher positive predictive value for HIV / AIDS. The incidence of malignant transformation of STD especially human papilloma virus infection viz. cervical intraepithelial neoplasia (CIN), cancer of penis or vulva or perianal area are higher in HIV seropositive individuals. The interaction of STD and HIV/AIDS is discussed in detail in a separate chapter.

Systemic Involvement in HIV Infection

Diseases of the Respiratory System[8] (P VI, Fig. 22-24)

Acute bronchitis and maxillary sinusitis are quite common. The most common manifestation of pulmonary disease is pneumonia. Both bacterial (pyogenic) and *P.carinii* pneumonia occur in AIDS. *P. carinii* is the most common life threatening opportunistic infection in most of the developed countries. The usual presentation is subacute with malaise, fatigue, weight loss, characteristic retrosternal chest pain which is typically worse on inspiration and non-productive cough. The chest radiograph may be normal or may show the classical finding of dense perihilar infiltrate (but which is rarely seen). The arterial oxygen tension is usually depressed. The diagnosis is usually confirmed by direct demonstration of the trophozoite or the cyst form in the sputum induced with saline or in bronchial lavage obtained by fibreoptic bronchoscopy.

Other causes of pulmonary infiltrates include mycobacterial infections, fungal infections, non-specific interstitial pneumonitis, Kaposi sarcoma and lymphoma.

Approximately one-third of all AIDS related deaths are due to tuberculosis. The clinical patterns of pulmonary tuberculosis in AIDS patients can vary depending upon the CD4 count. During the early phase of the disease with the CD4 count above 200 cell/mm^3, the disease has the classic upper lobe cavity changes whereas in the late stages, it characteristically affect the middle and lower lobe and cavitary changes are less frequently observed.

Atypical mycobacterial infections are also seen in AIDS patients especially with *M.avium*, *M.intracellulare* or *M.avium* complex (MAC). MAC infection is usually a late occurrence when the CD4 + T cell counts is < 50 cell/mm^3. The most common presentation is disseminated disease with fever, weight loss and night sweats. Other findings are abdominal pain, diarrhoea and lymphadenopathy. Chest x-ray will show bilateral lower lobe infiltrate suggestive of miliary spread and some times alveolar or nodular and hilar or mediastinal adenopathy may occur.

Disease of the Oropharynx and Gastrointestinal System[8] (P VI, Fig. 25, 26)

Most of the oropharyngeal and gastrointestinal diseases are due to secondary infection. The oral lesions are thrush, OHL and aphthous ulcers. Thrush is caused by *Candida albicans* and rarely by *C. krusei*. It appears as a white, cheesy exudate often on an erythematous mucosa in the posterior oropharynx. The soft palate is the commonest site but early lesions are seen along the gingival border. OHL caused by Epstein Barr virus (EBV), presents as white frond like lesions usually along the lateral borders of the tongue but sometimes in the buccal mucosa. Thrush and OHL usually occur in patients with CD4+ T cell counts of <300/cm^3.

Oesophagitis can be caused by candida, cytomegalovirus (CMV) or herpes simplex virus (HSV). CMV infection is associated with single large ulcer whereas herpetic infection presents with multiple small ulcers.

Infections of the small and large intestine with various bacteria, protozoa and viruses can cause diarrhoea and abdominal pain. Cryptosporidia, microsporidia and

Isospora belli are the most common opportunistic protozoa that infect the GIT and cause non-inflammatory diarrhoea. *Giardia intestinalis* and *E.histolytica* infections are common in homosexual men, among the bacterial, salmonella, shigella and campylobacter especially in homosexuals. CMV colitis presents as nonbloody diarrhoea, abdominal pain, weight loss, and anorexia. Endoscopic examination reveals multiple mucosal ulceration and the biopsy shows characteristic intranuclear inclusion bodies. In advanced disease MAC infection and various fungi like histoplasmosis, coccidioidomycosis etc may also cause diarrhoea. Besides these secondary infections HIV infection per se can cause AIDS enteropathy.

HIV and Nervous System[8]

Infections

Cerebral toxoplasmosis is the most frequent opportunistic infection of the central nervous system and it usually results from reactivation of toxoplasma cyst in the brain causing abscess formation. The abscess can be unifocal or multifocal and clinically it presents with features of a space occupying lesion. CT scan will show ring-enhancing abscess with surrounding oedema (**P VI, Fig. 27**).

Cryptococcal meningitis accounts for 5-10% of opportunistic infections in patients with HIV infection. The clinical presentation is subacute with headache, fever and cranial nerve palsies. Neck stiffness is relatively rare. CSF analysis will demonstrate the yeast in 70% of the cases and antigen detection is positive in 100% of the patients.

Progressive multifocal leucoencephalopathy is a demyelinating disease (slow virus disease)caused by JC virus. Clinically there may be focal deficits, ataxia and personality changes.

HIV Encephalopathy

Patients with this disorder have a form of dementia known as AIDS related cognitive motor complex. In the early stage there will be impairment of memory and concentration. Later motor signs appear such as hyper-reflexia, extensor plantar responses, in-coordination and ataxia.

Other neurological features in HIV infection are progressive vacuolar myelopathy (with spastic paraplegia, ataxia, loss of sphincter control), transverse myelitis (due to VZV, HSV and CMV infections), peripheral neuropathy and psychiatric manifestations (acute psychosis, depression).

Disease of the Liver, Gall Bladder and Pancreas[8] (P VII, Fig. 28).

The HIV / AIDS and hepatitis co-infection is the current topic of interest globally. There is paucity of epidemiological data on HBV or HCV infection in India viz. incidence, genotyping study and on natural history of infection, incidence of HIV and HBV / HCV co-infection.[32] It is believed that the effective mode of transmission for HBV or HCV in descending order would be transfusion > intravenous drug user > sexual > needle stick injury > unknown. There are ongoing studies to evaluate the effect of HIV infection on natural history of HBV or HCV infection, the effect of HBV or HCV infection on natural history of HIV infection, and the adverse effects of antiretroviral drugs or anti-tuberculous drugs on HIV and hepatitis co-infected individuals. The end stage liver disease is the commonest cause of mortality amongst such individuals especially if they are not treated with highly active antiretroviral treatment (HAART). As soon as HIV infection is brought under control, HCV or HBV infection should be appropriately treated for better quality of life.

Sclerosing cholangitis and papillary stenosis are reported in cryptosporidiosis, CMV infection and Kaposi's sarcoma. Pancreatitis usually occurs secondary to drug toxicity.

Diseases of the Kidney[8]

The kidneys can be involved in HIV infection and the most common presentation is with nephrotic syndrome and renal failure. Focal segmental glomerulosclerosis and mesangial proliferative glomerulonephritis account for most of the cases of HIV associated nephropathy. Renal disease can also occur as a side effect of therapy in HIV disease.

HIV and Tumours[8]

Kaposi's Sarcoma

Kaposi's sarcoma (KS) is usually seen in gay & bisexual men and also in women in Africa. It is extremely rare in intravenous drug users, blood transfusion recipients and haemophiliacs. This suggests that a transmissible agent is responsible for the development of KS and is found to be HHV 8. Clinically it is characterized by violaceous papules and nodules and it may be multifocal. Lesions may also occur in the mucous membranes especially in the hard palate and in the viscera mostly the lungs and gastrointestinal tract.

Non-Hodgkins Lymphoma

The CNS is the most common site. Most of the tumours are extralymphatic and histologically they are high grade

large cell immunoblastic or non-cleaved small cell tumours and they may be related to EBV. Clinically it presents with signs and symptoms of a space occupying lesion.

Other tumours which can occur in AIDS are Hodgkins lymphoma, squamous cell carcinoma of the anus especially in homosexual men and cervical cancer.

Opportunistic Infections in AIDS[8]

Most of the opportunistic infections in AIDS occur when the CD4 count falls below 200 cell/mm[3.] The various infections and their relation to the CD4 count are depicted in Figure 2.

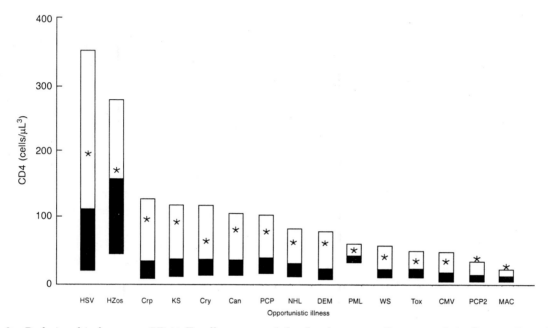

Fig. 2   Relationship between CD4+ T cell counts and the development of opportunistic diseases. Boxplot of the median (line inside the box), first quartile (bottom of the box), third quartile (top of the box), and mean (asterisk) CD4+ lymphocyte count at the time of the development of opportunistic disease. Can, candidal esophagitis; CMV, cytomegalovirus infection; Crp, cryptosporidiosis; Cyr, cryptococcal meningitis, DME, AIDS dementia complex; HSV, herpes simplex virus infection; HZos, herpes zoster; KS, Kaposi's sarcoma; MAC, *mycobacterium avium* complex bacteremia; NHL, Non-Hodgkin's lymphoma; PCP, primary *pneumocystis carinii* pneumonia; PCP2, secondary *Pneumocystis carinii* pneumonia; PML, progressive multifocal leukoencephalopathy; Tox, *Toxoplasma gondii* encephalitis; WS, Wasting syndrome.

(Adopted from Moore and Chaisson)

Immune Reconstitution Syndrome (IRS)[8]

This is also called as immune restoration syndrome or reversal phenomenon. It occurs following HAART. The incubation period for the development of such illness varies. This could involve any system of the

body. This illness is difficult to recognize. The various clinical manifestations are herpes zoster, reactivation of leprosy, tuberculosis (lymphadenopathy, pneumonia patch, tuberculoma of brain or liver), *P. carinii* pneumonia, hepatitis reactivation, CMV retinitis, fever, cyptococcosis. The management of immune reconstitution syndrome related illness is challenging.

Clinical Manifestation of HIV Disease in India[18]

HIV infected individual in India are exposed to various environmental factors like malnutrition & poverty and also to a host of tropical infections which are peculiar to this region. Striking similarities and certain differences exist between clinical presentation of AIDS in Indian population and the other countries. Slim disease or the wasting syndrome is the most common mode of presentation in Africa. Similar presentation was seen in 62% patients in a series from South India. *P. carinii* pneumonia is the most common opportunistic infection in most of the developed countries. By contrast PCP is unusual in Indian population and the most common opportunistic infection is tuberculosis. The rarity of PCP among the Indian patients may be due to the fact they have many other tropical infection diseases prior to reaching the severe immunosuppressed state and consequent relatively early mortality due to these infection.

Among the tuberculosis group *Mycobacterium avium intracellulare* is the most common of the mycobacterium isolated from patients in US, whereas *M. tuberculosis* is more frequently isolated in patients from India.

Candidiasis (oropharyngeal and oesophageal) is the second commonest opportunistic infection in India. Toxoplasmosis, histoplasmosis, Kaposi's sarcoma and CNS lymphomas are uncommon in Indian population compared to Western countries.

The Dermatological manifestations of HIV infection from two major centres in India are given in Table 4 & 5.

Table 4. Prevalence of Dermatological Manifestations in HIV patients

Dermatological manifestations	Prevalence
Intractable itching	46.7%
Oral candidiasis	45.0%
Multidermatomal herpes zoster	11.2%
Dermatophytosis of the skin	8.0%
Herpes genitalis	7.7%
Papular pruritic dermatitis	7.7%
Staphylococcal infection of the skin	2.9%
Alopecia	4.2%
Oral hairy leukoplakia	2.3%
Molluscum contagiosum	1.3%
Genital warts	1.2%
Scabies	0.5%

Adapted from Kumarasamy et al[16], Chennai, Tamil Nadu, India

Table 5. Mucocutaneous Markers of HIV Infection (n = 20,520)

Manifestation	Percent
Candidiasis	92%
Addisonian pigmentation	72%
Herpes simplex infection	68%
Hair changes	68%
Oral hairy leukoplakia	68%
Ichthyosis	65%
Herpes zoster	52%
Pruritic papular dermatosis	48%
Molluscum contagiosum	42%
Nail changes	28%
Seborrhoeic dermatitis	25%
Tinea incognito	21.5%
Scabies	14.5%
Pyoderma	14.5%
Endogenous eczema	7%
Drug reaction	4.5%
Cutaneous tuberculosis	5.5%
Photosensitivity	4.5%
Oral aphthosis	3.5%
Psoriasis	2.5%
Reiter's syndrome	1.5%
Cryptococcosis	1.5%
Leg ulcer	1.0%
Demodicidosis	1.0%
Skin infarcts	0.5%
Erythroderma	0.5%
Eosinophilic folliculitis	0.5%
Reactivation of leprosy	0.5%
Kaposi's sarcoma	0.25
Histoplasmosis	0.12%

Adapted from Maniar et al,[19] Mumbai, India

The clinical comparison of HIV patients from Latin America, Africa, Asia and India are depicted in Table 6.[20]

References

1. Dietrich U, Maniar JK, Rubsamen- Walgmann H. The epidemiology of AIDS in India. Trend Microbiol 1995; 3: 17-21.

2. Maniar JK, Saple DG. The HIV/AIDS epidemic in India. HIV & AIDS current trends 1998; 4: 3-6.

3. Maniar JK; Health Care Systems in Transition III: The Indian Subcontinent. JPHM-2000; 22: 33-37.

4. Joshi PJ, Maniar JK, Bhave GG. Profile of HIV Infection in India. In: S. Jameel L, Villarreal, eds. Advances in animal virology. New Delhi: Oxford & IBH Publishing; 2000 . p.371-381.

5. Clarke JR, Sahi DK, Maniar JK, Udwadia Z, Mitchell DM, Dual infection with HIV 1 and HIV 2. Thorax 1997; 52: 587-588.

Table 6. Spectrum of Clinical Disease Among HIV infected Adults in Africa, Latin America and Asia[20]

Region	Sub-Saharan Africa	Kenya	Latin America	Asia	Thailand
Country	Cote d'Ivoire Hospitalized HIV + patients	HIV+ medical ward admissions	Brazil Patients with AIDS, specialist clinic	India AIDS cases, national surveillance	Hospitalized patients with AIDS
No HIV + patient	349	95	111	3551	1553
Tuberculosis	28%	18%	32%	62%	37%
Bacteraemia	18%	26%	–	–	<1%
HIV wasting	11%	–	–	–	8%
Isoporiasis	7%	–	6%	–	0
Bacterial pneumonia	6%	16%	16%	–	<1%
Cerebral toxoplasmosis	6%	–	14%	3%	2%
Bacterial enteritis	5%	–	6%	–	–
Non-specific diarrhoea	5%	15%	–	–	–
Oesophageal candidiasis	3%	–	24%	57%	3%
Cryptoccosis	2%	1%	5%	4%	38%
Kaposi's sarcoma	1%	2%	5%	<1%	<1%
Cytomegalovirus	0	–	5%	1%	4%
PCP	0	–	22%	3%	5%
Cryptosporiodiosis	0	–	8%	4%	2%
Penicilliosis	0	–	–	–	3%
Histoplasmosis	0	–	–	–	2%

6. Maniar J. The natural history of HIV 2 infection in India. HIV & AIDS Current trends 2001; 7: 3-7.

7. Natural history and classification. In: Bartlett, edr. Medical Management of HIV infection. Baltimore: The Hopkins HIV report; 1999. p.1-16.

8. Fauci AS, Lane HC. Human Immunodeficiency virus (HIV) disease. In :Braunwald E, Fauci AS, Kasper DL, Hanser SL, Longo DL, James JL, eds. Harrisons Principles of Internal Medicine. 15th edn. New York: McGraw Hill; 2001. p. 1852-1913.

9. Acute HIV infection. In: Powderly WG, edr. Manual of HIV Therapeutics. 2nd edn. Philadelphia; Lippincott Williams; 2001.p.6-13.

10. Schacker T, Collier AC, Hughes J, Shea T, Corey L. Clinical and epidemiologic features of primary HIV infection. Ann Intern Med 1996; 125: 257.

11. Natural History. In: Powderly WG, edr. Manual of HIV Therapeutics. 2nd edn. Philadelphia. Lippincott Williams; 2001. p.14-19.

12. Singh S, Singh N, Maniar JK. AIDS associated toxoplamosis in India and its correlation with serum tumour necrosis factor-alpha. J of parasitic diseases 1996; 20: 49-52.

13. Epidemiology of communicable diseases. In: Park K, edr. Parks Text Book of Preventive and Social Medicine.

16th edn. Jabalpur: Banarsidas Bhanot; 2000.p. 257-266.

14. Centre for Disease Control. 1993 revised classification system for HIV infection. MMWR 1992; 41: 96.

15. Rajagopalan B, Jacob M, George S. Skin lesions in HIV-positive and HIV –negative in South India. Int J Dermatol 1996; 35: 489-92.

16. Kumarasamy N, Solomen S, Madhivanan P, Ravikumar B, Thyagarajan SP, Yesudian P. Dermatological manifestations among human immunodeficiency virus patients in South India. Int J Dermatol 2000 ;39 : 192-5.

17. Singh A, Thappa DM, Hamide A. The spectrum of mucocutaneous manifestations during the evolutionary phases of HIV disease: an emerging Indian scenario. J Dermatol 1999 ; 26: 294-304.

18. Chacko S, John TJ, Jacob M, Kaur A, Mathai D. Clinical profile of AIDS in India: a review of 61 cases. JAPI 1995; 43: 535-538.

19. Maniar JK. The HIV/AIDS epidemic in India - real challenge for Dermatovenereologists in the new millenium, 29th National Conferenve of IADVL, 1-4 February 2001, Agra.

20. Grant A. Clinical features of HIV disease in developing countries. Lepr Rev 2002; 73: 197-205.

Chapter 5

Laboratory Diagnosis of HIV Infection

Pradeep Seth

Introduction

Diagnosis of HIV infection can sometimes be intriguing as the infected persons may present with a spectrum of illnesses ranging from acute to chronic infection in adults, children and even in newborns or neonates. These infections may be confused with other febrile illnesses, for example, acute infectious mononucleosis or constitutional symptoms which appear in chronically infected patients may mimic pulmonary tuberculosis. Therefore, it is necessary to make correct utilization of appropriate diagnostic tests to confirm HIV infection. Although, the standard serological techniques make the diagnosis of HIV infection during chronic asymptomatic or symptomatic disease relatively straightforward, identification of HIV infection by these tests during the seroconversion period may be difficult.

It is therefore, imperative that those who are involved in the laboratory diagnosis of HIV must provide accurate and reliable results. To accomplish this, a better understanding of the biology of the virus[1], the natural history of HIV infection, immune response of the host and various tests currently available for the diagnosis of HIV infection including their principles, limitations and problems, their performance characteristics and proper use is needed.

Biology of the HIV

The HIV is an enveloped, RNA containing retrovirus that primarily infects CD4 receptor bearing lymphocytes, or helper T cells. The virus has the ability to integrate its RNA genome into the host cell genome by first transcribing this genome into DNA (HIV-provirus) with the help of an enzyme called reverse transcriptase. The provirus then is transcribed and translated along with the host-cell DNA resulting in the synthesis of specific virus components, which eventually assemble to produce complete virus particles.

The HIV is composed of an outer envelope and an inner core. The envelope consists of a bi-lipid membrane in which specific components of the virus are embedded. Each component is a mushroom shaped glycosylated protein or glycoprotein and consists of an external portion (gp 120) and a transmembrane portion (gp 41). These two envelope glycoproteins together are involved in the process of attachment of virus to the CD4 receptor on the host cell and subsequent fusion of the virus envelope with the cell membrane. The inner core components are bound by a protein coat encompassing RNA genome and three viral enzymes, reverse transcriptase, integrase and protease.

There are two types of HIV: HIV 1 and HIV 2. HIV 1 infections are prevalent world-wide. In contrast, HIV 2 is endemic primarily in West Africa. However, HIV 2 infections now are making their presence felt all over the world. HIV 2 genome shares 40-45% homology with HIV 1 and it causes similar pathological consequences. Diagnostically, HIV 1 and HIV 2 can present problems. Laboratory tests designed to detect HIV 1 infections do not always detect HIV 2 infections and vice-versa. Even then, antibodies to HIV 1 may frequently cross react with HIV 2 antigens and be detected in serological assays designed to detect antibodies to HIV 2. Similarly, HIV 2 antibodies may cross-react in HIV 1 serological tests. All the HIV serological assays available commercially detect both anti HIV 1 and anti HIV 2 antibodies.

Natural History of HIV Infection

After 1 to 3 weeks of initial entry of HIV into the body by any route, an infected individual may present with an acute infectious mononucleosis like syndrome characterized by sore-throat, fever, lymphadenopathy, hepatosplenomegaly, rash and other constitutional symptoms[2]. Although some patients may be asymptomatic, majority (40-60%) develop this mild to moderate illness which generally lasts for 1-3 weeks. Clinical laboratory studies show that during the first week, these patients may have lymphopenia and thrombocytopenia and elevated transaminases. In the second week, the CD4+ lymphocytes are reduced and CD8+ lymphocytes rise in number resulting in inversion of CD4+/CD8+ cell ratio. At the same time, atypical lymphocytes are also seen in the blood. After the acute infection, over the following months the CD4+ and CD8+ cell counts return to almost normal levels in most patients. These changes last for 1-3 weeks and the recovery is complete. Generally speaking, the patients usually become asymptomatic for many months to years after this primary HIV infection.

The infected individuals have high levels of infectious virus in the plasma in peripheral blood. This virus is relatively homogenous. Once the seroconversion takes place and the infected individual develops HIV specific immune response, virus variants emerge which results in heterogeneity or quasi-species. During the asymptomatic phase, the plasma viremia is markedly reduced.

The duration of asymptomatic HIV infection may vary from 5 years to greater than 15 years during which most patients experience relatively good health. However, viral replication is highly dynamic and continuous during this period of clinical latency. Evidently, there is profound reduction in CD4+ lymphocytes. The infected individual may develop minor ailments related to immune deficiency, which has been referred to as AIDS-related complex. With the continuous virus replication, there is a further fall in CD4+ T cell counts and the individual becomes further immuno-compromised. At this stage, the individual may develop a variety of opportunistic infections like *Pneumocystis carinii* pneumonia, generalized candidiasis, tuberculosis, cryptococcal meningitis, CMV retinitis, generalized herpes virus infection, toxoplasmosis, malignancies, etc. On the basis of CD4+ T cell count in the peripheral blood and clinical condition of the patient, the Centres for Disease Control and Prevention, Atlanta, USA proposed a classification system for identifying HIV infected individuals with or without AIDS for clinical management and antiretroviral therapy[3] (Table 1). This classification has since found universal acceptance.

Table 1. CDC Classification System for HIV Infection and Expanded AIDS Case Definitions

CD4+ T cell Categories (cells/µl)	Clinical categories[#]		
	A	B	C
500	A1	B1	C1
200-499	A2	B2	C2
< 200	A3	B3	C3

A: asymptomatic including acute primary HIV infection and persistent generalized lymphadenopathy (PGL); B: Symptomatic but not AIDS indicator conditions of group C; C: AIDS indicator conditions

Immune Response to HIV Infection

Following HIV infection, both humoral and cellular immune responses develop. Although, the initial antibody response is of IgM class, it is usually transient and not consistent. IgG antibodies to envelope and gag proteins appear first followed by antibodies to all other proteins of the virus. It is, therefore, important to understand the kinetics of the immune response in order to formulate the strategy of testing an individual infected with HIV. The antibodies are usually produced between 6 to 12 weeks following infection. In rare instances the antibodies may not be detected until 45 months after infection. Meaning thereby, any individual soon after acquiring infection will test negative, as he may not have antibodies to HIV. Antibodies to envelope antigens (particularly gp 41) will persist throughout the infection while antibody to core antigen (p 24) will decrease once the clinical disease develops and the concentrations of viral core antigen p 24 increases in the plasma.

HIV infection in newborn is closely linked to the maternal infection[4]. It occurs in the presence of maternally acquired antibodies. The risk of transmission is from 14.4% to 45% depending upon the severity of infection in pregnant mother. However, the diagnosis of congenital HIV infection presents enormous problems. Serodiagnostic tests are generally of not much help in the diagnosis of perinatal HIV infection especially in the presence of maternal IgG antibodies in the cord blood and IgM antibody production against HIV infection is very inconsistent and erratic. Maternal IgG has been reported to persist in infants for up to 18 months of age despite a reported half life for IgG of only 23 to 26 days.

Laboratory Tests

Laboratory tests employed for the diagnosis of HIVinfection may be classified into following groups (Table-2).

Table 2. Laboratory Tests for the Diagnosis of HIV Infection

(I) Tests for HIV-sepcific antibodies in serum/plasma
    a. Screening tests (i) ELISA
                  (ii) Rapid tests
    b. Supplemental tests (i) Western Blot assay
                      (ii) Immunofluorescence test
(II) Tests for HIV-specific antibodies in salive
(III) Confirmatory tests
    a. Virus isolation
    b. Detection of HIV-specific core antigen (p24)
    c. Polymerase chain reaction (RT PCR/b DNA)

1. Tests for HIV Specific Antibodies in Serum/Plasma

The test for detecting HIV specific antibodies are divided into screening and supplemental tests.

Screening Tests

These tests are rapid and inexpensive serological tests, which are used for screening antibodies against HIV in infected individuals. These tests possess a high degree of sensitivity but some false positive results do occur (i.e. some individuals will inevitably produce positive results even though they are not infected with virus). Therefore, these tests are used as presumptive tests.

Since a positive result may be obtained due to technical error, it is imperative that repeat testing is done in duplicate before the sample is considered reactive by the screening assay. Further, as these tests lack a sufficiently high degree of specificity, the positive results of these assays must be validated by supplemental tests. Screening tests include:

(a) Enzyme Linked Immunosorbent Assays (ELISA)
(b) Rapid tests

Enzyme linked immunosorbent assays (ELISA)

These assays use enzymes as the indicator system for the detection and quantitation of analyte present in the immune complexes formed as a result of reaction between solid surface bound HIV antigen and circulating antibody. These tests are highly sensitive and specific and take 60 to 90 min for completion. Although these tests require an initial investment of expensive instruments like plate washer, spectrophotometers etc., the running cost is rather low as compared to the supplemental test.

Rapid tests

These tests have a total reaction time of less than 30 minutes. They are more expensive per test than ELISA, though they do not require complex equipment. The results are read by naked eyes. Some of these tests may be completed within a few minutes and therefore, are best suited for emergency clinics, casualties or trauma clinics where immediate screening of a blood donor or a recipient may be required.

There are several formats of rapid tests available commercially but the most popular ones are the dot blot assays. In dot blot assay microscopic particles are coated with a synthetic peptide and then immobilized on a nitrocellulose membrane. Patient's serum containing antibodies, conjugate, developer and stop solutions are then added in sequence with usual incubation and washing steps. Then the colour develops which is in proportion to the amount of HIV antibodies bound to the peptide coated microparticles.

Supplemental Tests

These tests are also serological tests for detection of antibodies against HIV. These tests are recommended for validation of the positive results of the screening assays. There are two types of supplemental tests that are commonly used:

(a) Western blot assay
(b) Immunofluorescence test

Western blot assay

Western blot is a highly specific and equally sensitive assay. In this assay, specific viral proteins from whole virus lysate are separated by polyacrylamide gel electrophoresis according to their molecular weight and then are transferred onto a nitrocellulose membrane by a process called electroblotting. Following this transfer, the membrane is washed and cut into strips. A serum sample found positive by screening test is reacted with the HIV-proteins immobilized on the strip. An enzyme-conjugate and substrate are added to generate a colorimetric reaction. If the sample has antibodies, coloured bands will appear wherever human IgG binds to the viral protein on the strip. In the absence of coloured bands, western blot is interpreted as negative.

However, interpretive criteria for HIV 1 Western blot remain the subject of much discussion. There is no unanimity on this subject. Another problem with this assay is its prohibitive cost.

Immunofluorescence test

An alternative but seldom used assay for HIV diagnosis is indirect immunofluorescence assay as a supplemental test. In this test HIV infected cells are acetone fixed onto the glass slides and then reacted with test serum followed by fluorescein conjugated anti-human antibody. A positive reaction appears as apple-green fluorescence of the membrane. This test is very inexpensive to perform but requires expertize to conduct as well as for its interpretation.

2. Tests For HIV Specific Antibodies in Saliva

The immunoglobulins gain entry to the oral cavity by secretion from salivary glands and by transudation from blood capillaries beneath the gingival crevices. Since saliva contains low levels of IgG or IgM, sensitive and specific antibody assays with the class-specific antibody capture format have been designed for testing salivary specimens for the presence of anti HIV antibodies. Although these kits are efficacious, there is some concern about how early during seroconversion the anti-HIV antibody is detectable in saliva as compared to serum/plasma following primary infection. In addition, it is important to determine the minimum concentration of IgG at which each kit can be relied on to not to give a false negative result. Finally, role of supplementary/confirmatory testing on saliva specimens is not known. Studies on these important features of sensitivity of anti HIV assays applied to saliva are needed before they can be relied upon for diagnostic use.

3. Confirmatory Tests

These tests confirm the presence of virus in an individual who is either seropositive or has equivocal results from various serological tests.

Virus Isolation

The virus can be isolated from the blood of infected individuals by co-cultivating peripheral blood mononuclear cells (PBMC) with those from uninfected donors. It generally takes 4-8 weeks for virus isolation and identification of virus. This assay is 100% specific but its sensitivity varies with the stage of HIV infection. Therefore, virus isolation though confirms the diagnosis, a negative result does not rule out HIV infection in an individual. Moreover, both in adults and in children, virus cannot be cultured from PBMC for approximately 6 weeks following the time of transmission. However, this procedure is labour intensive and dangerous technique, which could be undertaken by the specialized laboratories only.

Detection of HIV Specific Core Antigen (p 24)

The antigen test detects HIV free antigen (p 24) in the serum. HIV antigenemia occurs during "window period" and during late disease when the patient is usually symptomatic. HIV antigenemia is also seen in HIV infected newborn. Therefore, an antigen test may be useful, (a) during "window period", (b) during late disease when the patient is symptomatic, (c) to detect HIV infection in a newborn because diagnosis is difficult due to the presence of maternal antibodies. (d) When HIV dementia and encephalopathy is suspected and the test is performed with the cerebrospinal fluid. However, only 30% patients during window period, 50-60% of AIDS patients, 30-40% of patients with AIDS related complex (ARC) and 10% of asymptomatic patients are antigen positive.

This test is relatively insensitive being able to detect 50-60 pg/ml of antigen. The reason for the lack of sensitivity of this test in AIDS patient is that the free antigen (p 24) in serum may be complexed with p 24 antibody. Another important point to note that this test detects soluble p 24 antigen and does not specifically identify live virus. Therefore, an antigen-negative test sample may still be infectious. Similarly, the presence of antigen does not by itself confirm that the sample is infectious.

This test employs indirect ELISA technology in which a specific antibody is bound to the solid phase and the serum containing free HIV antigen is made to react with this antibody. This is followed by addition of a conjugate (an antibody to core antigen coupled to an enzyme), substrate and stop solutions in sequence with usual incubation and washing steps. In this format the test is relatively insensitive being able to detect 50-60 pg/ml of antigen. The reason for the lack of sensitivity of this test is that the free antigen in serum may be complexed with anti core antibody. However, incorporating a step of preliminary acid hydrolysis of the serum sample to dissociate immune complexes to free p24 antigen, which can then be measured, has improved its sensitivity.

Polymerase Chain Reaction (PCR)

In this technique the target HIV RNA or proviral DNA is amplified enzymatically in vitro by chemical reaction. It is an extremely sensitive assay because a single copy of proviral DNA can be amplified and then be detected by the probe. This technique allows detection of HIV prior to the detection by antibody assays. In our experience, PCR can detect infection even before viral culture becomes positive. Presently it is the most sensitive known method for identification of HIV infection. However, it is technically demanding and is expensive and therefore it is not suitable for use in routine laboratories.

A modification of this assay, RT PCR is employed for quantitation of HIV present in plasma (plasma virus load). In this test HIV RNA from circulating plasma virus is first reverse transcribed to cDNA, which is then used as a template in PCR format for quantitation of HIV in plasma. This test has now become an important marker in assessing the risk of disease progression and monitoring anti-retroviral therapy. Three different techniques namely RT PCR, NASBA (nucleic acid sequence based amplification) and branched-DNA (b-DNA) assay have been employed to develop commercial kits. RT PCR and NASBA reactions are template (plasma RNA) amplification assays, whereas b-DNA assay amplifies the signal from the RNA-DNA hybridization reaction.

Selection of HIV Antibody Test

The selection of the most appropriate test or combination of tests for use depends on three criteria:

1. Objective of the HIV antibody testing,
2. Sensitivity and specificity of the test(s) being used
3. Prevalence of HIV infection in the population under study.

1. Objectives of HIV Antibody Testing

These are four main objectives for which HIV antibody testing is performed:

(i) Transfusion/blood or organ donation safety: Unlinked and anonymous screening of donated blood and blood products.

(ii) Sero-surveillance: Unlinked and anonymous testing of sera for the purpose of monitoring prevalence and trends in HIV infection overtime in a given population.

(iii) Diagnosis of HIV 1 infection : Voluntary testing of serum for asymptomatic persons or persons with clinical signs and symptoms suggestive of HIV infection/AIDS.

2. Sensitivity and Specificity of Antibody Tests

Sensitivity and specificity are two major factors that determine the accuracy and reliability of an assay in distinguishing an infected from an uninfected person. A test with high sensitivity will have very few false negative results. Therefore, only tests of the highest possible sensitivity should be used when there is a need to minimize the rate of false negative results (e.g. in transfusion/blood donation safety). A test with a high specificity will have very few false positive results. Therefore, it may be used when there is a need to minimize the rate of false positive results (e.g. in sero surveillance and in the diagnosis of HIV infection in an individual).

3. Prevalence of HIV Infection

The probability that a test will determine accurately the true infection status of a person varies with the prevalence rate or HIV infection in the population. It is expressed as predictive value. In general, higher the prevalence of HIV infection in a population, the greater is the probability that a person testing positive is truly infected (i.e. the greater the positive predictive value, PPV). Thus, with increasing prevalence, the proportion of serum samples testing false positve decreases.

The PPV of a test is very low when a population with low HIV prevalence is tested, even if the specificity of the test is very high. For this reason a supplemental test is necessary to enhance the PPV of HIV testing.

National HIV Testing Policy

The most popular algorithm for HIV antibody testing uses a highly sensitive enzyme-linked immunosorbent assay (ELISA) followed by the WB assay. This algorithm is expensive and produces indeterminate results of uncertain diagnostic significance quite often during early seroconversion. Studies have shown that combinations of EIAs (enzyme immunoassays) may provide results as reliable as and in some instances even more reliable than the ELISA/WB combination at a much lower cost.

On September 10, 1993 the National AIDS Control Programme Technical Advisory Committee of Ministry of Health and Family Welfare, Government of India recommended implementation of the following HIV antibody testing policy:

Testing Algorithm I

For transfusion purposes, only one highly sensitive, reliable, economically feasible and technically easy EIA for both HIV 1 and HIV 2 antibodies should be carried out by the Zonal Blood Testing Centres/Blood Banks and if the results indicate that antibodies are present, the blood should be discarded and no further test needs to be done on this blood sample. The HIV screening is anonymous and unlinked. The EIA test selected should be of a very high sensitivity and a good specificity to ensure almost negligible false negative reports and considerably reduced number of wasted blood units respectively.

Testing Algorithm II

For sero surveillance purposes, HIV 1 and HIV 2 combination kits conforming to the one used for the blood safety purposes, will be used by the surveillance centres. As in blood safety programme, the screening of the blood samples is anonymous and unlinked. All sera are first tested with one EIA. Any serum found reactive on the first assay is retested with a second EIA based on a different antigen preparation or principle. If it is found reactive by the second assay also, it is considered antibody positve. Any serum which is reactive on the first test but non-reactive on the second test is considered antibody negative. The selection of the EIA kits appropriate for serosurveillance testing purposes is very critical for the predictive value of this algorithm. The

first EIA should be of a very high sensitivity and a second EIA should be of a very high specificity. This algorithm will ensure almost negligible false negative reports and very few false positive reports.

Testing Algorithm III

HIV testing for diagnostic purposes depends on the clinical status of the patient. For asymptomatic persons, all samples are first tested with one EIA. Any reactive sample is tested further with a second EIA based on a different antigen preparation or principle. Samples found reactive by the second test are then subjected to a third EIA based on different antigen preparation or principle. The serum reactive on all three tests is considered HIV antibody positive. Serum that is non-reactive either in the first test or in the second test is considered negative. The serum that is reactive in the first and second tests but non-reactive in the third test is considered equivocal/borderline positive. Such serum samples should be subjected to retesting by the second and third EIA. In case of equivocal/borderline results on repeat testing, these sera should be tested by the western blot assay. In many cases, second blood sample from the same patient collected after 2 to 3 weeks later may be helpful. All patients with clinical signs and symptoms of HIV infection/AIDS should be tested by the same strategy which has been adopted for serosurveillance purposes mentioned above i.e. two EIA based on different antigens or based on different principle. The predictive value of this algorithm also depends on the selection of appropriate EIAs. The first EIA should be of a very high sensitivity, the second EIA should be of very high specificity and the third EIA should be of a good sensitivity and specificity to ensure negligible false negative as well as false positive reports.

Strategy for Laboratory Diagnosis of HIV Infection

Choice of laboratory tests employed to establish HIV infection in an individual depends on the stage of infection (see Table 3). In acute HIV infection during the window period in the absence of measurable antibody response the diagnosis rests upon (i) demonstration of viral nucleic acid in the PBMC by polymerase chain reaction (PCR) (ii) demonstration of HIV-specific P 24 antigen in plasma/serum, (iii) isolation of HIV from peripheral blood

Table 3. NACO Guidelines for HIV Antibody Testing Strategies

Objective of testing	Prevalence of HIV infection	Testing algorithm
Blood banks/transfusion safety	All prevalences	I
Serosurveillance	< 10%	II
	> 10%	I
Clinical sign and symptoms suggestive of HIV infection/AIDS.	All prevalences	II
Diagnosis/Identification of asymptomatic individuals	< 10%	III
	> 10%	II

Table 4. Laboratory Tests Employed for the Diagnosis and Monitoring of HIV Infected Individuals

Clinical Categories (Stages)	HIV serology	p24 antigen assay	PCR (qualitative)	Plasma HIV Load (quantitative)	Immunophenotyping CD 4+	CD8+	Ratio
Asymptomatic (A1-A3)							
Window period	–	40%	+	++	↓↓/N	↑↑/N	Inv
With/without PGL	+	–/±	+	– /±	↓	↑	Inv
Symptomatic (B1-B3)	+	+/ –	+	– /+	↓	↑	Inv
AIDS indicator illnesses (C1-C3)	+	++	+	++++	↓↓↓	↑↑	Inv
Paediatric HIV infection	+[a]	+	+	– /++	?[b]	?	?

Symbols used: +: positive; –: negative; ± : borderline positive; ↓: counts low; ↑: counts high; N: counts normal; Inv: CD4+/CD+8 ratio inverted.

a: maternal antibodies may be present until 17 months after birth in newborn.

b: role unknown in prediction or monitoring of HIV infection

mononuclear cells (PBMC). On the other hand during asymptomatic HIV infection, though the patients are apparently healthy, they have detectable anti HIV antibodies in their blood. Therefore the diagnosis of HIV infection is straight forward by demonstration of HIV specific antibodies in blood.

Laboratory diagnosis of HIV infection in patients with clinical manifestations suggestive of AIDS includes (a) demonstratrion of HIV specific antibodies in blood, (b) quantification of virus load in the plasma, and (c) demonstration of HIV-specific P 24 antigen in plasma/serum.

Diagnosis of HIV Infections in newborns depends on the route of infection.[5] Conventional commercial assays for detecting anti HIV antibodies are unable to diagnose HIV infection in infants born to HIV seropositive mothers owing to inability of these tests to distinguish between maternal IgG and infants own antibodies. Therefore, tests for identification of virus or

its constituents are the mainstay in the diagnosis of pediatric HIV infection. Isolation of virus by culture remains the 'gold standard' for the diagnosis of infection. In prenatal infections (that is, infants infected in utero) presence of virus may be established either by detection of HIV genome by PCR or by isolation of the virus from the cord blood lymphocytes within 48 hr of birth. In contrast, in perinatal infections (that is, intrapartum or infections acquired during passage through birth canal) viremia can only be detected 7 to 90 days later either by PCR or by virus isolation. Therefore, a practical algorithm for the diagnosis of HIV during infancy in a range of clinical settings is to identify HIV by culture or PCR in infants born to HIV seropositive mothers as close to birth as possible. If there is no evidence of virus at this time point, these -tests should be repeated at the age of 3 and 6 months. The presence of virus by either of these tests should be interpreted as probable infection.

References

1. Seth P, Arora A. HIV applied virology and vaccine implications. J Int Med Sci Acad 1998; 11: 131-134.

2. Wali JP, Handa R, Aggarwal P. Acute HIV infection. J Int Med Sci Acad 1998; 11: 139-142.

3. Castro KG, Ward JW, Slutsker L, et al. 1993 revised classification system for HIV infection and expanded surveillance case definition for AIDS among adolescents and adults. MMWR 1992; 41: 1-19.

4. Kabra SK, Singh A, Jain Y. HIV/AIDS in children. J Int Med Sci Acad 1998; 11: 179-183.

5. Wara DW, Luzuriaga K, Martin NL, Sullivan JL, Bryson YJ. Maternal transmission and diagnosis of human immunodeficiency virus during infancy. Ann N Y Acad Sci 1993; 693: 14-19.

Chapter 6

Antiretroviral Therapy

Jyoti Prakash Wali, Praveen Aggarwal, Rohini Handa

Introduction

Less than a decade ago, someone with HIV/AIDS had a little hope. The years 1996-1998 were turning point in the management of these patients due to three reasons: a new understanding of viral pathogenesis; new development of more powerful tools for measuring HIV levels in the blood and most importantly, introduction of new and effective antiretroviral treatment regimes. Measurement of HIV RNA using PCR techniques have shown that during the latent period, a patient with HIV infection could have 10,000 to 100,000 virus particles in 1 ml of blood. HIV RNA allows interventions prior to measurable evidence of further immunosuppression as evidenced by CD4 counts and is used in most studies to document the efficacy of antiretroviral strategies.

In this chapter, we shall discuss the standard recommendations for treatment of HIV infection followed by a section on treatment of HIV in a resource-poor country. Before putting down the details of treatment it is essential to know the life cycle of HIV so as to understand the mode and site of action of the antiretroviral drugs.

Replication Cycle of HIV

The human immunodeficiency virus is a retrovirus, which is a single stranded RNA virus. It can infect a number of different cells, including CD4 bearing macrophages and T-helper lymphocytes within the host. There are several steps in the viral replication cycle, which may be applied in developing antiretroviral therapies. HIV attaches to the target cells through binding of surface glycoprotein (gp)120 to cell surface CD4 molecules. Following CD4 binding, a centre material

change in the HIV gp120/gp 41 complex is induced by interaction of gp120 with the chemokine receptors CCR5. This change in confirmation exposes gp41 allowing it to initiate fusion of the membranes. The significant role of CCR5 in this process has been revealed upon the observation that individuals with homozygous for mutations within CCR5 are resistant to infection by HIV 1. Inhibition of this binding will inhibit viral replication. Drugs that act at this level are under investigation. One of the most promising agent which block fusion of HIV with the cell membrane is called T-20 (Enfuvirtide)and is in phase 3 clinical trial. The other fusion inhibitors are T-1249 and AMD-3100.

Another site is the viral reverse transcriptase (RT) enzyme. After the virus invades a macrophage or T lymphocyte, the RT enzyme initiates copying of the viral RNA into DNA, which gets integrated into the host's DNA. Drugs like nucleoside RT inhibitors diffuse into the infected cells and are converted to their active triphosphate forms by cellular kinases. These active nucleosides are incorporated into the growing viral DNA and cause premature chain termination. On the other hand, non-nucleoside RT inhibitors bind directly to the RT enzyme causing inhibition of its function.

The viral DNA migrates to and enters the host cell nucleus (a process facilitated by the HIV proteins vpr and MA) and becomes integrated into the cell DNA with the help of the enzyme integrase. The provirus can then remain latent or be active, generating products for the generation of new virions. A compound called S-1360, which targets integrase, is under trial.

Transcription and translation of viral DNA produces viral RNA. Drugs, which act at these steps, are being tested. The HIV genes, *gag* and *pol*, produce large polypeptides. Before budding of virus, these polypeptides undergo processing by the enzyme protease. Inhibition of protease using protease inhibitors results in production of immature defective virus particles.[1] The summary of HIV cycle and the action of antiretroviral drugs at different levels are shown in Figure 1.

The antiretroviral drugs currently available are given in Table 1.

Nucleoside Reverse Transcriptase Inhibitors (NRTI)

Zidovudine

The first antiretroviral (ARV) drug licensed for use was

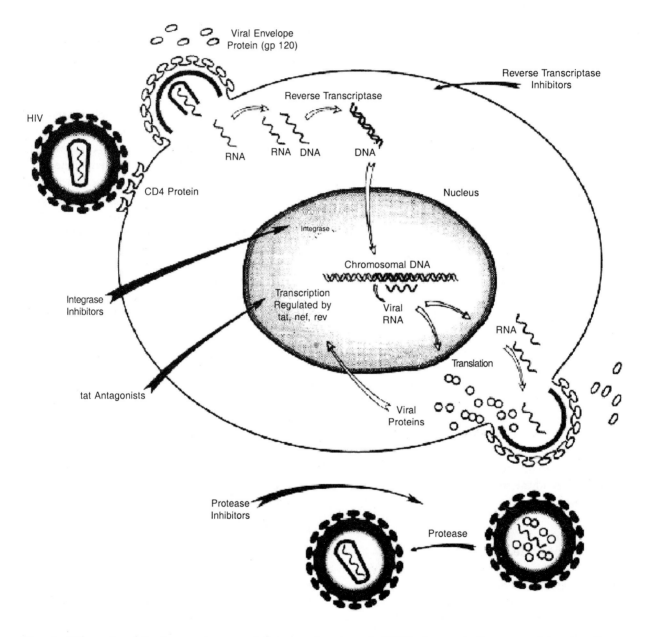

Fig. 1. Life cycle of the human immunodeficiency virus type 1 (HIV), demonstrating potential points for interference by antiviral agents. Adopted from JAMA HIV/AIDS Resource Centre www.ama.assn.org

Table 1. Antiretroviral Agents Currently Available (generic name/Trade name)

Nucleoside Analogues

Nucleoside Reverse Transcriptase Inhibitors

Zidovudine/*Retrovir* (AZT, ZDV)
Didanosine/*Videx, Videx EC* (ddI)
Zalcitabine/*HIVID* (ddC)
Stavudine/*Zerit* (d4T)
Lamivudine/*Epivir* (3TC)
Abacavir/*Ziagen* (ABC)

Non-Nucleoside Reverse Transcriptase Inhibitors

Nevirapine/*Viramune* (NVP)
Delavirdine/*Rescriptor* (DLV)
Efavirenz/*Sustiva* (EFV)

Nucleotide Analogue

Tenofovir DF/*Viread* (TDF)

Protease Inhibitors

Indinavir/*Crixivan* (IDV)
Ritonavir/*Norvir* (RTV)
Saquinavir/*Invirase, Fortovase* (SQV)
Nelfinavir/*Viracept* (NFV)
Amprenavir/*Agenerase* (APV)
Lopinavir/ritonavir, *Kaletra*

Adapted from 'The Hopkin's HIV Report' Sept. 2002. Life Cycle of HIV Infection [http://www.hopkins-aids.edu]

zidovudine (ZDV). Studies reported by the AIDS Clinical Trial Group in 1990 showed that a dose of 200 mg tid was as compared to effective in slowing the progression of HIV infection as higher doses.[2] However, long term studies published in 1992 and 1993 showed that the benefits of early treatment were not sustained and there was no difference in outcome whether ZDV was started early or late.[3]

Resistance

The duration of effectiveness of ZDV is however limited. This is due to emergence of resistance, which occurs because of mutations at 5 sites in RT gene.[4]

Side Effects

The most important adverse effect of ZDV is its toxicity on the bone marrow. Serious anaemia and neutropenia occur in nearly 30% patients. The risk of these adverse effects is more in AIDS patients than in asymptomatic HIV-infected patients. Macrocytosis occurs in almost all patients but it does not predict the occurrence of anaemia. Other side effects include nausea, anorexia, vomiting, headache, myopathy, fatigue and hyperpigmentation of the skin and nails.

Common Drug Interactions

Combination of ganciclovir and ZDV is poorly tolerated due to combined haematological adverse effects. ZDV should be stopped when the patient is on high dose of ganciclovir and may be restarted when the dose of ganciclovir is reduced during the maintenance phase. ZDV may decrease phenytoin levels, warranting monitoring.[5]

Other Nucleoside RT Inhibitors

Other nucleoside RT inhibitors include *didanosine (ddI)*, *zalcitabine (ddC)*, *stavudine (d4T)*, *abacavir (ABC)*, *lamivudine (3TC)*[6] and emtricitabine (investigational).[7] There is little cross-resistance between these agents and therefore, these agents can be used in combination.

Didanosine is inactivated by the low pH of stomach; therefore, it is available in combination with a buffer, which increases the gastric pH. ddC is less active clinically than ZDV. d4T and 3TC are well tolerated by most patients.

Side Effects

The most common side effect of these RT inhibitors is painful peripheral neuropathy.[6] This side effect is more common with ddC and d4T than with ddI. Therefore, these agents should be avoided in patients with pre-existing neuropathy. Hyperamylasemia and pancreatitis occur in 20% and 7% of patients treated with ddI. It is rare with other RT inhibitors. ddC may produce oral ulcers in as many as 10% of patients. NRTI may cause fatty change in the liver (hepatic steatosis) and lactic acidosis, a metabolic complication that is potentially fatal but very rare.[8,9] These two adverse effects are due to toxicity of the NRTI on cellular mitochondria. Changes in body fat distribution as well as derangements in the metabolism of fats have also been associated with the prolonged use of NRTI. Lipodystrophy, which usually occurs, with protease inhibitors (PI), has rarely been described with the use of NRTI.

Drug Interactions

In view of the possibility of development of pancreatitis, parenteral pentamidine should be avoided in patients on ddI. Ganciclovir increases the levels of ddI and therefore, the risk of pancreatitis is increased if both are combined. Certain drugs like dapsone, ketoconazole, itraconazole, pyrimethamine and trimethoprim require acidic pH in the stomach for their dissolution and absorption. Therefore, these drugs should be taken at least 2 hours before ddI. It has been hypothesized that zidovudine-5'-monophosphate (produced by the action of thymidylate kinase on ZDV) may inhibit the production of stavudine-5'-monophosphate, and therefore the combination of d4T and ZDV may be antagonistic.[5]

Non-Nucleoside Reverse Transcriptase Inhibitors (NNRTI)[10]

These analogues of RT inhibitors restrict the replication of the virus by binding to an active site of RT, which is different from that for the nucleoside RT inhibitors. Members of this class are highly active against HIV 1 but not HIV 2. Development of resistance and cross-resistance are the major problems with these agents. This group includes nevirapine (NVP), delavirdine (DLV) and efavirenz (EFV). Of these drugs, NVP is the most commonly used drug in India.

Nevirapine: This is the most commonly used NNRTI in India as it is cheap and is relatively well tolerated. In combination with 2 NRTI, it provides an effective treatment for HIV infection. The recommended dosage is 200 mg once a day for the first two weeks and then 200 mg twice a day afterwards. This dosage schedule reduces the chance of adverse effects associated with this drug. The most common side effects associated with this class of drugs are skin rash, nausea, headache and hepatic enzyme elevation. Skin rash develops in about 25% of people taking the drug. It is recommended

that if a patient develops a rash during the lead-in (lower dose) period, the dose should not be increased to the full dose. If the rash is uncomfortable, the drug, should be stopped. A rare side effect of NVP is Stevens Johnson syndrome. Patients should be carefully monitored during the first two months of taking NVP to watch for signs of skin or liver problems. Because of the risk of liver damage, NVP should not be used for post-exposure prophylaxis. NVP is metabolized by the liver and can interact with other drugs with predominant hepatic metabolism. These drugs include antihistamines, sedatives and anti-fungal agents. NVP also increases the metabolism of PI and therefore, should not be combined with them.

Nucleotide Reverse Transcriptase Inhibitors

Tenofovir, a nucleotide reverse transcriptase inhibitor prevents HIV from entering the nucleus of healthy T cells. It is now approved for the treatment of HIV infection by FDA. It is very similar to nucleoside analogues but the difference is that tenofovir unlike nucleoside analogues is chemically preactivated and thus requires less biochemical processing in the body. It must be used in combination with other drugs including NRTI and atleast one PI or NNRTI. The usual dosage is 300 mg once daily. The most common side effects are nausea, vomiting, diarrhoea and flatulence.

Adefovir is another new drug of nucleotide reverse transcriptase inhibitor. This is yet to be FDA approved, although phase III studies are near completion.[11]

Protease Inhibitors (PI)

Six PI, saquinavir (SQV), indinavir (IDV), ritonavir (RTV), nelfinavir (NFV), amprenavir (APV) and lopinavir-plus/ritonavir are in clinical use.[12,13]

Resistance

Development of resistance is a major limitation and this is related to the dose. Therefore, these agents must be used in full therapeutic doses. Also, cross-resistance among these agents, particularly indinavir and ritonavir, is common.

Side Effects

The main side effects of PI are nausea and vomiting. Indinavir can produce transient increase in indirect bilirubin. In 3–15% of patients, renal calculi can develop. Hence, patient should be asked to consume lot of fluids (48 ounces of water/day). Ritonavir has a bad taste and so produces more GI symptoms. Oral numbness is also seen in some patients.

PI have been associated with body fat redistribution, which manifests physically as thinning of arms, legs and face and/or deposition of fat in the abdominal and shoulder regions along with lipomas (lipodystrophy). It occurs in 6 to 80% of patients and develops after several months of therapy. The effects on fat metabolism may lead to raised levels of serum cholesterol and triglycerides, insulin resistance and rarely elevated blood glucose levels.[14] The overall cumulative incidence of these metabolic disturbances may be high (30%-60%) after 1 to 2 years of treatment.

Drug Interactions

Drugs like cisapride and metoclopramide, which increase gut motility, reduce the absorption of saquinavir. If indinavir is used in combination with ddI, it should be administered at least one hour before ddI, as buffer in latter increases gastric pH and thus reduces absorption of indinavir. Ritonavir is available both in solution and capsule forms. Oral solution contains 43% alcohol, while capsules also contain small amount of alcohol. Therefore, patients on ritonavir must avoid metronidazole and tinidazole. Saquinavir is available in 2 forms, hard gel (less oral bioavialability) and soft gel (3 times > than hard gel).

Hepatic microsomal enzymes metabolize PI and therefore, drug interactions are frequent. Enzyme-inducers like rifampicin, phenytoin, carbamazepine and phenobarbitone can reduce the concentration of PI. Inhibitors of microsomal enzymes like ketoconazole and itraconazole increase serum levels of these agents. This is most significant with saquinavir whose concentration is increased by 80% when combined with ketoconazole. Co-administration of rifampicin with IDV is contraindicated because of 89% decrease in IDV's availability concentration (AUC).[5]

A summary of various antiretroviral drugs is given in Table 2.

Table 2. Characteristics of Commonly Used Antiretroviral Drugs

Drug	Availability & Administration	Adverse effects	Common drug interactions	Cost/month (approximate)
Zidovudine (ZDV)	100 mg, 200 mg & 300 mg tab. 200 mg tid or 300 mg bid Take without regard to food	Bone marrow suppression, GI intolerance, headache, lactic acidosis	Avoid ribavarin, ganciclovir	Rs. 1150
Didanosine (ddI)	100 mg buffered tab. > 60 kg: 200 mg bid < 60 kg: 125 mg bid Take ½ h before or 2 h after meals	Pancreatitis, peripheral neuropathy, GI intolerance. lactic acidosis	Avoid intravenous pentamidine and ganciclovir	Rs. 2100
Zalcitabine (ddC)	0.75 mg tab. 0.75 mg tid Take without regard to meals Avoid administration of antacids	Peripheral neuropathy, stomatitis, lactic acidosis	——	——
Stavudine (D4T)	30 mg & 40 mg cap. > 60 kg: 40 mg bid < 60 kg: 30 mg bid Take without regard to meals	Pancreatitis, peripheral neuropathy, lactic acidosis stomatitis	Avoid combination with ZDV	Rs. 270
Lamivudine (3TC)	150 mg tab. 10 mg/ml solution 150 mg bid < 50 kg: 2 mg/kg bid Take without regard to meals	Well tolerated, lactic acidosis	——	Rs. 640

(Contd)

Table 2. *(Contd.)*

Drug	Availability & Administration	Adverse effects	Common drug interactions	Cost/month (approximate)
Nevirapine (NVP)	200 mg tab. 200 mg o.d. × 14 d and then 200 bid Take without regard to meals	Skin rash, hepatitis Do not restart after severe hepatitis or skin reaction	Avoid ketoconazole, rifampicin, oral contraceptives If used with IDV: IDV 1000 mg tid + NVP standard dose	Rs. 1070
Efavirenz (EFV)	200 mg cap. 600 mg at night Avoid taking after high fat meals	Skin rash, CNS effects (dizziness, insomnia, abnormal dreams, confusion, agitation, hallucinations), hepatitis	Avoid astemizole, cisapride, midazolam If used with IDV: IDV 1000 mg tid + EFV: standard dose If used with RTV: RTV 600 mg bid + EFV standard dose Not recommended with SQV	Rs. 3200
Indinavir (IDV)	400 mg cap. 800 mg tid Separate dosing with ddI by 1 h Take 1 h before or 2 h after meals	Nephrolithiasis, GI intolerance, headache, asthenia, blurred vision, dizziness, hyperglycemia, redistribution of fat and lipid abnormalities	Avoid lovastatin, simvastatin, rifampicin, astemizole, cisapride, midazolam Use atorvastatin with caution Reduce dose to 600 mg tid if on ketoconazole	Rs. 6500
Ritonavir (RTV)	100 mg cap. 600 mg/7.5 ml solution Day 1-2: 300 mg bid; Day 3-5: 400 mg bid; Day 6-13: 500 mg bid; Day 14 onwards: 600 mg bid Take with food Refrigerate capsules; do not refrigerate oral solution	GI intolerance, paraesthesias, hepatitis, hyperglycemia, redistribution of fat, lipid abnormalities, taste perversion	Avoid amiodarone, quinidine, lovastatin, simvastatin, astemizole, cisapride, midazolam, oral contraceptives Use atorvastatin with caution Ketoconazole dose 200 mg/day Monitor theophylline levels If used with IDV: IDV 400 mg bid + RTV 400 mg bid OR IDV 800 mg bid + RTV 100 or 200 mg bid	Rs. 27000
Nelfinavir (NFV)	250 mg tab. 750 mg tid Take with meal	Diarrhoea, hyperglycemia, redistribution of fat, lipid abnormalities, flatulence	Avoid lovastatin, simvastatin, rifampicin, rifabutin, astemizole, cisapride, midazolam, oral contraceptives Use atorvastatin with caution If used with SQV: NFV standard dose + SQV 1200 mg bid	Rs. 13000
Saquinavir (SQV)	200 mg cap. Hard gel cap.: 400 mg bid with ritonavir only. No effect of food 1200 mg tid/1800 mg bid Take with food Soft gel cap: store in refrigerator	GI intolerance, headache, hepatitis, hyperglycemia, redistribution of fat, lipid abnormalities, rhinitis,	Avoid lovastatin, simvastatin rifampicin, rifabutin, astemizole, cisapride, midazolam Use atorvastatin with caution If used with RTV: SQV 400 mg bid + RTV 400 mg bid	——
Lopinavir + Ritonavir	400 mg lopinavir + 100 mg ritonavir bid Take with food	GI intolerance, headache, hepatitis, hyperglycemia, redistribution of fat, lipid abnormalities	Avoid lovastatin, simvastatin, rifampicin, astemizole, cisapride, midazolam Use atorvastatin with caution	Not available in India

Goals of Therapy

(Adapted from DHHS draft document by R. Sherer and C. Baker)
Eradication of HIV infection is not possible due to the presence of latently infected CD4 Tcells during the very early stages of acute HIV infection that persists with an extremely long half life.

Clinical Goal

Prolongation of life and improvement of quality of life.

Virological Goal

To achieve maximal and durable suppression of viral load (20 copies/ml) so as to halt the disease progression.

Immunological Goal

To achieve immune reconstitution that is quantitative (CD4 count is normal range) and qualitative (pathogen specific immune response)

Therapeutic Goal

Rational sequencing of drugs is a fashion that not only achieves virologic goals, but also (1) maintains therapeutic options; (2) is relatively free of side effects; (3) is realistic in terms of probability of adherence.

Epidemiological Goal

To reduce HIV transmission

Indications for Antiretroviral Therapy[11]

It must be understood that eradication of HIV infection cannot be achieved with the currently available antiretroviral regimens. This is due to the establishment of a pool of latently infected CD4+ cells during the very early stages of acute HIV infection that persists with an extremely long half life. However, the use of highly active antiretroviral therapy (HAART) has been successful in reducing morbidity in HIV patients and improving the quality of life. The term HAART indicates use of 2 NRTI along with one NNRTI or a PI so as to achieve the goals of maximal and durable suppression of viral load, restoration and preservation of immune function, improvement of quality of life and reduction of HIV-related mortality and morbidity. CDC has formulated guidelines for initiation of HAART in HIV-infected patients (Table 3).[11] Role of antiretroviral therapy (ART) in patients with acute HIV infection is controversial.

HAART in Patients with CD4+ Cell Counts Above 200/mm³

While randomized clinical trials[15,16] have shown strong evidence for treating patients with CD4+ cell counts < 200/mm³, the optimal time to initiate HAART among

Table 3. Indications for Antiretroviral Therapy

Clinical category	CD4+ cell count	Plasma HIV RNA	Recommendations
Symptomatic HIV disease (wasting, unexplained fever for > 2 weeks or thrush) including patients with AIDS	Any value.	Any value	Start HAART
Asymptomatic	< 200/mm³	Any value	Start HAART
Asymptomatic	200-350/mm³	Any value	Offer HAART
Asymptomatic	> 350/mm³	> 55,000 (by RT-PCR or bDNA-version 3)★	Some experts recommend starting HAART
Asymptomatic	> 350/mm³	< 55,000	Most defer HAART

★With current bDNA assay (version 3), values are similar to those given by RT-PCR except when HIV-RNA levels are <1,500 copies/mm³. With older versions of bDNA (available in India), values are nearly 50% of those given by RT-PCR.

patients with CD4+ cell count >200/mm^3 is not clear. The Multicenter AIDS Cohort Study (MACS)[11] demonstrated that the 3-year risk of progression to AIDS was 38.5% among patients with CD4+ count of 201-350/mm^3 compared to 14.3% for patients with CD4+ counts >350/mm^3. However, the short term risk of progression was also related to the HIV-RNA levels as the risk of progression to AIDS over 3 years was 64.4% in those with HIV RNA >55,000/mm^3. Thus decision to start ART in asymptomatic patients with CD4+ cell count >200/mm^3 is complex and must be made after careful patient education and counselling.

Evaluation Before Initiating HAART

This includes the following:

- Complete history and physical examination
- Ophthalmologic examination
- Complete blood count, biochemistry profile and lipid profile
- CD4+ cell count
- Plasma HIV RNA measurement (load).
- Others tests including VDRL, Mantoux test, toxoplasma IgG serology, chest x-ray and serology for hepatitis C and B

Antiretroviral Regimens[11]

Most commonly used regimens include a PI with 2 NRTI, an NNRTI with 2 NRTI, or a 3 NRTI regimen. The goal of a class-sparing regimen is to preserve one or more than one class of drugs for later use. Viral load suppression and CD4+ cell responses similar to those achieved with PI containing regimens have been shown with selected PI sparing regimens such as efavirenz + 2 NRTI or abacavir + 2 NRTI; however it is not known whether such regimens will provide comparable efficacy with regard to clinical endpoints.

When initiating therapy, one should begin with an effective regimen. Consideration should also be given to the number of pills per day, frequency of dosing, food requirements, toxicity and drug interactions with other drugs being used by the patient.

Ritonavir increases the plasma levels of other PI by inhibiting both gastrointestinal and hepatic cytochrome P450, thereby reducing metabolism of other PI. This effect of ritonavir is increasingly being used to elevate the plasma levels of other PI. Standard doses of PI result in trough drug levels that are only slightly higher than the effective antiretroviral levels; this may allow the virus to replicate. Using ritonavir with other PI increases their trough levels, which markedly reduces the chances of viral multiplication and also enhances killing activity against viral strains moderately resistant to these PI. Thus ritonavir increases levels of saquinavir, lopinavir, nelfinavir and indinavir. Clinical efficacy has been shown with a combination of ritonavir with indinavir, saquinavir or lopinavir. When starting ART, all drugs should be started simultaneously at full dose with the exception of ritonavir and nevirapine where dose escalation is recommended.

Various combinations of drugs recommended are listed in the Table 4.

Factors Affecting Response to HAART

To maximize the benefits of ART, following factors should be ensured:

- Adherence to the drug regimen
- Adequate serum levels of antiretroviral drugs
- Rational sequencing of antiretroviral drugs so as to preserve future treatment options for as long as possible.

Adherence to HAART[11]

The ability of a patient to adhere to HAART is essential for successful treatment. Numerous reports have shown an association between poor adherence and virologic failure. In order to improve adherence to HAART, various strategies are listed in Table 5. Directly observed therapy (DOT): In DOT, a health care worker observes the ingestion of medication by the patient. Use of DOT in tuberculosis has shown highly encouraging results. In fact, both can be integrated in the same policy since both diseases are common in India. However, treatment for HIV requires at least two doses per day and is life-long therapy unlike tuberculosis where treatment is given on intermittent days and is for a few months only. Modified DOT is being studied in which the morning dose is supervised and evening and weekend doses are self-administered. The goal of this program is to improve *patient education and medication* self-administration over a period of about 3-6 months.

Table 4. Recommended Antiretroviral Agents for Initial Treatment of HIV infection (Choose one each from Column A and Column B)

Strongly recommended	Column A	Column B
	Efavirenz	Didanosine + Lamivudine
	Indinavir	Stavudine + Didanosine
	Nelfinavir	Stavudine + Lamivudine
	Ritonavir + Indinavir	Zidovudine + Didanosine
	Ritonavir + Lopinavir	Zidovudine + Lamivudine
	Ritonavir + Saquinavir	
	(SGC or HGC)	
Recommended as alternatives	Column A	Column B
	Abacavir	Zidovudine + Zalcitabine
	Delavirdine	
	Nelfinavir + Saquinavir (SGC)	
	Nevirapine	
	Ritonavir	
	Saquinavir (SGC)	
No recommendations	Hydroxyurea in combination with other agents	
Avoid	Column A	Column B
	Saquinavir (HGC)	Stavudine + Zidovudine
		Zalcitabine + Didanosine
		Zalcitabine + Lamivudine
		Zalcitabine + Stavudine

SGC = Soft-gel capsule; HGC = Hard-gel capsule;

Table 5. Strategies to Improve Adherence to HAART

Educate the patient about utility of HAART, possible side effects and drug interactions

Reduce dose frequency and number of tablets to minimum possible

Simplify food requirements

Emphasize the need for strict compliance at every visit

Educate family members to support treatment plan

Use of modified DOT

Monitoring of Therapy[11]

Decisions regarding initiation or changes in ART should ideally be guided by monitoring plasma HIV RNA and CD4+ T cell count, as well as clinical condition of the patient. These laboratory parameters should be repeated every 3-6 months in patients who have not been initiated on ART. If the first values of HIV RNA and CD4+ cell count indicate requirement to start ART, a repeat measurement of these parameters is recommended before initiating the treatment. After initiation of ART, HIV RNA should be measured at 4-8 weeks to assess the efficacy of treatment, as there should be a large decline in viral load during this period. The viral load should continue to decline after that and by 16-20 weeks, it should be undetectable (i.e., < 50 RNA copies/mL). The rate of viral load decline is affected by the initial viral load, baseline CD4+ cell count, potency of regimen used and presence of any opportunistic infections and prior exposure to ART. However, absence of decline of this magnitude should prompt the clinician to reassess the situation which includes reassessment of patient, check compliance of treatment, rule out intestinal malabsorption and confirm HIV RNA levels by repeating the test. If compliance and absorption can be assured, a change in the regimen should be considered. A minimally significant change in plasma HIV RNA is considered to be a 3-fold or 0.5 $\log_{10}$ increase or decrease. A significant decrease in CD4+ cell count is a decrease of > 30% from baseline for absolute cell numbers and a decrease of > 3% from baseline in percentage of cells.

Drug Resistance[11]

Testing for viral resistance to antiretroviral drugs may help to maximize the benefits of ART. Drug resistance can be identified by either genotypic or phenotypic assays. Genotypic assays detect drug resistance mutations present in the RT and protease genes of HIV and the results can be reported within 1-2 weeks. Phenotypic assays measure the ability of HIV to grow in different concentrations of antiretroviral drugs and the results are available in 2-3 weeks. However, phenotypic assays are costlier and more difficult than genotypic assays.

Drug resistance assays are potentially useful in acute HIV infection and in selecting active drugs when changing ART in the setting of treatment failure or in cases in which viral load suppression is suboptimal after initiation of ART.[17]

Changing Antiretroviral Treatment[11]

Change in ART is required if there is a suboptimal reduction in HIV RNA after initiation of treatment, re-appearance of viremia after initial suppression and decline in CD4 cell counts. Less than a 0.5-0.75 $\log_{10}$ reduction in HIV RNA at 4 weeks or less than 1 $\log_{10}$ reduction at 8 weeks of therapy or failure to suppress HIV RNA to undetectable levels at 4-6 months of therapy indicate inadequate response and warrant change of therapy. If the patient is unable to tolerate one of the agents, it should be changed with another agent while other agents should be continued. However, in case of failure of therapy, it is important to use at least two new drugs and preferably to change all the drugs and use an entirely new regimen. Ritonavir should not be changed to indinavir and vice versa since high level of cross-resistance is likely between these two drugs. Similarly, changing among NNRTI is not recommended for the same reason.

Interruption of HAART[11]

There has been recent interest in the area of stopping HAART temporarily. This is called supervised or structured treatment interruption (STI). It encompasses three major strategies: salvage STI, STI for auto-immunization and better immune control of HIV, and STI for reducing total time on HAART. Salvage STI indicates stopping HAART in patients who do not respond to ART. The idea is to allow replication of sensitive strains of HIV so that HAART can be restarted. Auto-immunization STI and STI to reduce total time on HAART are directed to patients who have maintained viral suppression below detection limit for a long time.

The theoretical goal is to allow several short bursts of viral replication to augment HIV-specific immune responses. However, at present none of these strategies are recommended.

Role of Hydroxyurea

Hydroxyurea inhibits the cellular enzymes ribonucleotide reductase resulting in reduced intracellular levels of deoxynucleoside triphopshates (dNTPs) that are necessary for DNA synthesis. This also results in incomplete reverse transcription of HIV genome in the infected cells. This action may enhance the antiretroviral effects of (ddI)and d4T. A few uncontrolled studies have shown some clinical utility of adding hydroxyurea to a regimen containing ddI+d4T.[18] In contrast, some controlled studies have not shown any benefit of adding hydroxyurea to a triple-drug regimen containing ddI and d4T.[19] In fact, the incidence of development of toxicity was higher in hydroxyurea group. However, since hydroxyurea is relatively cheap, it could be a part of ART regimens provided further studies show its efficacy in the treatment of HIV infection.

HAART and Antitubercular Drugs

PI and NNRTI are antiretroviral agents that may inhibit or induce cytochrome P-450 isoenzymes (CYP450). Rifampicin induces CYP450 and may decrease substantially the blood levels of antiretroviral drugs. The pharmacologic interactions are called "drug-drug" because, in addition to the effect, rifampicin has on PI and NNRTI, the antiretroviral agents may affect the blood levels of rifampicin. The other class of antiretroviral agents, NRTI is not metabolized by CYP450. Concurrent use of NRTI and rifampicin is not contraindicated and does not require dose adjustments. Rifampicin can be used for the treatment of active TB in three situations: (1) in a patient whose antiretroviral regimen includes the NNRTI efavirenz and two NRTI; (2) in a patient whose antiretroviral regimen includes the PI ritonavir and one or more NRTI; or (3) in a patient whose antiretroviral regimen includes the combination of two PI (ritonavir and saquinavir).

Rifabutin may be used in a dose of 300 mg/day in a selected group of patients on HAART i.e. those taking NRTI, NVP and SQV alone. However, its dose should be reduced to 150 mg two or three times per week when it is administered to patients taking ritonavir or ritonavir/lopinavir and to 150 mg once a day when used with IDV or NFV (dose of IDV and NFV is increased to 1000 mg tid). On the other hand, its dose should be increased to either 450 mg or 600 mg daily or 600 mg two or three times per week when rifabutin is used concurrently with efavirenz.

Management of HIV/AIDS in pregnancy is discussed in chapter 7.

Antiretroviral Therapy in Resource-Poor Nations

It is estimated that nearly 36 .million people in the developing countries are currently living with HIV/AIDS of which nearly 6 million people require ART. Unfortunately, due to resource limitations, only about 230,000 have access to these drugs. By the end of 2005, the developing world should be able to have 3 million people on ART so as to make an impact on the prevalence and transmission of HIV infection in these countries. Scaling up will not be possible in the absence of a clear public health approach that promotes the rational and safe use of antiretroviral agents. Drug access for the millions of poor people can be improved not only by guidance on the rational selection and use of ARV drugs, but also by providing accessibility to competent health services and cheaper drugs. Fortunately, at present most of the ARV drugs are available and the cost of these drugs has reduced remarkably over the past 2-3 years. Another limiting factor in a developing country is the high cost required for performing repeated HIV RNA tests and CD4+ cell counts. Important strategies for increasing the accessibility of antiretroviral agents in resource-limited settings include:

1. Scaling up of antiretroviral treatment programmes to meet the needs of people living with HIV
2. *Standardization* and simplification of ART regimens to support the efficient implementation of treatment programmes
3. Ensuring ART based on scientific evidence in order to avoid substandard treatment so as to avoid emergence of drug resistant virus

Indications for Initiating ART

The WHO recommends that in resource poor settings, HIV infected people should be offered treatment when they have:

1. WHO stage IV disease (clinical AIDS), regardless of CD4+ cell counts
2. WHO stage I, II or III of HIV disease with a CD4+ cell count below 200/mm^3
3. WHO stage II or III of HIV disease with total lymphocyte count <1200/mm^3

The countries are encouraged to use CD4+ cell counts instead of HIV RNA levels in monitoring the patients. If facilities to count CD4+ cells are not available, total lymphocyte count may be used to make decision regarding initiation of ART.

First Line Regimens

Antiretroviral treatment should be standardized in a developing nation. The country should select a single first line ART and a limited number of second line regimens so that large number of patients can be treated. Considerations in the selection of a regimen should carefully evaluate its potency, side effects, anticipated adherence, effects of co-existing conditions in the population (e.g., infections particularly tuberculosis), potential drug interactions, cost and the availability of health care facilities. Based on these considerations, the preferred first line ARV regimens are listed below:

Zidovudine + Lamivudine + Nevirapine

Stavudine + Lamivudine + Nevirapine

Zidovudine + Lamivudine + Efavirenz (should not be used in women of child-bearing age)

Zidovudine + Lamivudine + Nelfinavir

Zidovudine + Lamivudine + Ritonavir + Indinavir

Zidovudine + Lamivudine + Ritonavir + Lopinavir

Zidovudine + Lamivudine + Ritonavir + Saquinavir

It must be noted that use of only two NRT combination is not recommended even in resource limited areas since these regimens do not suppress viral replication adequately and are likely to produce resistance rapidly.

To enhance adherence, combination of drugs in a single pill is recommended. The family and community members should be asked to encourage the patient to take the pills regularly.

Second Line Antiretroviral Regimens

In a resource limited setting where viral loads are difficult to perform, treatment failure is evaluated primarily on the basis of clinical response and where possible CD4+ cell count. The second line regimens generally include a ritonavir enhanced PI combination. NFV can be considered as an alternative for PI component if RTV-enhanced PI is not available. The NRTI components in the regimen should also be changed, e.g., ZDV/3TC can replace d4T/3TC and vice-versa though there may be cross resistance among various NRTI. ABC/ddI can also be used in place of ZDV/3TC or d4T/3TC combination.

It is recommended that countries planning to implement ART programmes should also implement an HIV drug resistance surveillance programme so as to detect potential drug resistance at the population level and modify the recommendations as and when required.

Monitoring of Antiretroviral Treatment

A few baseline tests are mandatory before initiating ART. Haemoglobin level should be ascertained as zidovudine, one of the most frequently used NRTI, can produce anaemia as one of its side effects. Other tests include a white cell count and differential (to permit assessment of neutropenic side effects and to get baseline total lymphocyte count), serum transaminases (to assess the possibility of hepatitis), serum creatinine or blood urea (to assess baseline renal function), serum glucose and in women, pregnancy test. If facilities are available, CD4+ cell counts and lipid profile should be done. Follow up of patients on ART should include a detailed clinical examination and total lymphocyte counts.

Tuberculosis and Antiretroviral Treatment

Tuberculosis is common in patients from a resource limited country and this may complicate the use of ARV treatment. WHO recommends that people with tuberculosis and HIV should complete their treatment for tuberculosis prior to beginning ARV treatment unless there is a high risk of HIV progression and death during that period (i.e., CD4+ cell count <200/mm³ or disseminated tuberculosis). The recommendations for treating HIV infection in a patient with tuberculosis are shown in Table 6.

Post Exposure Prophylaxis

Refer to Appendix VI.

Table 6.   Treatment of Tuberculosis in HIV patients in a Resource-limited Country

Situation	Recommendations
Pulmonary tuberculosis and CD4+ cells >200/mm³ or total lymphocyte count >1200/mm³	Treat tuberculosis. Monitor CD4 cell counts if available. Start ARV after completion of antitubercular treatment (ATT)
Pulmonary tuberculosis with CD4+ cells 50-200/mm³ or total lymphocyte count < 1200/mm³	Start (ATT) After 2 months of ATT, add one of the following ARV regimens: ZDV+3TC+NVP ZDV+3TC+EFV ZDV+3TC+ABC ZDV+3TC+SQV+RTV
Pulmonary tuberculosis and CD4+ cells <50/mm³ or disseminated tuberculosis	Start ATT. As soon as patient can tolerate ATT, add one of the above-mentioned ARV regimens

Conclusion

Advances in pathogenesis of HIV and development of new, potent drug regimens have resulted in more effective therapies for HIV infection. Use of newer modalities (alone or in combination) of treatment may lead to the ultimate goal of curing HIV infection.

References

1. Powderly WJ. The pathogenesis of HIV infection. In: Powderly WJ, edr. Manual of HIV therapeutics. 2nd ed. Philadelphia: Lippincott William & Wilkins; 2001. p. 23-34.
2. Fischl MA, Richman DD, Hansen N, et al. The safety and efficacy of zidovudine (AZT) in the treatment of subjects with mildly symptomatic human immunodeficiency virus type 1 (HIV) infection. A double blind, placebo-controlled trial. AIDS Clinical Trial Group. Ann Intern Med 1990; 112: 727-737.
3. Hamilton JD, Hartigan PM, Simberkoff MS, et al. A controlled trial of early versus late treatment with zidovudine in symptomatic human immunodeficiency virus infection. Results of the Veterans Affairs Cooperative Study. N Engl J Med 1992; 326: 437-443.
4. Richman DD. Resistance of clinical isolates of human immunodeficiency virus to antiretroviral agents. Antimicrobial Agents Chemother 1993; 37: 1207-1213.
5. Safrin S. Antiviral agents. In: Katzung BG, edr. Basic and

Clinical Pharmacology. 8th ed. New York: Mc Graw Hill; 2001. p. 823-843.

6. Chaudry MN, Shepp DH. Antiretroviral agents. Current usage. Dermatol Clin 1997; 15: 319-329.

7. Ritche DJ. Antiretroviral agents. In: Powderly WJ, edr. Manual of HIV therapeutics. 2nd ed. Philadelphia: Lippincott Williams and Wilkins; 2001. p 33-47

8. Fortgang IS, Belitsos PC, Chaisson RE, Moore RD. Hepatomegaly and steatosis in HIV-infected patients receiving nucleoside analog antiretroviral therapy. Am J Gastroenterol 1995; 90: 1433-1436.

9. Harris M, Tesiorowski A, Chan K, et al. Lactic acidosis complicating antiretroviral therapy: Frequency and correlates. Antiviral Therapy 2000; 5 (Suppl 2): 31.

10. Guidelines for the use of Antiretroviral agents in HIV-infected adults and adolescents. Feb 2002. www.aidsinfo.com

11. Brown TJ, Straten MV, Tyring SK. Antiviral Agents. Dermatol Clin 2001; 19: 23-34.

12. Moyle G, Gazzard B. Current knowledge and future prospects for the use of HIV protease inhibitors. Drugs 1996; 51: 701-712.

13. Gazzard B, Moyle G. The role of HIV-protease inhibitors. Genitourin Med 1996; 72: 233-235.

14. Carr A, Samaras K, Thorisdottir A, et al. Diagnosis, prediction and natural course of HIV-1 protease-inhibitor associated lipodystrophy, hyperlipidemia and diabetes mellitus: a cohort study. Lancet 1999; 353: 2093-2099.

15. Gulick RM, Mellors JW, Havlir D, et al. Treatment with indinavir, zidovudine and lamivudine in adults with human immunodeficiency virus infection and prior antiretroviral therapy. N Engl J Med 1997; 337: 734-399.

16. Hammer SM, Squires KE, Hughes MD, et al. A controlled trial of two nucleoside analogues plus indinavir in persons with human immunodeficiency virus infection and CD4 cell counts of 200 per cubic milliliter or less. N Engl J Med 1997; 337: 7225-733.

17. Durant J, Clevenbergh, Halfon P, et al. Drug-resistance genotyping in HIV-1 therapy: The VIRADAPT randomized controlled trial. Lancet 1999; 353: 2195-2199.

18. Montaner JS, Zala C, Conway B, et al. A pilot study of hydroxyurea among patients with advanced human immunodeficiency virus (HIV) disease receiving chronic didanosine therapy: Canadian HIV trials network protocol 080. J Infect Dis 1997; 175: 801-806.

19. Weissman SB, Sinclair GI, Green CL, Fissell WH. Hydroxyurea-induced hepatitis in human immunodeficiency virus-positive patients. Clin Infect Dis 1999; 29: 223-224.

Chapter 7

HIV/AIDS in Pregnancy and Children

K Neeladri Raju

Introduction

HIV infection in pregnant women has become a serious health concern, as it has been associated with mother-to child transmission (MTCT). Our knowledge about HIV infection in pregnant women and children has been limited in the early period and the recent research with antiretroviral drug prophylaxis has shown tremendous potential for cutting down MTCT and reducing the load of childhood HIV infection.

Epidemiology

The first Acquired Immunodeficiency Syndrome (AIDS) case in the female was reported in 1981.[1] The global HIV pandemic affected thirty six million people by December 2000, half of them being women. Perinatal transmission of human immunodeficiency virus was first described in 1982,[2] and transmission through breast milk had been proposed in 1985.[3] UNAIDS and WHO in December 2000 estimated that 55% of women in Sub-Saharan Africa and 40% in North and Middle-East Africa, 35% in South and South East Asia and 13% in East Asia and Pacific have been infected with HIV. In India the HIV epidemic has shown varied distribution in women attending antenatal and STD clinics. Sentinel Surveillance of state-wise HIV prevalence in women attending antenatal clinics in 2000 showed highest rate of 2.6% in Andhra Pradesh and 2% in Mumbai. Tamil Nadu, Karnataka, Maharashtra and Nagaland have shown less than 2% prevalence rate. Kerala, Punjab, Sikkim and Meghalaya have shown zero percent prevalence. The States, in which antenatal prevalence is more than 1%, are called as high prevalence States. UNAIDS and WHO estimated that in India 0.6 million children

have been newly infected with HIV in the year 2000 and 1.4 million children were estimated to be living with HIV/AIDS. HIV/AIDS epidemic has spread in India among pregnant women and children with serious economic and psychological consequences.

HIV in Pregnancy

Effect of Pregnancy on HIV Status

There is a recent evidence that AIDS may be made slightly worse by pregnancy. Immune system is affected by physiological changes of pregnancy irrespective of the HIV status. The CD4 cell count reaches the nadir at 32 weeks of gestation followed by rebound in the postpartum period. Some studies have suggested that pregnancy may hasten the development of AIDS in those infected with the virus, but these findings are yet to be confirmed further.

Effect of HIV on Pregnancy

The outcome of pregnancy is also marginally affected by HIV seropositivity status. Some studies have reported links between HIV and poor obstetric outcome and are due to coexistent confounding factors (e.g., IV drug abuse, other STD). But some studies have reported slightly higher risk of pregnancy not leading to full term and increased risk of spontaneous abortion, still birth, perinatal mortality, intrauterine growth retardation (IUGR) and prematurity.

The earlier reports of AIDS defining opportunistic infections in pregnant women had shown that they have uniformly poor prognosis, but the population-based studies have not shown the same.

Perinatal Transmission of HIV

HIV transmission during the perinatal period occurs in intrauterine, intrapartum periods and through breast feeding. The rate of perinatal transmission of HIV has been observed to range from 13 to 40%. HIV has been isolated in foetal tissues as early as 8 weeks of gestation, from amniotic fluid, thymus, lung, spleen and brain of 15 to 20 weeks foetus but pathologic description of various foetal tissues and placenta was not well documented. Antibodies to HIV have been demonstrated in amniotic fluid at 24-27 weeks of gestation and it suggests the role of intrauterine transmission of HIV.

Transplacental infection occurs when the maternal virus or cell associated virus pass through trophoblasts and enter foetal circulation. HIV infects placental macrophages and trophoblasts which bear CD4+ on their surface and is likely to cause their dysfunction and contribute to immunological abnormalities seen in HIV/AIDS. It is likely that chorioamnionitis may increase the "leakiness" of trophoblast barrier and act as a risk factor for increased transmission of HIV. In spite of exposure of trophoblast cells to maternal blood, the rate (30%) of transmission of HIV is low, which may be due to the presence of neutralizing antibodies.

Intrapartum Transmission

HIV transmission at the time of delivery is through contact with blood and cervicovaginal secretions. International registry of HIV showed that first born twin was two times more likely to be infected, because the first twin comes in contact with cervix and maternal secretions for a longer duration compared to the second twin during labour. Prolonged exposure of infant's skin and mucous membrane to maternal blood during delivery would facilitate HIV transmission to infant.

Postnatal Exposure to Breast Milk

Breast milk contains both cell associated and cell free virus. Viruses can also be isolated from colostrum. Both colostrum and breast milk have been implicated in the transmission of HIV from mother to infant through breast feeding.

Risk Factors of MTCT

Several risk factors have been shown to contribute to MTCT. Maternal factors such as advanced stage, high viral load, low CD_4 count, decreased CD_4-CD_8 ratio, low titre of HIV specific antibody and low HIV specific cellular immunity may play a role in the transmission of the disease to the foetus. The role of monocytotropic or T-cell tropic HIV strains in the vertical transmission is unclear. Placental factors like a tear in the placenta, chorioamnionitis, placental cell susceptibility to HIV infection, presence of STD have been associated with increased transmission rates.

The obstetrical and foetal risk factors for MTCT are prolonged rupture of membranes, premature delivery, invasive foetal monitoring with exposure of foetus to microcirculation of maternal blood such as foetal scalp electrodes, scalp blood sampling and obstetric procedures episiotomy and operative vaginal delivery. It also appears that duration of ruptured membranes enhances the transmission rate to foetus. The perinatal transmission risk increases by 2% for every one hour increase in the duration of membrane rupture in an infected women with less than 24 hours of membrane rupture. The role of caesarean section needs further study. Preterm delivery before 34 weeks of pregnancy has two fold risk of transmission to foetus because of low levels of passively transferred maternal antibodies. Vitamin A deficiency is associated with increased rate of HIV transmission because of its effect on immune function, integrity of placenta and transfer of maternal antibodies to foetus. Further studies are needed to confirm these findings.

Prevention of Vertical Transmission

Prevention of vertical transmission can be aimed at intrauterine, intrapartum and postpartum period. This may be done through reduction of maternal viral load during pregnancy, chemoprophylaxis of infant during and after delivery and avoidance of breast feeding.

Chemoprophylaxis with antiretroviral therapy has shown promising results in preventing MTCT. PACTG 076 results on ZDV chemoprophylaxis reported that perinatal transmission rate for infants on placebo therapy was 22.6% when compared with 7.6% for infants who received ZDV, a 66% reduction in risk for transmission. Oral ZDV was recommended 100 mg orally five times daily or 200 mg orally three times or 300 mg twice daily between 14-34 weeks of gestation to HIV infected pregnant women during the antenatal period and intrapartum loading dose of ZDV 2 mg/kg IV over 1 hour followed by 1 mg/kg/hour until delivery plus oral therapy of ZDV to infant with 2 mg/kg every 6 hrs (total 8 mg/kg/day) for 6 weeks, beginning at 8-12 hrs after birth in asymptomatic ZDV-naive women with CD4 counts above 200/mm.[3] This therapy may be beneficial in women with advanced HIV disease and low CD4+ cell count <200/mm[3]. Intrapartum intravenous ZDV followed by 6 weeks of ZDV for the newborn can be recommended in women who have no prior antiretroviral therapy in pregnancy. A six-week neonatal ZDV therapy should be discussed with the mother who has not taken antiretroviral therapy during pregnancy or intrapartum period.

Clinical trials conducted in Thailand with a short course of ZDV to prevent MTCT in non breast feeding women, offered oral ZDV in a dosage of 300 mg twice a day from 36 weeks of gestation and 300 mg every 3 hours during labour and no zidovudine was given to the infant. Perinatal transmission of HIV was reduced by 50 percent with this therapy.[5] This regimen is cheap and can be used in developing countries. PETRA trial in Africa which was done in breast feeding women with a combination regimen of ZDV and 3 TC starting at 36 weeks gestation, orally intrapartum and one week postpartum for the mother and the infant reduced transmission by approximately 50% compared to placebo at age six weeks. In the same trial, it was also observed that, when the above combination was administered in intrapartum and postpartum period the reduction of transmission was 40%, but when administered only during intrapartum period there was no effect in reduction of transmission.[6]

A short course nevirapine regimen can be administered in pregnant women who are in labour and who have not received any antiretroviral therapy during pregnancy. HIV NET 012 trial which was again done in breast feeding population, demonstrated that a single dose of oral nevirapine 200 mg to the women at the onset of labour and single 2 mg/kg oral dose to the infant at age 48-72 hrs when compared to oral zidovudine given every 3 hours during labour and to the infant for 7 days reduced transmission by 50%. Nevirapine has a long half-life and appears to be more effective in reducing vertical transmission than short course of ZDV therapy. These two clinical trials have shown that the addition of single dose nevirapine regimen to short course ZDV may provide increased efficacy in reduction of perinatal transmission.[6]

It is apparent that several regimen can reduce the vertical transmission of HIV, the selection of regimen depends on drug availability, past history of treatment, period of gestation at diagnosis or reporting to health care provider. Single drug regimens carry the risk of development of resistant strains.

Correlation of HIV-1 RNA levels with risk for disease progression in non pregnant adult, warrant that HIV-1 RNA should be monitored during pregnancy at least as often as recommended for non pregnant states, i.e. approximately once in each trimester. In a cohort of 198 HIV-1 infected women, it was observed that HIV-I RNA levels were higher at six months post partum compared to ante-partum period, regardless of ZDV prophylaxis. There are conflicting datas regarding viral load and perinatal transmisson. But one important aspect from the studies like PACTG O76 and few smaller studies, showed that regardless of the HIV-1 RNA load, the perinatal transmission reduced with ZDV prophylaxis. Thus, at a minimum ZDV prophylaxis should be offered to all infected women, and RNA levels should not be a determining factor to use ZDV prophylaxis.[6]

Caesarean section may play a role in the prevention of intrapartum transmission of HIV. Transmission to foetus at a rate of 3.4% can occur even when maternal HIV-RNA levels are below the detectable levels (500 copies/ml or less). Scheduled caesarean section can be recommended when the viral load is above 1000 copies/ ml. ACOG has recommended scheduled caesarean delivery at 38 weeks of gestation to prevent HIV transmission. Several studies showed that elective or scheduled caesarean section performed before the onset of labour and rupture of membranes would reduce the transmission rate by 55-80%. But, it is also to be kept in consideration that risk of foetal lung immaturity is possible when delivered at 38 weeks. The risks and benefits of scheduled caesarean section should be weighed as well as the patient's option of whether to undergo a caesarean section or vaginal delivery, has to taken into consideration. Non elective caesarean section was not associated with significant reduction in transmission compared to vaginal delivery. The role of caesarean section among women with non-detectable viral load or with short duration of ruptured membranes has not been determined.[6]

The role of cleansing the vagina during labour with topical chlorhexidine solution in reducing genital tract viral load and perinatal transmission rate has been studied. This study did not show any significant benefit in reducing the transmission rate when compared to untreated group.[7] Several studies found that STD and genital tract infections more often have been associated with increase in vaginal viral load and enhanced the intrapartum transmission rate when compared with women without these infections.[6]

Post partum follow up of women is an essential part of management. All women should receive comprehensive health care services that continue after delivery for their own medical care and for family planning and contraception. Counselling regarding strict adherence to antiretroviral therapy, when required should be emphasized. In addition, it is an invaluable period to review immunization status and update vaccines schedules, assessing the need for prophylaxis against opportunistic infections, and re-emphasis on safer sex practices. And women who have received ZDV prophylaxis, should be reevaluated for ARV during postpartum period.[6]

Breast milk acts as a source of HIV, breast-feeding is not recommended in developed nations. However it is recommended in developing countries where the patients cannot afford expenditure on commercial infant formula. Modified breast milk can be made by boiling it to 62.5 degrees celsius for 30 minutes. Alternatively cow's milk can be given to the infant by adding 50 ml of water to 100 ml of milk with 10 g of sugar. Fifty ml of buffalo milk can be mixed with 50 ml of water and 5 g of sugar and can be used as an alternative. However home made formulas should be supplemented with micronutrients such as VitA, VitC, iron, folic acid and zinc.

Management

Detailed history and thorough physical examination should be carried out at the first visit for HIV positive pregnant women. Pelvic examination should be done to detect STD especially due to *N.gonorrhoeae*, *C.trachomatis*, syphilis and cervical cytology to document neoplasia. Tuberculin skin test should be offered to all HIV positive pregnant women if the test was not done within the past year. Laboratory tests that include complete blood picture, CD4 to CD8 T-lymphocyte ratio, absolute CD4+ count, CD4+ percentage, HIV-I RNA loads, antibody determination for toxoplasma, CMV, VDRL and HbsAg, Cryptococcal antigens should be obtained at the first visit.

During subsequent visits evaluate for STD especially for syphilis and perform CD4+ count in each trimester and offer ZDV if the CD4 count is above 200/mm[3] PCP prophylaxis is indicated if CD4 count is less than

200/mm[3]. The drug of choice is TMP-SMX, one double strength tablet daily. Aerosolized pentamidine 300 mg monthly is an effective prophylaxis. Oral dapsone 100 mg daily is considered to be an effective alternative.

Prophylaxis for opportunistic infections is a challenging issue in HIV positive pregnant women. Prophylaxis for toxoplasmosis is indicated when the CD4 count is less than 100 cells/mm[3] and the regimen includes TMP-SMX one double strength tablet daily. Chemoprophylaxis with isoniazid 300mg daily or twice weekly is recommended in HIV positive pregnant women with a positive tuberculin skin test or history of exposure to active TB, after active TB has been excluded. Pregnant women with salmonella gastroenteritis should be offered treatment as extraintestinal spread might lead to infection of placenta. The recommended treatment is with ampicillin, ceftriaxone or TMP-SMX. Chemoprophylaxis against oropharyngeal, esophageal or vaginal candidiasis with systemic azoles is contraindicated during pregnancy. Oral acyclovir prophylaxis for herpes genitalis in pregnant women is a controversial issue. VZIG can be recommended in VZV susceptible pregnant women within 96 hrs after exposure to VZV. Intrapartum and post partum management has been discussed earlier.

HIV in Children

Transmission in Children

Perinatal transmission is the predominant mode of transmission of HIV to children. The other less common routes of transmission are through blood transfusion and sexual abuse. Close child-to-child contact with extensive exposure to blood or body fluids may likely be a rare mode of transmission. Hence universal precautions need to be undertaken to prevent exposure of blood or body fluids. Isolation procedures are not recommended for HIV infected children in school or day care settings as no cases of HIV transmission have been reported.

Breast feeding has been accounted for 5-15% perinatal transmission in population with infant feeding practices. Some observational studies have found that, when the mother was infected prenatally the additional risk of transmission through breast milk would be 14% compared to 29% increased risk of transmission in woman infected with HIV postnatally. The risk of HIV to the breast fed infant was reported to be 0.7% per month during the first 6 months of life and decreased with the time and this could be due to immaturity of the immune system with high cellular content in early breast milk.

Colostrum intake may play a lesser role in the transmission of HIV through breast milk because of its contents like IgA, IgM and high levels of Vit A. These antibodies and Vit A has some neutralizing activity against HIV. It was demonstrated that epidermal growth factor in breast milk played a protective role by enhancing the maturation and integrity of gut epithelium and thus preventing the entry of HIV. Oral sores in newborns, neonatal hypochlorhydria, cracked nipple, mastitis may facilitate HIV transmission while breast feeding. Prolonged breast feeding may enhance the risk of HIV transmission to the infant. High HIV RNA viral load and lower CD4+ count in the breast milk may be a risk factor in the transmission of HIV to the infant.

Glycosaminoglycans found in breast milk could be protective, as it inhibits the binding of CD4+ to HIV envelope glycoprotiens.

Clinical Manifestations

HIV infected children show different pattern of clinical manifestations. CDC case definition for paediatric HIV classification was based on two parameters: clinical status and immunological status in developed countries.

Many children with HIV do not grow or gain weight normally. They usually suffer from childhood bacterial infections. These bacterial infections cause fever, diarrhoea, dehydration, pneumonia and seizures. Candidiasis that can cause oral thrush and diaper skin rash is frequently found in children with HIV. As the disease progresses neurological manifestation such as

Table 1. 1994 Revised Human Immunodeficiency Virus Infection-Paediatric Classification System

CLINICAL CATEGORIES

Category N: Not Symptomatic
Children who have no signs or symptoms considered to be the result of HIV infection or who have only one of the conditions listed in category A.

Category A: Mildly Symptomatic
Children with two or more of the following conditions but none of the conditions listed in categories B and C:

- Lymphadenopathy ($\geq$ 0.5 cm at more than two sites; bilateral-one site)
- Hepatomegaly • Splenomegaly • Dermatitis • Parotitis
- Recurrent or persistent upper respiratory infection, sinusitis, or otitis media.

Category B: Moderately Symptomatic
Children who have symptomatic conditions, other than those listed for category A or category C, that are attributed to HIV infection. Examples of conditions in clinical category B include but are not limited to the following:

- Anaemia (<8gm/dL), neutropenia (<1,000/mm^3), or thrombocytopenia (<100,000/mm^3) persisting $\geq$30 days. • Bacterial meningitis, pneumonia, or sepsis (single episode) • Candidiasis, oropharyngeal (i.e. thrush) persisting for >2 months in children aged >6 months •   Cardiomyopathy
- Cytomegalovirus infection with onset before one month of age
- Diarrhoea, recurrent or chronic • Hepatitis • Herpes simplex virus (HSV) stomatitis, recurrent (i.e. more than two episodes within one year) • HSV bronchitis, pneumonitis, or esophagitis with onset before age one month. • Herpes zoster (i.e., shingles) involving at least two distinct episodes or more than one dermatome. • Leiomyosarcoma • Lymphoid interstitial pneumonitis (LIP) or pulmonary lymphoid hyperplasia complex • Nephropathy • Nocardiosis • Fever lasting >1 month • Toxoplasmosis with onset before one month of age • Varicella, disseminated (i.e. complicated chickenpox)

Category C: Severely Symptomatic
Children who have any condition listed in the 1987 surveillance case definition for acquired immunodeficiency syndrome, with the exception of LIP (which is a category B condition).

Centres for Disease Control and Prevention. 1994 Revised classification system for human immunodeficiency virus infection in children less than 13 years of age (MMWR, 1994. 43 (No. RR-12): p. 1-10. Most of the HIV infected children are asymptomatic at birth.

difficulty in walking, seizures and other symptoms of HIV encephalopathy may be present. Motor skills and mental development such as speaking may be delayed.

CDC established a revised classification system of clinical manifestations in children in 1994, which is being used till date. Among the clinical categories, category N includes children with no signs or symptoms of HIV. Category A includes children with two or more of conditions listed in Table 1 and none of the conditions listed in category B or C. Category B is moderately symptomatic and the conditions listed are other than those in category A and C. Category C includes children with severely symptomatic AIDS-defining clinical conditions except lymphoid interstitial pneumonitis (LIP) which is included in category B. Paediatric AIDS diagnosis in developing nations are based on clinical criteria published by WHO where diagnostic facilities for HIV are limited.

WHO Case Definition for Paediatric AIDS

Major signs

- Weight loss or failure to thrive
- Diarrhoea more than one month
- Unexplained fever more than one month

Minor signs

- Generalized lymphadenopathy
- Oropharyngeal candidiasis
- Repeated common infections (otitis, pharyngitis etc)
- Persistent cough for more than one month
- Generalized dermatitis
- Confirmed HIV infection in mother

Paediatric infection is suspected when 2 major signs are associated with atleast 2 minor signs. The specificity of this definition is 80%, but the sensitivity is only 40%.

The association of HIV RNA copies with long term risk for death in HIV infected children have been determined. The risk is highest (71%) when viral load was more than 10^6 and low (24%) when the viral load is undetectable (< 4,000). Similarly association of baseline CD_4+T cell percentage to HIV RNA copies, found that death rate in children in HIV RNA levels of > 10^5 and CD_4+ > 15% was 36%, while it was 81% if the CD_4+ was < 15%. On the contrary, the death rate in children

with HIV RNA levels of < 10^5 and CD_4+ > 15%, while it was 63% if the CD_4+ was < 15%.[6]

Two different patterns of disease progression have been observed by researchers. In the first group about 20% of children develop serious infection in the first year of life. This group is characterized by rapid progression of the disease and most of the children die in the first 4 years of life. In the remaining 80% of HIV infected children, HIV related symptoms develop at a slower rate and many of them do not develop serious symptoms of AIDS until school age or even adolescence. Opportunistic infections are more often observed in HIV infected children with severe decline in CD4+ count. In children opportunistic infections present as primary infection whereas in adults they represent reactivation of a latent infection.

Variations in Clinical Features and Opportunistic Infections

Clinical manifestations of HIV in children may greatly vary from that of adults. Thrush is the most common manifestation and it occurs in more than 80% of HIV infected children. It frequently extends to oesophagus and also disseminates. In children recurrent bacterial infections, PCP and LIP are more commonly encountered opportunistic infections than in adults. Failure to grow and thrive may occur in children while adults may have HIV related wasting. CNS manifestations occur in the early stage of HIV infection in children while AIDS dementia complex occurs late in adults. Malignancies are uncommon in children. Children may develop opportunistic infections at higher CD4 cell counts than adults. Parotitis is a concern in paediatric HIV and children are more likely to have enlarged liver, spleen and lymphnodes.

The clinical profile of HIV infection among the children in Mumbai, India is given in Table 2.

Opportunistic Infections and Systemic Manifestions in Children

Opportunistic infections in HIV infected children have been associated with immunodeficiency and may be caused by bacterial, fungal, viral and protozoal pathogens. The commonly encountered systemic manifestation in paediatric HIV are discussed here.

Table 2. Clinical Profile of HIV Infection in Children Attending HIV Clinic in Mumbai

Clinical Features	Prevalence
Protein Energy Malnutrition	44.56%
Pulmonary & extra pulmonary tuberculosis	29.47%
Hepatosplenomegaly	28.77%
Lymphadenopathy	23.50%
Skin Lesions	22.10%
Chronic diarrhoea	15.08%
Oral thrush	14.73%
Pyrexia	12.63%
Chronic Lung disease	11.22%
Chronic hypertrophic parotitis	9.47%
Chronic ottorrhoea	9.12%
Recurrent lower respiratory tract	8.42%
Neurological manifestations (non tuberculosis)	4.56%
Pneumocystis carinii pneumonia	3.88%
Asymptomatic	16.84%
Death due to AIDS	10.52%

Adapted from Merchant RH, Oswal JS, Bhagwat RV, Karkare J. Clinical profile of HIV infection. Indian Pediatr 2001: 38: 239-246.

Bacterial Infections

Bacterial infections in HIV infected children are caused by *Streptococcus pneumoniae, H. influenzae, Salmonella spp.* Staphylococcus and *Pseudomonas aeruginosa.* These bacterial infections may be related to immune disturbances with altered T and B Lymphocyte functions. Abnormal B cell function results in disturbances in chemotactic and bactericidal function of neutrophils and macrophages. The common bacterial infections in children with HIV are sinusitis, pneumonia, skin and soft tissue infection, otitis media and bacteremia. Catheter related infections are most commonly encountered due to staphylococcus. It has been reported that antiretroviral therapy lowered the frequency of bacterial infections. Daily prophylaxis with TMP 150 mg/m^2/day in two divided doses may be given to prevent recurrent bacterial infections.

In HIV infected children with hypogammaglobulinemia intravenous immunoglobulin (IVIG) (IgG 400 mg/kg/day) should be used to prevent serious bacterial infections.

Tuberculosis

It is one of the most common opportunistic infections in HIV infected children. *M. tuberculosis* spreads via respiratory droplets. The clinical features are characterized by fever, cough, dyspnoea on exertion, night sweats and weight loss. Extrapulmonary tuberculosis may occur in various organs such as lymphnodes, central nervous system and bone. The other manifestations of tuberculosis are miliary tuberculosis, tuberculous meningitis, genitourinary tuberculosis and the other sites that can be affected are skin, soft tissues and viscera. Disseminated disease more commonly occurs in patients with low CD$_4$ count. Skin reaction with induration of >5 mm to a standard PPD is considered positive in HIV infected children. In patients with low CD$_4$ counts, cutaneous anergy to Mantoux test may give negative results and this cannot be used to rule out tuberculosis. The progression of HIV infection is more rapid in tuberculosis patients and the level of plasma viremia declines with treatment of tuberculosis. Sputum for acid-fast bacilli (AFB) positivity is more common in HIV positive children than in HIV negative children. Diagnosis of tuberculosis in children is difficult as they are not able to give sputum for demonstration of acid fast bacilli (AFB), tuberculin test may be negative and X ray film of the chest may be nonspecific. Diagnosis of tuberculosis in children needs high index of suspicion. Clinical and radiological clues for tuberculosis include history of adult contact suffering from tuberculosis, child getting cough, fever that is not responding to appropriate antibiotics and X ray film showing lymphadenopathy and parenchymal infiltrates unresponsive to antibiotics. For diagnostic purpose a tuberculin test showing induration of >5 mm is considered to be suggestive of tubercular infection. An attempt should be made to obtain sputum for AFB, if that is not possible than early morning gastric aspirate for 3 consecutive days may be obtained in young children. Radiometric culture technique isolates *M. tuberculosis* within 10-21 days. Drug susceptibility tests are available and can be used to detect drug resistance. Diagnosis of extrapulomnary tuberucolsis is made by examination of direct smears from tissues. PCR test can be used on sputum, pleural fluid and CSF to diagnose tuberculosis.

Treatment with antituberculous drugs shows similar response in both HIV positive and HIV negative patients. The four drug regimen consisting of isoniazid (5 mg/kg/day), rifampin (10-20 mg/kg/day), pyrazinamide (25-30 mg/kg/day) and ethambutol (15 mg/kg/day) or streptomycin (20-30 mg/kg/day) may prevent possible drug resistance in an individual patient. The duration of treatment for pulmonary tuberculosis is for 6-12 months and in extrapulmonary disease, the duration of treatment can be extended to further 12 months. Co-administration of rifampin with NNRTI and PI is contraindicated. As rifampin lowers the drug concentrations of PI and NNRTI rifampin may be replaced by rifabutin. Administration of rifabutin with antiretrovirals such as nevirapine and ritonavir is not recommended. The drug regimen in such cases is modified and recommeded as follows. Isoniazid, pyrazinamide and streptomycin daily for two months and then 2-3 times weekly for another 7 months. Directly observed therapy is preferred approach as it prevents multidrug resistant tuberculosis.

Prophylaxis to prevent the first episode of opportunistic disease in infants and children infected with HIV is given in Appendix IV.

Atypical Mycobacterial Infections

In immunocompetent children *Mycobacterium avium* complex (MAC) may be confined to respiratory tract. In HIV cases MAC may disseminate and cause multisystem disease. This rarely occurs until CD4+ count falls below 50 cells/mm^3. Clinical manifestations of disseminated MAC are characterized by recurrent fever, night sweats, weight loss, abdominal pain, diarrhoea, hepatomegaly, osteomyelitis, meningoencephalitis, intra abdominal abscess and rarely intestinal perforation. MAC is the most common intrahepatic opportunistic infection and may present with jaundice. The laboratory abnormalities include abnormal liver function tests with elevated alkaline phosphatase. Diagnosis is made by the identification of MAC from blood, tissue biopsy of lymphnode, bone marrow, liver or gastrointestinal tract. Positive culture results of sputum or stool may reflect colonization but do not confirm the diagnosis. Treatment can suppress the infection. The recommended therapy includes two agents. These drugs are either azithromycin (or clarithromycin) and ethambutol. The third drug is added in the form of either rifabutin, rifampin, ciprofloxacin or amikacin. In children receiving antiretroviral therapy, MAC infections are rarely reported. Drug prophylaxis can be offered to high risk children according to CD4+ counts. Oral suspensions of clarithromycin or azithromycin may be offered as prophylactic agents in children. Rifabutin liquid formulation is not available for children. Lifelong prophylaxis is recommended in children with a history of disseminated MAC to prevent recurrences (Appendix IV).

Pneumocystis Carinii Pneumonia (PCP)

It is one of the commonly identified opportunistic infection in children with HIV and occurs frequently during infancy. It can be prevented with antibiotic prophylaxis before 2 months of age. Its clinical course consists of cough, fever, tachypnoea, dyspnoea and severe hypoxia. Chest radiography findings demonstrate bilateral diffuse interstitial infiltrates. In a few cases nodular lesions, lobar infiltrates and pleural effusion may be seen. Initial presentation in patients receiving aerosolized pentamidine may manifest as upper lobe cavitatory disease. Diagnosis is made by identification of the organisms in either induced sputum or bronchoalveolar lavage fluid. Stains used for identification of *P. carinii* include methenamine silver, Giemsa, toludine blue and immunoflourescent technique. PCR technique is under evaluation for demonstration of the organism in induced sputum, bronchoalveolar fluid or peripheral blood.

The first choice for treatment of PCP is TMP-SMX. The recommended dosage is intravenous TMP 15-20 mg/kg/day and 75-100 mg/kg/day of SMX in four divided doses. Adjunctive therapy with intravenous methylprednisolone (2 mg/kg/24 hr in divided doses for every 6 or 12 hrs for 5-7 days) may decrease morbidity and be beneficial to the infant. Oral treatment with TMP/SMX is to be continued for a total of 21 days after clinical improvement with IV TMP/SMX. For PCP prophylaxis refer to Appendix IV.

Lymphoid Interstitial Pneumonitis (LIP)

LIP is an AIDS defining condition that is included in category B of revised paediatric classification. Its aetiology and pathogenesis are unknown. EBV may play a synergistic role with HIV or an exaggerated immunopathologic response to inhaled or circulating antigen which may contribute to LIP.[8] It generally presents as a chronic progressive interstitial lung disease in the second or third year of life. Clinical course in LIP includes insidious cough, digital clubbing, salivary gland enlargement, lymphadenopathy, hepato-splenomegaly, normal auscultatory findings and laboratory abnormalities with elevation of serum immunoglobulins. At present diagnosis can be confirmed by lung biopsy. Radiographic diagnosis of LIP is made by the demonstration of reticulonodular infiltrate with or without hilar adenopathy. Treatment with prednisolone 2 mg/kg day may improve the clinical condition of the child. Gammaglobulins and supportive care with oxygen and bronchodilators are needed.

Toxoplasmosis

Toxoplasma gondii, a coccidian protozoan, is a causative organism for toxoplamosis. It begins as an asymptomatic infection and reactivates in HIV immunocompromised children. The clinical manifestations are characterized by low birth weight, hepatosplenomegaly, icterus and CNS manifestations such as microcephaly, hydrocephaly, mental retardation, convulsions and intracranial calcification. The mechanism of transmission is by eating raw meat or undercooked meat. In pregnant woman transplacental transfer of *Toxoplama gondii* causes congenital infection in an infant. CT or MRI may show multiple ring enhancing lesions in the brain. Definitive diagnosis can be made by brain biopsy. The recommended treatment for congenital toxoplasmosis is as follows: Sulphadiazine 100 mg/kg as a loading dose followed by 85-120 mg/kg/day in two to four divided doses. Pyrimethamine 1-2 mg/kg/day for 2 days followed by 1mg/kg/day for 6 months and then 1 mg/kg/day thrice a week. Folinic acid is supplemented to this therapy to prevent anaemia. The duration of therapy for congenital toxoplasmosis is 12 months and it should be followed by life long prophylaxis. Alternate therapy with clindamycin, pyrimethamine and folinic acid may be recommended. In CNS toxoplasmosis pyrimethamine 2 mg/kg/day (maximum 50 mg/day) for 2 days followed by 1 mg/kg/day (maximum 25 mg/day); sulfadiazine 75 mg/kg/day as a loading dose followed by 5 mg/kg/day, folinic acid 5-20 mg/day thrice a week is indicated. The duration of the therapy is for 4-6 weeks beyond complete resolution of symptoms. The therapy should be followed by life long prophylaxsis (Appendix IV).

Viral Infections

Herpes simplex viruses (HSV) present as a primary or reactivation disease in HIV infected children. HSV stomatitis with recurrence (i.e. more than 2 episodes within a year) is included in category B of revised HIV paediatric classification. HSV lesions present as vesicles or ulcers on lips, tongue, gums, palate and oropharynx. It causes oesophagitis with ulceration, chest pain, odynophagia and may be complicated by local and cutaneous dissemination. AIDS patients with systemic HSV infections may present with pneumonitis, hepatitis, meningoencephalitis, shock and sepsis like syndrome.

The laboratory diagnosis is made by examination of Tzanck smear to detect multinucleated giant cells. The other laboratory tests to diagnose HSV infection include fluorescent antibody (FA) and culture. Culture takes 2-3 days and 95% of them are positive within 5 days. FA results are available within 24 hrs. The recommended treatment of HSV infection is with oral acyclovir (ACV) 80mg/kg/day in four divided doses for 10 days. ACV resistant cases may be treated with IV foscarnet 120mg/kg/day in 2-3 divided doses until the lesions are healed. Prophylaxis: Suppressive oral ACV 200 mg tid or 400 mg bid P.O is recommended for HIV patients with relapses.

Varicella zoster virus (VZV), the aetiologic agent of chicken pox manifests as a primary infection and it may be severe and prolonged and rarely has been documented to progress to visceral dissemination with involvement of lungs, liver, brain and pancreas. The course is fulminant in immunocompromised children. Diagnosis is made by clinical examination and laboratory tests that include demonstration of VZV antigens in skin lesions and cultures of the specimen. PCR is sensitive and specific test for diagnosis. The following regimens can be used to treat VZV infection. (i) iv. ACV 1500 mg/m^2/day in 3 divided doses for 7-10 days or until no new lesions appear. (ii) Oral Acyclovir 80 mg/kg/day in 4 divided doses. (iii) IV foscarnet 120-180 mg/kg/day in 2-3 divided doses in the treatment of ACV resistant VZV strains. HIV infected children who have been exposed to chicken pox should be given varicella zoster immunoglobulin (VZIG) within 96 hrs of exposure. Suppressive oral ACV is recommended in relapses.

In children herpes zoster occurs in early HIV disease and it appears soon after varicella. In the immunocompetent children it is dermatomal. It may be multidermatomal, recurrent or disseminated in HIV infected children. Systemic dissemination of zoster with constitutional symptoms, retinitis, hepatitis, pneumonitis and encephalitis may occur. Post-herpetic neuralgia is common. Diagnosis can be made clinically and laboratory diagnosis includes Tzanck test, FA and culture of the specimen. It can be treated with the following regimens. (1) Oral ACV 80 mg/kg/day in 4 divided doses (2) IV foscarnet 120-180 mg/kg/day in 2-3 divided doses in ACV resistant cases.

Cytomeglovirus (CMV) infections are endemic and occur without any seasonal variation. The spread of infection is through close contact with infected secretions. It may present as an acute infection, usually early in life after which it remains in a latent state. Disseminated CMV can occur when the CD4+ cell count falls below 50 cells/mm^3. Retinitis, oesophagitis, colitis, pneumonitis, hepatitis and encephalitis are the manifestations in disseminated CMV infection. The recommended therapy for CMV disease is IV ganciclovir 10mg/kg/day divided in 2 doses administered over 1-2 hrs for 21 days. Alternatively IV foscarnet 180mg/kg/day in 3 divided doses for 14-21 days can be used. Life long prophylaxis with IV ganciclovir 5 mg/kg/day for 5 days/week is indicated to prevent recurrence of CMV infection in patients with a history of CMV disease. Annual screening for retinitis in CMV infected children is recommended.

Fungal Infections

Candidiasis is the most common fungal infection and manifests as oral candidiasis or oesophageal disease in HIV infected children. The clinical manifestation of oropharyngeal candidiasis include white patches or plaques on an erythematous base on the tongue and buccal mucosa. When it extends to oesophagus, children may present with vomiting, dysphagia, substernal pain and weight loss. Diagnosis is made by demonstration of pseudohyphae on KOH preparation. Oesophageal candidiasis can be diagnosed by endoscopy and biopsy. Topical nystatin at a dose of 100,000 units/ml, 2-5 ml every six hours for 14 days, clotrimazole troches and amphotericin B solution may be effective for oral thrush. Oral fluconazole therapy at a dosage of 4-6 mg/kg/24 hrs for 14 days is recommended for oesophagitis. Itraconazole therapy can be given but there is limited experience with this drug. IV amphotericin B 0.5-1 mg/kg/day is recommended in refractory candidial esophagitis or disseminated candidiasis. Primary prophylaxis is generally not indicated in HIV infected infants. In severe recurrent mucocutaneous candidiasis particularly in infants with oesophageal candidiasis, suppressive therapy with systemic azoles should be considered. Deep fungal infections like disseminated histoplasmosis, cryptococcosis or coccidiodomycosis are not common in children.

Gastrointestinal Tract Disorders

Diarrhoea is a common gastrointestinal disorder in

children with HIV infection. It may be due to various organisms such as protozoa, bacteria, viruses and fungi. Clinical features are characterized by abdominal pain, watery stool, dehydration, fever and weight loss.

Protozoal Infections

Cryptosporidium is a coccidian protozoan that inhabits the microvillus region of epithelial cells. This was first identified in humans in 1976. In AIDS patients, cryptosporidiosis is characterized by bloating, intermittent abdominal cramps, diarrhoea, nausea and weight loss. It may cause biliary tract disease. Cryptosporidia have also been found in pulmonary specimen. Boiled water usage can prevent cryptosporidium infection.

Isospora belli is a coccidian protozoan, endemic in Asia, Africa, South America and Haiti and causes infection in the proximal small intestine with severe diarrhoeal manifestation. In AIDS patients cryptosporidium and isospora produce similar clinical manifestations. Diagnosis of crytosporidium or isospora is made by identification of the organism in stool specimen using modified acid fast stain. Intestinal mucosal biopsies usually confirm the diagnosis and these organisms are demonstrated on the surface epithelial cells which are arranged as clusters with little inflammation, ulceration or mucosal destruction. A few faecal white blood cells are seen in these infections. Cryptosporidium or isosporal infections are self limited in immunocompetent patients and usually do not require any treatment. The treatment of cryptosporidiosis consists of paromomycin 25-35 mg/kg/day PO in 3-4 divided doses, antimotility agents and fluid support. Recently nitazoxanide has been tried in some cases. Isosporiasis can be effectively treated with oral TMP-SMX 20 mg TMP/kg/day in 4 divided doses for 10 days and then bid for 21 days. Pyrimethamine alone or with folinic acid can be given in patients who are allergic to SMX. Maitenance therapy is indicated to prevent relapses.

Microsporidia are obligate intracellular protozoa and the disease presents with manifestations of chronic watery diarrhoea and malabsorption. Five genera have been identified as human pathogens in HIV (enterocytozoon, septata, nosema, pleistophora and encephalitozoon). Biliary tract may be involved in microsporidial infections. There is no effective therapy for microsporidiosis. Albendazole 400 mg bid can be tried. Symptomatic treatment with antidiarrhoeal agents and nutrtional support may be helpful in refractory cases. Diagnosis is based on modified trichrome staining of stool or small bowel biopsy specimens. Microsporidia have been noted in a variety of organs including eye, muscles and liver and can associated with conjunctivitis and hepatitis.

Giardiasis is water borne disease that infects the small intestine and it is often found in association with amoebiasis. The clinical features of giardiasis are characterized by abdominal cramps, diarrhoea, bloating and nausea. The organisms can be identified by multiple stool examinations. Trophozoites and cysts can be identified in stool and duodenal aspirates. Confirmation of the diagnosis is made by small bowel biopsy. Giardia antigen in the stool may be demonstrated by immunoassay. Treatment of giardiasis is with oral metronidazole 15 mg/kg/day in 3 divided doses for 5 days

Bacterial Infections

Campylobacter jejuni infection present with self limiting watery or bloody diarrhoea with fever and abdominal pain. Mucous or frank blood may be present in the stool. Campylobacterial infections may be more severe, persistent or recurrent and often associated with bacterial infections outside the bowel in HIV infected patients. Diagnosis is made by isolation of the organism from the stool by culture on selective media in a microaerophilic atmosphere. The recommended treatment for campylobacter infections is oral azithromycin 10 mg/kg on 1st day, followed by 5 mg/kg/day once a day for 4 days (or) oral erythromycin 30-50 mg/kg/day in 3-4 divided doses for 7 days or oral ciprofloxacin 20 mg/kg/day for 5 days.

Salmonella have been associated with four clinical types of presentation. Enteric (typhoid) fever, acute gastroenteritis, septicaemia with or without focal systemic lesions and asymptomatic carrier state. Salmonella bacteremia is transient in immunocompetent host. Salmonella bacteraemia in an HIV infected individual is diagnostic of AIDS. Diagnosis is made by the isolation of organism from the stool culture on selective media. The following antimicrobial therapy is recommended for 10-14 days to treat salmonella infection (1) oral ciprofloxacin 15-30 mg/kg/day or IV in 2 divided doses (2) IV cefotaxime 150-200 mg/kg/day in 3-4 divided doses (3) IV ceftriaxone 100 mg/kg/day in 1-2 doses. Cotrimoxazole can be used to prevent recurrent salmonella bacteria and isospora infections.

Shigella species are the cause of dysentery. *S. sonnei* and *S. flexneri* are responsible for most of the infections in U.S. Shigella are highly infectious, transmission of the oganism occurs rapidly and localized outbreaks are commonly attributed to contaminated food and water. The clinical features of shigellosis are characterized by an abrupt onset of diarrhoea, the stool may be frankly bloody or mucoid, abdominal cramps, tenesmus and fever. The infection may have complications such as toxic megacolon. These infections tend to be prolonged and recurrent in AIDS patients. Diagnosis is established by culture of the stool on selective media. Treatment is usually supportive. Antimotility drugs are not recommended. The following drugs may be recommended to treat shigella infections (1) Oral ampicillin 100 mg/kg/day for 10 days (2) Oral cefixime 8 mg/kg/day in two divided doses for 5 days (3) Ceftriaxone IV 50 mg/kg/day once daily for 5 days. Tab ciprofloxacin in a bid dosage is usually effective.

Clostridium difficile was demonstrated in 1935 from the faeces of infants and it has been associated with antibiotic associated colitis. Antibiotics such as ampicillin, tetracyclines and clindamycin have been found to be responsible for pseudomembranous colitis. Metronidazole is recommended to treat *C. difficile* infection.

Viral Infections

The viral infections that cause diarrhoea in HIV patients include rotavirus and adenoviruses. The treatment is generally supportive. Nutritional support and treatment of dehydration are indicated.

Fungal infections have been discussed earlier.

Haematologic Disorders

Erythrocytes, platelets, neutrophils and lymphocytes are affected by HIV infection. Most of the children may be present with anaemia. The anaemia is normocytic or microcytic. It may be due to iron deficiency, chronic infection, autoimmune phenomenon or side effects of drugs. Subcutaneous recombinant erythropoietin is recommended to treat children with low erythropoietin level.

Neutropenia occurs in 10% of patients which may be due to drugs used to treat HIV or opportunistic infections. It is benign and responds to bacterial infections when compared with neutropenia that develops after chemotherapy or radiation. Treatment with intravenous immunoglobulin (IVIG) or subcutaneous granulocyte colony stimulating factor offers some benefit in neutropenia or leukopenia. Lymphopenia is present in 30% of cases and it is a marker for advanced disease. Thrombocytopenia occurs in 10-15% of patients. Diminished platelet levels are present and the count may be 20,000/mm^3 to 45,000/mm^3. The cause may be unknown, drug induced or immunologic with platelet associated antibodies. AZT therapy for HIV associated thromobocytopenia improves platelet count. The counts rise from 100,000 to 400,000 platelets/mm^3 on therapy with AZT, but they usually fall if the drug is withdrawn. Treatment with IVIG, anti-D and corticosteroid shows improvement in some cases.

Polyclonal hypergammaglobulinemia, thrombotic thrombocytopenic purpura and diffuse infiltrative CD8 lymphocytosis syndrome have been associated with HIV infection.

Central Nervous System Disorders

CNS involvement in HIV infected children may present as progressive encephalopathy and is characterized by cognitive deterioration, motor and behavioural impairment with loss of developmental milestones. Older children may have learning disabilities or behavioural problems. CT scan shows cerebral atrophy, decreased attenuation of the white matter and basal ganglia calcification. Seizures and focal neurological signs are not common and they may represent tumour, opportunistic infections or other pathologic processes. Differential diagnosis includes CNS lymphomas, toxoplasmosis, CMV, JC Virus and HSV infections.

Cutaneous Manifestations

The cutaneous manifestations in children with HIV are more severe and more frequently recurrent than in immunocompetent children. Oral and oesophageal candidiasis, herpetic gingivo stomatitis, herpes zoster, molluscum contagiosum, anogenital warts, staphylococcal skin infections are common cutaneous manifestations in children with HIV infection. Seborrhoeic dermatitis, atopic dermatitis, drug eruptions, nutritional deficiencies are other cutaneous disorders in paediatric population with HIV infection. Kaposi's sarcoma is less frequently reported in children than in adults.

Diagnosis

Detection of HIV infection in a woman before or during pregnancy allows identification of HIV exposed infants and children and ensures care for the infected woman and HIV exposed or HIV infected childern. The serologic tests include enzyme-linked immunosorbent assays (ELISA) and supplemental tests such as western blot or immunofluorescence assay used to confirm the positive ELISA tests. Passive transfer of maternal HIV antibodies across the placenta to foetus may give rise to positive antibody tests in all new born infants. As the HIV antibody is present in uninfected infants upto the age of 18 months, a positive test for HIV antibody cannot be used as a definitive diagnosis in infants younger than 18 months. HIV infection can be identified by demonstration of IgA or IgM anti-HIV antibodies in the infants because these maternal immunoglobulins do not cross the placenta. HIV-IgA antibody assay is insensitive for the detection of infection in the first 3 months (17% at one month, 67% at 3 months) but it is a very sensitive assay in infants 6 months of age (94% detected at 6 months, 100% detected at 9 months). Hence the use of IgA assay in diagnosis of HIV infection in infants is limited.

Viral diagnostic tests (PCR, viral culture) can be used to definitely diagnose HIV infection. Definitive diagnosis can be made in most cases by age one month and possibly in all cases by age 6 months. A positive virologic test indicates possible HIV infection and as soon as possible should be confirmed by a second virologic test. Virologic tests in HIV exposed infants should be performed within the first 48 hrs of age and at 14 days as the test sensitivity is rapidly increased during the second week. Repeat testing is recommended at age one to two months and at age three to six months if the initial tests are negative. HIV infection in children may be reasonably excluded with two or more negative virologic tests performed at age greater than 4 wks, and one of those being performed at age greater than 16 wks.[9]

Perinatally exposed infants may be considered as "seroreverters" if they have become antibody negative after 6 months of age, have no other laboratory evidence of infection and have not met any AIDS defining condition. The median age of seroreversion in uninfected children is 10 months, but in a few cases presence of HIV antibody can be demonstrated until 18 months of age. Hence definitive diagnosis cannot be established before 18 months of age with HIV antibody tests.

Acquisition of HIV infection occurs during intrauterine and intrapartum periods. Early (i.e., intrauterine) infection is considered in infants with a positive virologic test at or before age 48 hrs. Late (i.e., intrapartum) infection is considered in infants who have a negative virologic test during the first week of life and subsequent positive tests in the later period. Infants with early infection may tend to have more rapid disease progression and need more aggressive therapeutic approach than those with late infection.

HIV infection in infants and children can be detected by several laboratory methods and include HIV culture, HIV DNA or RNA by PCR, HIV p24 antigen and immune complex dissociated p24 antigen (ICD-p24). HIV DNA PCR is the preferred virologic method as it is sensitive to diagnose HIV infection during the neonatal period. HIV RNA PCR method can be used in HIV exposed infants but the data regarding sensitivity and specificity are more limited when compared to HIV DNA PCR for early diagnosis.

HIV culture has sensitivity similar to that of DNA PCR but it is more expensive and results may not be available for 2-4 weeks. The sensitivity of immune complex dissociated p24 antigen is less and is not considered for routine use. The p24 antigen assay in infants less than a month is not recommended because of high frequency of false positive tests.

Treatment

The ideal antiretroviral therapy (ART) should provide a clinical, immunological and virologic benefit in children. Adherence to therapy is important and lack of adherence to recommended regimen may lead to subtherapeutic levels of antiretroviral drugs with subsequent development of drug resistance and virologic failure.

Antiretroviral drugs are classified into 3 categories:

NRTI	NNRTI	PI
• Zidovudine (AZT)	• Nevirapine (NVP)	• Saquinavir (SQV)
• Didanosine (ddi)	• Delavirdine (DLV)	• Ritonavir (RTV)
• Zalcitabine (ddc)	• Efavirenz (EFV)	• Lopinavir (LPV)
• Stavudine (d_4T)		• Indinavir (IDV)
• Lamivudine (3TC)		• Nelfinavir (NFV)
• Abacavir (ABC)		• Amprenavir (APV)

Indications for Initiation of ART in Children

Antiretroviral therapy in HIV infected children should be initiated to provide improvement in neurodevelopment, growth, immunologic and virologic parameters. A paediatric working group has proposed following guidelines for the treatment of HIV-infected children.

- Clinical symptoms associated with HIV infection (i.e. clinical categories A, B or C).
- Evidence of immune suppression, indicated by CD4+ T-lymphocyte, absolute number or percentage (i.e. immune category 2 or 3). Table 3.

Table 3.   Revised Human Immunodeficiency Virus Infection Paediatric Classification System. Immune Categories Based on Age-Specific CD4+ T-lymphocyte and Percentage

Immune category	<12 mos		1-5 yrs		6-12 yrs.	
	No./µ L	(%)	No./µ L	(%)	No./µ L	(%)
Category 1 No suppression	≥ 1,500	(≥25%)	≥1,000	(≥25%)	≥500	(≥25%)
Category 2 Moderate suppression	750-1,499	(15%-24%)	500-999	(15%-24%)	200-499	(15%-24%)
Category 3: Severe suppression	<750	(<15%)	<500	(<15%)	<200	(<15%)

- Modified from: CDC 1994 Revised classification system for human immunodeficiency virus infection in children less than 13 years of age. MMWR 1994; 43 (No. RR-12): 1-10

- Age < 12 months regardless of clinical, immunologic, or virologic status.
- For asymptomatic children aged ≥ 1 year with normal immune status, two options can be considered.

  1. Preferred Approach: Initiate therapy regardless of age or symptom status.
  2. Alternative Approach: Defer treatment in situations in which the risk for clinical disease progression is low and other factors (e.g., concern for the durability of response, safety, and adherence) favour postponing treatment. In such cases, the health-care provider should regularly monitor virologic, immunologic, and clinical status. Factors to be considered in deciding to initiate therapy include the following.

- High or increasing HIV RNA copy number.
- Rapidly declining CD4$^+$ T-lymphocyte number or percentage to values approaching those indicative of moderate immune suppression (i.e. immune category 2).
- Development of clinical symptoms.

Initial Recommended ART for Children

Strongly Recommended

Clinical trial evidence of clinical benefit and or sustained suppression of HIV replication in adults and or children.

- One highly active protease inhibitors (nelfinavir or ritonavir) plus two nucleoside analogue reverse transcriptase inhibitors.
- Recommended dual NRTI combinations: the most data of use in children are available for the combinations of ZDV and ddI, ZDV and lamivudine (3TC) and stavudine (d4T) and ddI. More limited data are available for the combinations of d4T and 3TC and ZDV and ddc.
- For children who can swallow capsules: the non-nucleoside reverse transcriptase inhibitor (NNRTI) efavirenz (Sustiva TM) plus two NRTI, or efavirenz (Sustiva TM) plus nelfinavir and one NRTI.

Recommended as an Alternative

Clinical trial evidence of suppression of HIV replication, but (1) durability may be less in adults and or children than with strongly recommended regimens or may not yet be defined; or (2) evidence of efficacy may not outweigh potential adverse consequences (i.e. toxicity, drug interactions, cost, etc): (3) experience in infants and children is limited.

- NVP and two NRTI.
- ABC in combination with ZDV and 3TC
- Lopinavir/ritonavir with two NRTI or one NRTI and NNRTI
- IDV or SQV soft gel capsule with two NRTIs for children who can swallow capsules.

Offered Only in Special Circumstances

Clinical trial evidence of either (1) virologic suppression that is less than for the strongly recommended or alternative regimes; or (2) data are preliminary or inconvlusive for use as initial therapy but may be reasonably offered in special circumstances.

- Two NRTI.
- APV in combination with two NRTI or ABC.

Not Recommended

Evidence against use because (1) overlapping toxicity may occur; and/or (2) use may be virologically undesirable.

(a) Any monotherapy
(b) d4T and ZDV·
(c) ddc and ddI
(d) ddc and d4T
(e) ddc and 3TC.

Monitoring of Paediatric HIV

Laboratory tests and clinical evaluation should be done to monitor disease progression in HIV infected children. These include (1) Immunologic criteria (2) Plasma Viral load (3) Clinical aspects.

Immunologic Criteria

In HIV infected children CD4 + T cell absolute count and percentage are the markers of disease progression. In healthy infants higher CD4 + T cell absolute count and percentage have been observed when compared to healthy adults, and these counts reach adult values by age 6 yrs. CD4+ T cell percentage in each immunologic category doesn't change with age. CD4+ T cell absolute count has been found to change with age. Hence CD4+ percentage is taken into consideration in identifying disease progression in children. Altered or transient decrease in CD4+ cell count and percentage may occur in the presence of mild illness or vaccinations and those values should be measured when the patients recover from illness. Due to higher CD4+ counts in children, age adjusted CD4+ values are taken into account in identifying the disease progression. CD4+ values should be measured as soon as possible in HIV infected child. Two CD4+ measurements are needed with a minimum of one week between measurements when modification in therapy is recommended (Table 3).

Plasma Viral Load

Quantitative HIV RNA assays can determine viral load in peripheral blood. Primary infection in adults show high HIV RNA levels. Immune response to HIV may lead to decline in HIV RNA levels to about 2-3 $\log_{10}$ copies and reaches a virologic set point approximately within 6-12 months following primary infection.[10,11] Some studies have shown that low HIV RNA levels were found at birth and reached peak values at about 2 months of age and then slowly declined. The mean HIV RNA level within 1yr. of age was 185,000 copies/ml. In contrast to the adult pattern, HIV RNA levels have shown decreased levels after one year of age and these levels would continue to fall in the next few years of life. And this pattern may be due to an immature immune system in controlling viral replication in infants.

Interpretation of HIV RNA Assays

Plasma HIV RNA can be measured by three different assays.

These include

(1) Qauantitative RNA assays (Amplicor HIV-1 Monitor ^{TM})
(2) Branched DNA assay (Quantiplex)
(3) Nucleic acid sequence based amplification assay (NASBA)

Amplicor and NASBA assays yeild approximately twice the values obtained by Quantiplex. Therefore one method should be used consistently to estimate the viral load. Biological variation in viral load tends to occur and greater in infected infants and young children then in infected adult. This variation in a stable infected adult may vary as much as 3 fold in a day or on different days. This variation in children should be taken into account while interpreting changes in HIV RNA load as an average decline of 0.6 $\log_{10}$ per year occurs between 12-24 months of age and these values further decrease by about 0.3 $\log_{10}$ per year until 4-5 yrs. of age. Further viral load changes greater than five fold in children under 2 yrs. of age and those greater than 3 fold in children aged >2 yrs. of age should be considered as a significant change. Two HIV RNA measurment should be taken before a change in therapy is considered.

Changing ART in Children

Change in antiretroviral therapy is warranted in disease progression, viral and immuologic failures.

The assessment of treatment failure is based on the following criteria in HIV infected children.

Virologic Consideration

- Less than 10 fold decrease from baseline RNA levels who receive ART with two NRTI and one PI or less than 5 fold decrease in HIV RNA levels from baseline who receive less potent ART (i.e. dual NRTI combinations) after 8-12 weeks of therapy.
- HIV RNA not suppressed to undetectable levels after 4-6 months of therapy.
- Repeated detection of HIV RNA in children who responded to therapy with undetectable levels.
- Increase in HIV RNA levels with initial HIV RNA response but still have HIV RNA detectable levels.

Immunologic Criteria

- Change in immunologic classification.
- For children with CD4+ T cell percentage of <15% (i.e. immunecategory 3), a persistent decline of 5 or more percentiles in CD_4 + T cell percentage (i.e. from 15% to 10%).
- A rapid and significant decrease in absolute CD4+ T cell count i.e. > 30% decline in 6 months.

Clinical criteria

- Progressive neuro developmental deterioration
- Growth failure

- Disease progression from one paediatric clinical cateogory to another.

The dose and side effects of antiretroviral therapy is summarized in Table 3.

Table 3. Anti Rertroviral Drugs Used in Paediatric HIV

Drug	Dose	Side Effects
NRTI		
Zidovudine (AZT, ZDV)	Neonatal dose (Infants aged <90 days) oral 2 mg/kg every 6 hrs. Paediatric dosage range: 90-180 mg/m^2 every 6-8 hrs.	Anaemia, neutropenia myopathy, GI intolerance
Didanosine (ddi)	90-150 mg/m^2 every 12 hrs.	Pancreatitis, peripheral neuropathy, diarrhoea, abdominal pain, vomiting
Zalcitabine (ddc)	0.01 mg/kg every eight hours	GI disturbance, peripheral neuropathy, pancreatitis and oral oesophageal ulcers.
Lamivudine (3TC)	Neonatal dose: 2 mg/kg twice daily Paediatric dose: 4 mg/kg twice daily	Headache, nausea, diarrhoea, skin rash, pancreatitis, peripheral neuropathy.
Stavudine (d$_4$T)	1 mg/kg every 12 hrs (upto 30 kg)	Headache, GI upset, skin rashes, peripheral neuropathy, pancreatitis.
Abacavir (ABC)	Paediatric/adolescent dose: 8 mg/kg twice daily Max. dose 300 mg twice daily	Headache, GI disturbances, fatal hypersensitivity reaction
NNRTI		
Nevirapine (NVP)	Neonatal dose: (through age 2 months) 120 mg/m^2 once daily for 14 days followed by 120 mg/m^2 every 12 hrs. for 14 days followed by 200 mg/m^2 every 12 hrs. Paediatric Dose: 120-200 mg/m^2 every 12 hrs Note: Inititate therapy with 120 mg/m^2 once daily for 14 days Later 120-200 mg/m^2 every 12 hrs.	Skin rashes, Stevens Johnson Syndrome
Protease Inhibitors		
Amprenavir (APV)	Paediatric/adolescent dose (<50 kg) for children 4-12 yrs. or 13-16 yrs. (<50 kg) Oral solution 22.5 mg/kg twice daily or 17 mg/kg three times daily (max. 2800 mg/day) Cap. 20 mg/kg twice daily or 15 mg/kg three times daily (max. 2,400 mg/day)	GI disturbances, perioral paraesthesias, rash, Stevens Johnson syndrome
Ritonavir (RTV)	Dose range: 350-400 mg/m2 every 2 hrs. start with 250 mg/m^2 every 12 hrs. and increase to full dose over 5 days	Nausea, vomiting, diarrhoea, circumoral paraesthesia
Nelfinavir (NFV)	25-30 mg/kg three times a day	Diarrhoea, abdominal pain, asthenia
Indinavir (IDV)	500 mg/m^2 every 8 hrs.	Asymptomatic hyper bilirubinaemia, nephrolithiasis
Saquinavir (SQV)	50 mg/kg every 8 hrs.	Nausea, diarrhoea Skin rash, paraesthesias

NRTI: Liquid formulations are available for ZDV, ddI, 3TCd$_4$ T & ABC except DDC.
NNRTI: Nevirapine liquid formulation is available. Delavirdine is not approved for children over 3 years of age. Efavirenz is available as capsule formulation and is approved for children over 3 yrs of age.
Protease Inhibitor: PI that can be used in children who cannot swallow capsules are Nelfinavir, Ritonavir, Amprenavir and Lopinavir/Ritonavir.

Immunization in HIV Infected Children

HIV infection has been associated with immunosuppression and progressive deterioration in children and made them susceptible to various types of infections. Use of live vaccines can result in severe vaccine associated illness in children. The immunization recommendation for HIV infected children are shown in Table 4.[12]

Table 4.   Recommendation for Immunization in HIV Infected Children

Vaccine	Known asymptomatic		Known symptomatic	
	WHO	ACIP/AAP	WHO	ACIP/AAP
BCG	Yes★	No	No	No
DPT/DtPa	Yes	Yes	Yes	Yes
OPV	Yes	No	No	No
Measles/MMR	Yes	Yes	Yes	Yes
IPV	–	Yes	–	Yes
Hepatitis B	Yes	Yes	Yes	Yes
Hib	–	Yes	–	Yes
Pneumococcal	–	Yes	–	Yes
Influenza	–	Yes	–	Yes
Varicella	–	Consider	–	Consider
Hepatitis A	–	Yes	–	Yes

★For regions where risk of tuberculosis is high.

Conclusion

An effort to identify HIV in pregnant mother ensures early recognition of HIV infection in the infant. HIV counselling of all pregnant women and education about prevention of mother to child transmission with antiretroviral prophylaxis regimen and risks about breast milk feeding will drastically reduce the number of HIV infected children in the future. The management of HIV infected children is to be carried out in close cooperation with paediatrician or physicians dealing with HIV infected cases.

References

1. Centres for Disease Control: Follow up on Kaposi sarcoma and pneumocystis pneumonia. MMWR 1981; 30: 277.
2. Centres for Disease Control: Unexplained immuno-deficiency and opportunistic infections in infants - New York, New Jersey, California. MMWR 1982; 31: 665.
3. Zeigler JB, Cooper DA, Jhohnson RO, et al: Postnatal transmission of AIDS-associated retrovirus from mother to infant. Lancent 1985; 1: 896–898.
4. Connor EM, Sperling RS, Gelber R, et al. Reduction of Maternal-infant transmission of Human immunodeficiency virus type I with zidovudine treatment. Pediatric AIDS clinical Trials group protocol 076 Study Group. N Engl J Med 1994; 331: 1173-1180.
5. Administration of zidovudine during late pregnancy and delivery to prevent perintal HIV transmission-Thailand, 1996-1998. MMWR 1998; 47: 151-154.
6. Perinatal HIV guidelines. Living document. HIV/AIDS Treatment information websites Aug 2002. www.aidsinfo.org.
7. Biggar RJ, Miotti PG, Taha TE, et al: Perinatal intervention trial in Africa: Effect of a birth canal cleansing intervention to prevent HIV transmission. Lancet 1996; 347: 1647-1650.
8. Connor EM. Lymphocytic interstitial pneumonitis. Wilfert C, edr. Pediatric AIDS. 2nd edn. Baltimore: Williams & Wilkins; 1994. p. 467-481.
9. Centres for Disease Control: 1995 Revised guidelines for prophylaxis against PCP for children infected with or perinatally exposed to HIV. MMWR 1995; 44: 1-11.
10. Katzenstein TL, Pedersen C, Nielson C, et al. Longitudinal serum HIV RNA quantification: correlation to viral phenotype at seroconversion and clinical outcome. AIDS 1996. 10: 167-173.
11. Henrard DR, Philips JF, Muenz LR, et al. Natural History of HIV-1 cell-free Viremia: JAMA 1995; 274: 554-558.
12. Parthasarathy A. Reply (Measles and MMR Immuniza-tion). Indian Paediatrics 2002; 39: 108-111.

Chapter 8

Counselling in HIV/AIDS

Dinesh Mathur, Veena Acharya

Counselling

"Confidential dialogue between a client and a care provider aimed at enabling the client to cope with stress and take personal decision related to HIV/AIDS. The counselling process includes an evaluation of personal risk of HIV transmission and facilitation of preventive measures." This includes information, education and psychosocial support and allows individuals to make decisions that facilitate coping and preventive behaviours (WHO).

Counselling has become an integral part of prevention, diagnosis, management, care and support of people living with HIV/AIDS. Since the diagnosis of HIV/AIDS, or even a suspicion of the possibility of having infection brings profound emotional, social, behavioural and medical consequences and one has to deal with each one of them and there subsequent effects in different fields of life. Counselling enables a person's coping capacity to come out of the difficult situations during the course of HIV disease. Since HIV infection is a dynamic, evolutionary and lifelong process it makes new and changing demands on the patients, relations and community. Counselling takes into account not only the immediate medical requirements, but also their social relationships and attitudes about HIV/AIDS. It also provides information and education relevant to the day to day life of the person concerned including the patient's sexual and occupational needs and general aspirations.

Both health education and counselling aim at changing risk behaviour and both use two way interaction, however education is emotionally neutral whereas counselling has strong emotional overtones despite the detachment of the provider who augments the coping capacity of the client.

Basic Purpose of Counselling

1. To enable the person to prevent the spread of infection by helping in change of behaviour and life style.
2. To provide psychosocial support to individual and family.

The Counselling Process

The process of counselling differ from place to place, however risk assessment is essential element. The counsellor should not pre-judge the risk factors of any person, nor should be biased and use all the available information. The "appearance" of a patient or area where they come from should not be taken as an indication of a risk factor.

In view of the many variables in defining risk, it is essential for the counsellor to carry out a comprehensive sexual and lifestyle history of the patient covering sexual behaviour of the individual. The history of intravenous drug abuse, past history of blood transfusions, use of blood products for the treatment of haemophilia, sickle cell anaemia, operations prior to the introduction of HIV screening of donors or intensive procedures carried out under non-sterile conditions such as traditional rituals like circumcision, cosmetic procedures and repeated infections.

In all counselling situations, there are some basic principles to be observed such as:

- Welcoming the patient & using acceptable traditional greeting practices depending on the local customs in that area.
- The room should be as comfortable as possible with diffuse light.

- The counsellor should be seated facing the patient and not behind a table.
- The patient should be given a chance to pause or ask questions.
- The counsellor should ask open ended questions which would offer them a chance to answer or not to answer.
- Tell the patient directly, without evasion. Listen carefully.

Basic Micro-Counselling Skills

Active attending and listening, reflection of feeling, effective questioning, paraphrasing and interpretation are essential skills in counselling.

Qualities of An Effective Counsellor

- Positive regard or respect for people.
- Open, non judgemental and high level of acceptance.
- Caring and empathetic.
- Self aware and self disciplined.
- Knowledgable and informed about the subject.
- Culturally sensitive
- Patient and a good listener
- Ability to maintain confidentiality
- Objective and having clarity.

Effective Feedback

For getting effective feedback, sentences should start with "I", as these are only your subjective feelings and views. Some one else may feel differently about the same issue. So make statements beginning with "I feel", "I think" etc.

Give positive comments and offer alternatives or suggestions. Use simple words and short sentences. Do not interrupt or side-talk during the interaction.

Essential Stages of Counselling

Stage One: Forming rapport and gaining the client's trust
Stage Two: Definition and understanding of roles, boundaries and needs.
Stage Three: Process of ongoing, supportive counselling.
Stage Four: Closure or ending the counselling relationship.

Elements of Counselling

The fundamental elements of any counselling programme can be summarised by a mnemonic "GATHER" which is used in other counselling situations like family planning.

The GATHER approach can be understood as follows.

G — Greet the client politely
A — Ask about their needs, doubts, concerns
T — Tell the client about the facts, side effects and give options
H — Help the client to choose
E — Explain about the different issues
R — Return for follow-up

Different Types of HIV/AIDS Counselling

1. Pre test counselling: Counselling before the test for HIV
2. Post test counselling: Counselling after the HIV test is done, whether positive or negative
3. Risk reduction assessment
4. Counselling after a diagnosis of AIDS has been made
5. Family and relationship counselling.
6. Bereavement counselling
7. Outreach counselling
8. Crisis counselling
9. Telephone and hotline counselling

Who Can Provide Counselling?

Counselling can be provided by any dedicated person who has got basic information and training in different issues of HIV/AIDS and counselling skills e.g. health care providers viz. doctors, nurses, para-medical staff, psychologists, psychotherapists and social workers. Non health care providers such as teachers, health educators, religious and community leaders, youth workers and traditional healers can also provide counselling after suitable training

Setting

Counselling can be provided in any setting where discussion about HIV AIDS can take place such as out patient departments of hospitals, STD, ANC, family planning clinics, blood banks, drug deaddiction centres, prisons, community health centres, schools etc.

Indications

People who are candidate for testing of STD and HIV, identified patients of HIV disease and people seeking help/assistance because of their current or past high risk behaviour, should be given counselling. (Table 1).

Table 1. Indication for HIV Counselling and Testing

Clinical indications

Signs and symptoms of HIV (eg, unexplained weight loss, fever, atypical pneumonia, or oral thrush)

Acute HIV seroconversion symptoms

Confirmation, if prior reported positive test is not documented

Prior risk behaviour

Multiple sexual partners, sexual partner at risk, prior or recent STD diagnosis, injection drug use and transfusion with blood and its products before screening for HIV was introduced, haemophiliacs who received factor VIII before screening for HIV, men who have sex with men (MSM)

Pregnant women

Exposure to HIV

Occupational

Sexual or drug abuse

Persons who request HIV testing

Pre test counselling: Counselling is very much needed when a person is offered a test to know about an individual's HIV status. Pre test counselling (Table 2) should include accurate and updated information about transmission and prevention of HIV and other sexually transmitted diseases. Inform about the window period of the HIV test i.e. a period of 12 weeks since the last possible exposure to HIV should have elapsed by the time of testing. Explain clearly about what a test can do i.e. it looks for the antibodies to HIV and it is not a test for AIDS, the difference between HIV positive status and full blown AIDS, prepare mentally to whom to disclose/share if test is positive and how would the client cope personal resources, support network of friends, family members and community. Inform about the partner notification issues that the HIV positive status has to be disclosed to the sexual partner under the course of law. Inform from where the results of test are to be collected in person from the physician or the counsellor.

Table 2. Components of HIV Pretest Counselling

Ascertain risk

Discuss likelihood and meaning of positive, negative, and indeterminate test result

Assess understanding of HIV transmission and natural history; psychological stability; social support; impact of a positive result

Discuss confidentiality provisions and anonymous testing

Ensure that follow-up is available (especially important when testing occurs in urgent care settings)

Emphasize the importance of obtaining test results

Discuss risk reduction plan and referral to other services if needed

Obtain informed consent for HIV antibody testing

Post test counselling: The results of HIV testing should always be given in person and under all precautions of keeping confidentiality. If a person is HIV negative with a possibility of window period, he should be asked to come again and get his test done after some time. He should also be given all information regarding safer sexual practices, so that in future chances of contracting HIV/STD become less (Table 3).

If a person is HIV positive, then the results should be given in appropriate manner to break the bad news. Recommended manner of breaking a bad news is: eliciting the person's understanding, exploring his knowledge and breaking the news at persons pace in manageable chunks. Acknowledge immediate reactions and allow time to absorb initial shock. Counsellor has to deal with emotional reactions and offer support as appropriate. Counsellor has also to give correct information about future management and refer to appropriate agency required to manage his clinical or social problems. It has been observed in cases of HIV disease that before accepting the fact of life, the client invariably denies the bad news and this denial is a valid mechanism of coping which may be total (rare) or ambivalent. Sometimes relatives may also encourage the denial. The other psychological events encountered are:

- Initial shock of diagnosis and a hopelessness for the future.
- Anxiety and fear of uncertain prognosis, incurability of the disease and reactions of family members.
- Anger and frustration of becoming infected and development of sense of guilt.
- Depression due to possible, social, occupational and sexual rejection.

Table 3. Components of HIV Post Test Counselling

Ensure that client is ready to receive results

Disclose test results and provide interpretation (positive, negative, indeterminate) in the context of that person's risk of infection

HIV seronegative persons

Readdress and reinforce risk reduction plan

Discuss the need for repeat testing for those with recent (<6 months) exposure or ongoing risk behaviour

Persons with indeterminate HIV 1 Western blot

Discuss prevalence of and risk factors for indeterminates, for persons with p24 bands and or those with risk behaviour discuss the possibility of acute HIV infection and need for serologic follow up at 1, 3, and 6 months; discuss safe sexual and drug use behaviour until indeterminate is resolved

Consider performing supplemental assays (e.g., polymerase chain reaction) to more quickly identify seroconverters and reassure those with HIV infection, particularly for pregnant women

HIV seropositive persons

Counsel about the meaning of a positive HIV test (HIV infected and thus potentially infectious)

Differentiate between being HIV infected and having AIDS (review natural history of HIV and immunosuppression)

Emphasize the importance of early clinical intervention (ability to alter disease progression through antiretroviral therapy and prophylaxis against opportunistic infections)

Discuss ways to avoid transmitting HIV to others (abstinence, condoms, not sharing needles if IDU)

Assess need for psychological support

Provide referrals for medical, psychological, or social services, if necessary

Confirm HIV antibody test, if positive test is not consistent with risk history

Schedule follow up visit to assess psychological status, and to address partner notification issues

Counselling About Future Management

Since significant developments have occurred in the field of therapeutics of HIV, a detailed information about the available drugs should be given to the patient. Knowledge about opportunistic infections and drugs to prevent them should be imparted to the patient alongwith side effects of antiretroviral therapy be clearly told to the patient. Importance of taking regular treatment, adherence, signs and symptoms of possible drug resistance and failure should also be told.

Confidentiality

Confidentiality has always been an ethical and legal requirement for the health professionals such as nurses and doctors and one should always take all precaution to keep confidentiality in dealing with HIV/AIDS patients. Health care providers have to share information with colleagues to ensure proper care of the client. Doctors may need to discuss relevant health care information with the patient and or their family. The nurse has an obligation to document observations and care given (charting/report writing) to the patient. The "private" information may be disclosed with the patients consent only.

The legal and ethical issues are discussed in chapter on Sexual Assault and STD.

References

1. HIV/AIDS Counselling Training Manual for Trainers - A Document of NACO, Ministry of Health and Family Welfare, Govt. of India.
2. HIV Counselling and the psychosocial management of patients with HIV or AIDS - Sarah Chippindale, Lesley French. BMJ 2001; 322: 1533–1535.
3. Counselling about HIV/AIDS - Role of Dermato-venereologists - Dr. Dinesh Mathur - Abstract from Oration in the 27th National Conference of IADVL, 1999, Bhuvaneshwar.

Chapter 9

Interaction of Human Immunodeficiency Virus and Sexually Transmitted Diseases

H K Kar

Introduction

Globally the majority of human immunodeficiency virus (HIV) epidemic is through heterosexual transmission; HIV infection is thus by definition is one of the sexually transmitted infections (STI) or diseases (STD). The complex interaction between STD and the HIV has been demonstrated in many epidemiological, in vitro and clinical studies over the last number of years.

The explosive spread of HIV 1 in areas where classic STD are epidemic (e.g., sub-Saharan Africa, Thailand) has encouraged a remarkable number of studies designed to examine the association between these STD (urethritis, cervicitis, and genital ulcers) and HIV 1 infection.[1,2] Proving that STD were indeed a cofactor was initially difficult, because HIV 1 and STD share same sexual mode of transmission, so associations seen in epidemiological studies may well have resulted from the confounding effect of risky sexual behaviour. In cross sectional studies, the time sequence of infections is difficult to establish. But longitudinal studies provided strong evidence, and showed substantial relative risks for HIV 1 infection associated with various STD. Classic STD could facilitate HIV 1 transmission by increasing either the infectiousness of the index case, the susceptibility of the partner, or both.[1,2]

Relationship between STD and HIV Infection

The complex relationship between STD and HIV infection is infact manifold:

1. The predominant mode of transmission of both HIV infection and other STD is through sexual route.
2. STD are biological cofactors for acquisition, transmission of HIV infection.
3. Concurrent HIV infection alters the natural history of classic STD.
4. STD are markers for high risk behaviour for HIV infection.
5. Many of the measures for prevention of sexual transmission of HIV and STD are the same as are the target audiences for these interventions.
6. STD clinical services are important access point for persons at high risk not only for diagnosis and treatment but also for education on prevention and counselling for HIV infection.
7. Management of STD may reduce HIV transmission, particularly in developing countries.
8. Trends in STD incidence and prevalence can be useful indicators of changes in sexual behaviour and are easier to monitor than trends in HIV seroprevalence and therefore valuable for determining the impact of HIV/AIDS control programme.

STD as a Cofactor for HIV Transmission

There is a strong association between the occurrence of HIV infection and the presence of other STD. During the last decade, from different epidemiological, clinical and biological and in vitro studies, overwhelming evidence has accumulated that both ulcerative and non-ulcerative STD promote HIV transmission by augmenting HIV infectiousness and HIV susceptibility via different biological mechanisms.[3]

There is increased risk of HIV infection associated with common STD (Table 1). Six out of ten studies in Kenya and Zaire found that people with genital ulcers caused mainly by chancroid were more likely to be infected with HIV than people without ulcers. Their the risk is two to five times greater. Nine out of 11 studies of syphilis and HIV found an association. Syphilis increased the risk of HIV infection three to nine fold for heterosexual men. In three of six studies of genital herpes and HIV infection, herpes doubled the risk of HIV infection for women and heterosexual men. Besides the genital ulcer diseases (GUD), other studies found that many non-ulcerative STD like chlamydia infection, gonorrhoea and trichomoniasis could increase the risk of HIV transmission to women by three to five fold. Few studies from India shows increasing prevalence of HIV infection among STD clinic attendees, prevalence was found higher among GUD patients than non-ulcerative STD patients.[4,5] The relative importance of ulcerative and non-ulcerative STD appears to be complex. Owing to the greater frequency of non-ulcerative STD in many populations, these infections may be responsible for more HIV transmission than genital ulcers.[3]

The possible mechanisms of cofactor effect of ulcerative and non-ulcerative STD on HIV transmission by augmenting HIV infectiousness and HIV susceptibility are as follows:

1. Lack of mechanical skin/mucous membrane/ endocervical epithelium barrier makes an easy viral exit and entry due to ulceration or microulceration.[6-10]
2. Among HIV seronegative individuals, genital ulcers may increase susceptibility to HIV by not only disrupting mucosal and skin integrity but also by increasing the presence and activation of HIV susceptible cells in the genital tract (the susceptibility cofactor effect). *Haemophilus ducreyi*, for example, evokes a cell mediated immune response which attracts HIV susceptible cells to the ulcer surface.[11] In fact, *H. ducreyi* may contain specific T cell stimulating antigens, which may further predispose T cells to infection by HIV. In addition, with viral STD such as herpes, there may be interactions between viruses in genital tract, which promote the establishment of HIV infection. For example, in tissues co-infected with HSV-1, HIV 1 virions are able to infect keratinocytes despite the lack of CD4 receptors. In gaining access to cells, HIV may also take advantage of changes in cellular chemokine receptors that result from infection with other viruses, as shown recently in studies of cytomegalovirus.

3. Genital ulcers bleed frequently during sexual intercourse, resulting in potential increases in HIV infectiousness (the infectivity cofactor effect).
4. Presence of HIV in genital ulcer exudate in HIV infected individuals confirmed by culture and PCR[12] (the infectivity cofactor effect).
5. Increased number of HIV containing white blood cells, in both ulcerative and inflammatory genital secretions (the infectivity cofactor effect).
6. Increased shedding of HIV virus in the genital tract (the infectivity cofactor effect) particularly in non-ulcerative STD, probably by recruiting HIV infected inflammatory cells as part of the normal host response. Investigators have noted a significant increase in detection of HIV 1

Table 1.   Association of STD and HIV Infection

STD	Increased risk for HIV acquisition		Clinical Exacerbation
N. gonorrhoeae infection	+\-	3 to 5 times	+\-
Chlamydia trachomatis infection	+	3 to 5 times	+\-
Trichomonas vaginalis infection	+	3 to 5 times	–
Chancroid	+	2 to 5 times	+
Syphilis	+	3 to 9 times	+
Genital herpes	+	2 times	+
Granuloma inguinale	+		+\-
Human papillomavirus infection	+		+
LGV	+		+\-
Hepatitis B	—		+

DNA in cervicovaginal fluids of patients with gonorrhoea, chlamydia infection.[13]

7. Increasing HIV replication by certain ulcerative STD pathogens, (e.g. *Treponema pallidum* lipoproteins)[14] and/or increasing number of receptors expressed per cell receptive to HIV 1, (e.g. *H. ducreyi* lipo-oligosaccharide may increase the number of CCR5 receptors on a macrophage cell line).[1]

9. For cervicitis specifically, three potential mechanisms have been suggested to explain the observed relationship of cervicitis and HIV infection:[15]

   (a) Recruitment of inflammatory cells to the cervical mucosa results in increased concentration of HIV-infected CD4 lymphocytes and infected monocytes-macrophages.

   (b) In the presence of an inflammatory milieu, HIV replication is enhanced, perhaps through the generation of reactive oxygen products secreted by granulocytes[16] and secondary to cell activation which is mediated by inflammatory cytokines (interleukin-1 or tumour necrosis factor-alpha).[15]

   (c) Cervicitis is associated with micro-ulceration and friable mucosal tissue that can provide a portal of exit for HIV infected cells or a portal of entry for virus or infected cells.

10. Bacterial vaginosis (BV) may facilitate HIV transmission.[17,18] It requires special mention, since it is a common vaginal infection in women and the relative risk of transmission of HIV is 2 to 5 times in the presence of BV infection. Schmid et al[19] have summarized all possible mechanisms, from research studies of different workers:

   (a) Lactobacilli produce lactic acid that maintains vaginal pH and inhibits the growth of many organisms, including those associated with BV. Some lactobacilli particularly those that posted against development of BV produce hydrogen peroxide which is toxic to a number of organisms including HIV.

   (b) A low vaginal pH may inhibit CD4 lymphocyte activation and therefore decrease HIV target cells in the vagina. Therefore, a high vaginal pH due to presence of BV may make the vagina more conductive to HIV survival and adherence.

   (c) BV has also been shown to increase intravaginal levels of interleukin-10, which increases susceptibility of macrophages to HIV.

   (d) A heat stable protein elaborated by *Gardnerella vaginalis* increases the production of HIV by HIV infected cells by as much as 77 fold. *Mycoplasma hominis* is the most potent inducer of HIV 1 expression among several vaginal bacterial species studied.

Effect of STD Management on HIV Transmission

If STD cofactor effects are strong and STD are highly prevalent, STD control, via improvement of STD management, can be a strong strategy for HIV prevention.[20]

In a study conducted in Malawi, the results showed that HIV 1 positive men with urethritis had HIV 1 concentrations in the seminal plasma eight times higher than those in seropositive men without urethritis. After urethritis patients were treated for their STD, the concentration of HIV 1 RNA in semen decreased significantly.[21] Ghys and coworkers[14] found a significant increase in detection of HIV 1 DNA in cervicovaginal lavage samples from patients with gonorrhoea, chlamydia infection, cerviovaginal ulcer, or cervical mucopus. A week after STD treatment, detection of HIV 1 in these secretions decreased from 42% to 21%; changes in detection rate were not observed in women whose STD were not cured.

A compelling body of evidence shows that prevention, early diagnosis and treatment of STD can be important for HIV prevention strategy. This is particularly true when treatment of symptomatic STD are addressed. The syndromic approach is endorsed by WHO and National AIDS Control Organization (NACO), Government of India, Ministry of Health and Family Welfare as an effective means to treat symptomatic STD promptly when rapid and sensitive laboratory tests are not available. A randomized control trial was done to evaluate the impact of improved STD case management as per the WHO recommended syndromic STD management guidelines at primary care level on the incidence of HIV infection in rural Tanzania, over a two years period. The trial demonstrated a 42% reduction in new sexually transmitted HIV infection in the intervention communities compared with the control communities.[22]

However, in another community-based randomized trial conducted in the Rakai district, Uganda between 1994 and 1998 no effect on HIV incidence was seen, either overall or in subgroups including initially discordant couples or pregnant women. Some reductions in curable STD were seen in both the studies. The unexpected result from Rakai studies might be due to several factors.[23]

Possible explanations include:

(a) Differences in the stage of HIV 1 epidemic (16% in Rakai and 4% in Mwanza population),

(b) Potential difference in frequency of incurable STD like genital herpes (45% of all genital ulcers in Rakai where as it is less than 10% in Mwanza),

(c) Perhaps greater importance of symptomatic than asymptomatic STD for HIV 1 transmission and,

(d) Possibly greater effectiveness of continuously available services (Mwanza) than of intermittent mass treatment to control rapid STD re-infection in Rakai.

Clearly, the two trials tested different intervention, and used different methods for effect evaluation, in different epidemiological environments; therefore the divergent results may be complementary rather than contradictory.[23]

Even if STD cofactor effects on HIV transmission would be weaker than previously thought, improving STD management remains an important component of HIV prevention programme.[20] An association between STD and HIV, whether casual or not, indicates that STD patients are at high risk of contracting and transmitting HIV. The education, counselling, condom promotion and provision, contact tracing and treatment that is part of comprehensive STD management can therefore be an effective mean of targeting the HIV prevention strategies to those most in need.

II. Impact of HIV Infection/AIDS on Other STD

The natural history, manifestations and treatment of classic STD is altered by concurrent HIV infection. The impact of HIV and its resulting immunosuppression, on the classic manifestations and management of STD, has been noted from the beginning of the AIDS epidemic.

Syphilis

The interaction of syphilis in HIV positive patients is not clear. HIV appears to affect the epidemiology, clinical manifestations and treatment of syphilis (Table 2). Although the incidence of syphilis rose dramatically in the United States in the late 1980s, especially among the inner city African-American communities, no such trend was reported from India.[24-26]

Unusual or severe manifestations of syphilis have been reported increasingly in HIV-infected patients due to some degree of immunodeficiency and there is reduced response to conventional therapeutic regimens in these individuals. In the HIV infected patients with moderate to advanced immunodeficiency, who becomes infected with *T. pallidum*, the following variations from the expected course of syphilis (Table 2) have been noted:

Table 2. Variation in Syphilis Occurring in Individuals with HIV-infection

Clinical finding	Primary lesions	Painless ulcer becomes painful due to super infection; giant chancre
	Secondary lesions	Lues maligna- secondary syphilis with vasculitis manifested by fever, malaise, headache, nodules, indurated plaques with or without hyperkeratoses and/ or ulceration, sclerosis
	Course of the disease	Shorter latent period with rapid progression to tertiary disease within first year of infection, i.e. meningovascular syphilis
Serological response to syphilis		Limited or absent antibody response to syphilis with repeatedly negative reagin and treponemal antibody testing in serum or CSF
Diagnosis		In the absence of negative serological tests dark field microscopy, biopsy of the lesion, direct fluorescent antibody staining of material from lesion may be helpful
Treatment		Greater likelihood of treatment failure, relapse without re-exposure despite adequate treatment

Antibody Response

Limited or absent antibody response to infection with repeatedly negative reagin and treponemal antibody testing due to defective B and T cell function leading to abnormal immune response, thus making serological diagnosis of syphilis unreliable. A delayed serologic serum titre response found in HIV infected patients after treatment of diverse stages of syphilis in four studies, while three other studies showed a normal serologic response.[27]

Clinical Manifestations

(i) Primary lesion- the usually painless chancre becoming painful due to secondary infection, risk of multiple chancres in primary syphilis[29], development of giant primary chancre.

(ii) Secondary lesion- Lues maligna (malignant syphilis)[29,30] characterized by nodulo-ulcerative lesions with systemic symptoms, with florid cutaneous and mucocutaneous lesions, pustular, nodular necrotizing secondary lesions, hyperkeratotic verrucous plaque type lesion[31]; rapid progression to secondary syphilis with persistence of the primary chancre[32] and thus HIV enhancing its own transmission.

(iii) Latent period- shorter latent period before development of meningovascular syphilis, increasing the incidence of early neurosyphilis even along with primary and secondary lesions[33], rapid progression to tertiary syphilis within first year of infection.

Diagnosis

When the clinical findings suggest syphilis, but serological tests are negative or inconclusive, alternative tests such as dark field microscopy, biopsy of the lesion for histopathological examination and direct fluorescent antibody staining of materials obtained from the lesions may be needed in these cases. The diagnosis of neurosyphilis is especially difficult in HIV seropositive patients, because both HIV and syphilis can cause a mononuclear pleocytosis and elevated protein in CSF and CSF VDRL can be negative in persons with neurosyphilis.[34] However, CSF examination of HIV-infected patients with late latent syphilis or latent syphilis of unknown duration is mandatory, preferably as a part of initial diagnostic program before treatment according to CDC.[28] WHO guidelines (2001) and NACO

guidelines for STD treatment (2002) suggest that all patients with syphilis should be strongly encouraged to undergo testing for HIV because of the high frequency of dual infection and its implications for clinical assessment and management. Neurosyphilis should be considered in differential diagnosis of neurological diseases in HIV infected individuals. In cases of congenital syphilis, the mother should be encouraged to undergo testing for HIV infection; if her test is positive, the infant should be referred for follow up.

Treatment

There was lack of response to penicillin therapy and relapse without exposure despite adequate treatment in many studies.[35-37] Immunodeficiency induced by HIV appears to render the benzathine penicillin G treatment ineffective in a substantial proportion of cases.[25] Jarisch-Herxheimer reaction in syphilis is more frequently among HIV infected early syphilis patients compared to non-HIV infected controls.[28]

As per the current WHO, CDC and NACO guidelines (2002) for the management of STD, recommended therapy for early syphilis in HIV infected patients is no different from that in non-HIV infected patients. Penicillin regimens should be used whenever possible for all stages of syphilis in HIV: Single dose of benzathine penicillin G 2.4 million IU IM as for HIV sero-negative individuals for early syphilis and three weekly doses of benzathine penicillin G 2.4 million IU IM for late syphilis. However, some authorities advise examination of the CSF and/or more intensive treatment (e.g., benzathine penicillin G administered at weekly intervals for 3 weeks, as recommended for late syphilis), a regimen appropriate for all patients with dual infections of *T. pallidum* and HIV, regardless of clinical stage of syphilis. In all cases, careful followup is necessary to ensure adequacy of treatment with quantitative VDRL at 1,2,3,6,9, and 12 months after treatment. Patients with early syphilis whose titres increase or fail to decrease four fold within six months should undergo CSF examination and be re-treated. In such patients, CSF abnormality could be due to HIV-related infection, neurosyphilis, or both. *T. pallidum* may persist in the CNS of HIV-infected patients in spite of adequate antibiotic therapy.

The treatment of syphilis in immunocompromised patients remains an unresolved issue.[38] Failure to respond to treatment of early syphilis and subsequent progression to neurosyphilis in HIV positive patients,[39] difficulty in diagnosing neurosyphilis and subsequent recommendations for treatment with higher and more prolonged dose[40] in patients with HIV make syphilis management an area yet to be fully delineated.

Chancroid

Chancroid, caused by *H. ducreyi* may be both a marker for increased risk of HIV infection and a cofactor for HIV transmission. Since the advent of HIV infection in Africa, several studies suggest a change in the natural history of chancroid.

The following variations are noticed in natural history and therapy of chancroid (Table 3):

(a) Genital ulcers tend to be larger and persist longer.[41]

(b) Chacroid with multiple inguinal buboes.

(c) Frequent occurrence of giant and phagedenic ulcer.

(d) Less responsive to standard antibiotic therapy. Single dose therapies such as azithromycin and ceftriaxone, also have been associated with a three to four fold higher failure rate in the treatment of chancroid among HIV seropositive when compared with seronegative men.[42, 43]

In patients infected with HIV, treatment may appear less effective, but this may be due to co-infection with genital herpes or/and syphilis. Since chancroid and HIV infection are closely associated and therapeutic failure is likely to be seen with increasing frequency, WHO guidelines for the management of STD (2001) suggest that all patients should be followed up weekly until there is clear evidence of improvement or cure. Increased dose and a more prolonged duration of therapy might be necessary in patients with concomitant HIV infection.

Because data is limited concerning the therapeutic efficacy of the recommended single dose regimens (ceftriaxone, 250 mg IM and azithromycin 1 g orally) in HIV infected patients, these regimens should be used for such patients only if follow up can be ensured (CDC, 2002). Some specialists suggest using erythromycin 7-days regimen for treating HIV- infected persons (CDC, 2002).

Herpes Genitalis

Herpes simplex virus (HSV) infections occur more frequent and severe in immunocompromised patients secondary to HIV infection (Table 3).[44-46] There is a synergistic relationship between HSV and HIV leading to enhanced replication of viruses and potentiation of HIV transmission.[47]

Clinical Presentation

It ranges from those described in immunocompetent patients to life-threatening disseminated infection. The severity and frequency of recurrence increase over time as HIV-induced immunosuppression progresses. The lesions may persist or progress to produce erosions that enlarge into painful ulcers with raised margin involving larger areas of perianal, scrotal or penile skin. The ulcer may bleed. Nonhealing perianal ulcerative herpes simplex was initially opportunistic infections described in homosexual men with HIV infection. Chronicity parallels with immunosuppression.

Treatment

Most lesions of herpes in HIV infected persons respond to acyclovir, but dose has to be increased and treatment given for a longer than the standard recommended period. WHO (2001) and NACO guidelines (2002) have recommended acyclovir 400 mg orally five times daily until complete clinical resolution or 5 to 10 mg/ kg IV 8 hourly until clinical healing of the lesions. Subsequently, the patients may benefit from chronic suppressive therapy to decrease in frequency of recurrence. Recommended regimens for daily suppressive therapy in persons infected with HIV are acyclovir 400-800 mg orally bd or tid (CDC, 2002).

In some cases the patients may develop thymidine-kinase deficient mutants for which standard antiviral therapy becomes ineffective. It should be replaced by alternate antiviral. Early virus culture, if available, allows for prompt sensitivity testing.[48] All acyclovir resistant strains are resistant to valacyclovir and most are resistant to famciclovir. Foscarnet, 40 mg/kg body weight IV every 8 hours until clinical resolution is attained, is often effective for the treatment of acyclovir resistant genital herpes (CDC, 2002).

Granuloma Inguinale

In the presence of HIV infection with moderate to severe immunodeficiency, clinically the lesion of granuloma inguinale may be larger, extensive and the pseudobubo may burst producing ulceration and there is slow response to treatment (Table 3).

Persons with both granuloma inguinale and HIV infection should receive the same regimens, as those who are HIV negative. Recommended regimens are doxycycline 100 mg orally bd or erythromycin 500 mg orally qid for atleast 2-3 weeks (CDC-2002, WHO-2001, NACO-2002). Addition of gentamycin 1 mg/kg IV every 8 hours to the above regimen is suggested if improvement is not evident within the first few days of therapy (CDC, 2002 and WHO, 2001).

Lymphogranuloma Venereum

There may be an acute inflammation with bilateral inguinal bubo, which may burst into ulceration with moderate to severe immunodeficiency due to HIV infection (Table 3).

Persons with both LGV and HIV infection should receive the same regimens as those who are HIV negative. Prolonged therapy may be required, and delay in resolution of symptoms may occur (CDC-2002).

Urethritis and Cervicitis

Gonococcal urethritis, chlamydial urethritis, and nongonococcal, nonchlamydial urethritis may facilitate HIV transmission. Patients who have NGU and also are infected with HIV should receive same treatment regimen as those who are HIV negative urethritis.

Similarly patients who have mucopurulent cervicitis and also infected with HIV should receive the same treatment regimen as those who are HIV negative.

Bacterial Vaginosis and Trichomoniasis

Patients who have either of the above infections and also are infected with HIV should receive the same treatment regimen as those who are HIV negative.

Vulvovaginal Candidiasis

Vaginal candida colonization rates in HIV infected women are higher than among seronegative women with similar demographic characteristics and high risk behaviours and colonization rates correlate with increasing severity of immunosuppression. Symptomatic vulvovaginal candidiasis (VVC) is more frequent in seropositive women and similarly correlates with severity of immunodeficiency. In addition, among HIV infected women, systemic azole exposure is associated with the isolation of non-albicans Candida species from vagina.

Therapy for VVC should not differ from that for

Table 3. Variations in Other STD Occurring in Individuals with HIV Infection

Chancroid	Clinical finding	Genital ulcers tend to be larger and persist longer. Multiple inguinal buboes. Frequent occurrence of giant and phagedenic ulcer.
	Treatment	Less responsive to standard therapy, 3 to 4 fold higher failure rate with single dose therapy with azithromycin and ceftriaxone.
Herpes genitalis	Clinical findings	As immunosuppression progresses lesion may persist or progress to chronic enlarged painful ulcers with raised margin, ulcer may bleed.
	Treatment	Higher dose and longer period treatment with acyclovir, 400 mg orally 5 times daily until complete clinical resolution or 5 to 10 mg/kg IV 8 hourly until clinical healing (WHO guideline, 2001).
		Suppressive therapy includes acyclovir 400-800mg bid or tid (CDC, 2002)[63]
Granuloma inguinale	Clinical findings	Lesion may be larger, extensive, pseudobubo formation which may burst producing ulceration, slow response to treatment
	Treatment	Doxycycline 100mg orally bid or erythromycin 500 mg orally qid for 2-3 weeks(CDC-2002, WHO-2001, NACO-2002)
		If no improvement, addition of gentamycin 1mg\kg IV suggested
LGV	Clinical findings	Acute inflammation with bilateral inguinal bubo which may burst into ulceration
	Treatment	Same regimen(doxycycline, 100mg orally bd or erythromycin, 500mg orally qid for 14 days (WHO, 2001), but prolonged therapy may be required

seronegative women. Although long term prophylactic therapy with fluconazole at a dose of 200 mg weekly has been effective in reducing *C. albicans* colonization and symptomatic VVC, it is not recommended for routine primary prophylaxis in HIV infected women in the absence of recurrent VVC.

Human Papilloma Virus Infection

Human papillomavirus (HPV) infection, as one of the very common STD, presents as genital warts to carcinoma in HIV positive patients. The causal link between invasive cervical squamous cell carcinoma and cervical intraepithelial neoplasia (CIN) in women is well demonstrated.[49] Women who are HIV positive have the double edged sword of having higher incidences of both HPV infection and CIN changes than HPV negative women.[50, 51] The immune status of women with HIV has been shown to influence the progression of CIN.[52] The association between HPV and anal carcinoma in both men and women with HIV is almost as certain.[37] The incidence of anal carcinoma in homosexual men with AIDS was 40 times that of general population and significantly higher than that of seronegative homosexual men.[53]

In immunocompromised patients the genital warts may be more florid, disseminated and often refractory to treatment. Squamous cell carcinomas arising in or resembling genital warts may occur more frequently among immunosuppressed persons, thus requiring biopsy for confirmation of diagnosis. Because of increased incidence of anal cancer in HIV infected homosexual men, screening for a squamous intraepithelial lesion (SIL) by cytology in this population is advocated by some specialists, but not recommended by CDC.

After obtaining a complete history of previous cervical disease, HIV infected women should be provided a comprehensive gynaecologic examination, including a pelvic examination and Pap test, as part of their initial evaluation. A Pap test should be obtained twice in the first year after diagnosis of HIV infection and, if the results are normal, annually thereafter. If the results of the Pap test are abnormal, care should be provided according to the Interim guidelines for management of abnormal cervical cytology.[54] Women who have a cytological diagnosis of high grade SIL or squamous cell carcinoma should undergo colposcopy directed biopsy. HIV infection is not an indication for colposcopy in women who have normal Pap smear.

Molluscum Contagiosum

Molluscum contagiosum (MC) began to receive more attention with the advent of AIDS.[55-57] In AIDS patients, MC does not just occur in male homosexuals, but throughout all races and in all groups when sufficiently immunocompromised. Despite recalcitrant MC in HIV patients, all are not sexually transmitted. The lesions are usually in clusters, pearly with an umbilicated centre. Hundreds of lesions may be found between the umbilicus and the genitals in sexually active young adults. On the pubis and external genitalia, they often coexist with genital warts and thus may represent a therapeutic challenge.

Hepatitis B

Hepatitis B is caused by infection with HBV. HBV infection in HIV infected persons is more likely to result in chronic HBV infection. HIV infection also can impair the response to hepatitis B vaccine. Therefore, HIV infected persons antibodies should be tested for to HBs Ag 1-2 months after the third vaccine dose. Revaccination with three more doses should be considered for persons who do not respond initially to vaccination. Those who do not respond to additional doses should be counselled in the use of methods to prevent HBV infection.

Pelvic Inflammatory Disease

Difference in clinical manifestations of PID between HIV infected women and HIV negative women have not been well delineated. In recent, more comprehensive observational and controlled studies, HIV infected women with PID had similar symptoms when compared with uninfected control.[58-60] They were more likely to have a tubo ovarian abscess, but responded equally well to standard parenteral and oral antibiotic regimens when compared with HIV negative women.

The microbiologic findings for HIV positive and HIV negative were similar, except for (a) higher rates of concomitant *M. hominis*, candida, streptococcal, and HPV infection and (b) HPV related cytological abnormalities among those with HIV infection.

Whether the management of immunodeficient HIV infected women with PID requires more aggressive intervention (e.g., hospitalization or parenteral antimicrobial regimen) has not been determined (CDC, 2002).[61]

Ectoparasitic Infections

Pediculosis pubis patients who are also infected with HIV should receive same treatment regimen as those who are HIV negative (Permethrin 1% cream or Lindane 1% shampoo/lotion)

Crusted scabies is an aggressive infestation that usually occurs in HIV infected persons and other immunodeficient patients. Crusted scabies is associated with greater transmissibility than scabies. Substantial treatment failure might occur with single tropical scabicide or ivermectin treatment. Some specialists recommend combined treatment with a topical scabicide and oral ivermectin or repeated treatment with ivermectin. Lindane should be avoided because of risks of neurotoxicity with heavy applications and denuded skin. Patient's fingernail should be closely trimmed to reduce injury from excessive scratching.

Patients with uncomplicated scabies with HIV infection should receive the same treatment regimens as those who are HIV negative.

Conclusion

Effective treatment regimens are available for traditional STD and when promptly applied along with other STD control measures such as condom use and safe sex and counselling might be expected to have an impact on HIV control particularly when the population is still in early epidemic phase. Detection and treatment of classic STD must be undertaken in HIV positive patients to reduce their infectiousness and in their partners to reduce susceptibility to infection.[1]

References

1. Cohen MS. Sexually transmitted diseases enhance HIV transmission: a hypothesis no longer. Lancet 1998; 351 (suppl III): 5-7.
2. Wasserheit JN. Epidemiological synergy: interrelationships between human immunodeficiency virus infection and other sexually transmitted diseases. Sex Transm Dis 1992; 19: 61-77.
3. Fleming DT, Wasserheit JN. From epidemiological synergy to public health policy and practice: the contribution of other sexually transmitted diseases to sexual transmission of HIV infection. Sex Transm Inf 1999; 75: 3-17.
4. Kar HK, Jain RK, Sharma PK, et al. Increasing HIV prevalence in STD clinic attendees in Delhi, India: 6 year (1995-2000) hospital based study results. Sex Transm Inf 2001; 77: 393.
5. Kumar B, Gupta S. Rising HIV prevalence in STD clinic attendees at Chandigarh(North India)- A relatively low prevalence area. Sex Transm Inf 2000; 76: 59.
6. Moss GB, Kreiss JK. The interrelationship between human immunodeficiency virus infection and other sexually transmitted diseases (Review). Med Clin North Am 1990; 74: 1647-1660.
7. Laga M, Nzila N, Goeman J. The interrelationship of sexually transmitted diseases and HIV infection: implications for the control of both epidemics in Africa (Review). AIDS 1991; 5: S55-63.
8. Wasserheit JN. Epidemiological synergy: interrelationships between human immunodeficiency virus infection and other sexually transmitted diseases (Review). Sex Transm Dis 1992; 19: 61-77.
9. Mostad SB, Kreiss JK. Shedding of HIV 1 in the genital tract (Editorial review). AIDS 1996;10:1305-1315.
10. Vernazza PL, Eron JJ, Fiscus SA, Cohen MS. Sexual transmission of HIV: infectiousness and prevention. AIDS 1999; 13: 155-166.
11. Magro CM, Crowson AN, Alfa M, et al. A morphological study of penile chancroid lesions in human immunodeficiency virus (HIV)- positive and –negative African men with a hypothesis concerning the role of chancroid in HIV transmission. Human Pathol 1996; 27: 1066-1070.
12. Plummer FA, Wainberg MA, Plourde P, et al. Detection of human immunodeficiency virus type 1 (HIV 1) in genital ulcer exudate of HIV 1- infected men by culture and gene amplification (letter). J Infect Dis 1990; 161: 810-811.
13. Ghys PD, Fransen K, Diallo MO, et al. The associations between cervicovaginal HIV shedding, sexually transmitted diseases and immunosuppression in female sex workers in Abidjan, Cote d' Ivoire. AIDS 1997; 11: F85-93.
14. Theus SA, Harrich DA, Gaynor R, Radolf D, Norgard MV. *Treponema pallidum* lipoproteins and synthetic lipoprotein analogues induce human immunodeficiency virus type 1 gene expression in monocytes via NF-Kb Activation. J Infect Dis 1998; 177: 941-950.
15. Kreiss J, Willerford DM, Hensel M, et al. Association between cervical inflammation and cervical shedding of human immunodeficiency virus DNA. J Infect Dis 1994; 170: 1597-1601.
16. Ho JL, He S, Hu A, et al. Neutrophils from human immunodeficiency virus (HIV) seronegative donors induce HIV replication from HIV-infected patients mononuclear cells and cell lines: an in vitro model of HIV transmission facilitated by *Chlamydia trachomatis*. J Exp Med 1997; 181: 1403-1505.
17. Klebanoff SJ, Coomb RW. Virucidal effects of lactobacillus acidophilus on human immunodeficiency virus type-1: possible role in heterosexual transmission. J Exp Med 1991; 174: 289-292.
18. Cohen CR, Duer RA, Pruithithada N, et al. Bacterial

vaginosis and HIV seroprevalence among female commercial sex workers in Chaing Mai, Thailand. AIDS 1995; 9: 1093-1097.

19. Schmid G, Markowitz L, Joesoef R, Koumans E. Bacterial vaginosis and HIV infection. Sex Transm Inf 2000; 76: 3-4.

20. Korenromp EL, Sake J, Vlas DE, et al. Estimating the magnitude of STD cofactor effects on HIV transmission, how well can it be done? Sex Transm Dis 2001; 28: 613-621.

21. Cohen MS, Hoffman IF, Royce RA, et al. Reduction of concentration of HIV 1 in semen after treatment of urethritis: implications for prevention of sexual transmission of HIV 1. Lancet 1997; 349: 1868-1873.

22. Grosskurth H, Mosha F, Todd J, et al. Impact of improved treatment of sexually transmitted diseases on HIV infection in rural Tanzania: randomized controlled trial. Lancet 1995; 346: 530-536.

23. Grosskurth H, Gray R, Hayes R, Mabey D, Wawer M. Control of sexually transmitted diseases for HIV 1 prevention: understanding the implications of the Mwanza and Rakai trials. Lancet 2000; 355: 1981-1987.

24. Wald A, Corey L, Handsfield HH, Holmes KK. Influence of HIV infection on manifestations and natural history of other sexually transmitted diseases. Ann Rev Publ Health 1993; 14: 19-42

25. Chopra A, Dhaliwal RS, Chopra D. Pattern and changing trend of STD at Patiala. Indian J Sex Transm Dis 1999; 20: 22-25.

26. Raj Narayan, Kar HK, Gautam RK, et al. Pattern of sexually transmitted diseases in a major hospital of Delhi. Indian J Sex Transm Dis 1996; 17: 76-78.

27. Pieter C, Vader VV. Syphilis management and treatment. Dermatol Clin 1998; 16: 699-711.

28. Rolfs RT, Joesoef MR, Hendershot EF, et al. Randomized trial of enhanced therapy for early syphilis in patients with and without HIV infection. N Engl J Med 1997; 337: 307.

29. Schofer H, Imhof M, Thoma-Greber E, et al. Active syphilis in HIV infection: A multicentre retrospective survey. Genitourin Med 1996; 72: 176.

30. Mohan KK, Rao GRR, Lakshmi P, Babu A. Changing patterns of secondary syphilis (a clinical study). Indian J Sex Transm Dis 2000; 2: 75-78.

31. Thappa DM, Hemanth RH, Karthikeyan, Ravindran G. Unusual manifestations of secondary syphilis in a patient with human immunodeficiency virus infection. Indian J Sex Transm Dis 1999; 20: 29-32.

32. Hutchinson C, Hook EW, Shepard M, et al. Altered clinical presentation of early syphilis in patients with HIV infection. Ann Intern Med 1994; 121: 94.

33. Pavithran K, Beena S. Primary chancre – associated syphilitic meningitis during HIV infection. Indian J Sex Trans Dis 1999; 20: 55-56.

34. Feraru ER, Aronow HA, Lipton RB. Neurosyphilis in AIDS patients: initial CSF VDRL may be negative. Neurology 1990; 40: 541-543.

35. Dover JS, Johnson RA. Cutaneous manifestations of Human immunodeficiency virus infection. Arch Dermatol 1991; 127: 1549-1558.

36. Hook EW, Marra CM. Acquired syphilis in adults. N Engl J Med 1992; 326: 1060-1069.

37. Pavithran K. Chancre redux and tinea incognito in an HIV-infected person. Indian J Sex Transm Dis 1997; 18: 22-23.

38. Ormond P, Mulcahy F. Sexually transmitted diseases in HIV positive patients. Dermatol Clin 1998; 16: 853-857.

39. Johns D, Tierney M, Felsenstein D. Alteration in the natural history of neurosyphilis by concurrent infection with the human immunodeficiency virus. N Engl J Med 1987; 316: 1569-1572.

40. Goldmeier D, Murphy G. Neurosyphilis and HIV infection. Int J STD AIDS 1994; 5: 379.

41. Latif AS. Epidemiology control of chancroid, 8th Int Soc STD Res 1989 Copenhagen (Abstr. 66)

42. Tyndall M, Agoki E, Ombetti J, et al. A randomized, single blinded study of azithromycin in male patients with culture proven chancroid. 9th Int Soc STD Res 1991 Banff. (Abstr. A-041)

43. Tyndall M, Malisa M, Plummer FA, et al. Ceftriaxone in the treatment of chancroid. 9th Int Soc STD Res 1991 Banff. (Abstr. A-42)

44. Johnson R, Leef, Hadgu A, et al. Genital herpis trends during the first decade of AIDS: Prevalence increased in young whites and elevated in blacks. 10th International Meeting of the Int Soc for STD Res 1993 Helsinki (Abstract)

45. Norris SA, Kessler HA, Fife KH. Severe progressive herpetic whitlow caused by an acyclovir resistant virus in a patient with AIDS. J Infect Dis 1987; 157: 209-210.

46. Safrin S, Asseykeen T, Follansby, et al. Foscarnet therapy for acyclovir resistant mucocutaneous herpes simlex virus in 26 AIDS patients. J Infect Dis 1990; 161: 1078-1084.

47. Heng M, Heng S, Allen S. Coinfection and synergy of human immunodeficiency virus-1 and herpes simplex virus-1. Lancet 1994; 343: 255-258.

48. Barton SE. The management of chronic progressive anogenital ulceration in an HIV seropositive patient. Herpes 1997; 4: 47.

49. Nash JD, Burkar TW, Hoskin WJ. Biological course of cervical human papilloma virus infection. Obstet Gynaecol 1987; 69: 160-162.

50. Byrne MA, Taylor-Robinson D, Munday PE, Harris JR. The common occurrence of human papillomavirus infection and intraepithelial neoplasm in immunosuppressed women infected by HIV. AIDS 1989; 3: 379-382.

51. Vermund SH, Kelley KF, Klein RS, et al. High risk of human papillomavirus and cervical squamous intraepithelial lesions among women with symptomatic human immunodeficiency virus infection. Am J Obstet Gynecol 1991; 165: 392-400.

52. Silman J, Stanek A, Sedlis A, et al. The relationship between human papillomvirus and lower genital intraepithelial neoplasia in immunosuppressed women. Am J Obstet Gynaecol 1984; 150: 300-308.

53. Melbye M, Cote T, Biggar R, et al. High incidence of anal cancer among AIDS patients X International Conference on AIDS, 1993 Berlin. (Abstract po-b14-1636).

54. Kurman RJ, Henson DE, Herbst AL, Noller KL, Schiffman MH, National Cancer Institute Workshop. Interim guidelines for management of abnormal cervical cytology. JAMA 1989; 262: 931-934.

55. Gottlieb SL, Myskowski PL. Molluscum contagiosum. Int J Dermatol 1994; 33: 453-461.

56. Myskowski PL. Molluscum contagiosum: New insights, new directions. Arch Dermatol 1997; 133: 1039-1041.

57. Meadows KP, Tyring SK, Pavia AT, et al. Resolution of recalcitrant molluscum contagiosum lesion in human virus infected patients treated with cidofovir, Arch Dermatol 1997; 133: 987-990.

58. Cohen CR, Sinei S, Reilly M, et al. Effects of human immunodeficiency virus 1 infection upon acute salpingitis: a laparoscopic study. J Infect Dis 1998; 18: 1352-1358.

59. Bukesi EA, Cohen CR, Stevens CE, et al. Effects of human immunodeficiency virus 1 infection on microbial origins of pelvic inflammatory disease and on efficacy of ambulatory oral therapy. Am J Obstet Gynecol 1999; 18: 1374-1381.

60. Irwin KL, Moorman AC, O'Sullivan MJ, et al. Influence of human Immunodeficiency virus infection on pelvic inflammatory disease. Obstet Gynecol 2000; 95: 525-534.

61. CDC, Sexually transmitted diseases treatment guidelines, MMWR, 2002; 51: RR-6.

PART III
Basics of Anatomy and Clinical & Laboratory Methods

Chapter 10

Applied Anatomy of Male and Female Reproductive Tract

Gurvinder P Thami

Introduction

A basic knowledge of anatomy is of paramount importance in all the fields of clinical medicine. Conversely, an ignorance of anatomy of a particular region is a serious handicap in understanding the disease process affecting that anatomical region. Besides building up a differential diagnosis based upon the structures involved in an anatomical region, it also helps in making an accurate clinical diagnosis of various disorders.

Sexually transmitted diseases (STD) in particular, affect the so called private parts of human anatomy for which patients are often hesitant to reveal the relevant information about their illness. Similarly, a good clinical examination may not always be possible due to reluctance of patient for a reasonably good genital exposure. As such, a majority of symptoms and signs of STD can easily be traced to their anatomical origin. A sound knowledge of anatomy of male and female genitalia can thus be of extreme benefit for reaching an accurate diagnosis and instituting prompt treatment of STD.

Male Genitalia

The Male Urethra (Fig. 1)

The male urethra is a 18-20 cm long membranous canal for the external discharge of urine and seminal fluid, which starts proximally at the neck of urinary bladder and ends up distally at external urethral meatus. It is a commonly involved structure in urethral syndromes of gonococcal and non-gonococcal origin. It is divided into three parts starting distally; spongy, membranous and prostatic urethra. The spongy or penile part of male

urethra is often regarded as anterior urethra by the clinicians while the membranous and prostatic parts together constitute posterior urethra. The spongy part of urethral mucosa is lined by pseudostratified columnar epithelium except in its distal (fossa navicularis) 10-12 mm where it is lined by stratified squamous epithelium. The membranous and the prostatic urethra are lined by transitional epithelium. The gonococci have a predilection for columnar epithelium while stratified squamous epithelium and transitional epithelium are relatively resistant to infection with *Neisseria gonorrhoeae*. Inflammation of urethra is known as urethritis and anterior urethritis is by convention, regarded as sexually transmitted unless proved otherwise. Gonococcal and non-gonoccal urethritis (due to chlamydia and mycoplasma) often present with urethral discharge and dysuria. Spongy or the penile urethra can be felt running deep within corpora spongiosum along the median raphe of penis and scrotum ventrally. Palpation of urethra in this location can detect urethral strictures and milking of urethra in proximal to distal direction helps to bring out the urethral discharge for the laboratory diagnosis of gonococcal and non-gonoccal urethritis

Penis (Fig. 2)

(i) **Shaft or body of penis** consists of erectile tissue, constituted by corpora spongiosum penetrated by urethra throughout its length ending up in a bulb like projection known as glans penis and two corpora cavernosa lying side by side.

(ii) **Glans penis** is the distal end of corpora spongiosum ending up in a bulb like projection. It has a rim like raised surface at its proximal end which is

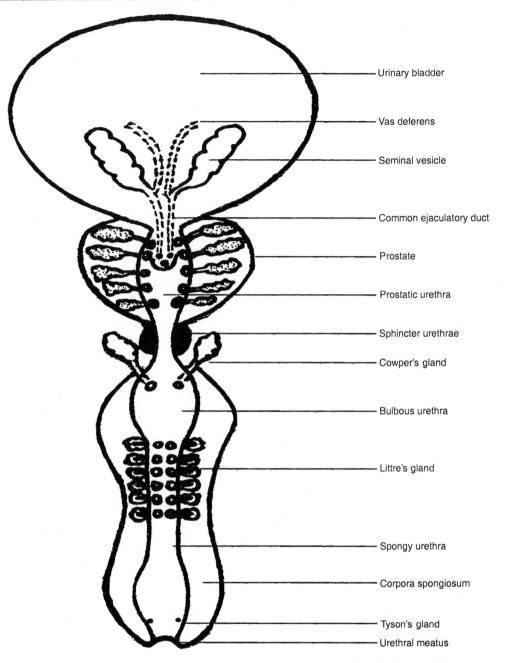

Urinary bladder

Vas deferens

Seminal vesicle

Common ejaculatory duct

Prostate

Prostatic urethra

Sphincter urethrae

Cowper's gland

Bulbous urethra

Littre's gland

Spongy urethra

Corpora spongiosum

Tyson's gland

Urethral meatus

Fig. 1   Diagrammatic Representation of Coronal Section of Male Genital Organs.

termed as corona glandis. A circular groove, coronal sulcus runs along corona glandis and separates it from the shaft of penis. Small pin head sized projections studded over corona glandis in one or two rows are known as pearly penile papules which may be confused with condyloma acuminata.

(iii) **Prepuce** is a specialized fold of skin, which marks the junction between cutaneous and mucocutaneous areas of penis. This fold of skin covers the glans penis to form a potential space known as preputial sac. Mobility and loose character of prepuce makes it a vulnerable tissue for trauma during coitus. Majority of the genital ulcer disease affects the mucocutaneous area of prepuce primarily and makes it non-retractable over glans penis. Preputial sac itself, due to its occlusive effect over the glans and undersurface of prepuce, makes this sac and the glans penis vulnerable for inflammation, which is termed as balanoposthitis.

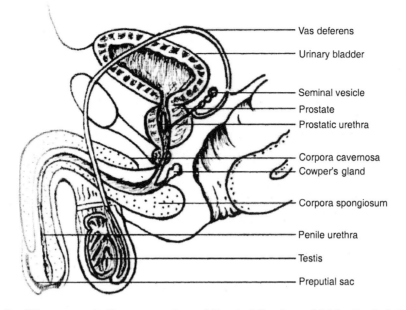

Fig. 2 Diagrammatic Representation of Saggital Section of Male Genital Organs.

Prepuce is attached to the glans penis at its ventral surface near external urinary meatus with a fold of skin known as frenulum. A tight frenulum is often predisposed to trauma during sexual intercourse and serves as another portal of entry for STD.

Scrotum

Scrotum is a loose sac of skin, which contains testes, epididymis, vas deferens and loose areolar tissue. Scrotal skin is vulnerable to genital ulcer disease due to its close proximity with penis. Genital ulcer disease at penoscrotal junction often points towards STD following the use of condom. Ulcers over penoscrotal junction and scrotum are also observed in Behcet's disease. Acute or chronic epididymitis can be a manifestation of gonococcal or non-gonococcal infections. Scrotal skin is predisposed to develop nodular scabies and persistent pruritic nodules of scabies while *Phthirus pubis* (pubic louse) enjoys the habitat of scrotal and pubic hair.

Glands (Fig. 1 and 2)

(i) **Prostate** is a racemose type of branched glandular tissue with one middle and two lateral lobes, which encircles the prostatic urethra throughout its length starting from the neck of bladder. The glandular tissue is lined by columnar epithelium and opens with multiple ducts into the prostatic urethra. The common ejaculatory ducts formed by joining the vas deferens and seminal vesicles opens up in the prostatic urethra over verumontanum. The branching character of prostatic glandular tissue along with columnar epithelium makes it especially vulnerable for gonococcal and non-gonococcal infections often leading to chronicity with consequent difficulty to eradicate the infection. Prostate can be felt through per rectal examination (feel of prostate is like tip of the nose) and prostatic massage is a useful tool to bring about prostatic secretions for examination in cases of non-gonococcal infections. This procedure is however, avoided in the presence of acute infections.

(ii) **Cowper's glands** or bulbourethral glands of Cowper are two in number, lying one on either side of the membranous urethra, which is surrounded by the sphincter urethrae muscle. The gland and its duct are lined by columnar epithelium. Gonococcal infection can lead to acute cowperitis or abscess formation in the gland, which is usually unilateral and points towards perineum. It leads to frequency of micturition, throbbing pain, fullness in the perineum and rarely acute retention of urine due to reactive spasm of sphincter urethrae. Chronic cowperitis can be a manifestation of non-gonococcal infection presenting as scanty morning urethral discharge with or without mild dysuria. Enlarged Cowper's gland can be felt one each on the side, just below the prostate on per rectal examination.

(iii) **Littre's glands** are group of mucous glands,

which are present in the roof and sides of penile urethra. These glands are also lined by columnar epithelium, hence a site of predilection for infection with gonococcus. Infection of these glands as such does not produce any specific symptoms but threads in first glass of a two or three glass test signify infection of Littre's glands. Rarely small abscesses may develop in the wall of urethra as a sequel to infection of these glands.

(iv) Tyson's glands are sebaceous glands present one each on the side of frenulum in a parafrenal distribution and on superior surface of corona of glans penis. Gonococcal tysonitis and abscess formation may be observed as a swelling on one side of the frenulum.

Female Genitalia (Fig. 3-5)

Vulva

Vulva constitutes the external genitalia of the female consisting of labia majora and minora, mons pubis, clitoris, vestibule, Skene's glands and greater vestibular (Bartholin's) glands.

(i) **Labia majora** are two folds of skin and subcutaneous tissue, which cover the vaginal opening and other structures of external genitalia. These folds join anteriorly to form mons pubis, a rounded bulge of pad of subcutaneous fat covered with hair. Posteriorly, these join to form a small transverse fold called as posterior commissure. Labia majora are the female counterparts of scrotum.

(ii) **Labia minora** are smaller folds interior to labia majora with inner mucosal and outer cutaneous surface. Labia minora fuse anteriorly to form a fold of skin that is known as clitoral prepuce and posteriorly they join at the posterior commissure or fourchette. The fourchette is quite predisposed to trauma during sexual intercourse, hence, a common site for the genital ulcer diseases.

(iii) **Clitoris** is an erectile tissue analogous to penis in the male. It has a small rudimentary glans and a prepuce.

(iv) **Vestibule** is the space between two labia minora

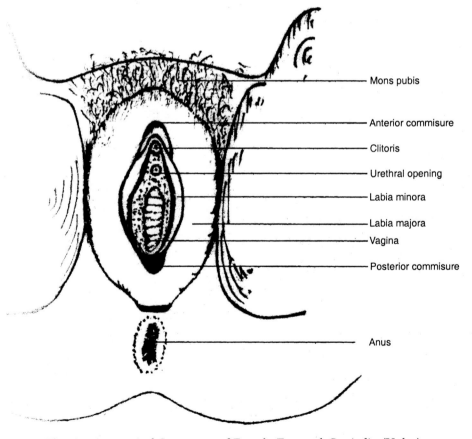

Fig. 3 Anatomical Structures of Female External Genitalia (Vulva).

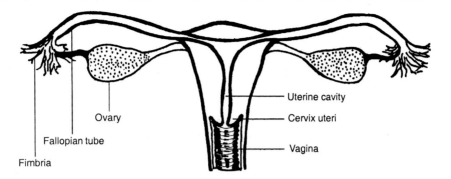

Fig. 4 Coronal Section of Female Genital Organs.

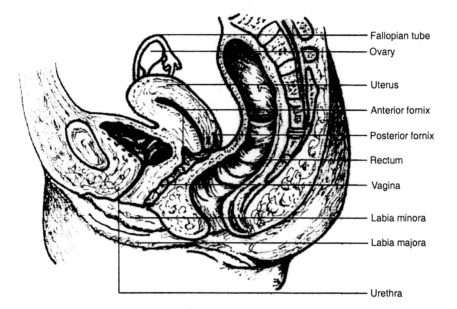

Fig. 5 Saggital Section of Female Genital Organs.

that is penetrated by openings of urethral meatus, vaginal introitus, paraurethral glands of Skene and ducts of Bartholin's gland. A thin translucent membrane called hymen covers the vaginal introitus during childhood and adolescence and is usually ruptured due to trauma, physical exercise or sexual intercourse.

(v) **Bartholin's glands**, also known as greater vestibular glands homologous to Cowper's glands in male lie in the lower third of labia majora on either side and their duct open at the side of the hymen, between the hymen and labia minora. These are compound racemose types of glands lined with columnar epithelium. Bartholin's glands get acutely inflamed with gonococcal infection (bartholinitis) and rarely may lead to bartholin abscess, which manifests as a unilateral, swelling of lower end of labia majora with consequent difficulty in walking.

(vi) **Skene's glands** or paraurethral glands are analogous to prostate in the male and lie adjacent to urethral meatus and open either directly in the vestibule or just inside the urinary meatus. Rarely, these glands can also be involved in various STD.

Female Urethra

Female urethra is quite short (3.5 cm-4 cm) as compared to the male urethra and is lined by stratified squamous epithelium in its distal part and transitional epithelium in its proximal part. Many mucosal glands, analogous to Littre's glands in the male open in the roof and the sides of female urethra. Lack of columnar epithelium makes female urethra relatively resistant to gonococcal infection.

Vagina

Vagina is a muscular tube, which starts at vestibule and continues proximally with cervix uteri. It's length is variable anteriorly (9 cm) and posteriorly (11.5 cm). Vaginal mucosa is rugose and is lined by stratified squamous epithelium, which is rich in glycogen and helps in keeping the vaginal environment acidic (pH-4.5) and thus less susceptible to penetration by sexually acquired pathogens.

Uterus

(i) **Cervix uteri** or the neck of uterus is an important organ for STD and its involvement is termed as cervicitis. Cervical canal is lined by columnar epithelium quite susceptible for gonococcal and non-gonococcal infections. Its projection into vagina divides upper vaginal space into vaginal fornices where pooled secretions serve as an important sample for isolation of sexually transmitted pathogens. It serves as a good site for collecting diagnostic samples, as it is invariably involved in gonococcal and non-gonoccal infections.

(ii) **Body of uterus** is lined by thick endometrium and may get affected in ascending infection from lower genital tract leading to endometritis and parametritis, which are common manifestations of pelvic inflammatory disease (PID) along with features of salpingitis.

(iii) **Fallopian tubes** arise from side of uterus as tortuous structures, which end up laterally as fimbriae, opening into peritoneal cavity in the vicinity of the ovaries. The tubes have different diameter at isthmus, ampulla and infundibulum. The ciliated columnar epithelium of fallopian tubes arranged in longitudinal folds is quite susceptible to infection with gonococcal and non-gonococcal pathogens resulting in acute salpingitis or acute pelvic inflammatory disease. Communication of fallopian tubes through fimbriae to the peritoneal cavity can lead to periappendicitis or perihepatitis due to either direct spread of sexual pathogens or as a sequel of PID.

Lymphatic Drainage of Genitalia

Superficial structures of genitalia drain chiefly into inguinal group of lymph nodes, constituting superficial and deep inguinal lymph nodes. (Fig. 6)

Superficial Inguinal Lymph Nodes

These are group of lymph nodes, which lie superficial to deep fascia of thigh and have two subgroups; horizontal and vertical. Horizontal subgroup lies along the inguinal ligament and is further divided into medial and lateral chains. Medial chains are 2-3 nodes in number. They drain external genitalia except glans penis or clitoris, lower parts of vagina below hymen and anal canal below the pectinate line. Some lymphatics from superolateral angle of uterus also pass through inguinal canal to drain into medial chain. Lateral chain of horizontal group of superficial inguinal lymph nodes drains lymphatics from the abdominal wall below umbilicus. Vertical group of superficial inguinal lymph nodes (4-5 nodes) lies along great saphenous vein and drain lymphatics from thigh and leg. All efferents from superficial inguinal lymph nodes ultimately drain into deep inguinal lymph nodes and external iliac lymph nodes.

Deep Inguinal Lymph Nodes

These are usually 1-3 in number with one of them usually lying within femoral canal (node of Cloquet) deep to the deep fascia medial to femoral vein. Glans penis and clitoris directly drain into deep inguinal lymph nodes. Deep lymphatics of lower limb and efferents from superficial inguinal lymph nodes drain into deep inguinal lymph nodes. Ultimately all lymphatics from inguinal lymph nodes drain through external and internal iliac lymph nodes to common iliac and paraaortic lymph nodes.

Different parts of genitalia drain their lymphatics into different lymph nodes:

(i) **Penis**: Lymphatics from the skin of the penis drain into the medial chain of horizontal group of superficial inguinal lymph nodes while deep structures including anterior urethra drain into the deep inguinal lymph nodes and posterior urethra drain into deep iliac nodes. Lymphatics from glans penis drain directly into the deep inguinal lymph nodes.

(ii) **Scrotum**: Lymphatics from the skin of scrotum drain into the medial chain of horizontal group of superficial inguinal lymph nodes, while testes and epididymis drain into the pre and para aortic group of lymph nodes.

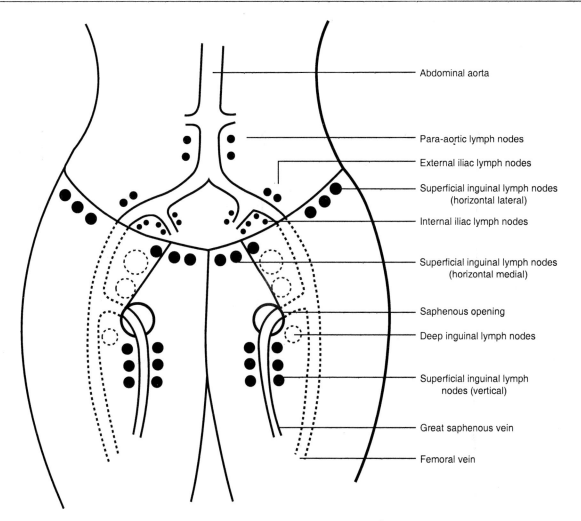

Fig. 6 Lymphatic Drainage of Genital Organs.

(iii) **Prostate**: Lymphatics from prostate drain into the internal iliac and sacral lymph nodes and partly into the external iliac lymph nodes.

(iv) **Vulva**: Lymphatics from vulval structures drain into medial chain of horizontal group of superficial inguinal lymph nodes and also femoral nodes. Some of the lymphatic vessels from vestibule also drain into the common iliac and sacral lymph nodes.

(v) **Vagina**: Lymphatics from upper third of vagina drain into the external iliac, middle third into internal iliac and lower third into medial chain of horizontal group of superficial inguinal lymph nodes.

(vi) **Cervix**: Lymphatics from cervix drain into the external and internal iliac and sacral lymph nodes. Some

of the lymphatics pass directly to the common iliac and lower paraaortic nodes.

(vii) **Uterus**: Lymphatics from uterus are divided into upper lymphatics which drain into paraaortic group of nodes, middle group to the external iliac lymph nodes and lower lymphatics running along the round ligament pass through inguinal canal to drain into medial chain of horizontal group of superficial inguinal lymph nodes.

(viii) **Fallopian tubes**: Lymphatics from the fallopian tubes drain predominantly into paraaortic lymph nodes. The lymphatics from the isthmus drain into the superficial inguinal lymph nodes

(ix) **Ovaries**: Lymphatics from ovaries drain into para and preaortic lymph nodes.

Enlargement of regional lymph nodes is invariably observed in all STD and is of considerable clinical significance in the diagnosis of genital ulcer disease. Variable morphology of inguinal lymphadenopathy in genital ulcer disease forms the basis of various inguinal syndromes or buboes. Separation of enlarged superficial inguinal lymph nodes from the deep seated femoral lymph nodes by inguinal ligament or fascia is basis of the genesis of 'groove sign of Greenblat' initially regarded to be characteristic of lymphogranuloma venereum. Similar groove sign has, however, been observed to be the manifestation of other infections and malignancy affecting inguinal lymph nodes.

Consequences of Lymphatic Blockade

Inguinal lymph nodes are by far the most important lymph nodes from the viewpoint of STD. Destruction of these lymph nodes through any process like infection, carcinoma, irradiation etc. leads to blockage of lymphatic drainage of external genitalia and lower limb. Long-term sequelae of genital lymphoedema and subsequent elephantiasis are not uncommon in infections like lymphogranuloma venereum, donovanosis, filariasis, carcinoma, tuberculosis or irradiation. Pseudoelephantiasis is condition where lymphatics rather than lymph nodes are destroyed due to local infiltration of tissues with the offending pathogen.

Perineum: It is the diamond shaped space at the lower end of the trunk and situated between the two thighs. The boundaries are outlined by scrotum in males and mons pubis in females anteriorly, posteriorly by the buttocks and laterally medial side of thighs. This site commonly overlooked and lesions like condylomata lata, genital warts or ulcers can occur in this region. Lymphatics of the perineum drain into the superficial medial group of inguinal lymph nodes.

Anorectal Mucosa and Sexually Transmitted Diseases

Anorectal mucosa has a complex lining epithelium. The perianal area up to anal verge is lined by keratinized stratified squamous epithelium similar to other mucocutaneous junctions. This is followed by conversion of squamous epithelium to stratified cuboidal epithelium of anal canal and true columnar epithelium of rectum.

Almost all the pathogens capable of producing STD over genitalia can affect anorectal mucosa and perianal skin. Lesions of STD within the anal canal and perianal area are extremely painful and produce tenesmus and painful spasm of anal sphincter due to rich nerve supply in this area. Similar lesions in the rectum are usually painless but may produce bleeding per rectum and mucopurulent discharge.

Anorectal mucosa is quite vulnerable to infection with sexually transmitted pathogens in females due to close proximity of vulva and anal orifice. Rectal mucosa is predisposed to infection with gonococcus in females and rectal involvement has been observed in 50-60% of cases of genital infection. Lymphatics from perianal skin and anal canal below the pectinate line drain into medial chain of horizontal group of superficial inguinal lymph nodes while those from rectal mucosa drain into internal iliac lymph nodes.

Oral Mucosa and Sexually Transmitted Diseases

Oral mucosa lined with stratified squamous epithelium is equally vulnerable to sexually transmitted agents as anorectal mucosa. Pharynx and tonsils are common sites affected by sexual pathogens and most of the infections in these areas are asymptomatic. Presence of lymphoid tissue in the oral mucosa in the form of tonsils makes these infections less amenable to treatment with same regimen as used for a similar infection in the genital area. Lymphatics from the oral mucosa drain into submandibular, submental, jugulodiagastric, jugulo omohyoid and other groups of superficial and deep cervical lymph nodes.

Normal Anatomical Variations In the Genital Region

Some of the anatomical variations within normal limits can mimic STD. These include:

(i) **Pearly penile papules** are small monomorphous, fibromas, which are present in a row or two over the corona glandis. They are most common in uncircumcised men. These are asymptomatic but may cause apprehension in an individual patient and mimic genital warts.

(ii) **Vestibular papillomatosis** is characterized by raised small papillae over the mucous membranes of introitus. These are normal variants and may be an incidental finding with any other symptoms over the genitalia. Like pearly penile papules these may also be mistaken for genital warts.

(iii) **Fordyce spots** are ectopic sebaceous glands present over the prepuce or inner aspect of labia minora. These lesions are often mistaken for genital warts.

(iv) **Physiological hyperpigmentation:** It is observed primarily in dark skinned individuals. The hyperpigmentation is around edges of labia minora in females, scrotum and penile skin in males and perianal skin in both sexes. Therapy is unnecessary.

References

1. Hollinshead WH. Anatomy for surgeons. (The thorax, abdomen and pelvis). New York: Harper and Row and John Weatherhill; 1966. p. 749-909.
2. McMinn RMH. Last's Anatomy: Regional and applied. Edinburgh: Churchill Livingstone; 1991. p. 385-412.
3. Williams PL. Gray's Anatomy. The anatomical basis of medicine & surgery. London: Churchill Livingstone; 1995. p. 1813-1876.
4. Agur AMR. Grant's Atlas of Anatomy. Philadelphia: Williams & Wilkins; 1991. p. 147-198.
5. Moore KL. Clinically oriented anatomy. Philadelphia: Williams & Wilkins; 1992. p. 295-322.
6. Snell RS. Clinical anatomy for medical students. London: Little, Brown and Company; 1995. p. 347-379.
7. Graney DO, Vontver LA. Anatomy and physical examination of the female genital tract. In: Holmes KK, Sparling PF, Mardh PA, et al, eds. Sexually Transmitted Diseases. New York: McGraw Hill; 1999. p. 685-698.
8. Krieger JN, Graney DO. Clinical anatomy, histology and physical examination of male genital tract. In: Holmes KK, Sparling PF, Mardh PA, et al, eds. Sexually Transmitted Diseases. New York: Mc GrawHill; 1999. p. 699-710.
9. Orient JM. Sapira's Art and Science of Bedside Diagnosis. Philadelphia: Lippincott Williams & Wilkins; 2002. p. 157-162.
10. Tindall VR. Jeffcoate's Principles of Gynaecology, Oxford: Butterworth-Heinmann; 1997. p. 16-52.

Chapter 11

Examination of the Patient in STD Clinic

K P Narender

Introduction

The patients should be explained and counseled regarding the steps of examination. The clinical examination should be conducted in a private and well-lit room. Gloves should be worn. Before proceeding to genital examination one should examine the skin and other relevant systems.

Skin

One should look for generalized maculopapular rash which can be seen in secondary syphilis, acute HIV seroconversion syndrome, acute hepatitis B, infectious mononucleosis etc. In disseminated gonococccal infection pustular lesions are seen mainly on the limbs particularly around the joints. Psoriasiform plaques are features of Reiter's disease. Burrows, excoriated papules and pustules in the web spaces of the hands are features of scabies. Special attention should be given to the palms and soles. Keratoderma blenorrhagicum of Reiter's diseases are classically seen in the palm & soles. The rash of secondary syphilis is more often seen on the palms and soles. Erythema nodosum, a feature of lymphogranuloma venereum (LGV), may be seen on the shins. Cutaneous features of HIV infection like atypical viral, bacterial and fungal infections, generalized dermatitic rash, Kaposi's sarcoma, etc should be looked for.

Oral Mucosa

Extragenital primary syphilitic chancre and oral warts can be seen in patients experiencing oral sex. Syphilitic chancre may be present on the lips, buccal mucosa or tongue. Mucous patches and snail track ulcers of secondary syphilis are seen in the oral mucosa. In late syphilis, patients can have leucoplakia, chronic superficial glossitis and gummatous perforation of the palate. Rhagades and Hutchinson's teeth are features of congenital syphilis. Oral manifestations of HIV infection include oral hairy leucoplakia, oral thrush, aphthous ulcers, gingivitis, etc.

Eyes

Patients with congenital syphilis can have iritis, interstitial keratitis and chorioretinitis. Argyll-Robertson pupil is a feature of neurosyphilis. Conjunctivitis can be seen in chlamydial, gonococcal and herpetic infections and also in Reiter's disease. Iridocyclitis may be seen in Reiter's disease, secondary & late syphilis, Behcet's disease and HIV infection. Retinal exudate and haemorrhage is seen in HIV infection.

Joints

Painful joint swellings are seen in disseminated gonococcal infection and Reiter's disease. Charcot's joints are painless, deformed and hypermobile, seen in tabes dorsalis. Clutton's joints are bilateral painless joint effusions seen in congenital syphilis.

Lymph Nodes

Generalized lymphadenopathy is usually seen in secondary syphilis and HIV infection.

Abdomen

Abdomen should be examined for evidence of pelvic inflammatory disease (PID) due to gonococcal and non gonococcal infections.

Pubic Region and Groin

Pubic region should be examined for pediculosis (pubic louse and nits) and pearly white umbilicated papules of molluscum contagiosum.

Groin should be examined for lymphadenopathy. Tender suppurative lymphadenopathy is usually seen in LGV, chancroid and herpes genitalis. 'Sign of groove'-Inguinal lymphadenopathy both above and below the inguinal ligament is suggestive of LGV. However, it may also be seen in chancroid. Syphilis usually gives rise to discrete painless rubbery nodes. Inguinal bubo is not seen with donovanosis but pseudobubo due to subcutaneous granulomata can occur. True lymphadenopathy in donovanosis suggests secondary infection or malignant transformation. Anal, penile and vulvar carcinoma can give rise to hard lymphadenopathy.

Genital Examination

Inspect the penis and scrotum for any obvious lesions or urethral discharge. If there is urethral discharge note whether it is mucoid or mucopurulent or thick pus. Urethral discharge may occur either due to urethritis or secondary to sexually transmitted ulcerative lesions or non STD ulcerative lesions in the under surface of the prepuce or on the glans penis. In uncircumcised males, retract the prepuce by gently withdrawing it over the glans penis and determine that the discharge is due to STD related urethritis or ulcer or non STD. If there is scanty urethral discharge, then milking of urethra should be done from the root of the penis towards urethral orifice.

If there are genital ulcers one should examine whether they are elevated or depressed ulcers. Elevated ulcers are seen in syphilis and donovanosis. Syphilitic ulcer is usually a single small button like ulcer seen in the coronal sulcus. Donovanosis has large granulomatous destructive ulcers. Depressed ulcers are seen in herpes genitalis, chancroid and LGV. The classical herpetic ulcers are painful superficial polycyclic erosions and in chancroid the ulcers are multiple, deep, tender and circular with necrotic slough. In LGV the ulcers are herpetiform but are rarely seen. Traumatic ulcers are usually seen on the frenulum of the penis.

Examine the penis for any growth. Lesions of Bowenoid papulosis are usually seen on the shaft of the penis. Uniform inflammation of the glans penis and the undersurface of the prepuce with pustular lesion is seen in candidal balanoposthititis. Some times only intense erythema is seen suggestive of candida hypersentivity reaction. Circinate balanitis of Reiter's disease manifests as erythematous eroded lesions with polycyclic edge.

Scabetic excoriated papules and burrows are usually seen on the shaft of the penis. In Peyronie's disease there may be induration or fibrotic lump inside the penile shaft. Urethral meatus should be examined carefully for syphilitic chancre or any other ulcers, discharge, narrowing and warts.

One should be aware of some of the physiological condition, which might pose diagnostic dilemma. Pearly penile papules otherwise known as hirsute papillomas are tiny regular papules arranged in rows around the coronal sulcus. These may be mistaken for warts. Multiple small yellow or white submucous ectopic sebaceous glands which are known as Fordyce's spots may be seen on the inner surface of the prepuce.

Scrotum should be examined for swelling, erythema and ulcers. Ulcers are most often due to Behcet's disease. However, it can also result from syphilitic gumma or fungating testicular cancer. Tiny dark red papules are seen in angiokeratoma whereas firm whitish nodules are seen in sebaceous cysts. Erythematous pruritic nodules are seen in scabies.

Testes and Epididymis

Testes and epididymis should be examined. The normal testes are equal in size varying between 3.5 and 4 cm in length. Look for any tenderness, swelling, nodularity and testicular sensation. The epididymis has head and tail ends. The head end is present at the upper pole of the testes on its posterior aspect and is a soft nodular structures about 1 cm in length. The tail is found on the posterolateral aspect of the inferior pole of the testes. It is a soft coiled tubular structure. Tender enlargement is seen in acute gonococcal and chlamydial infection.

Genital examination is incomplete without anorectal examination. It should be done in both homosexual and heterosexual men. The patient should lie down in the left lateral position with the knee drawn up or in the knee-elbow position. 'Funnel' shaped and lax anus is suggestive of homosexuals. One should look for ulceration, warty growth, fissures and tags. Syphilitic chancre and herpetic infection can be confused with an anal fissure. Anal tags may resemble that of warts or condylomata lata of secondary syphilis. Rectal mucosae should be examined for ulceration, warty lesions or any other inflammation after inserting the proctoscope lubricated with KY gelly or liquid paraffin.

Examination of Female Genitalia

Women should be examined with their consent and in the presence of a female attendant. The best position is lithotomy. One should examine the perineum, vulva, labia majora and labia minora for discharge, redness, swelling, excoriation, ulcers, warts and any other skin lesions. The approach to the genital ulcer is same as in men. Swelling of the vulva erythema and excoriation are suggestive of either candidiasis or trichomoniasis.

Separate the labia and look for any discharge, wipe away any excessive discharge and insert a bivalve Cusco speculum after moistening with water. Look for evidence of vaginitis. If there is vaginal discharge, note the colour, consistency, and odour of the discharge. Curdy white discharge is suggestive of candidiasis. Frothy greenish yellow and malodorous discharge is characteristic of trichomoniasis. In bacterial vaginosis, the discharge is non-inflammatory and whitish. Also look for any other lesions. After careful examination of the vagina, one should examine the cervix. Wipe the cervix with a cotton swab and look for any discharge from the os, ulcers/erosion, warts and cervicitis. For cervical cytology smear can be taken from the cervix. Once the examination is over then remove the speculum and see the uretheral orifice for inflammation, discharge or warts. If there is no obvious discharge and milk urethra gently forward.

Examination of the anal and perianal region is done as in men.

Bimanual examination is performed to detect PID or abnormalities of the upper genital tract. It is customary to use the fingers of the right hand in the vagina and to place the left hand on the abdomen. In virgins and children only a rectal examination should be performed. For per vaginal examination, separate the labia with the left hand to expose the vestibule and insert the examining finger of the right hand. The cervix is palpated and any hardness or irregularity is noted. The examining left hand is placed over the abdomen just below the umbilicus and the fingers of both hands are then used to palpate the uterus. The size, shape, position, mobility and tenderness of the uterus is noted. The tips of the vaginal fingers are then placed into each lateral fornix and the adnexae are examined on either side. Tender uterus, fallopian tubes and positive cervical motion tenderness is suggestive of PID.

The various lab diagnostic procedures including collection of samples for urethral and vaginal discharge are discussed in a separate chapter.

The details of history taking and the proforma are given in Appendix I.

References

1. Genitalia and sexually transmitted diseases. In: Swash M, edr. Hutchison's Clinical Methods. 21st edn. London: ELBS; 2002. p. 407–419.
2. The Gynaecological history and examnation. In: Campbell S, Monga A, eds. Gynaecology by ten teachers. 17th edn, London: ELST; 2000. p. 1–5.

Chapter 12

Side Laboratory Procedures in Sexually Transmitted Diseases

Vinod K Sharma, G Sethuraman

Introduction

Sexually transmitted diseases (STD) are a group of communicable diseases, which are acquired during heterosexual or homosexual intercourse. STD still remain an important major public health problem not only because of their complications, sequelae and the social stigma but also because they increase the risk for transmission of human immunodeficiency virus. Hence a good clinical assessment and the appropriate laboratory tests are mandatory for the diagnosis and management of different STD. A number of bacteria, spirochaetes, viruses, fungi, chlamydiae and protozoa are known to cause STD. Identification of these different group of organisms needs skilled laboratory personnel and a good laboratory infrastructure. In this chapter the common laboratory diagnostic procedures which can be done in an outpatient department are described (Table 1).

Table 1. Side Lab Procedures in STD

1. Dark field microscopy
2. Gram stain
3. Giemsa stain
4. Wet mount
5. KOH wet mount
6. Whiff or sniff test
7. Bubo aspiration
8. Acetic acid test
9. Two and three glass test

Dark Field Microscopy[1]

Dark field microscopy commonly referred to as dark ground illumination (DGI) is the only method of demonstrating *Treponema pallidum*, the causative agent

for syphilis. The organism is not stained by ordinary reagents and is so thin that it cannot be visualized under the normal light microscope.[2] In dark field microscopy, only light rays hitting the organisms at an oblique angle enter the microscope objective giving rise to a luminous appearance against a black background. Hence visualization of *T. pallidum* becomes much easier.

Requirements

- Dark field microscope
- Thin glass slides (1 mm)

Collection of Specimen for Dark Field Microscopy

T. pallidum can be identified in serous fluid from the lesions of primary and secondary syphilis and early congenital syphilis. Rarely, it can be identified in lymph node aspirate.

- Clean the lesion carefully with sterile gauze soaked in saline.
- Gently abrade the lesion with dry gauze, wipe off any blood stained serum and squeeze to produce clear serous exudate.
- The serous exudate is transferred on to the glass slide either by pressing the cover slip directly on to the serous exudate or by Pasteur pipette.
- If serous exudate is sufficient, cover with cover slip and examine.
- If the material is not sufficient then it is mixed with a drop of saline to give a homogenous suspension.

- Seal the edges of the cover slip with petroleum jelly.
- Examine immediately.

Setting the Microscope for the Examination

- Bring down the condenser of the dark field microscope.
- Put a drop of liquid paraffin on the condenser of dark field microscope.
- Place the slide on the microscope stage.
- Raise the condenser until there is good contact between the oil and bottom of the slide.
- Avoid trapping of air bubbles in the oil.

Focussing

Bring the specimen into focus by means of the low power objective (x10). Centre the light in the field by adjusting the centering screws located on the condenser and focus the condenser by raising and lowering it until the smallest possible diameter of light is obtained. Recentre the light if necessary. Put a drop of liquid paraffin on coverslip and examine under 100x oil immersion lens. Bring the specimen into focus and examine the slide carefully. The contrast will be better when the microscopy is carried out in the dark. Avoid bright daylight. If Brownian movements can be seen clearly, the slide is focussed.

WHO[1] claims that *T. pallidum* can be seen under dry x40 lens but it is not a common practice in India.

Reading

T. pallidum appears white, illuminated on a dark background. The organism is identified by its typical morphology, size and movements. It is a thin spiral organism 6-14 μm long. It has 8-14 spirals which are regular and pronounced. It rotates relatively slowly about the longitudinal axis (like a corkscrew). The rotation is accompanied by sudden bending at acute angle which is most typical or twisting in the middle of the organism. Other movements which may be observed are lengthening, shortening and distortion in tortuous convolutions. Obstruction of the treponemes by heavier objects might distort the coil. The pathogenic *T. pallidum* can be differentiated from other non-pathogenic spirochaetes in which the movements are different unlike the corkscrew, they take the form of a writhing motion with marked flexion and frequent relaxation of the coils.

The presence of *T. pallidum* confirms the diagnosis of syphilis. Ideally the test should be done on 3 consecutive days as a single dark field microscopy has a sensitivity of no more than 50%. Dark field microscopy is less useful for lesions in the oral cavity as it is colonized by other spirochaetes.[1,3]

Reasons for Negative Test

- Non-syphilitic ulcer
- Natural resolution of the lesion
- Treated patients
- Prior topical application of antiseptics or antibiotics
- The number of organisms present in the specimen is insufficient

Gram Staining[4,5]

Gram staining is useful for the diagnosis of gonococcal and non-gonococcal urethritis, mucopurulent cervicitis, chancroid, bacterial vaginosis and candidal infections.

Requirements

- Crystal violet
  Dissolve 2 gm of crystal violet (methylrosanilinium chloride) in 20 ml of 96% ethanol and then add 80 ml of 0.08 mol/L (1%) ammonium oxalate.
- Iodine solution
  2 gm of iodine crystals are dissolved in 10 ml of 1mol/l NaOH solution: make up to 100 ml with distilled water.
- Decolourizing solution
  10 ml of analytical grade acetone is mixed with 50 ml of 96% ethanol.
- Counter stain solution (either fuschsin or safranin)
  Fuschsin
  0.3 gm of basic fuschsin is dissolved in 10 ml of 96% ethanol. 5 gm of phenol is dissolved in 95 ml of distilled water. Mix the solutions slowly with vigorous stirring. Add 950 ml of distilled water. Allow the mixture to stand for 2-3 days. Filter through a 0.22 μm filter before use.
  Safranin
  1 gm of safranin O is dissolved in 20 ml of 96% ethanol and 10 ml of this solution is diluted with 90 ml of distilled water.

Collection of Specimen for Gram Staining

Sterile cotton, calcium alginate or polyethylene terephthalate (PET) swabs can be used for collecting the specimen. In India sterile cotton wool swab is routinely used.

Gonorrhoea

Gonorrhoea caused by *Neisseria gonorrhoeae* produces lower urogenital tract infection and pelvic inflammatory disease (PID) in women, urethritis and epididymitis in men and proctitis, pharyngitis, conjunctivitis and disseminated infections in both the sexes. The appropriate site for specimen collection will depend on the age, sex, sexual practices and the clinical symptoms.

Site for Collection of Specimens

The primary collection site in heterosexual men is the urethra and in homosexual men the urethra, rectum and oropharynx. In women the material is collected from the endocervical canal. The secondary sites of specimen collection in women include urethra, vagina, rectum and oropharynx. Direct microscopic examination is generally not recommended for the diagnosis of rectal and pharyngeal infection.

Method of Collection of Specimen

Urethra: Urethral specimen is collected at least 1 hour after the patient has urinated. Retract the prepuce, clean the tip of the meatus with normal saline and collect the pus directly onto the swab. If no discharge is seen, milk the urethra from root of penis towards glans to express the pus. If no pus is obtained, insert a thin sterile swab 2-3 cm into the urethra and gently scrape the mucosa by rotating the swabs for 5-10 seconds. The organisms can be also be demonstrated in the sediment of early morning first voided urine sample. In women, massage the urethra against the pubic symphysis and use the same technique as for men.

Endocervical specimen: The routine use of antiseptics, analgesics or lubricants should be avoided. The vaginal speculum is inserted after moistening with warm water. Clean the exocervix using forceps with sterile cotton swab. Insert another sterile swab 2 cm into the cervical canal, rotate and move from side to side for 5-10 seconds and withdraw.

Vagina: Vaginal specimens are collected for prepubertal girls and women who have had a hysterectomy. The material is taken from the posterior fornix with a swab either with or without a speculum.

Nongonococcal Urethritis and Mucopurulent Cervicitis

Specimen is collected in the same manner as in gonorrhoea but as discharge in NGU may be scanty, the samples are collected after holding the urine for 3-4 hours.

Chancroid

In chancroid the specimen is usually collected from the edge of the ulcer. First, clean the ulcer with a saline soaked gauze and then with dry gauze, take a sterile swab and roll it in one direction on the edge of undermined ulcer. After doing so, reroll the swab in the reverse direction on a glass slide and stain it. The organisms may be demonstrated from the material aspirated from an intact bubo.[3]

Bacterial Vaginosis

It is caused by replacement of the lactobacilli of the vagina by the characteristic group of bacteria. Here the specimen is collected from the posterior or lateral wall of vagina with a sterile swab soaked in saline.

Procedure

A. Preparation of Smear

- Take a clean glass slide, wipe it with gauze piece and pass it through the flame twice or thrice and wipe it again.
- Draw 2 vertical lines 2.5 cm apart with a glass marking pencil on the central part of the slide.
- Roll the swab with the specimen over the marked area and spread it to make a smear of 2 × 1 cm size.
- Label the smear on the right or left corner of the slide.

B. Fixing of Smear

- Fixing kills the organism, fixes it to the slide, prevents autolytic changes and makes the organisms permeable to dye and harmless to the person handling the smear.

- Hold the slide with the smear facing upwards.
- Pass the slide over the flame of a Bunsen's burner or spirit lamp twice or thrice.
- Allow the fixed smear to cool.
- Heating should be appropriate and tolerable to the back of the hand.

C. Staining

- Cover the fixed smear with crystal violet for 1 minute and then rinse it with tap water.
- Flood the slide with Gram's iodine solution for 1 minute. Drain off the solution and gently rinse with running water.
- Decolourize with acetone-ethanol until the drops falling off the slide are no longer blue. This usually takes 10 to 20 seconds depending on the thickness of the smear. Excessive decolourization must be avoided. Rinse quickly under running water to stop decolourization and drain off excess water.
- Counterstain with safranin or fuschsin for 1 minute. Gently wash in running water and blot the slide with absorbent paper.

Smear Reading

Examine the slide using a light microscope. Scan the smear first and focus a good field. Put a drop of liquid paraffin without air trapping and examine under 100x oil immersion objective. Push the condenser up and open the iris diaphragm so that maximum light passes through the slide.

Identification of gonococcus which appear as intracellular gram negative kidney or coffee bean shaped diplococci, 0.6-0.8μm in size confirms the diagnosis of gonorrhoea. Sometimes organisms may be extracellular. In addition clumps of pus cells are also seen. Non-pathogenic Neisseria other than *N. meningitidis*, which are morphologically indistinguishable from *N. gonorrhoeae* are generally not cell associated. Acinetobacter species are bipolar staining gram negative bacilli.[6]

Presence of 5 or more polymorphonuclear leucocytes (PMN) in the absence of intracellular gram negative diplococci is suggestive of non-gonococcal urethritis.[7] Cervical gram stain with more than 30 PMN/high power field in women of menstruating age is suggestive

of mucopurulent cervicitis.[8]

Haemophilus ducreyi, the causative agent of chancroid appears as small gram negative bacilli grouped in chains or "school of fish" or "railroad track" appearance. The sensitivity of gram staining in chancroid is less than 50% as the typical arrangement is seen only infrequently on smears. Often, the ulcers harbour polymicrobial flora due to contamination resulting in false positive diagnosis.

Presence of "clue cells" are highly diagnostic of bacterial vaginosis (BV). Clue cells are squamous epithelial cells coated with many small coccobacillary organisms giving a stippled or granular appearance. The edge of the cells are usually indistinct. In BV, a mixture of normal exfoliated vaginal epithelial cells and 20% or more clue cells are seen. The organisms are usually *G. vaginalis* which are gram variable to gram negative small rods (1.5-2.5μm × 0.5μm) showing pleomorphism. Sometimes other anaerobes like Prevotella spp and Mobiluncus spp are seen as slender (0.3-0.4μm) slightly curved rods either singly or in pairs with the appearance of gull wings.[9]

Gram staining may also be used in the diagnosis of vulvovaginal candidiasis and balanoposthitis which will show gram positive budding yeast cells looking like "figure of 8" and yeast hyphae. However KOH wet mount examination may improve the diagnostic sensitivity.[9]

Tzanck Smear or Giemsa Stain[10,11]

Tzank smear or Giemsa stain is a simple bed side test which can be used in the diagnosis of various STD, like genital herpes, molluscum contagiosum, donovanosis and chancroid.

Requirements

- Giemsa stock: It can be prepared by dissolving 4 gm Giemsa powder in 250 ml glycerol at 60°C and then add 250 ml methanol.
- 4 ml of stock solution is added to 96 ml of distilled water or buffered water at pH 7.0-7.2.

Collection of Specimen in Various STD

Herpes Progenitalis

The intact roof of the vesicle or blister is opened along

one side and folded back. Scrape the under surface of roof of vesicle and the floor of ulcer with a curette or scalpel and smear the obtained material on a clean glass slide.[12,13]

Donovanosis

Clean the granulomatous ulcer at the edge with gauze soaked in saline and then with dry gauze. A small piece of tissue is removed with forceps or a curette. Local anaesthesia may be required. Alternatively, the ulcer can be scraped with a scalpel. Place the tissue specimen over a clean glass slide. Keep another slide over the specimen and press it firmly so that the tissue is crushed between the two slides. Spread the crushed tissue and allow the smear to dry. Direct impressions on a glass slide are not usually adequate because surface debris and other bacteria are liable to obscure the picture.[14]

Molluscum Contagiosum

Central semisolid core is removed and stained.

Procedure

- Initial preparation of the slide is same as in Gram's stain.
- The smear is fixed in methanol. Dip the slide for 5 minutes in Coplin jar containing methanol.
- Allow the smear to dry.
- Dilute the Giemsa stain 10 times or 1ml of Giemsa stain is added to 9 ml of distilled water.
- Cover the slide with the diluted Giemsa stain and leave it for 20-30 minutes.
- Wash the slide with distilled water or buffer.
- Allow the smear to dry.

Smear Reading

The smear is examined under the low power and then under the oil immersion objective. Herpes progenitalis will show the characteristic multinucleated giant keratinocytes. The cells show ballooning degeneration sometimes reaching a diameter of 60-80 μm. The nuclei show blurring of chromatin pattern and loss of staining. Intranuclear inclusion bodies surrounded by a subtle halo are highly diagnostic of herpetic infection but difficult to find in the smear.[12]

The demonstration of intracellular donovan bodies is the gold standard for the diagnosis of donovanosis. They appear as coccobacilli within the large vacuoles (80-90 μm in diameter) in the cytoplasm of large histiocytes and rarely in plasma cells and PMN. They are blue purple in colour and resemble "safety pins". A wide variety of stains may be used for demonstrating the donovan bodies viz. Leishman or Wright's stain, Delafield's haematoxylin with a small amount of eosin.[14]

Molluscum contagiosum will show the characteristic molluscum or Henderson–Patterson's bodies. They are the largest inclusion bodies (30-35 μm). They are basically virus transformed keratinocytes that appear as ovoid deeply basophilic bodies with a hyaline homogenous structure surrounded by a membrane.[12] Although molluscum bodies can be identified in the smear, the diagnosis is generally made on clinical grounds.[15]

Wet mount (direct microscopy without staining)[5]

This is mainly used for the diagnosis of trichomoniasis, BV and candidiasis in women and occasionally in men with urethral discharge in whom trichomoniasis is suspected.

Collection of Specimens

Vaginal discharge is obtained with cotton tipped swab from the posterior fornix. In men, the sample is collected by inserting a sterile swab into the urethra for 1-2 cm.

Procedure

The sample is placed on a clean glass slide, diluted with a drop of saline, and then a coverslip is placed. It is examined under the light microscope immediately under low power (X40) with reduced illumination.

Reading

In trichomoniasis, *Trichomonas vaginalis* is identified by its typical jerky movements. They are clear pear shaped organisms about the size of a pus cell with four anterior flagellae and an axostyle that traverses the body to end in a spine. They have a lateral undulating membrane. In addition, large number of leucocytes are seen in most of the patients.

Though clue cells of bacterial vaginosis can be seen in wet mount, they are better visualized with gram stain. Yeast cells of candidiasis can also be seen in wet mount but 10% KOH mount is better.

KOH Wet Mount[16]

KOH wet mount is used for the diagnosis of candidal infection of the genital tract.

Requirement

10 or 20% KOH

Specimen Collection

In females, the discharge is collected from the posterior fornix. In men with balanitis, a swab moistened in saline is rubbed against the glans penis.[9]

Procedure

- Take a clean microscopic slide.
- Place the specimen on the slide.
- Add 2 drops of 10% KOH to the specimen.
- Put a clean cover slip over the specimen. Ensure that no air bubble is trapped under the coverslip.
- The prepared smear is examined under the light microscope first scanning the material under low power (10x) and then using 40x magnification.

Reading

Identification of yeast usually confirms the diagnosis of candidiasis. Yeasts are round to ovoid cells, 4μm in diameter showing typical budding (blastoconidia) and the pseudohyphae.

Acetic Acid Test[17]

The acetic acid test is used to detect the subclinical genital human papilloma virus (HPV) associated infection.

Requirements

- Acetic acid 3 to 5%.
- Swab sticks

Procedure

- Clean the area to be tested with gauze soaked in saline and then with dry gauze.
- Apply the acetic acid with the swab.
- Wait for 2 to 3 minutes for lesions of vulva and penis. In uterine cervix the reaction appears within 1 minute.

What to look for ?

The affected area becomes whitish, distinctly demarcated and thickened sometimes with elevated borders and centrally located epithelial fissures. In men, the surface of the affected areas may look red because of hypervascularization. The whitish appearance of the epithelium is due to over expression of cytokeratin 10 in the HPV infected suprabasal cells. The epithelial cells of HPV infected areas are undifferentiated containing large nuclei and their protein content is very high. Acetic acid application causes denaturation of these proteins which results in whitish appearance of the epithelium.

Limitation

The test is not specific for HPV infection as acetic acid induced whitish reaction of the genital epithelium can occur in other nonspecific inflammation. But in HPV infection the reaction occurs much slower.

Whiff Test or Sniff Test[5]

Whiff test is diagnostic of BV. Addition of 1 or 2 drops of 10% KOH solution to the specimen of vaginal discharge on a glass slide causes enhancement of typical fishy odour.

Aspiration of Bubo

Aspiration of bubo is carried out for fluctuant bubo associated with chancroid and LGV. Once bubo becomes fluctuant it may continue to progress despite antimicrobial therapy.

Procedure

Patient is made to lie on the couch in supine position. Skin is sterilized with iodine and bubo is aspirated with 16-18G needle with 10 or 20 ml syringe. Aspiration is done from the non-dependent fluctuant part of the bubo. The aspiration is continued till all parts of the swelling are reduced. The material is collected and sent for culture for *H. ducreyi*, chlamydia and anaerobes and smear for gram stain and direct immunofluorescene for chlamydia.

Two and Three Glass Test[18]

This test is mainly used to differentiate anterior urethritis from posterior urethritis or infection of the bladder. The patient is asked to pass urine into two separate glasses. In case of anterior urethritis the first specimen is cloudy or hazy with pus or mucous threads and the specimen in the second glass is clear. Haziness in the second specimen suggests involvement of the posterior urethra. If both the specimens are hazy then bacterial cystitis should be suspected. For greater accuracy it is necessary to apply the three glass test, in which the anterior urethra is irrigated with colourless antiseptic solution (such as 1:8000 oxycyanide of mercury) until the washings contained in the first glass seem to be clear. The patient then passes urine into two other separate glasses. If the first sample of urine contains pus, the posterior urethra is infected. If there is pus in the second glass, then infection has extended into the bladder. But these days, it is used infrequently.

References

1. Dyck EV, Meheus AZ, Piot P, eds. Syphilis. In: Laboratory diagnosis of sexually transmitted diseases. Geneva: World Health Organization; 1999. p. 36-49.
2. Young H. Syphilis-serology. Dermatol Clin 1998; 16: 691–698.
3. Arndt KA, Bowers KE, eds. Sexually transmitted diseases. In: Manual of dermatologic therapeutics. Philadelphia: Lippincott Williams and Wilkins; 2002. p. 196-208.
4. Dyck EV, Meheus AZ, Piot P, eds. Gonnorrhoea. In: Laboratory diagnosis of sexually transmitted diseases. Geneva: World Health Organization: 1999; 1-21.
5. Management of patients with sexually transmitted diseases. Geneva: World Health Organization, 1991.
6. Hook EW, Handsfield HH. Gonococcal infections in the adult. In: Holmes KK, Mardh P, Sparlin FP, et al, eds. Sexually transmitted diseases. New York: McGraw Hill; 1999. p. 407-422.
7. Stary A. Urethritis: Diagnosis of nongonococcal urethritis. Dermatol Clin 1998; 16: 723-726.
8. Stamm WE. *Chlamydia trachomatis* infection of the adult. In: Holmes KK, Mardh P, Sparling PF, et al, eds. Sexually transmitted diseases. New York: McGraw Hill; 1999. p. 407-422.
9. Dyck EV, Meheus AZ, Piot P, eds. Vaginitis in adults. In: Laboratory diagnosis of sexually transmitted diseases. Geneva: World Health Organization; 1999:70-80.
10. Dyck EV, Meheus AZ, Piot P, eds. Media, reagents, stains (Annex 2). In: Laboratory diagnosis of sexually transmitted diseases. Geneva: World Health Organization; 1999: 102-112.
11. Dyck EV, Meheus AZ, Piot P, eds. *Chlamydia trachomatis* infection. In: Laboratory diagnosis of sexually transmitted diseases. Geneva: World Health Organization; 1999: 22-35.
12. Ruocco V, Ruocco E. Tzanck smear, an old test for the new millennium: when and how. Int J Dermatol 1999: 38: 830-834.
13. Yeung-Yue KA, Brentjens MH, Lee PC, Tyring SK. Herpes simplex viruses 1 and 2. Dermatol clin 2002; 20: 249-266.
14. Richens J. The diagnosis and treatment of donovanosis (granuloma inguinale). Genitourin Med 1991; 67: 441-452.
15. Perna AG, Tyring ST. A review of the dermatological manifestations of pox virus infection. Dermatol Clin 2002; 20: 343-346.
16. Warren NG. Taxonomy and introduction. Dermatol Clin 1996; 14: 1-7.
17. Strand A, Rylander E. Human papilloma virus. Subclinical and atypical manifestations. Dermatol Clin 1998; 16: 817-822.
18. King A, Nicol, Rodin P, eds. 'Non specific' urogenital infections; Non gonococcal genital infections in children; Non gonococcal ophthalmia. In: Venereal diseases. 4th edn. London: ELBS; 1980. p. 274-293.

PART IV
Sexually Transmitted Diseases

Chapter 13

Syphilis : Clinical Features and Natural Course

R S Misra, Joginder Kumar

Syphilis simulates every other disease. It is the only disease necessary to know. One then becomes an expert dermatologist, an expert laryngologist, an expert alienist, an expert oculist, an expert internist and an expert diagnostician,

Sir William Osler

Introduction

With its protean manifestations syphilis is not an exclusive domain of the venereologists. The disease is systemic right from its inception. In fact occasionally it has been transmitted by blood transfusion even during its incubation period in the donor. Early world literature talks of genital ulcers or chancres, skin rashes and bone pains as its clinical manifestations. The disease was known to occur after coitus and through surgical instrumentation. The redoutable experiment of John Hunter[1] (1728-1793) gave rise to misconcept of common aetiology of syphilis and gonorrhoea. He had inoculated himself or a patient's urethra with discharge from a prostitute. The development of chancre as well as gonorrhoea made him propagate this concept. Later, Philip Ricord[2] in 1838 proved the concept to be erroneous and established syphilis and gonorrhoea as two distinct disease entities. John Hunter's patient had probably been suffering from both the diseases. John Hunter, a keen observer, had noticed the occurrence of two types of genital chancres—hard ones and soft ones. He referred the latter as non-specific. Another worker Bassereau in 1852 detected that patients with hard or soft chancre passed similar lesions to their contacts and separated both as two different venereal diseases.[3] To link some of the systemic symptoms and signs to syphilis had been difficult. Syphilitic origin of aortic aneurysm had been suspected in early eighteenth century but consensus could only be reached on this aspect

two centuries later in 1903, when the histopathological picture had become clear.[4] Clustering of tabes patients and patients with general paresis of insane among past sufferers of syphilis led to the suggestion of their relationship with syphilis.

The clinical picture of syphilis now has become clear. The disease presents in a congenital or an acquired form. The acquired form may be early or late depending upon whether the infection was acquired within the last two years or earlier than that. The most accepted classification of syphilis is as below:

A. Acquired Syphilis

Early Syphilis

- Primary syphilis
- Secondary syphilis
- Early latent syphilis

Late Syphilis

- Late latent syphilis
- Tertiary syphilis
  Benign tertiary
  Cardiovascular syphilis
  Neurosyphilis

The term tertiary syphilis is used to include benign tertiary, cardiovascular and neurosyphilis.

B. Congenital Syphilis

Early congenital syphilis
Late congenital syphilis
Stigmata of congenital syphilis

Biology of *Treponema pallidum*

Treponema pallidum is a member of the order spirochaetales. *Treponema pallidum* subspecies *pallidum* is 6-20 μm in length and 0.10 to 0.18 μm in breadth. Unstained organism can only be visualized in the dark field microscope. Silver impregnation technique makes the organism visualized easily when examined under the microscope. The electron microscopic examination reveals that the organism has regular tight spirals with a coil length of 1.1μm and an amplitude of 0.2 to 0.3μm. The spirochaete lacks the capsule. It is composed of an outer membrane, and inner cytoplasmic membrane. The thin cell wall is also composed of an outer membrane, and inner cytoplasmic membrane. The cell wall is composed of peptidoglycans. The outer membrane lacks lipopolysaccharide,[5] which makes the organism susceptible to disruption by routine physical manipulation like centrifugation, washing in vitro, incubation and treatment with detergent.[3,6] The outer membrane contains only rare integral membrane protein, some of which are integral membrane protein referred to as treponemal rare outer membrane protein (TROMP).

The movement of the *T. pallidum* depends on the flagella that are located in the periplasmic space.[3] The spiral structure of the organism and unique location of flagella enables the spirochaete to retain motility in the viscous fluid like synovial, eye and extracellular matrix of the skin.[7] The three periplasmic flagella originate at each end of the *T. pallidum* and entwine the protoplasmic cylinder extending towards the centre. The periplasmic flagella are composed of hook-basal body complex and flagellar filament made up of multiple protein that are arranged into outer sheath and central core. The motility related genes play a role in dissemination.

The organism can't be grown in vitro for a extended period. For the experimental purpose *T. pallidum* is grown in the rabbit testicles.[7,8] Limited growth of *T. pallidum* in tissue culture of Sf1Ep cottontail rabbit epithelial cells is obtained under microaerobic condition (1.5% O_2) at 34 to 35°C. The generation time in vivo is 30-33 hours.

Several animal model of *T. pallidum* infection have been investigated but only the infection in the rabbit results in the infection similar to the human beings. The primary lesion developed at the site of inoculation; but the lesion did not develop in the older rabbit. In case of animal model like hamsters[9] and guinea pigs[10] there was no skin lesion but the systemic infection like lymphadenopathy, humoral and cellular immunity took place. Since these animals were susceptible to the *T. pallidum* subspecies *endemicum*, it also serves as animal model for endemic syphilis and yaws.

Incubation Period

The primary syphilitic lesions appear within 9 to 90 days as an ulcer (chancre) at the site of inoculation. In the majority, the chancre appears at 2-6 weeks with a median incubation period of about 3 weeks. The incubation period is inversely proportional to the number of treponemes inoculated. The disease manifests when the organisms multiply to a density of 10^7 per gram of tissue.[11] The three weeks incubation period corresponds to an inoculum containing 500 to 1000 organisms. Trauma during sexual intercourse is the other factor that can decrease the incubation period.

Transmission of the Disease: Mode of Infection

The organism *T. pallidum* does not occur in the environment and man is the only natural host and reservoir. The organism is very sensitive to temperature and drying. It is the moist skin or mucosal lesion which transmits the disease. The prime route of acquiring infection is sexual contact. Majority of the patients are heterosexual acquiring infection through peno-vaginal intercourse. The efficiency of this route to infect the contacts is around 30%. With the changing sexual norms, oral sexual contact is also emerging to be important mode especially among homosexuals. In a recent outbreak, as many as one third of the patients had oral sex as the only risk factor.[12]

The primary chancre and secondary syphilitic mucosal or moist cutaneous lesions are the sources of treponemes to pass the disease onto the contacts. The 50% infectious dose has been worked out to be 57 organisms using Nichol's strain of the treponeme.[13]

Apart from sexual route other modes of transmission include vertical transmission from infected mother to the foetus (congenital syphilis). Kissing, fondling an infant having early congenital syphilis, accidental inoculations among medical personnel by needle pricks on the digits or spill of syphilitic material in the eye have also caused the disease. Improved modern blood storage techniques have almost eliminated the possibility of transmission by blood transfusion as the organism soon loses its virulence outside the body.[14]

Handling of inanimate objects can transmit the disease if it had moist infected body fluids. An out-break of syphilis in the medieval cities of Europe could be traced to a ritual of cupping (a procedure to exude 'bad fluids') in the social bathhouses. The primary lesions had been restricted to the sites of cupping. No fresh cases were seen after the closure of these bath-houses.[15]

Progression of the Disease: Course of Untreated Syphilis (Fig. 1)

Philip Ricord in 1838 had classified syphilis into primary, secondary and tertiary stages but exact progression of the disease could be known only when report of Oslo study became available. Professor Caeser Boeck had

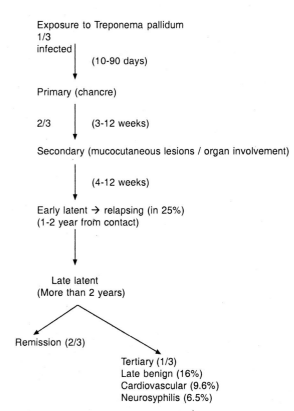

Exposure to Treponema pallidum
1/3 infected | (10-90 days)

Primary (chancre)

2/3 | (3-12 weeks)

Secondary (mucocutaneous lesions / organ involvement)

| (4-12 weeks)

Early latent → relapsing (in 25%)
(1-2 year from contact)

Late latent
(More than 2 years)

Remission (2/3)

Tertiary (1/3)
Late benign (16%)
Cardiovascular (9.6%)
Neurosyphilis (6.5%)

Fig: 1 Natural Course of Untreated Syphilis

withheld the treatment of 1978 patients of primary and secondary syphilis during the period between 1891 to 1910, with the belief that treatment available was inadequate. The outcome had been analyzed by some workers.[16] The limitation of the study was that the basis of diagnosis was only clinical criteria. Clark and Danbolt re-studied the available clinical material and concluded that the great majority of these patients had early syphilis.[17] The other studies dealing with the natural course, Tuskegee[18] and Rosahn[19] are said to be biased for some or the other reason and have shown spontaneous cure in some patients.

After an incubation period of about 3 weeks, about 30% of people having unprotected sex with infected partners develop the chancre of primary syphilis. These lesions heal in about 3 to 8 weeks.

After 2 to 8 weeks of appearance of primary chancre, lesions of secondary syphilis appear. About 25% of the patients in secondary syphilitic stage do not give history of primary lesion. Almost all patients undergo secondary phase though the manifestation may be mild and subtle to be noticeable.[20] The lesions of secondary syphilis heal in about 3 months but may show waxing and waning up to 9 months before complete disappearance.

The patient thereafter enters into the phase of latency. There are no active lesions at this stage. About 25% of the patients in latent phase experience one or more self-remitting relapses conforming to lesions of secondary syphilis. In the Oslo study, mouth, throat and anogenital lesions predominated in these relapses. Over 75% patients had relapsed within 6 months and 93% within one year. No relapses were seen after 5 years.

Still further along the time scale about two thirds of the latent syphilitics either remit spontaneously or persist in latent phase without any symptom throughout the life. Only the remaining one third develop tertiary syphilis (late benign, cardiovascular and neurosyphilis).

Late benign syphilis develops in about 15% of the total syphilitic patients. In the Oslo study, the majority had developed this form within first 15 years (one to 46 years). The lesions of benign tertiary syphilis remitted and relapsed at one or the other place. About 25% of males and 34.7% females had 2 to 7 such episode. Solitary, single structure lesions were seen in 90%. About 70% lesions were on the skin.

Cardiovascular syphilis manifests about 10-40 years after the initial infection and neurosyphilis is seen after about 3-35 years.

In the Oslo study, cardiovascular syphilis developed

in 10.4% and neurosyphilis in 6.4%. The patients infected before the age of 15 years did not develop cardiovascular syphilis and patients infected after 40 years of age did not get neurosyphilis. The risk of cardiovascular complications was twice in males as compared to females. Untreated syphilis was the cause of death in about 11% of the total syphilitics. More importantly it was found that 60%-70% of the patients lived without any major problem attributable to syphilis.

In the present era of antibiotics the course of syphilis is likely to be changed. Late syphilis has almost disappeared from the scene possibly due to effective treatment of early syphilitic stage. Use of penicillin or other antibiotics for treating some other disease also could be a probable cause of this reduced morbidity of late syphilis. However one can also think of a situation where use of these antibiotics are not adequate for elimination of treponemes because of inadequate dosage or duration. In these cases, the disease may run a subclinical course and manifest later on or are detected by serology. Authors are already seeing an increase in patients of secondary syphilis without any history of primary lesion. Latent syphilis is also being detected with increased frequency. These findings have been corroborated by other workers.[21] By the same analogy one can expect resurgence of late syphilis in near future though expression of the disease may change. Some subtle and atypical forms of neurosyphilis have already been reported[22] thereby retaining its title of 'greatest imitator' of all diseases. The whole picture may be further confused by emergence of HIV infection.

Early Syphilis

Pathogenesis

The early syphilis is said to be infectious while late syphilis to be non-infectious but there is no strict dividing line. The exact pathogenetic mechanisms in the evolution of the disease are still being elucidated. Sequencing of *T. pallidum* genome so far has not revealed any ortholog for a known virulence factor.[23] The appearance and disappearance of the lesions, inactivity of the organisms after primary stage or during the phase of latency are the questions yet to be answered.

After inoculation the treponemal proteins help it to adhere to the host cell receptors especially the surface fibronectin.[24] Subsequent multiplication and migration

of *T. pallidum* across the anatomical barrier is still an unsettled issue. The cork-screw motility of the treponemes is useful but is not the only factor for its penetration into the host tissues.[25] Once inside the tissues the organisms not only multiply but also disseminate rapidly. The experiments have shown the presence of treponemes in the blood as well as lymphatics within few hours of inoculation.[14] *T. pallidum* enter the circulation by their capacity to penetrate through the intercellular junctions of the endothelial cells of the blood vessels[26] and soon disseminate throughout the body. Antibody response at this stage is undetectable. At about 3 weeks time the multiplication of *T. pallidum* at the site of inoculation reaches the required density to cause a local tissue reaction with the formation of the typical ulcer (chancre). The organisms are cleared from the lesions by the process of phagocytosis and the lesions heal by themselves within three to six weeks time, even without treatment.

This is followed by two to eight weeks later, by the appearance of secondary stage. How some treponemes escape from destruction by the immune system of the body, to cause the secondary stage, is not known. That the immune system is active against *T. pallidum* is evidenced by (1) spontaneous healing of the lesions without any form of treatment, (2) the patients harbouring *T. pallidum*, in active or latent phase, are immune to re-infection (however this immunity is lost after treatment) and (3) presence of high levels of the treponemicidal antibodies in the host. The possible mechanisms of their survival include rapid dissemination before immune system incapacitates them at inoculation site. After dissemination, they escape from immune system by lodging in some anatomic sites, which are rather not amenable to the immune mechanisms. These sites may be central nervous system, eyes, bones, lymph nodes and perilymph of the middle ear. By some protective covering their antigens remain hidden from immune system. This protective covering may be a characteristic of their surface or could be acquired from the host or inhibition of cell mediated immune responses of the host by *T. pallidum*. The major manifestations during secondary stage are mucocutaneous and skin lesions and lymphadenopathy. Since there is dissemination of the treponemes, the other organs may also be involved. The secondary stage lesions also show a tendency towards healing even without treatment. The patient usually becomes asymtomatic in 2 to 12 weeks after appearance of the secondary lesions and passes into the stage of latency. However some recurrences of secondary syphilitic lesions can keep on occurring during this period of latency especially during the first year.

Primary Syphilis

(Primary sore or chancre, Hard sore or chancre, Hunterian chancre)

As expected the disease occur in the reproductive age group, most commonly involving people of 20-30 years age but old age also does not escape because of Freudian lust. Children are unfortunate victims of child abuse or due to the prevailing concept that sex with a child may cure the sexually transmitted diseases. It is more commonly seen among males because they have more opportunities to venture out.

The primary syphilis presents as an ulcer or chancre usually situated on genitalia. The lesion starts as a dusky red, painless, non-itchy macule of about 0.5-1 cm in size. The patient usually fails to notice this. It soon becomes elevated to form a papule that increases in size and ulcerates. The resulting chancre or ulcer is variable in size but rarely exceeds 2 cms. It is painless causing only little discomfort to the patient and often the patient keeps on postponing his visit to the clinician. The chancre is rounded with well-defined regular edges that may be raised, rolled out or may imperceptibly merge with the surrounding tissue. The floor is clean looking with dull red granulation tissue. The chancre is non-tender (**P VII, Fig. 29–31**). The most characteristic feature appears to be the induration of its base, which sometimes is hard enough to feel like a button justifying to be called a hard chancre. A hard chancre on the inner surface of prepuce may result in the snapping back of a retracted prepuce (Dory flap sign). However the induration of lesions on coronal sulcus should be cautiously interpreted as any other lesion here, may, also feel indurated. Non-indurated chancre can also occur. In the majority, the chancre tends to be single but multiple lesions can occur simultaneously or soon after the appearance of initial chancre. The manipulation of the chancre leads to exudation of serous fluid, which is highly contagious.

At times the prepuce may not be retractable due to associated oedema or phimosis. On deep palpation one may feel a localized indurated area underneath the prepuce, which represents the chancre. The chancre in pregnant women is often larger and more indurated due to increased vascularity.

Non-chancre presentations include multiple erosive lesions especially on glans penis and balanoposthitis. The authors have seen primary lesions in the form of about 1-2 cm, localized, non-ulcerated plaques on the genitalia from which they could recover treponemes. Rarely, a unilateral firm oedema having rubbery consistency develops without visible chancre, which may 'represent a deep-seated chancre.[27] The regional lymph nodes become enlarged within 7-10 days, initially unilateral but soon other side also becomes involved. In case of ano-genital chancre there is bilateral enlargement in a majority of cases at the time of presentation. Characteristically the lymph nodes appear small, discrete, non-tender, firm, rubbery in consistency and they do not suppurate.

Morphology of the chancre could be modified due to drying of exudates or formation of scab. The tissue around the chancre may become oedematous. The chancre may become tender due to secondary infection and so do the regional lymph nodes. The application of certain indigenous products, not necessarily medicated ones, may also confuse the picture.

Due to mode of its transmission the prime sites of the primary chancre are genitals. In males the common sites are coronal sulcus, glans penis, prepuce, frenum and shaft of penis. Intrameatal chancre cannot be visualized without urethroscope, and suspicion rests on the presence of scanty, serous urethral discharge with the palpation of indurated area in the line of urethra near external urinary meatus.

In women the common sites of primary chancre are labia, fourchette, around urethra, clitoris, cervix, perineum and vaginal wall. A cervical chancre is often not detected by the woman and she may present in secondary stage.

Extragenital Sites of Primary Chancre

Virtually any part of the body can be involved especially the erogenous zones. Many of these may be painful. Lymphadenopathy is usually unilateral in these cases except in ano-rectal lesions. Oral, ano-rectal, breast, digital lesions rank next to genital sites. Lip, (**P VIII, Fig. 32, 33**) tongue and other oral sites can be involved by kissing or oral sex. Oral lesions have also been reported to have occurred by drinking vessels, pipes, toothpicks etc. when used immediately after their use by a syphilitic having oral lesions. Anal chancres are being seen among homosexuals with increasing frequency. They may be painful and may have an atypical appearance. Chancres on fingers can occur due to accidental exposure among the medical personnel, especially the dentists, and present as classical chancre or a chronic whitlow. Fingers can also become involved due to sexual foreplay practices.

The term 'syphilis d'emblee' denotes those cases where primary syphilitic stage is absent and patient directly presents with the features of secondary syphilis. It can happen when treponemes have been deeply inoculated as in the case of a puncture wound or transmission by blood transfusion.

Healing of Primary Chancre

The spontaneous healing of the chancre is rather slow without treatment. It takes about 3-8 weeks leaving behind a thin, atrophic scar in some patients. With adequate treatment the ulcer heals in one to two weeks time. Enlargement of the lymph nodes may persist for an indefinite time.

Diagnosis

Diagnosis is based on demonstration of the treponemes from the chancre and serological tests for syphilis. The organisms in the lesions are demonstrated by doing a dark-ground microscope examination of the exudates. The ulcer is cleaned by normal saline and it is manipulated to exude fluid, which is collected on a cover slip. The cover slip is inverted on a thin glass slide and the preparation is examined by dark-ground microscope. In case of likely delay in the examination, the preparation is sealed by vaseline. However in a hot weather the vaseline may seep through the cover slip and may cause confusion. The organisms can be demonstrated in the chancre in about 80% of the cases. In case of dry lesions or inaccessibility of the chancre, one can demonstrate the organism by aspiration of enlarged lymph node. For this a lymph node is fixed and overlying skin is made taut with one hand and 0.05-0.1ml normal saline is injected into the lymph node. After some manipulation of the needle the lymph is sucked out. The fluid is spread on a thin glass slide, covered with a cover slip and subjected to dark-ground microscopy.

Serological tests become positive 5-6 weeks after infection or 2-3 weeks after appearance of primary chancre. Reaginic tests are positive in about 80% of the patients with primary syphilis. Positivity is generally in dilution of less than 1:32.

Differential Diagnosis

Ulcers of venereal origin–chancroid, donovanosis, lymphogranuloma venereum (LGV) and herpes genitalis. Other ulcers—traumatic ulcers, Behcet's disease, and a malignant ulcer. The details are discussed in chapter 42.

Secondary Syphilis

The secondary stage begins 2-8 weeks after the appearance of primary chancre. One fourth of the patients are probably still recovering from the primary chancre when the secondary stage becomes manifest. Secondary stage represents the dissemination of the disease involving many organs of the body. Commonest involved tissues are skin, mucous membranes and lymph nodes. A small number have involvement of the bones, eyes, nervous system and abdominal organs. Many patients develop constitutional symptoms in the form of low-grade fever, malaise, headache and anorexia. Persistent severe headache may signify nervous system involvement. More often the patient with secondary syphilis lands up in a dermatology clinic with skin rash.

Muco-cutaneous Involvement

Cutaneous involvement takes the form of different types of eruptions. Characteristically these eruptions are (1) non-vesicular (2) non-pruritic (3) wide-spread and bilaterally symmetrically distributed but few patients do complain of pruritus and at times the rash may be confined to only one anatomical area as palms and soles or genitalia. The rash may show polymorphism in the same patient. A good daylight is essential to visualize the rash which at times may be faint enough to be missed. Tilting the patient to change the angle of incident light sometimes may be helpful. If not treated the rash may persist for many weeks or even months. The rash may become much more intense after starting the treatment. The eruptions of syphilis can be macular, papular, pustular or a combination of these.

Macular syphilide

Appearing at about 8 weeks it is the earliest eruption to become noticeable and may be evanescent. The eruption may be, pinkish or coppery red but more frequently it is grayish among Indians. The macules are discrete, non-scaly round or oval in shape usually less than one cm in size. They are concentrated on trunk, shoulders and flexor aspects of upper arms. Palms and soles are more frequently involved sites and rash here appears more dramatic in dark skinned individuals as skin in these areas is lighter in colour. (PVIII, Fig. 34–36). Rash may be sparse and often overlooked by the patient. It may disappear in few days or evolves into papular rash. Occasionally it may persist as such.

Papular syphilide

This is the most characteristic rash of syphilis. It evolves from macular rash through a maculopapular phase or manifests as such. In fact the maculopapular rash is the commonest rash of secondary stage but frequently goes unnoticed. The papular syphilide appears around 3 months post-infection. The papules are dull red and measure less than one cm. In dark-skinned patients they are skin coloured or grayish. The eruption is non-scaly initially but lesions can be scaly afterwards. The papules are firm to feel. Lichenoid, acneiform and nodular lesions can occur. Lichenoid lesions may itch. (**P VIII, Fig. 34, 36**). The rash is wide spread with a distribution on trunk, extremities, face and genitals. The papules are usually discrete but may be arranged in circinate, annular or a corymbose pattern (**P VIII, Fig. 37**). Their linear arrangement along the forehead hairline has been referred to as 'corona veneris'. Annular syphilides are seen on the face. The corymbose syphilide resembles a spatter of a liquid with a large papule in the centre and a few small ones around it.

The papules on the moist intertrigenous areas tend to become large and coalescent to form large fleshy masses with flat tops and broad bases. Due to maceration they appear grayish white and may be eroded. These are 'condyloma lata' or flat lesions of syphilis, which are highly infectious because of the fluid they continue to exude. Many accept their evolution from direct spread of treponemes from the primary chancre, as at times they are seen independent of appearance of skin rash.[28] The common sites of condyloma lata are perianal, between thigh and scrotum, vulva and perineal regions (**P IX, Fig. 38, 39**). These have also been seen at the angles of mouth, axillae and other moist areas of the body. Rarely lesions between toes and upper eyelid have been described.[29,30]

The acuminate follicular papular lesions are responsible for the 'moth eaten' alopecia, which appear as irregular patches of non-scarring hair loss on the occipital and parietal regions of the scalp. The alopecia can involve other hairy parts of the body. The appearance of small clusters of miliary follicular eruption on the trunk and extremities has been known as 'lichen syphiliticus'.

Nail involvement can occur in late secondary stage. Nail bed or nail matrix can be involved by papular syphilide. The nails loose luster and become brittle. Pitting, splitting, onycholysis, shedding and distortion of the nail can occur in secondary syphilis. Nailfold involvement can result in paronychia.

Papulosquamous syphilide is essentially a papular eruption in which scaling is prominent and lesions may form plaques. Presence of scaly plaques may resemble the clinical picture of psoriasis.

Pustular syphilide

This evolves from papular lesions, which have undergone central necrosis due to endarteritis obliterans. Rarely seen these days, pustular syphilitic lesions tend to develop in patients who are debilitated. (**P X, Fig. 40–42**). The lesions may be rupioid with heaped up crusts. 'Malignant syphilis' is a rare form of pustular syphilide with deep cutaneous ulcerations, visceral involvement and severe toxemia, which could prove fatal.

Healing of cutaneous lesions: pigmentary changes

Cutaneous rashes may be a part of early relapsing syphilis in which the rash comes and goes. Macular lesions heal without any trace. Papular lesions may leave behind hyperpigmented or hypopigmented areas. Hyperpigmentation usually fades up with time. The terms 'leukoderma colli' or 'collar of venus' denote a residual depigmentation of the neck area. Depigmentation may be confused with vitiligo. Sometimes atrophic macules may persist at the place of papular rash. The pustular lesions, especially of malignant syphilis develop due to tissue necrosis, and they heal by scarring. Secondary anetoderma can occur.

Mucous membrane lesions

These are painless lesions and take the form of dull red erythematous macules, mucous patches and condyloma lata. So called mucous patches are erosive lesions of the mucosa that appear at the same time as papular syphilide. A mucous patch starts as grayish-white plaque, its surface gets eroded forming a sharply defined superficial erosion (**P X, Fig. 43**). It is surrounded by a dull red areola. These are highly infectious lesions. Confluence of these lesions form irregular, serpiginous erosions or ulcers that have been called 'snail track ulcers'. Mucous patches are seen on the oral as well as genital mucosa. Lips, buccal mucosa, palate, tongue, fauces, are the common oral sites and glans penis, prepucial and vulvar mucosa, vaginal orifice, posterior commisure and cervix are genital sites. On the tongue they are seen as smooth areas with loss of papillae. The patient may have a sore throat or hoarseness with the pharyngeal or laryngeal involvement respectively. On the genitals mucous patches can be confused with primary chancre.

Condyloma lata can involve oral commissures and have similar characteristics as the same lesions elsewhere.

Malignant Syphilis or Lues Maligna[31,32]

Malignant syphilis, also known as Lues maligna, is an explosive form of syphilis that was first described before the turn of the 20th century. This rare form of syphilis is characterized by a prodrome of fever, headache, and muscle pains followed by a papulopustular eruption that soon becomes necrotic, resulting in sharply marginated ulcers with a thick, rupioid crust. Mucous membranes are involved in more than one third of patients and hepatitis may be associated. Histologic study shows an intense plasma cell and histiocyte infiltrate obscuring blood vessels and obliterative vasculitis of medium sized vessels at the dermal subcutaneous junction with associated necrosis of the overlying skin. It has become more prevalent after the advent of HIV infection.

The most of the clinical data of early syphilis is based on old studies and in a recent study Kumar et al from India in a analysis of 53 cases (34 males, 19 females) (1990-1999) reported that skin rash was found in 38 (71.7%), lymphadenopathy in 26 (49%), persistent chancre in 4 (7.5%), nodular syphilide in 2 (3.8%), lues maligna in 2 (3.8%), mucous patches in 6 (11.3%), condylomata lata in 14 (26.4%), split papules in 2 (3.8%) and healed scar of primary chancre in 5 (9.5%).[33] Three patients were HIV positive and one patient each had lues maligna, lichenoid and nodular syphilide.

The histopathology of secondary syphilis was studied in 40 biopsies of mucocutaneous lesions by Pandhi et al[34] and a spectrum of changes ranging from minimal infiltrate to granulomatous inflammation throughout the dermis was seen. The pattern of inflammation correlated well with type of skin lesions, with macules showing the least and nodules the most prominent changes. The predominant cell type in infiltrate was the mononuclear cells, lymphocytes. Plasma cells were seen infrequently except in condylomata lata. Endothelial proliferation, the classical features of histopathology of syphilis, was noted infrequently.

Lymphadenitis

The lymhadenopathy is one of the common finding of secondary syphilis. It is said to be generalized, though one or the other groups of the lymph nodes are involved more frequently. Bilateral inguinal involvement is the commonest, followed by axillary, cervical, epitrochlear and femoral in order of frequency.[35] Other groups can rarely be involved. Characteristically the involved lymph nodes are non-tender, discrete, mobile, nonsuppurative and are bilateral symmetrical. Their consistency is firm and rubbery with a size usually less than one cm, often appearing as 'lead shot' like.

Systemic Manifestations

Secondary syphilis is a systemic disease. Involvement of other organs occurs mainly through blood stream.

Ophthalmologic involvement is rare. It is seen during late phase of secondary syphilis and patient complains of pain in the eye, photophobia, excessive lacrimation and redness of one or both the eyes. There is unilateral or bilateral anterior uveitis or iritis. Rarely choroidoretinitis and occlusion of retinal vessels may occur. In a study, the syphilitic uveitis accounted for about 4% of total uveitis cases.[36]

Musculoskeletal system involvement is rarely seen clinically. The involvement includes periostitis, joint effusion, bursitis, osteomyelitis and myopathy. Tendon sheaths may be involved. Patient presents with local aching pains over bones especially over tibia with signs of inflammation. Joint effusion may limit the movements. Radiologically the bones show destructive or productive lesions. The lesions may take one year to resolve completely. Muscle involvement causes generalized muscle weakness and pains. Muscles become tender.

Gastro-intestinal system involvement include hepatitis and stomach lesions. Hepatitis can be observed among 10% of cases and in a small numbers the treponemes can be recovered.[37] It is usually subclinical though jaundice may manifest in some patients and liver enzymes may be raised. Stomach lesions are even rarer and endoscopy reveals erosions, ulcers or nodular lesions.[38] The patient complains of abdominal pain, vomiting and loss of weight. Hepatitis as well as stomach lesions respond to anti-syphilitic therapy.

Renal involvement is rare and may results in nephrotic syndrome due to acute membranous glomerulonephritis. Its pathogenesis appears to be immune complex deposition.[39]

Cardiac involvement is rare and causes conduction defects.

Neurological involvement may be asymptomatic with abnormalities of cerebrospinal fluid (CSF) or is symptomatic with signs and symptoms pertaining to meningitis, raised intracranial pressure and cranial nerve palsies. The patient presents with headache, vomiting and papilloedema. Signs of acute meningeal involvement are usually absent. Damage to eighth cranial nerve can cause deafness. The CSF abnormalities include high cell count, raised proteins and positive reagin and specific tests for syphilis.

Haematological abnormalities include mild to moderate anaemia, raised erythrocyte sedimentation rate and leukocytosis.

Diagnosis

The diagnosis is established by demonstration of *T. pallidum* from moist lesions, mucous membrane lesion or in the lymph node aspirate and by serological tests. Dark ground microscopy from oral lesion is not reliable because of presence of *T. microdentium*, a commensal in the mouth. However fluorescent staining can be used. Reaginic and specific tests are invariably positive in secondary syphilis.

Differential diagnosis

- Macular syphilide-viral exanthemata, drug rash, pityriasis rosea, glandular fever.
- Papular syphilide-pityriasis rosea, lichen planus, papular urticaria, pityriasis lichenoides, drug rash.
- Papulosquamous syphilide- psoriasis, seborrhoeic dermatitis, drug rash.
- Follicular lesions-lichen scrofulosorum, lichen spinulosus, lichen planus, pityriasis rubra pilaris,
- Condylomata lata-condyloma acuminata, prolapsed hemorrhoids.
- Oral mucosal lesions-aphthous ulcers, pemphigus, Behcet's disease, Stevens-Johnson syndrome, lichen planus, Vincent's angina, tonsillitis.
- Genital mucosal lesions-herpes genitalis, primary chancre, Behcet's disease, fixed drug eruptions.

Viral exanthemata usually start with fever and a flu-like illness. They are self limiting and rarely persist beyond 15–20 days. Drug rashes are itchy eruptions preceded by a variable interval after drug intake. Lymph node involvement is uncommon. Pityriasis rosea can be most confusing. There is a larger herald patch and rash is aligned along the skin creases on the back. Generalized lymphadenopathy can occur. The rash usually resolves within 6 weeks.

Early Latent Syphilis

After healing of secondary syphilitic lesions and occasionally directly after primary stage the patient enters into the long phase of latency. Detection of latent syphilis within two years of infection is referred to as early. The dividing line of two years between early and late latent syphilis is rather an arbitrary one and CDC puts the limit at one year. There are no clinical symptoms and signs and diagnosis is based on finding positive reaginic and specific tests of syphilis. A common problem with regards to latent syphilis is the exact categorization of early or late syphilis due to lack of information regarding the incriminating sexual intercourse. It is better to treat these 'difficult to categorize' patients as late latent syphilis.

Early Relapsing Syphilis

Relapses occur in about 25% of the patients during latent phase among untreated syphilitics. About 75% relapses are observed during the first six months, 90% within the first year and none after five years. In the Oslo study on natural course, 18.5% had experienced two and 22.5% patients had experienced four relapses. Some of the cases relapse after inadequate treatment. The relapse may be clinical or only serological. Clinical relapses conform to a picture of secondary syphilis though the disease is less extensive. Predominantly there are oral and ano-genital mucocutaneous lesions, which at times may be the only manifestations. Skeletal, visceral, ophthalmic and nervous system lesions can also be seen.

Occasional occurrence of a relapsing lesion resembling a primary chancre at the site of initial primary chancre has been referred as 'monorecidive' or 'chancre redux'. It is the result of the proliferation of the residual treponemes at the initial site.

The serological relapse without clinical manifestations may precede clinical relapse. It is defined as rising titres of antibodies or a negative serological test turning into a positive one.

Infectivity of Early Syphilis

Infection has been known to be transmissible by the process of blood transfusion during incubation period but such cases might be only few. The primary chancre, moist and ulcerated lesions of secondary syphilis are contagious, while dry, healing non-ulcerated lesions are not. Condylomata and mucous patches are highly infectious. Body fluids as saliva, blood and semen may contain enough treponemes during secondary stage to be infective.[40] The disease could be transmitted by CSF in animal models.[41] Lesions of relapsing secondary syphilis are infectious in a similar way. Even after the lesions of secondary syphilis have disappeared in their natural course, the body fluids remain infective during the latent phase usually upto two years. However the patient's infectivity potential declines even in untreated disease with the passage of time especially after two years. No infectivity has been observed after 10 years. Treatment aborts infectivity.

Late Syphilis

After 2 years the disease enters the non-infective stage. For the majority of untreated patients it remains latent without any clinical manifestations and can be suspected only during blood testing for blood donation, ante-natal check up or check ups for immigration purposes. Since in all these cases the VDRL serology is positive in low dilutions it needs to be confirmed by specific tests for syphilis and in all such cases more serious asymptomatic neurosyphilis needs to be excluded by CSF examination. The tell-tale signs of early syphilis like a penile scar of healed primary sore or leukoderma of neck or macular atrophy of earlier secondary syphilis may be evident.

The lesions of tertiary syphilis start appearing 3-10 years after primary infection. The tissues most commonly involved during this stage are:

- Covering structures: skin, mucous membranes, subcutaneous tissue.
- Supporting structures: bones, joints, muscles, ligaments.
- Visceral involvement: gastro-intestinal tract; liver, spleen and other abdominal organs.

Incidence

The incidence of late benign syphilis had considerably decreased to the point of becoming non-existent except for occasional case-reports in the literature. The increased incidence of HIV with concomitant immuno-suppresion has enhanced the fear of rise in incidence of late syphilis. A critical review of 1147 untreated patients of Boeck-Brussgaard study in 1955 reported that 15.8% of these individuals sooner or later developed late benign lesions of the skin, mucous membranes, bones or joints. These were seen more in women (17.3%). Of these about a quarter or more had 2-7 episodes of these manifestations with more than one tissue involvement in some.

Pathogenesis

The characteristic lesion in late syphilis is gumma, which may be single or multiple and varying size from pin-head to a few centimeters in diameter. It has a central area of tissue necrosis resembling caseous material surrounded by a zone of granulation tissue with a narrow zone of tough fibrous tissue at the outer and peripheral margin. The intima of the blood vessels shows cellular hypertrophy due to endarteritis. The *T. pallidum* are rarely demonstrated due to supervening local tissue allergy in the host. The gummatous lesion heals with central scarring but spreads peripherally. In contrast to localized gummatous lesions the diffuse gummatous reaction is seen in tongue and testis with diffuse interstitial fibrosis.

Gummatous Lesions of Covering Structures

1. Nodular lesions: Nodular lesions are seen as deep indurated nodules varying in size from pin-head to pea-size. The multiple nodules adopt an arciform pattern with predilection for face, scapular, interscapular area and extremities. Nodular lesions break down to become nodulo-ulcerative form, which lead to atrophic noncontractile scarring. Under treatment they heal promptly.
2. Psoriasiform or scaly lesions: Here the tissue reaction is more intense leading to waxy scaling. Such lesions are seen on palms and soles. On scraping in contrast to psoriasis the Auspitz sign is negative, i.e., no capillary pinpoint bleeding is seen after removing scales.
3. Subcutaneous gumma: Single or multiple painless subcutaneous lesions over which the overlying skin gradually gets attached taking a dull-red hue. They break down to form punched out

ulcers with rounded or polycyclic margin (**P XI, Fig. 44, 45**). The walls of the ulcer are vertical giving the appearance of a well punched out ulcer with wash leather slough on the walls and floor. Such subcutaneous gummata are seen on legs, scalp and face along with involvement of sternum and sterno-clavicular joints. These subcutaneous nodules may originate from or extend to periosteum of the underlying bone which may form the floor. These gummatous ulcers heal by tissue paper scarring.

4. Mucosal surface involvement: The involvement of the mucosal surface may be localized, or diffuse. The localized gumma are seen in mouth, throat, palate, pharynx, larynx or nasal septum. On breaking down they leave behind a characteristic punched out ulcer (**P XI, Fig. 46**). The destructive lesions may cause dysfunction in the area involved and over long period of time, are prone to malignant changes. The tongue has diffuse gummatous involvement and as a result the tongue becomes swollen leading finally to chronic superficial glossitis. Such patients may complain of discomfort on taking hot, spicy food with large tongue. Due to interstitial fibrosis there may be deep, irregular furrowing of tongue and patches of necrotic epithelium may lead to leukoplakia. Thirdly due to loss of filiform papillae the sides and tip of the tongue may look smooth and glazed.

The gummatous lesions of skin and mucous membranes need to be differentiated from other granulomatous conditions, like tuberculosis, leprosy, deep fungal infections and non-granulomatous conditions, like psoriasis, seborrheic dermatitis, superficial dermatophytes, squamous cell epithelioma as per involvement of area and surface. The leg ulcers need to be differentiated from stasis ulcers, sporotrichosis and erythema induratum.

Gummatous Lesions of Supporting Structures

1. Bones: The bones are affected in tertiary syphilis 5-25 years after the original infection. It is more commonly seen in men. The bones commonly involved are long bones, bones of skull and shoulder girdle. There is deep-seated boring pain at the site of involvement in 50% cases, which is worse at night. The involvement of the skull bones at times gives rise to continuous severe headache. In case the subcutaneous bone is involved there may be a tender swelling at site. Disability due to bone involvement is rare. The overlying subcutaneous tissue and skin may get involved giving rise to gummatous ulceration and necrotic bone. The hard palate and nasal septum involvement may lead to perforation at site, which is obvious on examination.

Etiopathogenesis: There is involvement of fibrous layer of periosteum with infiltration of lymphocytes, plasma cells and a few epithelioid cells and occasional giant cells with large number of fibroblasts. The inflammation in turn stimulates osteoblastic activity leading to new bone formation; but the new bone is laid in irregular fashion and lacks usual cortical pattern and is sclerotic in nature. The bone involvement is patchy and the transition from healthy to diseased bone is abrupt. Due to new bone formation there is no tendency to bending or pathological fractures. The gummatous involvement of medullary cavity leads to syphilitic osteomyelitis. In contrast to long bones, in membranous bones of skull, nasal septum, hard palate destruction outpaces the new bone formation and periosteal reaction is slight leading to rounded areas of destruction starting from outer table and extending on to inner table. This destructive process falls short of duramater and thus cerebral cortex is spared. The gummatous osteo-periostitis of skull bones is local and is termed as worm-eaten skull.

A radiological study of 115 bones of 67 patients showed the following patterns of bone involvement:

- Periosteitis, periosteal thickening with increased density in laminated layers: 27 bones.
- Gummatous osteitis, destructive or osteomyelitic lesions, usually with periosteal or endosteal changes and sclerosis of the surrounding bones: 72 bones.
- Sclerosing osteitis, in which the increased density and periosteal changes hide the gummatous lesion: 16 bones.

2. Muscles: Primary muscle involvement is rare but they may get involved due to gumma in subcutaneous tissue or underlying bone.

3. Joints, bursae and tendon-sheath: They are rarely involved in tertiary syphilitic lesions. Hard fibrous nodules found along tendon-sheaths or subcutaneously near joints called juxta-articular nodes of late syphilis disappear after anti-syphilitic treatment.

Gummatous Lesions of Viscera

1. Gastro-intestinal Involvement

In an analysis of 200 patients of syphilis, 87% patients gave 'stomach trouble' as their chief complaint. Of them only 8 (4%) had true symptoms of the stomach. Neurosyphilis is primarily the cause of gastric complaints.

2. Liver, Spleen and Other Organ Involvement

Liver involvement used to be the most common abdominal organ involvement in syphilis. This is either in form of (i) diffuse interstitial cirrhosis or (ii) focal gumma of the liver progressing to irregular fibrosis (hepar lobatum).

The portal cirrhosis was found in equal frequency in syphilitics as well as non-syphilitics.

The patient with syphilitic liver involvement presents with complaints of loss of weight, jaundice, pain or tenderness in right hypochondrium. In some cases symptoms, like vomiting, haematemesis due to varicosity of oesophageal venous plexus; and abdominal mass may be palpated. On clinical examination besides hepatic enlargement, ascites may be found with portal hypertension. Abnormal LFT and positive serological test for syphilis confirms the diagnosis. The condition needs to be differentiated from other causes of acute abdomen.

Other organ involvement e.g., the lung, urinary tract, reproductive organs are rarely reported to be involved in syphilitic gumma.

Cardiovascular Syphilis

Manifestations of cardiovascular syphilis, like other forms of tertiary syphilis are likely to be due to an immunological response and manifest quite late, ranging from 10 to 40 years from the onset of infection. Its incidence in untreated patients ranged from 10% in caucasians to 25 to 50% in the Negroes. The cardiovascular system is not affected in early syphilis but evidence of infection is present in upto 80% of patients with tertiary syphilis though most do not have clinical disease. In the post antibiotic era, cardiovascular syphilis is considered a rarity, even in patients with AIDS.[43,44] Yet it has been considered to be the cause of death in 1492 persons between 1976 to 1985.[45] It has been suggested that a late stage of syphilis should be considered in the differential diagnosis of cerebrovascular lesions in young patients. Men have a more frequent and earlier age of onset than women. History of a primary or secondary stage may not be available in all cases and about 40% cases may have associated involvement of the nervous system. Depending on the site of involvement, it can be broadly categorized as syphilis of the heart, syphilis of the great vessels and syphilis of the medium sized vessels.

Syphilis of the Heart

Myocardial disease is rare and accounts for 2.4% cases of cardiovascular syphilis. It may take the form of diffuse myocarditis or gumma. Gumma commonly involves the left ventricle and the septum and present as ventricular arrythmias and valve dysfunction.

Syphilis of the Great Vessels

Lesions may occur in the aorta, in the pulmonary artery or in the great vessels emerging from the aorta. Spirochaetes reach the aorta in the early stage of the disease, lodge there in a dormant state for many years and cause gradual changes of endarteritis, commencing from the vasovasorum to the proximal part of the aorta. Subsequently all three layers of aortic wall are affected by the same process. Medial destruction causes dilatation of the aortic wall with different sequelae; minimal dilatation causes uncomplicated aortitis, extension of the dilatation to the aortic ring causes aortic regurgitation, gross dilatation at any point causes aortic aneurysm. The damaged intima becomes the site for atherosclerotic patches and calcification and presence of such changes coupled with fibrotic changes near the openings of the coronary ostia leads to coronary ostial stenosis.[43]

Uncomplicated Aortitis

It accounts for 27 to 36 percent cases of cardiovascular syphilis. The ascending part of the aorta is involved in most cases, less than 10% cases show involvement of the abdominal aorta; only 2 percent involve the portion below the renal artery.[45] Clinical suspicion can be made when a loud and *tambour* like second sound (bruit de Tabourka) is heard in a patient who has neither hypertension nor atherosclerosis. Radiological suspicion can be made when linear calcifications can be seen on the anterolateral wall of the ascending aorta.[43]

Aortic Aneurysms

They comprise 20% cases of cardiovascular syphilis. Saccular and fusiform aneurysms are characteristic; dissecting aneurysm does not occur. Over 60% of aneurysms involve the ascending portion of the thoracic aorta and 25% involves the transverse arch. They remain asymptomatic for many years and commonly present as a palpable pulsating mass on the chest wall (PXI, Fig. 47). They may manifest with host of other features like chest discomfort, dyspnoea, cough, haemoptysis, hoarseness, backache, drowsiness, seizures, flushing and features of superior vena caval syndrome. If neglected, one third of patients may die due to spontaneous rupture.

- On auscultation, heart sounds are found to be tambouric.
- Chest X-ray may show typical egg shell calcification which is characteristic.

Coronary Artery Disease

The coronary ostia or the most proximal part of the coronary arteries are preferentially involved in cardiovascular syphilis; coronary artery stenosis accounts for 25 to 30% cases of cardiovascular syphilis. Patients commonly present with congestive cardiac failure and angina pectoris; acute myocardial infarction almost never occur. When a patient with either a history of syphilis or other presenting feature of cardiovascular syphilis show evidence of isolated right or left main coronary ostial narrowing on angiography without atherosclerotic changes, the diagnosis of a syphilitic pathology should be considered.

Aortic Valve Disease

Aortic valvular incompetence is a relatively late manifestation occurring mostly in patients who are 50 years or older. If there is associated aortic stenosis, the possibility of a syphilitic cause is almost excluded. On auscultation, soft diastolic blowing murmur is heard along the lower left sternal border. A ventricular diastolic gallop with tambour like quality or a 'Austin flint' murmur may be heard at the apex.

Syphilis of the Medium Sized Vessels

The cerebral and spinal arteries are affected in cardiovascular syphilis, but as the clinical manifestations are neurological, they are categorized under neurosyphilis. Rarely, the hepatic, carotid, mesenteric, renal, iliac or femoral arteries may be involved by the syphilitic process. But except for occasional cases of gangrene of the extremities, diagnosis is mostly at autopsy.

Neurosyphilis

In the pre-penicillin era, physicians were well conversant with the manifestation of neurosyphilis, accounting for about 29% of cases in some hospitals. The common forms were asymptomatic neurosyphilis and tabes dorsalis. In the antibiotic era, prior to and during the early years of HIV epidemic, penicillin and incidental antibiotic therapy brought down these cases considerably. Number of admissions with symptomatic syphilis came down from 4.3 cases in 100,000 population in 1946 to 0.4 cases per 100,000 population in 1960. However, with the upsurge of HIV infection in the population, the incidence of an early form of neurosyphilis, 'acute syphilitic meningitis' has gone up and also presence of later forms of the disease like paresis, gumma, ophthalmic disease and otologic complications have become more familiar.[44] Development of meningovascular syphilis even after therapy for primary syphilis necessitates the need for appropriate serologic follow up.[46] A relatively high incidence of neurosyphilis (17.5%) was observed in men with neurological symptoms and multiple sexual partners in a study from India, in the absence of any associated HIV infection.[47]

Despite the re-emergence of neurosyphilis in the acquired immunodeficiency syndrome (AIDS) era, a consideration of neurosyphilis is often neglected in patients with aseptic meningitis and mental changes who are negative for HIV culminating in high mortality rates. Hence, a high index of suspicion and early inclusion of young patients with cognitive decline in the differential diagnosis of neurosyphilis is mandatory.[48] Haematogenous invasion of the meninges by *T pallidum* occurs early. There may be spontaneous resolution, some may develop acute symptomatic meningitis while few others remain asymptomatic to manifest 5 to 35 years later with meningovascular, parenchymatous and gummatous disease in the brain and spinal cord respectively. Classification is difficult because of the various anatomical sites involved with variable histological reactions; manifesting in the form of various clinical syndromes and significant overlap. The following classification for neurosyphilis is commonly followed:

Classification of Neurosyphilis

Asymptomatic

- Early
- Late

Meningeal

- Acute syphilitic meningitis
- Meningovascular
- Cerebral
- Spinal form

Parenchymatous

- General paresis
- Tabes dorsalis
- Taboparesis (mixed)
- Optic atrophy

Gummatous

- Cerebral form
- Spinal form

Asymptomatic Neurosyphilis

It refers to a state of finding abnormalities in the CSF in the absence of any clinical symptoms and signs. The levels of CSF abnormalities peaks at 12-18 months from onset of infection and is also a predictive indicator of development of neurosyphilis; absence of abnormalities beyond 2 years almost rules out chances of developing neurosyphilis. Persistence of CSF abnormalities beyond 5 years of infection (late asymptomatic neurosyphilis) increases the chances of neurosyphilis upto 87%. CSF picture shows cells in the range of 10-100 WBC/mm^3 (predominantly lymphocytes), or protein content of 50-100 mg/dl, a reactive non treponemal antibody test and positive blood serology in most cases. Treated or untreated, this stage may progress to neurosyphilis.[44]

Meningeal Neurosyphilis

This may occur early or late. Meningitis may be the first clinical manifestation in one fourth of patients with neurosyphilis. Acute syphilitic meningitis occurs at a time when secondary rash may still be present, in less than 1 year from infection. The symptoms are like any other aseptic meningitis and may manifest as headache, fever, photophobia, nausea, vomiting, stiff necks (Kernig's sign) and confusion. Acute syphilitic hydrocephalus may occur, between 3 months to 6 years of primary infection in one third of cases. Papilloedema is a principal finding of hydrocephalus.

Syphilitic meningitis with cerebral changes account for one fourth of the cases of early neurosyphilis. Forty percent cases present with cranial nerve palsies, unilateral or bilateral due to basal meningitis. Frequently involved cranial nerve are 3rd, 6th, 7th and 8th. Reversible sensorineural deafness is a common accompaniment (20%) of cranial nerve involvement, and may develop abruptly within 1 or 2 weeks or may develop gradually.[44] Involvement of the meninges of the vertex and underlying cortex present in the form of convulsions, aphasias, mental confusion, papilloedema with normal pupillary reaction and mono or hemiplegia. Subependymal gliosis may disrupt the fibres of the light reflex, pupillary light reflex is lost, and accommodation reflex is preserved.

Involvement of the meninges of the spinal cord may lead to involvement of the pyramidal tract and other motor tracts, producing lower motor neurone lesions. Meningitis in the dorso lumbar and cervical regions may manifest as:

- Erb's syphilitic spastic paraplegia
- Hypertrophic cervical pachymeningitis
- Syphilitic amyotrophy

The current serum RPR is positive in most cases of acute syphilitic meningitis. CSF examination shows elevated intracranial pressure, mononuclear pleocytosis of 10-200 cells/mm^3 (may be as high as 1000-2000 cells/mm^3), protein content as high as 200 mg/dl, elevated globulin level and or reduction in the glucose content. The CSF VDRL is positive in most cases.

Histopathology shows inflammatory changes not only in the meninges, but also in the ependyma (granular ependymitis), cells predominantly being lymphocytes and plasma cells. Progressive inflammation produces endarteritis, with subsequent vascular thrombosis, occlusion and cerebral infarction.[44]

Meningovascular Neurosyphilis

It constitutes 10% of all cases of neurosyphilis and may involve both the cerebrum (cerebrovascular) or the spinal cord (spinal meningovascular).

Cerebrovascular Syphilis

It is caused by endarteritis of the medium and large arteries (Heubner's arteritis) or small arteries and arterioles (Nissl's arteritis).[45] More than 12% of patients have involvement of more than one cerebral artery, commonest being middle cerebral artery. Symptoms may begins as early as 2 years but onset after 4 to 7 years is more common. Manifestations may be sudden or there may be prodromal signs like headache, dementia, dizziness and sleep disturbances. Various neurological features may be seen, depending on the vessel involved. Commoner presentations are hemiparesis or hemiplegia, aphasia and seizures. Other presentations like homonymous hemianopia, cerebellar ataxia, and various syndromes like Horner's syndrome, Walkenberg's syndrome, Weber's syndrome and Dejerine-Roussy syndrome may be encountered. Such features are more prevalent in untreated patient; the present era is more conversant with atypical manifestations like 'drop attacks' suggestive of vertebrobasilar artery disease. Blood and CSF tests for syphilis are positive.[44,49]

Angiography shows diffuse irregularity and 'beading' of anterior and middle cerebral arteries and segmental dilatation of the pericallosal artery. Computed tomography shows low density areas with variable degrees of contrast, suggestive of multifocal infarction. Magnetic resonance imaging show focal regions of high signal density, suggestive of foci of ischaemia. Histology shows inflammatory changes and occlusive pathology to the vasovasorum, medium and small sized arteries.[44]

Spinal Meningovascular Syphilis

Comprises of two forms, syphilitic meningomyelitis and spinal vascular syphilis (acute syphilitic transverse myelitis). The basic pathology is chronic spinal meningitis, which leads to parenchymatous degeneration of the cord directly or due to a vascular thrombosis. Syphilitic meningomyelitis is more common and manifests insidiously after a latency of 20-25 years with paraesthesia and weakness of the legs, sensory loss, sphincter disturbances, pain and muscular atrophy. Abdominal reflexes are absent, deep reflex are hyperactive and extensor plantar response can be elicited. Acute transverse myelitis or spinal vascular syphilis produce sudden paraplegia, sensory loss and urinary retention simulating the Brown-Sequard syndrome[44,45]. Blood and CSF tests are positive for syphilis.

Parenchymatous Neurosyphilis

It can be categorized under 3 headings–general paresis of the insane, tabes dorsalis and optic atrophy.

General Paresis of the Insane (GPI)

Paretic neurosyphilis or dementia paralytica is a meningoencephalitis associated with direct cerebral invasion by *T. pallidum* and accounts for 10% cases of neurosyphilis.[44,49] Cerebrocortical function is severely affected due to degenerative changes, gross atrophy of the frontal and temporal lobes occur. The symptoms are either psychiatric, neurologic or both. Early complaints are of a psychiatric nature and manifest as memory loss, delusion (mostly of grandeur), megalomania, disinhibition, emotional lability, erratic behaviour, deterioration of personal habits and hygiene and disintegration of symbolic thoughts resulting in professional disaster and social catastrophy. Paresis may manifest with adult onset seizures in 15 to 20 percent of patients, without any accompanying mental aberrations.[50] Most common neurologic signs are pupillary abnormalities (Argyll Robertson pupil), flattening of facial lines, impaired writing and speech, tremors of lips, tongue, facial muscles and fingers. More extensive involvement may lead to apathy, hypotonia, dementia, cranial nerve palsies, long tract signs, clumsiness, in co-ordination and sphincter incontinence.[49] Blood and CSF tests are positive for syphilis. Computed tomography shows decreased attenuation in the cerebral white matter of the frontal and parietal lobes, with enlarged cortical sulci and ventricular dilatation. Histopathology shows granular ependymitis, formed by whorls of subependymal astrocytes.

Tabes Dorsalis

Locomotor ataxia is a late manifestation of syphilis due to parenchymatous involvement of the spinal cord. It is commoner in men and occurs later than GPI, approximately 20-25 years after the primary infection. The early features are those of posterior root and posterior column dysfunction, manifesting as lightening pain, paraesthesia, diminished deep tendon reflexes, and poor pupillary responses to light. Lancinating or stabbing types of repeated, clustered pain develops for several days or longer, primarily affecting the legs and less frequently, the trunk and arms. Visceral crises occur concurrent with lightening pain, manifesting as severe abdominal pain, vomiting, paralytic ileus, and bladder and bowel crises. Hypotonia follows loss of deep tendon reflexes and hypermobility of joints sets in; this combined with sensory impairment leads to grossly swollen and disorganized joints, known as Charcot's joints. Postural ataxia, unsteady gait and painless, penetrating trophic ulcer on the base of the toe (mal perforans) are some other features. Optic atrophy occurs commonly; as also occulomotor palsies resulting in a characteristic 'tabetic' facies. Other forms of neurosyphilis frequently co-exist. CSF and blood show positive changes of syphilis, except in advanced 'burnt out' cases.[44]

Syphilitic Optic Atrophy may occur as an isolated manifestation of neurosyphilis or as an accompaniment of tabes dorsalis. It occurs due to damage to the optic nerve fibers from chronic inflammatory changes and manifests as progressive visual loss involving first one and then both eyes.[45]

Gumma of the Brain and Spinal Cord

Gumma of the brain are rare lesions and may involve the meninges by virtue of extension from skull bones. They are rubbery nodules, single or multiple and usually produce space occupying signs and symptoms.

Gumma of the spinal cord is essentially a granuloma with features of spinal cord compression manifesting as root pain, spastic paraplegia, urinary and faecal incontinence and sensory loss below the lesion.

Syphilitic Osteitis

Syphilitic osteitis of the skull and vertebra is more of a historical entity now, and signs are secondary to pressure changes on the spinal cord and brain.[49]

Congenital Neurosyphilis

Asymptomatic neurosyphilis is encountered in upto one-fourth of the patients with congenital syphilis, over the age of 2 years. Symptomatic neurosyphilis is much rarer and once it develops, it manifests after adolescence with juvenile paresis and other adult onset features like tabes dorsalis, syphilitic encephalitis (general paresis) and local gummata.[51]

Neurosyphilis and HIV

HIV infection has had a significant impact on the manifestation of neurosyphilis. Some authors are of the opinion that HIV infected patients have a greater chance of developing secondary syphilis, atypical manifestations of neurosyphilis and atypical serological tests including false positive tests for syphilis.[49] Both the processes affect the neurological system and can hence produce confounding clinical manifestations. Others believe that the disease is not 'atypical' but in fact, present with manifestations that are typical of early neurosyphilis. Amongst the manifestations, acute syphilitic meningitis was found to be the commonest.

Cardiovascular syphilis is exceedingly rare and has not been reported except for occasional case report.[55,56] Neurosyphilis is also becoming progressively uncommon, however, cases are still occurring especially in HIV positive cases. Neurosyphilis has also been described in HIV carriers.[57] In a recent study at Madurai, a cohort of 40 patients (34 males, 6 females) presenting with neurologic symptoms and history of multiple sexual exposures was evaluated.[47] Seven (17.5%) males were found to have neurosyphilis. None of them were HIV positive. It suggests that there are still pockets of infection where late syphilis is still present. Similarly benign tertiary syphilis has become uncommon but cases are still occurring but are not being reported.

The interaction of syphilis and HIV is discussed in a separate chapter.

Immunological Hypothesis of Syphilis[52,53]

Syphilis immunology is an enigma and despite 400 years of its occurrence we are unable to decipher it completely. The part of difficulty is inability to culture the organism and cumbersome procedures of animal inoculation and their maintenance. Both cell mediated immunity (CMI) and humoral immunity play a role in development of different stages of syphilis. After the inoculation of *T. pallidum* the tissues are initially infiltrated by polymorphonuclears which are later replaced by lymphocytes macrophages and plasma cells. The ratio CD4+ to CD8+ T-lymphocyte is high in skin and serum at this time and Th_1 cytokines can be detected. It results in the development of indurated chancre due to massive infiltrate by the lymphocytes and plasma cells. In due course of time the *T. pallidum* reach the draining lymph nodes which starts an antibody response. The combined cell mediated and humoral immunity is unable to clear the infection and even though the primary sore subsides, the treponemas continue to proliferate and produce secondary syphilis. It has been demonstarated that serum of syphilis patients has immunosuppressive factor that can be removed by treatment with hyaluronidase. It was proposed that it is the capsular mucopolysacchride that may be immunosuppressive. Similar findings have been documented in experimental syphilis.[54] The secondary syphilis has a rash, lymphadenopathy, hepatosplenomegaly and can have arthritis and nephritis, a clinical picture of immune complex disease. It is associated with high level of antibodies to cardiolipin and treponemal antigens and CMI is suppressed temporarily though there is resistance to newer infection. There is waxing and waning of immunological response as secondary rash slowly disappears but there may be relapse. Gradually most of organisms are eliminated and a state of balance is reached. In this stage antibodies are still demonstrable and person is infectious especially in first two years. During secondary stage *T. pallidum* are widely distributed, reach almost all the organs and continue to persist in protected sites like central nervous system, eyes, aorta, bones, lymph nodes, perilymph of middle ear. In late syphilis this equilibrium is disturbed and organism again elicit CMI and cellular infiltrate and granuloma develop resulting in tertiary syphilis. *T. pallidum* have been demonstrated in gummas by polymerase chain reaction.

References

1. Power DA. Hunterian oration 1925. John Hunter: a martyr to science. In: selected writings. 1877-1930. Oxford: Clarendon pres, p. 1-28.
2. Ricord P. In: letters sur la syphilis. 2nd edition. Paris: 1856. p. 348.
3. Bloomfield AL. A Bibliography of internal medicine. Chicago: University of Chicago Press; 1958. p. 309-310.
4. Bloomfield AL. A Bibliography of internal medicine. Communicable diseases. Chicago University of Chicago press. 1958. p. 318.
5. Hardy PH Jr, Levin J. Lack of endotoxin in Borrelia hispanica and *Treponema pallidum*. Proc Soc Exp Biol Med 1983; 174: 47–52.
6. Stamm LV, Hodinka RL, Wyrick PB, Bassford PJ Jr. Changes in cell surface properties of *Treponema pallidum* that occurs during in vitro incubation of freshly extracted organism. Infect Immun 1987; 55: 2255–2261.
7. Charon NW Greenberg EP, Koopman Mb, Limberger RJ. Spirochete chemotaxis, motility and the structure of the spirochetal periplasmic flagella. Res Microbiol 1992; 143: 597–603.
8. Turner TB, Hollander DH. Biology of the treponematoses.

Geneva: World Health Organization, 1957.
9. Schell R.F. Rabbit and hamster models of treponemal infection in pathogenesis and immunology of treponemal infection. Schell R.F, Musher DM (eds). New York Mariel Dekkar 1983; 121-135.
10. Wicher K, Wicher V. Experimental syphilis in guinea pig. Crit Rev Microbiol 1989; 16: 181–324.
11. Lukehart SA, Holmes KK. Spirochaetal diseases: syphilis. In: Isselbacher KJ, Braunwald E, Wilson JD, et al eds: Harrison's principles of medicine. 13th Ed. New York: McGraw-Hill; 1994. p. 720-726.
12. Poulton M, Dean GL, Williams DI, et al. Surfing with spirochaetes; on ongoing syphilis outbreak in Brighton. Sex Transm Dis 2001; 77: 319-321.
13. Magnuson HJ. Inoculation syphilis in human volunteers. Medicine 1956; 35: 33-82.
14. Willcox RR. Early acquired venereal syphilis. In: Textbook of venereal diseases and treponemtoses. 2nd Ed. London: William Heinmann Medical Books Ltd; 1964. p. 166-187.
15. Oriel JD. The French disease In: The scars of Venus: a history of venereology. London: Springer-Verlog Ltd; 1994. p. 11-23.
16. Gjestland T. The Oslo study of untreated syphilis. Acta Derm Venered (Stockh). 1955; (suppl 34): 35.
17. Clark EG, Danbolt N. The Oslo study of natural course of untreated syphilis: An epidemiologic investigation based on a restudy of Boeck-Bruusgard material. Med Clin North Am 1964; 48: 613-623.
18. Talbot MD; Morton RS. The Tuskegee study of untreated syphilis. Eur J Sex Transm Dis 1984; 125-32.
19. Roahn PD. Autopsy studies in syphilis. U.S. Public Health Service, venereal disease division. J Vener Dis Inf 1947; 21(suppl).
20. Sanchez MR. Infectious syphilis. Seminars Dermatol 1994; 13: 234-242.
21. Gurvinder PT, Sukhjot K, Amrinder JK. The changing face of syphilis: from mimic to disguise. Arch Dermatol 2001; 137: 1373-1374.
22. Hooshmand H. Neurosyphilis: A study of 241 patients. JAMA. 1972; 219: 726.
23. Radolf Jd, Steiner B, Shevchenko D. Treponema pallidum: Doing a remarkable job with what It's got. Trends Microbiol 1999; 7: 7-9.
24. Baseman; Hayes EC. Molecular characterization of receptor binding proteins and immunogens of Virulent *Treponema Pallidum*. J Exp Med 1980; 151: 573-586.
25. Fitzgerald JJ, Repesh LA. Toxic Activities of *Treponema pallidum* In: Schell R.F, Musher DM, eds: Pathogenesis and immunology of treponemal infection. New York: Marcel Dekker And Basel Inc; 1983. p. 173-193.
26. Thomas DD, Navab M, Haake DA, et al. *Treponema pallidum* invades intercellular junction of endothelial cell monolayers. Proc Natl Acad Sci. USA 85: 3608-3612.
27. Sanchez MR. Syphilis. In: Freeberg IM, Eisen AZ, Wolff K, et al eds: Fitzpatrick's Dermatology in General Medicine. 5th Ed. New York: McGraw-Hill; 1999. p. 2551-2581.

28. Mushel DM. Early syphilis. In: Homes KK, Marth PA, Sparling, PF et al eds: Sexually Transmitted Diseases. 3rd eds. New York: McGraw-Hill, 1999. p. 479-485.

29. Sharma VK, Chander R, Kumar B, Radotra BD. Condylomata lata of eyelids. Genitour Med 1989; 65: 124-125.

30. Rosen T, Hwong H. Pedal interdigital condylomata lata: a rare sign of secondary syphilis. Sex Trans Dis 2001; 28: 184-186.

31. Sharma VK, Kumar B. Malignant syphilis or syphilis simulating malignancy. Int J Dermatol 1991; 30: 676.

32. Kumar B, Muralidhar S. Malignant syphilis: a review AIDS patient care STDS 1998; 12: 921-925.

33. Kumar B, Gupta S, Muralidhar S. Mucocutaneous manifestations of secondary syphilis in north Indian patients: a changing scenario? J Dermatol 2001; 28: 137-144.

34. Pandhi RK, Singh N, Ramam M. Secondary syphilis: clinicopathologic study. Int J Dermatol 1995; 34: 240-243.

35. Chapel T. The Signs and symptoms of secondary syphilis. Sex Trans Dis 1980. 7: 161-164.

36. Barile GR, Flynn TE. Syphilis exposure in patients with uveitis. Ophthalmology 1997; 104: 1605-1609.

37. Fehr J Feher J, Somogyi T, Timmer M et al. Early syphilitic hepatitis. Lancet 1975; 2: 896-898.

38. Winters H A, Notar-Francescov, Bromberg K, et al. Gastric Syphilis: Five recent cases and a review of literature. Ann Intern Med 1992; 116: 314-319.

39. Gamble C N, Reardan J B. Immunopathogenesis of syphilitic glomerulonephritis. N Eng J Med 1975; 292: 449-454.

40. Willcox RR. Syphilis: history and experimental infection. In: Textbook of venereal diseases and treponematoses. 2nd ed. London: William Heinemann Medical Books Ltd; 1964. p. 127-147.

41. Tuner T B. Infectivity Tests in Syphilis. Br J Vener Dis 1969; 45: 183-196.

42. Stokes JH, Beerman H, Ingraham NR. Modern clinical syphilology. WB Saunders Co, Philadelphia & London, 1945.

43. Cardiovascular syphilis. In: King A, Claude Nicol C, Rodin P, eds. Venereal disease. 4th edition. London: ELBS; 1980. p. 67-80.

44. Swartz MN, Healy BP, Musher DM. Late syphilis. In: eds. Holmes KK, Mardh PA Sparling PF, et al. Sexually Transmitted Diseases. 3rd edition. New York: McGraw Hill 1999. p. 487-509.

45. Sanchez MR. Syphilis, In: Fitzpatrick, et al. Dermatology in General Medicine, 5th edition, Vol II, 2551-2581.

46. Moskovitz BL, Klimek JJ, Goldman RL. Meningovascular syphilis syphilis after 'appropriate' treatment of primary syphilis. Arch Intern Med 1982; 142: 139-140.

47. Ganesh R, Stanley A, Ganesh N. Prevalence of neurosyphilis at Government Rajaji Hospital, Madurai, India. Int J STD AIDS. 1994; 5: 290-292.

48. Schiff E, Lindberg M. Neurosyphilis. South Med J 2002; 95: 1083-1087.

49. Milne A. Encephalitis and other brain infections. In: Donaghy M eds Michael Donaghy Brain's Diseases of the Nervous System 11th edition. London: Oxford University Press; 2001. 1118-1180.

50. Dorson-Buttervorth K, et al. Review of hospitalized cases of general paralysis of the insane. Br J Vener Dis 1970; 46: 295.

51. Wile V, Mundt LK. Congenital syphilis. A statistical study with special regard to sex incidence. Am J Syph Gon Vener Dis 1942; 26: 70.

52. Turk JL. Contribution of modern immunlogical concepts to an understanding of diaeases of skin. Br MJJ 1970; 3: 363-368.

53. Fitzgerald JT. Pathogenesis and immunology of *Treponema pallidum*. Ann Rev Microbiol 1981; 35: 29-54.

54. Centurion-Lara A, Castro C, Shaffer JM, et al. Detection of *Treponema pallidum by* sensitive reverse transcriptase PCR. J Clin Microbiol 1997; 35: 1348-1352.

55. Hemdevarajan, Williams J, Gopikishanan. Syphilitic abdominal aortic aneurysm in middle aged married villager. Int J STD AIDS 2000; 11): 485-486.

56. Rathore AS, Ray K, Ramesh V, Mukherjee A. Periodic syphilis profile in a New Delhi hospital. J Commun Dis 1998; 30: 153-157.

57. Tien RD, Gean Marton AD, Mark AS. Neurosyphilis in HIV carriers. MR findings in six patients. Am J Roentgenol 1992; 158: 1325-1328.

Chapter 14

Congenital Syphilis

O P Singh

Introduction

Transmission of syphilitic infection from the mother to the foetus via the placenta is congenital syphilis. It may occur when an infected woman becomes pregnant or when a pregnant woman becomes infected.[1,2] The disease may or may not appear at birth. Hence many prefer the term prenatal syphilis. Syphilis seems not to cause abortion in the first 4 months of pregnancy and it has been supposed that the Langhans cell layer provides a barrier against the infection of the foetus.

Congenital syphilis has been recognized for several centuries and still continues to be a major problem in certain countries of Eastern Europe, the former Soviet Union and sub-Saharan Africa despite effective penicillin treatment being available for over a half a century.[3] The occurrence of congenital syphilis is one of the indicators of sexually transmitted diseases in a given population. The prevention of congenital syphilis is more cost-effective than the prevention of mother-to-child transmission of HIV infection.

Outcome of Pregnancy

The following may happen to an untreated syphilitic pregnant woman:

1. Miscarriage may ensue at some period later than the 12-16 weeks, following the formation of the placenta.
2. In about 30% of the cases, the foetus may die *in utero* late in pregnancy resulting in a stillbirth/macerated foetus.[4]
3. In a few cases, the foetus may be born apparently normal, but develops signs of early congenital syphilis during the first few weeks or months **(Profeta's law)**.

4. In a few cases, the foetus may be born showing signs of congenital syphilis.
5. The infant with early congenital syphilis subsequently may or may not show signs of late congenital syphilis.
6. The child may not show early congenital syphilis but may develop late congenital syphilis in later years.
7. The foetus may escape the infection. This may occur with increasing probability with longer duration of the disease in expectant mother. The observation that the untreated syphilitic mother tends to improve on past performances; that is to have later and later miscarriages, then syphilitic and finally non-syphilitic children. **(Diday's or Kassowitz's law)**.

Colles (1837) had made an observation that the syphilitic infant did not infect its own mother but is capable of infecting others **(Colles' law)**. It is now clear that it is because the mother is probably having latent form of syphilis and has a degree of immunity to super infection from her own child.

Prophylaxis

The prevention of congenital syphilis depends on adequate follow-up during pregnancy. An ideal routine for antenatal clinic would be to examine the pregnant woman and take blood for VDRL checkup as early and as late in pregnancy as possible. The control of congenital syphilis depends on adequate treatment being given to the infected pregnant woman at the earliest.

Congenital syphilis is a preventable disease. Adequate therapy before the fourth month of pregnancy almost always prevents the infection in the newborn. Treatment after 18 weeks usually brings about an *in utero* cure, though it may not prevent bone or joint involvement, neural deafness or interstitial keratitis in the newborn.[5]

Incidence

The incidence of congenital syphilis varies from time to time and place to place in different countries and populations. It largely depends upon the prevalence of infectious syphilis in the concerned population at the relevant time and the availability of the treatment to the infected pregnant woman. The incidence of congenital syphilis is quite low, though the reported incidence in India varies from 0.5% to 5%.[6,7] In Bulgaria, great political, social and economic changes reflected the increase in the incidence of congenital syphilis from 1 in 1990 to 35 in 1998.[8]

Pathology

Gross placental changes are found only when pregnancy ends in stillbirth. If the foetus survives, it owes its life to the fact that the placental lesions were minimal. Diseased placenta is bulky, heavy, pale and greasy. Syphilitic endarteritis produces alterations in the chorionic villi with a subsequent decrease in the blood vessels, with an increase of connective tissue and infarcts. The weight of the placenta is usually greater than one quarter that of the foetus. Demonstration of *T. pallidum* in the placenta clinches the diagnosis.[9]

Once the treponema have entered the foetal circulation, dissemination to all the tissues occurs at once, thereby provoking the characteristic cellular inflammatory response of small lymphocytes and plasma cells.[10] The foetus may be overwhelmed by the infection and may die. The stillborn foetus may have the macerated appearance with collapse of the skull and protuberant abdomen. The skin may be of livid red colour with hemorrhagic bullae. At autopsy, the liver and spleen are enlarged with cellular inflammatory response in other organs, including bones. Erythroblastosis is more common in stillborn infants with congenital syphilis. Placental histopathology may reveal necrotizing funisitis, villous enlargement and acute villitis.[11]

If the treponemal infection does not prove fatal, it may still interfere with normal development at various stages of intrauterine and extrauterine life.

Certain characteristic manifestations at a later life, such as interstitial keratitis and Clutton's joints, are possibly not direct effects of treponemal activity, but believed to be phenomenon of hypersensitivity.

Clinical Manifestations

There are usually no signs of the disease at birth. The presence of hemorrhagic bullae and muco-cutaneous lesions at the time of birth signifies a severe infection. Usually, a period of 2-6 weeks elapses before signs of infantile congenital syphilis appear. By the time such signs appear, the serum reactions to tests for syphilis are positive. There is no primary stage in the infant as the disease is already blood borne. Sometimes there are no clinical signs apart from a positive serum reaction.

For the purpose of convenience, congenital syphilis has been classified into early, late and the stigmata. An arbitrary division between the early and late stages of the disease is customary to place this at the end of second year of life. Early lesions of the first two years of life are comparable to those of secondary syphilis in the acquired form. Vesicobullous lesions called as pemphigus syphiliticus (a misnomer) arise predominantly on palms and soles.[12] Bullous lesions seen in the early congenital syphilis are characteristically absent in acquired syphilis. The lesions of the first two years of life are contagious. Many of the late lesions are gummatous and are not contagious. The stigmata are the scars or deformities resulting from early or late healed lesions.

Early Congenital Syphilis

As already mentioned, there is no primary stage and signs are similar to those of secondary stage of acquired syphilis. If a lesion resembling primary chancre is seen in an infant, it may be due to acquired syphilis from genital lesion of very recent infection in the mother. Condylomata lata lesions at mucocutaneous and intertriginous areas of perianal skin are the markers of untreated congenital syphilis, which show recurrences.[12]

Blood taken from the umbilical vein (cord blood) or from the infant may give positive results, but these positive results do not necessarily indicate infection of the infant with syphilis. The positive results may be due to the presence of reagin and specific antibodies, which have passed from the maternal to the foetal circulation. It has been suggested that reliable information of an active infection can be obtained in these cases from an FTA-Abs test using fluorescent-labeled IgM conjugate in place of an ordinary fluorescent labeled anti-human globulin. A negative blood test at birth does not exclude infection, as it may become positive later in a few weeks or months. This also applies to the FTA-IgM test, so that, when congenital syphilis is a possibility, follow up of an infant for at least 3 months is essential before the infection can be excluded.[13]

General

These include marasmus and 'old man' appearance. Weak infants are prone to intercurrent infections and failure to regain the birth weight.[9]

Skin Lesions

The earliest type of lesion is the bullous rash distributed symmetrically on palms and soles and occasionally on other parts of the body. The floor of the lesion is dull red and when the bulla is ruptured and discharges its infectious fluid. Other rashes are similar to those described in secondary syphilis and usually appear some weeks after birth. The rash may be very profuse, specially so on the lower part of the face, where it may be confluent. Movement of the lips is apt to produce radiating fissures at the angles of the mouth, which when secondarily infected may leave linear scars (rhagades). They may also be found around the nares and the anus.

Hair may be brittle and sparse. Infantile alopecia affecting the eyebrows is suggestive of syphilis.[14] Paronychia particularly affects the fourth and the fifth digits, which usually leads to a narrow atrophic nail and produces a claw nail deformity.

Mucous Membrane Lesions

Syphilitic rhinitis produces a nasal discharge (snuffles), which is highly infectious. It is watery initially and later becomes thicker, purulent and bloody. Mucous patches and moist erosions may be present in the buccal mucosa and genital mucosa. Syphilitic rhinitis may lead to ulceration and perforation of the nasal septum with flattening of the nasal bridge forming the characteristic saddle nose.[5] The nasal obstruction due to the discharge may cause breathing and suckling difficulties. Throat lesions may cause pharyngitis and laryngitis, leading to a characteristic hoarse cry and cough.[15]

Bone Lesions

In the first six months of life, osteochondritis of the long bones is a characteristic finding. There is a periosteal reaction with deposition of new bone under the periosteum appearing on the surface of the cortex. In severe cases, the mother may have noticed loss of movement of the affected limbs, the syphilitic pseudoparalysis. The child screams while handling due to severe pain and tenderness. In some cases the symptoms and signs may be absent and the bone changes are seen only on radiological examination. The more rapidly growing bones show the most marked changes, particularly in the upper end of the tibia and the distal end of the radius and the ulna. **Wimberger's sign** is a loss of density on the medial side of the upper end of the tibia, which is characteristic of congenital syphilis (**P XII, Fig. 48**).[10]

The signs of osteochondritis disappear in the second six moths of life, but periosteitis persists and becomes more marked. The radiographic examination shows 'onion-peel' periosteum as successive layers of the bone are laid down on the surface of the cortex in a regular fashion. In the second year of life the characteristic lesion of the bone is the osteochondritis of phalanges, the 'syphilitic dactylitis'.[16] It is the proximal phalanges which are likely to be affected and the fingers are involved more frequently than the toes. One digit or several digits may be involved. Syphilitic dactylitis is a painless, fusiform swelling, which unlike the equivalent tubercular dactylitis almost never breaks down.

Lymph Nodes

Generalized lymphadenopathy is found in 20%-50% of the cases. The nodes are firm, discrete, rubbery and non-tender. Epitrochlear lymphadenopathy which is characteristic, is found in 20% of cases of lymphadenopathy.[17]

Liver and Spleen

The infant's abdomen may be grossly protuberant owing to hepatosplenomegaly. Enlargement is due to diffuse increase in fibrous tissue and to abnormal persistence of the foetal blood forming tissues. The patient may show a slight icteric tint, but marked jaundice is uncommon.

Kidneys

Involvement of the kidneys is only of slight degree. In some cases, the urine shows albumin and a few or many hyaline and granular casts. Either proliferative or membranous glomerulonephritis may be found.[14]

Lungs

Infants who die of early congenital syphilis are some times found to have wide spread infiltration of the lungs, so called 'white pneumonia.'

Eyes

Choroidoretinitis, glaucoma and uveitis are the three ocular lesions associated with early congenital syphilis. Choroidoretinitis may remain unrecognized in the early months of life but it is likely that the residual evidence, may be found as stigmata in later life as pepper and salt fundus showing black pigment and white atrophic patches.[15]

Central Nervous System

The neurological involvement ranges from asymptomatic neurosyphilis to acute syphilitic leptomeningitis. Forty to sixty percent of the infected infants have abnormal CSF findings although the incidence of clinical involvement is much lower.[14] Symptomatic syphilis due to meningitic or meningoencephalitic changes may present as convulsions, bulging fontanelles, stiffness of the neck and hydrocephalus.[5] Most infants with *T. pallidum* infection of the central nervous system can be identified by physical examination, conventional laboratory tests and radiographic studies. However, the identification of all such infants requires the use of additional tests including IgM immunoblotting and P.CR assay. In a study conducted on 76 infants of congenital syphilis who had no prior antibiotic exposure, 17 (22%) showed spirochetes in their CSF.[18]

Identification of infants with *T. pallidum* infection of the nervous system remains difficult.

Other Clinical Features

Syphilitic diarrhoea due to involvement of pancreas and intestines, myocarditis, anonychia and paronychia have been reported.[4, 14, 15]

Hematological Manifestations

Anaemia, leucocytosis or leucopenia, monocytosis, thrombocytopenia and raised ESR may occur. Anaemia is probably due to autoimmune hemolysis and it may be associated with cryoglobulinemia. The anaemia, which is Coomb's test negative, is often associated with reticulocytosis and erythroblastosis.[14]

Late Congenital Syphilis

The late stage of congenital syphilis is beyond the 2nd year of life. The early stage may go unnoticed in about 80% of the cases of late congenital syphilis. The late manifestations correspond to the tertiary phase of acquired syphilis. The classic syndrome of late congenital syphilis is now rare because of concomitant antibiotic treatment of other intercurrent infections.[19] The clinical manifestations may be due to hypersensitivity or inflammatory reaction to *T. pallidum*.

Interstitial Keratitis

It is the most common late manifestation which is more common in females. It appears first as circumcorneal vascularization, followed by vascular infiltration extending from the sclera into the deep layers of the cornea and cellular exudation into the deep corneal structures. It usually starts in one eye but the other eye is likely to be involved, irrespective of the antisyphilitic treatment. It has a self limited or relapsing course that ends in corneal ground glass appearance. If the corneal vascularisation is quite intense, it may be clinically obvious as a dull pink patch at the periphery of the cornea, the so called "Salmon patch". The condition is usually associated with iridocyclitis. The symptoms are photophobia, pain, excessive watering of the eyes and blurred vision.[19]

Teeth

Hutchinson's teeth: The permanent upper central incisors are shorter than the lateral incisors and widely spaced, have a notch in the biting edge as a result of defective enamel formation and assume a barrel or peg shape (**P XII, Fig. 49**). They usually appear at the age of 6 years or later. X-ray findings permit the diagnosis even when unaffected deciduous teeth are in place. Other incisors may also be affected.[20]

Mulberry or Moon's molars: The other characteristic dystrophy is that of the first molar teeth. The first lower molars, which are developing at the same time as the incisor teeth, are most often affected. Moon has first described that the cusps are under developed and poorly enameled. The biting surface looks dome-shaped, with small projections of the ill-developed cusps. This deformity is less common than the incisor teeth. The affected molars are very prone to caries and are usually lost early in life, due to poor development of enamel, the teeth are predisposed to cavity formation.[21]

Neural Deafness

It is often preceded by tinnitus and vertigo followed by loss of hearing, first in one ear and then in the other. The primary lesion is osteochondritis affecting the otic capsule causing cochlear degeneration. The prognosis is poor but the condition is rare in congenital syphilis. Nerve deafness generally takes its course irrespective of antisyphilitic treatment but may be modified by steroid therapy.[10]

Neurosyphilis

Like acquired syphilis, the clinical manifestations may be asymptomatic or symptomatic. Juvenile paresis has been observed more frequently than juvenile tabes.

Hutchinson's Triad

It is considered as a pathognomonic sign of late congenital syphilis. It includes

1. Interistitial keratitis
2. Hutchinson's teeth
3. Eighth nerve deafness

Skin and Mucous Membrane Lesions

Gummata may lead to nasal septum perforation and palatal perforation (**P XII, Fig. 50**). This may cause nasal voice and regurgitation of food. Other clinical features are similar to those seen in acquired syphilis.

Bone Lesions

Most of the lesions result in sclerosis and considerable new bone formation, but destructive lesions occur in the palate and nasal septum. All patients with syphilis should be examined by shining a torch into one nostril while observing through the other to see whether the light shines through to the other half of the nasal cavity. Tibia is most frequently involved and the thickening of the middle third of the bone may give the appearance called "sabre tibia". Localized osteo-periostitis of the bones of the vault of the skull may lead to the formation of rounded, bony swelling, called Parrot's nodes. The areas of thickening may give the impression of the thinning of the rest of the bones, but it is a false impression, occasionally seen in early congenital syphilis. Thickening of the inner end of the clavicle (*Higoumenaki's sign*) and dactylitis are occasionally found in cases of late congenital syphilis.[19]

Clutton's Joint

Hydro-arthrosis due to perisynovitis has been described by Clutton. The patient may suffer from diffuse arthralgia. Usually both knee joints are involved, often simultaneously, but occasionally there may be a lapse of months or even years before the second joint is affected. There is little impairment of function and X-ray shows enlargement of the joint spaces but no bony changes. Rarely, elbow joints are involved.[22] The onset is commonly painless and insidious, and the course is chronic, and does not respond to antisyphilitic treatment as *T. pallidum* has never been found in the tissues or joint fluid in these cases. Clutton's joint, like interstitial keratitis, is due to hypersensitivity. Recovery is slow, but steady.

Paroxysmal Cold Haemoglobinuria

This is a rare manifestation seen in congenital and also in acquired syphilis in which the affected patient on exposure to cold will, within a few minutes, develop chills, malaise, headache, pain in the back, fever and urticaria. The urine passed during or just after the attack is red or brown. In a day or two the urine returns to normal but the patient may show jaundice. The serum of these patients contains a hemolysin which, in the presence of complement, first sensitizes the red cells during the period of chilling, then hemolyses them when the body temperature returns to normal. This is known as *Donath-Landsteiner reaction*, which can be performed in vitro as a diagnostic test.[10] The test may be positive without the patient having haemoglobinuria. Antisyphilitic treatment usually cures the condition.

Other Organs

Liver is occasionally involved but visceral involvement

is rare and similarly cardiovascular syphilis is quite rare in late congenital syphilis.

Stigmata

Stigmata are the scars or deformities resulting from early or late congenital syphilis lesions which are often characteristic and remain as permanent evidence of the infection. The stigmata are diagnostic of congenital syphilis, if they present with positive serological tests for syphilis. Stigmata suggestive of congenital syphilis are saddle nose (**P XII, Fig. 50**), frontal and parietal bossing, short maxillae, bull dog jaws, a high arched palate, sabre tibia, scaphoid scapulae, Hutchinson's teeth, Moon's molars, corneal opacities salt and pepper fundus, optic atrophy, 8th nerve deafness, and rhagades. Certain other findings have been described as stigmata, but they are not in themselves diagnostic as they may occur in normal people.

Diagnosis

Demonstration of *T. pallidum* by direct examination from the early lesions of congenital syphilis is confirmatory. A positive non-treponemal test titre being significantly higher than the mother suggests a prenatal infection and the infant should be treated. In any controversial situation it is better to give treatment as the delay may be unnecessarily detrimental for an early cure.

Evaluation and Treatment of Congenital Syphilis (CDC)[23]

Routine screening of newborn sera or umbilical cord blood is not recommended. Serologic testing of the mother's serum is preferred over testing infant serum, because the serologic tests performed on infant serum can be non-reactive if the mother's serologic test result is of low titre or if the mother was infected late in pregnancy. No infant or mother should leave the health care facility unless the maternal serologic status has been documented at least once during pregnancy and preferably again at delivery.

Evaluation and Treatment of Infants in the First Month of Life

The transplacental transfer of maternal nontreponemal and treponemal immunoglobulin G (IgG) antibodies to the foetus complicates the diagnosis of congenital syphilis and it makes the interpretation of reactive serologic tests for syphilis in infants difficult. Treatment decisions often must be made on the basis of a) identification of syphilis in the mother, b) adequacy of maternal treatment, c) presence of clinical, laboratory, or radiographic evidence of syphilis in the infant and d) comparison of maternal (at delivery) and infant nontreponemal serologic titers utilizing the same test and preferably the same laboratory.

All infants born to mothers who have reactive nontreponemal and treponemal test results should be evaluated with a quantitative nontreponemal serologic test (RPR or VDRL) performed on infant serum, because umbilical cord blood can become contaminated with maternal blood and could yield a false-positive result. A treponemal test (i.e., TPHA or FTA-ABS) on a newborn's serum is not necessary. Currently, no commercially available IgM test is reliable.

All infants born to women who have reactive serologic tests for syphilis should be examined thoroughly for evidence of congenital syphilis (e.g., nonimmune hydrops, jaundice, hepatosplenomegaly, rhinitis, skin rash, and/or pseudoparalysis of extremity). Pathologic examination of the placenta or umbilical cord using specific fluorescent antitreponemal anti-body staining is suggested. Darkfield microscopic examination or direct fluorescent antibody staining of suspicious lesions or body fluids (e.g., nasal discharge) should also be performed.

The following scenarios describe the evaluation and treatment of infants for congenital syphilis.

Scenario 1. Infants with proven or highly probable disease

(a) An abnormal physical examination that is consistent with congenital syphilis

(b) A serum quantitative nontreponemal serologic titre that is fourfold greater than the mother's titre or

(c) A positive darkfield or fluorescent antibody test of body fluid(s).

Recommended evaluation

- CSF analysis for VDRL, cell count, and protein.
- Complete blood count (CBC) and differential and platelet count.

- Other tests as clinically indicated (e.g., long-bone radiographs, chest radiograph, liver function tests, cranial ultrasound, ophthalmologic examination and auditory brainstem response).

Recommended Regimens
Aqueous crystalline penicillin G 100,000– 150,000 units/kg/dose iv every 12 hours during the first 7 days of life and every 8 hours thereafter for a total of 10 days *or* Procaine penicillin G 50,000 units/ kg/ dose lm. in a single daily dose for 10 days.

If more than 1 day of therapy is missed, the entire course should be restarted. Data are insufficient regarding the use of other antimicrobial agents (e.g., ampicillin). When possible, a full 10-day course of penicillin is preferred, even if ampicillin was initially provided for possible sepsis. The use of agents other than penicillin requires close serologic follow-up to assess the adequacy of therapy. In all other situations, the maternal history of infection with *T. pallidum* and treatment for syphilis must be considered when evaluating and treating the infant.

Scenario 2. Infants who have a normal physical examination and a serum quantitative nontreponemal serologic titre the same or less than fourfold the maternal titre and the

(a) Mother was not treated, inadequately treated, or has no documentation of having received treatment
(b) Mother was treated with erythromycin or other nonpenicillin regimens
(c) Mother received treatment ≤ 4 weeks before delivery or
(d) Mother has early syphilis and has a nontreponemal titre that has either not decreased fourfold or has increased fourfold.

Recommended Evaluation
- As for Scenario 1

Recommended Regimens
Aqueous crystalline penicillin G 100,000– 150,000 units/kg/day, administered as 50,000 units/ kg/dose IV every 12 hours for the first 7 days of life and every 8 hours thereafter for a total of 10 days, or Procaine penicillin G 50,000 units /kg/dose lm. in a single daily dose for 10 days, or Benzathine penicillin G 50,000 units /kg/dose IM in a single dose.

A complete evaluation is not necessary if 10 days of parenteral therapy is administered. However, such evaluation may be useful; a lumbar puncture may document CSF abnormalities that would prompt close follow-up. Other tests (e.g., CBC, platelet count, and bone radiographs) may be performed to further support a diagnosis of congenital syphilis. If a single dose of benzathine penicillin G is used, then the infant must be fully evaluated (i.e., through CSF examination, long bone radiographs, and CBC with platelets), the full evaluation must be normal and follow up must be certain. If any part of the infant's evaluation is abnormal or not performed, or if the CSF analysis is rendered uninterpretable because of contamination with blood, then a 10-day course of penicillin is required.

Scenario 3. Infants who have a normal physical examination and a serum quantitative nontreponemal serologic titre the same or less than fourfold the maternal titre and the

(a) Mother was treated during pregnancy, treatment was appropriate for the stage of infection and treatment was administered >4 weeks before delivery
(b) Mother's nontreponemal titres decreased fourfold after appropriate therapy for early syphilis or remained stable and low for late syphilis and
(c) Mother has no evidence of reinfection or relapse.

Recommended Evaluation
- No evaluation is required.

Recommended Regimen
Benzathine penicillin G 50,000 units/kg/dose IM in a single dose.

Scenario 4. Infants who have a normal physical examination and a serum quantitative nontreponemal serologic titre the same or less than fourfold the maternal titer and the

(a) Mother's treatment was adequate before pregnancy and
(b) Mother's nontreponemal serologic titre remained low and stable before and during pregnancy and at delivery (VDRL ≤ I:2 ; RPR ≤ I:4).

Recommended Evaluation

- No evaluation is required.

Evaluation and Treatment of Older Infants and Children

Children who are identified as having reactive serologic tests for syphilis after the neonatal period (> 1 month of age) should have maternal serology and records reviewed to assess whether the child has congenital or acquired syphilis. Any child at risk for congenital syphilis should receive a full evaluation and testing for HIV infection.

Recommended Evaluation
- As for scenario 1
Recommended Regimen
No treatment is required; however, some specialists would treat with benzathine penicillin G 50,000 units/kg as a single IM injection, particularly if follow-up is uncertain.

Follow Up

All seroactive infants (or infants whose mothers were seroactive at delivery) should receive careful follow up examinations and serlogic testing (a nontreponomal test) every 2-3 months until the test becomes non reactive or the titre has decreased fourfold. Nontreponemal antibody titres should decline by 3 months of age and should be nonreactive by 6 months of age if the infant was not infected (if the reactive test result was not caused by passive transfer of maternal IgG antibody) or was infected but adequately treated. The serologic response after therapy may be slower for infants treated after the neonatal period. If these titres are stable or increase after 6-12 months of age, the child should be evaluated (given a CSF examination) and treated with a 10 day course of parenteral penicillin G.

Treponemal tests should not be used to evaluate treatment response because the results for an infected child can remain positive despite effective therapy. Passively transferred maternal treponemal antibodies can be present in an infant until age 15 months. A reactive treponemal test after age 18 months is diagnostic of congenital syphilis. If the nontreponemal test is nonreactive at this time, no further evaluation or treatment is necessary. If the nontreponemal test is reactive at age 18 months, the infant should be fully (re) evaluated and treated for congenital syphilis.

Infants whose initial CSF evaluations are abnormal should undergo a repeat lumbar puncture approximately every 6 months until the results are normal. A reactive CSF VDRL test or abnormal CSF indices that cannot be attributed to other ongoing illness requires retreatment for possible neurosyphilis. Follow-up of children treated for congenital syphilis after the newborn period should be conducted as is recommended for neonates.

Control

Effective prevention and detection of congenital syphilis depends on the identification of syphilis in pregnant women and, therefore, on the routine serologic screening of pregnant women during the first prenatal visit. Serologic testing and a sexual history also should be obtained at 28 weeks of gestation and at delivery in communities and populations in which the risk for congenital syphilis is high. Moreover, as part of the management of pregnant women, who have syphilis, information concerning treatment of sex partners should be obtained to assess the risk for reinfection. All pregnant women who have syphilis should be tested for HIV infection.[23]

For the control of congenital syphilis the current antenatal screening of syphilis should continue.[24] The success of therapy in preventing congenital syphilis was almost 100%, except in secondary syphilis in which 4 failure out of 75 (p = 0.03) have been reported.[25] This suggests the higher risk of foetal treatment failure with maternal secondary syphilis showing high VDRL titres at treatment and delivery and/or infant born at less than 36 weeks.[26]

Though penicillin remains the treatment of choice, since its introduction in 1940, uncertainty regarding the optional treatment regimens still remains. Congenital syphilis is an increasing problem in developing countries due to the transitional economy compounded by aggravation when associated with HIV/AIDS. Wallen GJ in the Cochrane data base analysis tried to identify the most effective antibiotic treatment with consideration of above mentioned factors in syphilitic pregnant women with or without concomitant HIV infection. Only 26 studies met the criteria for detailed scrutiny, but none of them met the predetermined criteria. In the reviewers' conclusion it was observed that penicillin is effective in the treatment of syphilis in pregnancy and in prevention of congenital syphilis, but doubt regarding optional treatment was still persisting. So the effectiveness of various antibiotics regimens for the same in pregnant women has to be assured carried out with randomized controlled trails with the existing recommendations.[27]

References

1. Wicher V, Wicher K. Pathogenesis of maternal – foetal syphilis revisited. Clin Infect Dis 2001; 33: 354-363.

2. Peihong J, Zhiyong L, Rengui C et al. Early Congenital Syphilis. Int J Dermatol 2001; 40: 191-209.

3. Walker DG, Walker GJ. Forgotten but not gone: the continuing scourge of congenital syphilis. Lancet Infect Dis 2002; 2: 432-436.

4. Mavrov GI, Goubenko TV. Clinical and epidemiological features of syphilis in pregnant women: the course and outcome of pregnancy. Gynecol Obstet Int 2001; 52: 114-118.

5. Sanchez M. Syphilis, In: Fitzpatric TB, Eisen AZ, Wolf K, Freedberg IM, Austen FK, eds. Dermatology in general medicine. 4th ed. New York: Mc Graw-Hill; 1999. p. 2551-2581.

6. Garg BR, Sardarilal. Changing pattern of sexually transmitted diseases. Indian J Sex Transm Dis 1982; 3: 41-42.

7. Darkfman DM, Glaser JH. Congenital syphilis presenting in infants after the newborn period. N Eng J Med 1990; 323: 1299-1302.

8. Dencheva R, Spirov G, Gilina K et al. Epidemiology of syphilis in Bulgaria, 1990-1998. Int J STD AIDS 2000; 11: 819-822.

9. Willcox RR. Textbook of venereal diseases and treponematoses. 2nd ed. London: William Heinemann Medical Books Ltd; 1964. p. 231.

10. King A, Nicol C, Rodin P. Congenital syphilis. In: Venereal diseases. 4th ed. London: ELBS 1980. p. 104-132.

11. Sheffield JS, Sanches PJ, Wendel GD jr, et al. Placental histopathology of congenital syphilis. Obstet Gynecol 2002; 100: 126-133.

12. Thappa DM, Karthikeyan K. Late diagnosis of early congenital syphilis. Indian J Sex Transm Dis 2002; 23: 43-45.

13. Johnston NA. Neonatal syphilis. Diagnosis by the absorbed fluorescent treponemal antibody (IgM) test. Brit J Vene Dis 1972; 48: 464-469.

14. Wendel GD Jr. Early and congenital syphilis. Obstet Gynecol Clin North Am 1989; 16: 479-494.

15. Arya OP, Osab AD, Benatt FJ. Syphilis. In: Tropical venereology. 2nd ed. Edinburgh: Churchill Livingstone, 1988. p. 39-132.

16. Levin TL, Schulman M, Zieba P, Goldman HS. Absence of lower extremity ossification centres in term infants with congenital syphilis. J Perinatal 1994; 4: 106-109.

17. Michelle L, Bennett HD, Annette W, et al. Congenital syphilis: Subtle presentation of fulminant disease. J Am Acad Dermatol 1997; 36: 351-354.

18. Michello IC, Wendel GD jr, Norgard MV, et al. Central nervous system infection in congenital syphilis. N Engl J Med 2002; 346: 1792-1798.

19. Siddappa K, Ravindra K. Syphilis and nonvenereal treponematoses. In: Valia RG, Valia AR, eds. IADVL Textbook and Atlas of Dermatology. Mumbai: Balani Publishing House; 2001. p. 1390-1422.

20. Sood VK, Dogra A, Minocha YC. Congenital syphilis stigmata. Indian J Dermatol Venereol Leprol 1995; 61: 358-39.

21. Pavithran K. Clutton's joints. Indian J Dermatol Venereol Leprol 1990; 56: 236-237.

22. Anandam K, Srijaya R. Clutton's joint – case report. Indian J Dermatol Venereol Leprol 1970; 36: 160-163.

23. Centres for Disease Control. Sexually Transmitted diseases Treatment Guidelines. MMWR. 2002; 51 (RR. 6): 26-28.

24. Connor N, Roberts J, Nicoll A. Strategic options for antenatal screening for syphilis in the United Kingdom: a cost effective analysis. J Med Screen 2000; (7): 7-13.

25. Alexander JM, Sheffield JS, Sanchez PJ, et al. Efficacy of treatment for syphilis in pregnancy. Obstet Gynecol 1999; 93: 5-8.

26. Sheffield JS, Sanchez PJ, Morris G, et al. Congenital syphilis after maternal treatment for syphilis during pregnancy. Am J Obstet Gynecol 2002; 186: 569-573.

27. Walker GJ. Antibiotics for syphilis diagnosed during pregnancy. Cochrane Database Syst Rev 2001; (3): CD001143.

Chapter 15

Laboratory Diagnosis of Syphilis

Madhu Vajpayee

Introduction

Syphilis, caused by the spirochaete *Treponema pallidum* subsp. *pallidum,* is a chronic infection with many diverse clinical manifestations that occur in distinct stages. As *T. pallidum* cannot be readily cultured[1] or stained with simple laboratory stains, other laboratory methods to identify infection in various stages of syphilis have been developed. Tests for syphilis fall into four categories: (i) direct microscopic examination, used when lesions are present; (ii) nontreponemal tests, used for screening; (iii) treponemal tests that are confirmatory; and (iv) direct antigen detection tests currently used in research settings and as gold standards for test evaluation.

Direct Detection Methods

Dark Field Microscopy

The most specific and easiest means of diagnosing syphilis is by direct detection of organism if lesions are present. A positive result on microscopy is definitive evidence of syphilis, if infection with other pathogenic treponemes can be excluded. Darkfield examination must be accomplished immediately after the specimen is obtained because viability of the treponemes is necessary to distinguish *T. pallidum* from morphologically similar saprophytic spirochaetes within and near the genitalia. Dark field examination is most productive during primary, secondary, infectious relapsing and early congenital syphilis when moist lesions containing large number of treponemes are present.

The lesions should be cleaned only if encrusted or obviously contaminated and only tap water or physiological saline (without antibacterial additives) should be used. A minimum amount of liquid should be used for cleaning because large amounts may dilute organism and hinder the ability to recover treponemes. Antiseptics or soaps should not be used because they may kill the treponemes and invalidate interpretation of the dark field examination. After cleaning the lesion, abrasion should be done with gentle pressure and clear serum exudate should be collected. The material can be collected directly on the cover slip, which is then placed on glass slide and examined while organism is still motile. The specificity of dark field examination is dependent on the skill of the microscopist in distinguishing *T. pallidum* from other commensal spirochaetes (Table 1). Positive findings on dark field examination permit a specific and immediate diagnosis of syphilis. However, a negative dark field finding does not exclude the diagnosis of syphilis. The sensitivity of dark field examination approaches 80%.[2]

Direct Fluorescent Antibody (DFA) Test for *Treponema Pallidum*

Lesion samples for the DFA for *T. pallidum* (DFA-TP) examination are collected in the manner described for dark field examination. The test detects and differentiates pathogenic treponemes from non-pathogenic treponemes by an antigen antibody reaction; thus the organism is not required to be motile in the DFA-TP. It is applicable to samples collected from oral, rectal or intestinal lesions because the conjugates used are specific for pathogenic strains of Treponema spp. However the test cannot distinguish between the pathogenic strains of Treponema spp. Smears are stained with FITC labeled anti *T. pallidum* globulins prepared from the sera of humans or rabbit with syphilis and that have been absorbed with Reiter's treponemes. More recently, mouse monoclonal antibody to *T. pallidum* has been used in the DFA-TP.[3]

Table 1.   Morphology and Motility of *T. pallidum* subsp. *pallidum* and Related Non-pathogenic Species

Organism	Location	Coils	Length (µm)	Width (µm)	Wave length (µm)	Wave depth (µm)	Translation	Rotation	Flexion
T. pallidum Subsp. *Pallidum*★	Skin and mucosal lesions	Spiral shape 10-13 coils	Medium, 10	Very thin 0.13-0.15	Tight, 1.1 (1.0-1.5)	Deep, 0.5-0.7	Slow, deliberate	Slow to rapid; like a cork-screw	Soft bending in middle; pops back into place with spring
T. refringens	Normal genital flora	Spiral shape 2-3 coils	Short, 5-8	Thick, 0.20-0.50	Loose, 1.8 (1.5-2.5)	Shallow 0.4-0.6	Rapid	Very rapid; serpentine-like	Marked bending, relaxed coils
T. phagedenis	Normal genital flora	Spiral shape 10-12 coils	Medium long, 10-12	Thick, 0.20-0.25	Loose, 1.4-1.6 (1.5-2.0)	Shallow, 0.4-0.6	Slow, jerky; deliberate	Slow to rapid; rotates without changing place	Jerky; twists or undulates from side to side
T. denticola	Normal oral flora	Spiral shape 6-8 coils	Medium, 8	Very thin 0.15-0.20	Tight 0.9 (0.8-1.2)	Deep, 0.4-0.6	Slow, deliberate	Slow to rapid, jerky	Soft bending; bends, twists, or undulates

★Reiter's treponeme

Animal Inoculation

The oldest method for detecting infection with *T. pallidum* is animal infectivity testing. This technique probably is the most sensitive method for detecting infectious treponemes and is used as a gold standard for measuring the sensitivity of methods such as PCR.[4]

Serological Diagnosis of Syphilis

Except during the very early stage of infection, serology remains the mainstay of laboratory testing for syphilis, and certain characteristics of syphilis make it amenable to serological screening. There have been several developments in serological tests for syphilis in recent years, particularly the advent of enzyme immunoassays (EIA), and lately the commercial availability of recombinant antigen-based tests.

Natural History of Infection and Immune Response

The natural history of syphilis is very variable; the course of the infection spans many years and may lead to a variety of clinical presentations including primary, secondary, latent and late syphilis, and may be further divided into early (infectious) and late (non-infectious) stages. The immune response to syphilis is complex and involves production of antibodies to a broad range of antigens, including non-specific antibodies (cardiolipin or lipoidal antibody), and specific treponemal antibodies. The first demonstrable response to infection is the production of specific anti-treponemal IgM, which may be detected towards the end of the second week of infection, whilst anti-treponemal IgG appears later, at about 4 weeks.[5] By the time the symptoms are present, most patients have both detectable IgG and IgM antibody.[6] The immune response can be affected by treatment and by HIV infection. The titres of non-specific antibody and specific IgM decline rapidly after adequate therapy of early syphilis but specific IgG antibody generally persists. HIV infection may lead to a reduced or delayed antibody response in primary syphilis but in most cases the response is normal or exaggerated.[7]

Serological Tests for Syphilis and Their Application

Serological tests for syphilis may be classified into two groups: *non-treponemal* tests, which detect non-specific treponemal antibody, eg. the Venereal Diseases Research Laboratory (VDRL) or rapid plasma reagin (RPR) tests, and *treponemal* tests, which detect specific treponemal antibody, eg. *Treponema pallidum* haemagglutination assay (TPHA), fluorescent treponemal antibody-absorbtion (FTA-abs) and enzyme immunoassay (EIA) tests (Tables 2 and 3)

Table 2.　Basis of Non-Treponemal Tests

Capture system	Test	Comments
Liposomes in suspension producing visible flocculation with lipoidal antibodies	VDRL	
Liposomes in suspension + unattached charcoal particles producing dark coloured flocculation due to trapping of charcoal particles in lattice formed by antigen-antibody complex	RPR	USR (Unheated Serum Reagin) TRUST (Toluidine Red Unheated Serum Test)
VDRL antigen coated onto wells of microtitre plates and attached antibody detected by enzyme immunoassay	EIA (Reagin)	

Table 3.　Basis of Treponemal Tests

Antigen	Capture System	Test
Intact Treponemes	Treponemes fixed onto microscope slides	FTA-ABS
Purified and sonicated treponemes	Attached to red blood cells	TPHA
	Attached to gelatin particles	TPPA
	Attached to microtitre plates	EIA
	Proteins separated by PAGE and transferred to filter paper by Western blotting	Immunoblots
Recombinant antigens	Attached to microtitre plates	EIA
	Attached to latex particles	Latex agglutination

PAGE – Polyacrylamide gel electrophoresis

Non Treponemal test

In 1906, Wassermann et al adapted the complement fixation test, previously introduced by Bordet and

Gengou in 1901, for serologic testing of syphilis.[3] The antigen used in the Wassermann test for syphilis was an extract of liver from newborns, who had died of congenital syphilis and later beef heart extracted in alcohol, served equally well as an antigen.[8] Although the complement fixation tests contributed immensely to the diagnosis of syphilis, they were too complicated to perform and required many reagents and as long as 24 hours to complete. Kahn in 1922[9] introduced a flocculation test without complement that could be read macroscopically in a few hours but the antigen, a crude extracts of tissue, varied in quality. Pangborn in 1941[10] successfully isolated from beef heart the active antigenic component, a phospholipid, cardiolipin. Cardiolipin, when combined with lecithin and cholesterol, forms a serologically active antigen for the detection of syphilitic antibody. In contrast to the crude tissue extract antigens, the pure cardiolipin-cholesterol-lecithin antigens could be standardized chemically as well as serologically, thus ensuring greater reproducibility of test results both within and between laboratories.[11]

Non-treponemal tests can be used as qualitative tests for initial screening or as quantitative tests to follow treatment. All four tests are based on an antigen composed of alcoholic solution containing measured amount of cardiolipin, cholesterol and sufficient purified lecithin to produce standard reactivity. The nontreponemal (reagin) tests measure IgM and IgG antibodies to lipoidal material released from damaged host cell as well as to lipoprotein like material and possibly to cardiolipin released from treponemes. The antilipoidal antibodies are produced not only as a consequence of syphilis and other treponemal diseases but may also be produced in response to non treponemal disease of an acute and chronic nature in which tissue damage occurs. Without some other evidence for the diagnosis of syphilis, a reactive nontreponemal test does not confirm *T. pallidum* infection. Serum is the specimen of choice for both treponemal and non treponemal tests. However plasma samples may also be used in the RPR card test and TRUST. Plasma cannot be used in the VDRL test since the samples must be heated before testing and it cannot be used in the treponemal test for syphilis. The VDRL is the only test that can be used for testing CSF. The CSF is not heated before the test is performed.[3]

False Positive Reaction

Antibodies against cardiolipin may also occur in the absence of treponemal infection and give what has been referred to as biological false positive(BFP) reactions. BFP reactions are defined as those present in patients whose serum gives positive cardiolipin antigen test but negative specific treponemal antigen test in the absence of past or present treponemal infection. False positive reaction can be divided into two groups: those that are acute false positive reactions of less than 6 month in duration and those that are chronic false positive reactions that persist for more than 6 month. Acute false positive nontreponemal reactions have been associated with hepatitis, infectious mononucleosis, viral pneumonia, chicken pox, measles, other viral infections, malaria, pregnancy and laboratory or technical error. Chronic false positive reactions have been associated with connective tissue diseases such as SLE or diseases associated with immunoglobulin abnormalities which are more common in women. Other conditions associated with chronic false positive reactions are narcotic addiction, aging, leprosy and malignancy.[5]

Treponemal Test

In 1949, Nelson and Mayer developed the first treponemal antibody test, the *T. pallidum* immobilization (TPI) test.[12] The TPI test uses *T. pallidum* (Nichol's strain) grown in rabbit testes as the antigen and is based on the ability of patient's antibody and complement to immobilize living treponemes, as observed by dark-field microscopy. The TPI test was rapidly accepted as a specific test for syphilis. However, because the TPI test was complicated, technically difficult, time-consuming and expensive to perform, a simpler procedure was sought. In addition, studies[13] in the 1970's found that the TPI test was less sensitive and specific than the treponemal test that appeared in the 1960s.

In 1957, a major breakthrough in treponemal antigen tests occurred with the development of the fluorescent treponemal antibody (FTA) test.[14] The original FTA procedure used a 1:5 dilution of the patient's serum in saline solution, reacting with a suspension of killed treponemes. A flourescein-labeled anti-human immunoglobulin was used as the conjugate, and the test was read under a microscope with a UV light source. When an improved flourescein compound, flourescein isothiocynate (FITC) was used to prepare the labeled anti-human globulin conjugate, nonspecific reactions were encountered in approximately 25% of normal serum specimens. To eliminate these false-positive, reactions, the test was modified by diluting the patients serum 1:200, the FTA-200.[15] However, the FTA-200 test, although highly specific, was not very sensitive. The nonspecific reactions of the original FTA test were found to arise because of shared antigens common to *T. pallidum* and the nonpathogenic treponemes that occur as part of the normal bacterial flora of humans.[16] Deacon and Hunter, by preparing a sonicate from cultures of the Reiter's spirochaete, removed the common antigens by absorption: their work led to the development of the more specific and sensitive FTA absorption (FTA-ABS) test.[17] The FTA-ABS and its counterpart, the FTA-ABS double-staining test, used with incident light microscopes, remain the standard treponemal tests for syphilis today.

In 1965, Rathlev[18] reported the first reliable application of haemagglutination techniques to the serologic diagnosis of syphilis. The antigen used in her procedure was formalinized, tanned sheep erythrocytes sensitized with ultrasonicated material from *T. pallidum* (Nichol's strain). The presence of treponemal antibody in the patient's serum was detected by indirect agglutination of the sensitized erythrocytes and the subsequent formation of a mat of erythrocytes upon their settling.

Testing Strategy

An important principle of syphilis serology is the detection of treponemal antibody by a screening test, followed by confirmation of a reactive screening test result by additional testing. The confirmatory test, or tests, should have equivalent sensitivity and ideally greater specificity compared to the screening test and should be methodologically independent, where possible, so as to reduce the chance of coincident false-positive reactions. A quantitative non-treponemal test and/or detection of specific treponemal IgM may be useful for assessment of the stage of infection and to monitor the effect of therapy. Serology cannot distinguish between the different treponematoses (syphilis, yaws, pinta and bejel or non-venereal 'endemic syphilis').

The testing strategy employed varies; either a non-treponemal test alone, or a treponemal test alone, or both in combination may be used, depending on a number of factors including whether it is intended to detect all stages of syphilis or only infectious syphilis. In the United States, India and certain countries in Europe, e.g. France and Belgium, non-treponemal tests are used for screening.[19]

One advantage of this approach is that it does not detect most adequately treated cases, thus simplifying patient assessment. The disadvantages with this approach is screening undiluted specimens with a non-treponemal test alone can give rise to false-negative reactions in the presence of high titres of antibody, the prozone phenomenon. This phenomenon may occur in early infection and with concomitant HIV infection. In addition, non-treponemal tests lack sensitivity in late stage infection and screening with a non-treponemal test alone may also give rise to false-positive reactions in a variety of acute and chronic conditions in the absence of syphilis (biological false positive reactions). In some countries in Europe, eg. Germany and the Netherlands, the TPHA is used for screening.[19] This provides a good screen for all stages of syphilis beyond the early primary stage but, because more primary infections are detected by a combination of VDRL and TPHA tests, the use of the TPHA alone has found limited favour in diagnostic laboratories in UK, where screening with both VDRL and TPHA tests in combination has been common practice for many years.[20] The combination of VDRL and TPHA tests provides sensitive and specific screening for all stages of syphilis other than very early primary infection but it is more labour intensive than a single screening test, requires subjective interpretation and cannot be readily automated.[20] With these practical disadvantages, and with the recent commercial availability of EIA, the VDRL and TPHA combination for screening is increasingly being replaced in various diagnostic microbiology laboratories by the use of EIA tests detecting treponemal IgG, IgM or both. The advantages of the EIA format include the production of objective results, the ability to link EIA plate readers directly to laboratory computer systems, hence reducing the potential for errors transcribing results, and the facility for automation. These factors make EIA attractive for laboratories with large workloads.

The development of commercial EIA tests has occurred since the WHO recommended the use of a combination of a non-treponemal test and a treponemal test for screening and diagnostic purposes.[21] Although the treponemal IgG EIA is still regarded as an investigational test in the United States[3], there are published data showing both that screening with a treponemal IgG EIA gives comparable results to the VDRL and TPHA combination[22] and that it may be a useful method for detecting treponemal antibody in patients who are infected with HIV.[23]

Confirmatory tests

The FTA-abs is still generally regarded as the 'gold standard', but in fact it has a number of limitations. It is a subjective test and difficult to standardize. The TPHA is more sensitive, than FTA-abs except in the 3rd to 4th week of infection; and is also more specific.[5] In addition, false negative FTA-abs results have been described in HIV infection[24] and in association with autoimmune disorders. Thus the TPHA is the most appropriate test for confirming reactive EIA results at present; equally, if TPHA is used for screening, an EIA can be used as the confirmatory test.[20] Although immunoblotting has been suggested as a possible confirmatory test,[25] further evaluation is required in order to define its precise role.

Assessment of the Stage of Infection and Monitoring the Effect of Therapy

In treponemal infection, a quantitative non-treponemal test and/or a test for specific anti-treponemal IgM helps with the assessment of the stage of infection, and provides a baseline for monitoring the effect of therapy. In general, IgM becomes undetectable within 3 to 9 months after adequate treatment of early syphilis, although it may persist for 1 to 1.5 years after treatment of late disease. Detection of specific anti-treponemal IgM in patients without a history of recent treatment suggests active disease and the need for therapy. Quantitative non-treponemal tests such as the VDRL/RPR remain the method of choice for follow-up testing, the object being to demonstrate a decline in titre, depending on a range of factors including the initial titre, stage of infection when treated, treatment regimen and HIV status.[20]

To monitor the efficacy of treatment, quantitative nontreponemal test should be performed on the patient's serum samples, which are drawn at 3 months intervals for at least 1 year. Following adequate therapy for primary and secondary syphilis, there should be at least fourfold decline in titre by the third or fourth month and an eightfold decline in titre by the sixth to eight months. Patients treated in the latent or late stages, or who have had multiple episodes of syphilis, may show a more gradual decline in titre.[26] As far as can be determined, this persistent seropositivity does not signify treatment failure or reinfection, and these patients are likely to remain serofast even if they are retreated.

The failure of nontreponemal test titres to decline after treatment with standard therapy has been documented for HIV-seronegative persons treated during latent stage or late-stage syphilis and in persons treated for reinfection. Therefore, the failure of titres to decline with treatment for syphilis in HIV-infected person is probably related to the stage of syphilis rather than to HIV status.

Summary

1. Follow-up of seronegative patients at recent risk of acquiring a sexually transmitted infection is essential because of the seronegative window in early primary syphilis.
2. Screening with a non-treponemal test alone is not recommended because of the potential for false-negative results.
3. A treponemal EIA alone (IgG or IgG/IgM), or a combination of a non-treponemal test (VDRL/RPR) and a treponemal test (TPHA), is most appropriate for screening.
4. Specimens that are reactive on screening require confirmatory testing with a different treponemal test of equal sensitivity and, greater specificity.
5. Specimens giving discrepant treponemal test results on confirmatory testing need additional testing.
6. Following confirmation of a reactive specimen, a second specimen should be tested to confirm the results and the correct identification of the patient.
7. In treponemal infection, a quantitative non-treponemal test, and/or a test for specific treponemal IgM, should be performed as part of the assessment of the stage of infection and to monitor the efficacy of therapy.

Polymerase Chain Reaction

PCR based tests have been developed by several laboratories either as potential diagnostic tests or to identify *T. pallidum*-infected animals in experimental animal systems.[27,28] Most of the tests have been based on membrane lipoproteins, of which a large number have been cloned and sequenced. Two PCR-based techniques were described almost simultaneously in 1991.[27,28] Since sensitive and inexpensive serologic tests are available for most stages of syphilis in adults, the investigators in these two articles concentrated on problem areas in which definitive diagnosis is beyond the abilities of most clinical laboratories. The first of these was based on the amplification of a 658-bp segment of the gene for the 47-kDa surface antigen: this is a lipoprotein that is antigenically dominant in the human immune response to *T. pallidum*.[3]

Several studies have indicated that *T. pallidum* can persist for long periods in the central nervous system, even apparently in patients who have received what was considered adequate antibiotic treatment.[29] Thus, a method that could detect the presence of *T. pallidum* in small samples of CSF could prove extremely valuable, especially in determining whether treatment was sufficient in cases where neurosyphilis is suspected or known to have occurred. Noordhoek et al[28] used as their target the gene coding for a 39-kDa basic membrane protein.

PCR could be extremely valuable in diagnosing infection in congenital syphilis, in diagnosis neurosyphilis (the serologic test available presently is only 50% sensitive), in diagnosing early primary syphilis (the only tests available currently are microscopic) and finally in distinguishing new infections from old infections (presently only a rise in titre can be used).[3]

Laboratory Diagnosis of Different Stages of Syphilis

Early Syphilis

The finding of treponemes with characteristic appearance by dark field microscopic examination of fluid obtained from the surface of chancre is the most specific and sensitive method for verifying the diagnosis of primary syphilis. The dark field examination is actually the only test that specifically establishes the diagnosis of primary syphilis. Antibody to cardiolipin, as measured by the non treponemal test is present, often at a relatively low level in about 80% of patients at the time they come to medical attention for primary syphilis (Table 4). In early syphilis, non treponemal test reactivity reflects activity of disease. This reactivity is expected to disappear with treatment. The non treponemal test is generally requested even when the dark field examination is positive, in order to provide a baseline for follow-up after therapy.

Tests that measure antibody to surface proteins of *T. pallidum* by treponemal tests are positive in about 90% of patients at the time they seek medical attention for a chancre (Table 5). Thus a negative result does not

Table 4.   Sensitivity and Specificity of Nontreponemal Tests

TEST	% Sensitivity at given stage of infection				% Specificity
	Primary	Secondary	Latent	Late	(nonsyphilis)
VDRL	78(74-87)	100	95 (88-100)	71 (37-94)	98 (96-99)
RPR	86 (77-100)	100	98 (95-100)	73	98 (93-99)
USR	80 (72-88)	100	95 (88-100)		99
RST*	82 (77-86)	100	95 (88-100)		97
TRUST	85 (77-86)	100	98 (95-100)		99 (98-99)

*Reagin Screen Test

Table 5.   Sensitivity and Specificity of Treponemal Tests

TEST	% Sensitivity at given stage of infection				% Specificity
	Primary	Secondary	Latent	Late	(nonsyphilis)
FTA-ABS	84 (70-100)	100	100	96	97 (94-99)
MHA-TP	76 (69-90)	100	97 (97-100)	94	99 (98-100)
FTA-ABS Double Staining	80 (69-90)	100	100		99 (97-100)

exclude the diagnosis. Once *T. pallidum* infection has caused the treponemal test to be positive, these tests remain positive for life. Thus a positive result does not establish a diagnosis of primary syphilis in someone who has a lesion that might be syphilitic, since antibody may be present as a result of some earlier infection.[30] For these reasons, the search for treponemes by dark field examinations should be undertaken, even though it is time consuming and requires trained personnel.

Secondary Syphilis

Treponemes can be easily found by dark field examination of material obtained from moist wet lesions in secondary syphilis. This test is usually not done on dry skin lesions. Serological tests give far more distinctive results in secondary than in primary syphilis. Antibody to cardiolipin is always present, usually at a high dilution (VDRL more than 1:32). Rarely, a prozone phenomenon occurs, in which a blocking antibody obscures a positive reading in undiluted serum, but the positive reaction is readily apparent with dilutions. In doing the non-treponemal test, most laboratories do not perform serum dilutions if the undiluted serum gives a negative result unless the physicians specifically indicates that the diagnosis of syphilis is suspected clinically; therefore in ordering a non treponemal test in a case of suspected secondary syphilis, a request for dilutions should be specifically made. In secondary syphilis, the treponemal tests are always positive.[31]

Latent Syphilis

At the present time, patients are diagnosed as having latent syphilis if they have a reactive non treponemal test in the absence of any apparent signs of the disease and the treponemal test is positive. If a patient admits to having had a chancre or a skin rash for which he did not seek treatment and he now has a reactive non treponemal with a positive treponemal test, the diagnosis of latent syphilis is apparent. However this would not always be the case. More often the serological findings are present without any useful information on the medical history. Such patients are regarded as if they have latent syphilis from the public health point of view. It is worth mentioning however, that such a diagnosis is difficult. On the one hand, these serological abnormalities may have persisted after adequate treatment (serofast state) so that it may be difficult, to be certain whether the patient has partially treated syphilis, latent syphilis, or an adequately treated syphilis in which the serological abnormalities persist. On the other hand, the positive serological test may indicate unrecognized active disease after unrecognized chancre or lesion has healed and manifest late syphilis is not present. In this scenario, the patient may have asymptomatic neuro-syphilis which can only be excluded by documenting a normal cerebrospinal fluid. This leads to recommendations that a spinal tap be done and the CSF be negative in order to establish the diagnosis of latency.[31]

Syphilis and HIV infection

The problems in the diagnosis of syphilis with HIV are (i) confusing clinical signs and symptoms[32]; (ii) lack of serologic response in a patient with a clinically confirmed case of active syphilis[33]; (iii) failure of nontreponemal test titres to decline after treatment with standard regimens; (iv) unusually high titres in nontreponemal test[34], perhaps as the result of B-cell activation; (v) rapid progression to late stages of syphilis and neurologic involvement even after treatment of primary or secondary syphilis[34]; and (vi) the disappearance of treponemal test reactivity over time.

Aberrant results in the serological tests for syphilis appear to be related to abnormally low absolute CD4 cell counts and are relatively rare.[35] The diagnosis of syphilis in these cases was supported either by an observation of *T. pallidum* in material from typical lesions or by the appearance of serologic reactivity after treatment. The delay in development of a response to syphilis theoretically should be expected in persons with abnormal lymphocyte counts; however, the frequency of this occurrence is unknown.

Late Syphilis

The serum non treponemal test is positive in most cases of acute syphilitic meningitis. The CSF changes include elevated pressure, mononuclear pleocytosis of 10 to 200 cells per cubic millimeter, elevated protein concentration (200 mg/dl), elevated globulin level and a modest reduction in glucose in 45 percent of cases. The VDRL test on CSF is reactive in most, but not all cases. It has been noted that patients who present with isolated involvement of the eighth cranial nerve are likely to have a normal CSF with a nonreactive VDRL test. Serum non treponemal test is positive in meningovascular syphilis. The CSF changes are those usually seen in neurosyphilis, in keeping with a smouldering low grade meningitis owing largely to vascular occlusive disease. The CSF VDRL test is positive in most, but not all cases. Nontreponemal serological tests of blood and CSF are nearly uniformly positive in cases of paresis. Other CSF findings are typical of those in neurosyphilis. The CSF may be normal in a patient, whose neurosyphilis has been arrested by treatment, leaving persistent mental changes. A positive serum VDRL often is a clue to presence of neurosyphilis. Specific anti treponemal antibody tests of CSF, such as FTA-ABS or MHA-TP have been studied as a tool to diagnose neurosyphilis in the occasional case in which the CSF VDRL is non reactive.[36] These test may be reactive as a result of diffusion of serum immunoglobulin into the CSF or as a result of contamination of CSF by small amount of blood rather than because of local antibody synthesis in the CNS. Hence a careful collection of CSF sample, free of contamination by blood is essential.[37] Another approach is to examine intrathecal antibody synthesis using the CSF–IgG index,[37] obtained by dividing the CSF to serum IgG ratio by the CSF to serum albumin ratio. A result of more than 0.7 is indicative of IgG synthesis within the CNS, but this finding is consistent with a variety of infectious or inflammatory processes.[38] Specificity is provided by demonstrating that the antibody is produced intrathecally, as determined by an intrathecal *T. pallidum* antibody index >100,[39] defined as

$$\text{CSF-TPHA titre} = \frac{\text{CSF albumin (mg/dl)} \times 10^3}{\text{serum albumin (mg/dl)}}$$

Better evidence for intrachecal antitreponemal antibody synthesis may be obtained if the serum: CSF ratio of TPHA is at least four times lower than the corresponding ratio for some other unrelated but ubiquitous antibody, such as adenovirus haemagglutination antibody.[40]

The potential usefulness of the MHA-TP index has been confirmed , but tests for antitreponemal IgM antibodies in CSF are rarely performed. There is much research going on for use of polymerase chain reaction (PCR) test for *T. pallidum* as a means of diagnosing neurosyphilis, but the sensitivity and specificity are still under investigation.[41]

Neurosyphilis in HIV Infected Persons

Neurosyphilis can usually develop rapildly when there is concomitant infection with HIV.[42] CSF examination is necessary when there is evidence of clinical relapse or a four fold rise is noted in the titre of follow up serological test on serum. It is generally agreed that the CSF should be examined in all patients with clinical neurosyphilis and in all syphilitic infections of more than 2 years, in order to exclude asymptomatic neurosyphilis. It is unnecessary to perform routine tests for syphilis on the CSF of patients with central nervous system symptoms in whom there is no suspicion of syphilis. A negative *T. pallidum* antigen such as the TPHA, on serum will virtually exclude active neurosyphilis and is a better screen for the detection of all forms of late syphilis than examination of the CSF. The latter should be reserved for cases selected on clinical grounds and backed by positive TPHA test on serum. A negative TPHA test on CSF excludes neurosyphilis. A negative VDRL test on CSF does not exclude neurosyphilis as a third to half of patients with clinically active neurosyphilis will give a negative VDRL result on the CSF.

Cardiovascular Syphilis

Screening serological tests are helpful because they are usually reactive, especially where there is extensive involvement of soft tissue. The serological test result may be of high titre. The prozone phenomenon has been a problem in some case, with serological tests shown to be positive upon retesting in appropriate dilutions of serum. On the other hand a negative reaction may accompany a localized lesion, as of bone.

References

1. Fieldsteel, AH, Cox DL, Moeckli. RA. Cultivation of virulent Treponema pallidum in tissue culture. Infect Immunol 1981; 32: 908-915.
2. Romanowski B, Forsey E, Prasad E, Lukehart S, Tam M, Hook EW. Detection of *Treponema pallidum* by a fluorescent monoclonal antibody test. Sex Transm Dis 1987; 22: 156-159.
3. Larsen SA, Steiner BM, Rudodph AH. Laboratory diagnosis and interpretation of tests for syphilis. Clin Microbiol Rev 1995; 8: 1-21.
4. Grimprel E, Sanchez PJ, Wendel GD, et al. Use of polymerase chain reaction and rabbit infectivity testing to detect *Treponema pallidum* in amniotic fluid. J Clin Microbiol 1991; 29: 1711-1718.
5. Luger AFH. Serological diagnosis of syphilis: Current

methods. In:Young H, McMillan A, eds. Immunological diagnosis of sexually transmitted diseases. New York: Marcel Decker; 1988: p. 249-274 .

6. Baker-Zander SA, Hook EW, Bonin P, Handsfield HH, Lukehart SA. Antigens of *Treponema pallidum* recognized by IgG and IgM antibodies during syphilis in humans. J Infect Dis 1985; 151: 264–272

7. Rufli T. Syphilis and HIV infection. Dermatologica 1989; 179: 113-117.

8. Eagle H. The laboratory diagnosis of syphilis, St. Louis. The C.V. Mosby Co. 1937: 21-28.

9. Kahn. RL. A simple quantitative precipitation reaction for syphilis. Arch Dermatol Syphilol 1922; 5: 570-578, 734-743; 6: 332-341.

10. Pangborn MC. A new serologically active phospholipid from beef heart. Proc Soc Exp Biol Med 1941; 48: 484-486.

11. Rudolph A H, Larsen SA. Laboratory diagnosis of syphilis, In: Demis DJ ed. Clinical Dermatology. Lippincott Co: Philadephia. 1993: 1-16.

12. Nelson RA Jr, Mayer MM. Immobilization of Treponema pallidum in vitro by antibody produced in syphilitic infection. J Exp Med 1949; 89: 369-393.

13. Rein MF, Banks GW Logan LC, et al. Failure of the *Treponema pallidum* immobilization test to provide additional diagnostic information about contemporary problem sera. Sex Transm Dis 1980; 7: 191-105.

14. Deacon WE, Falcone VH, Harris A. A fluorescent test for treponemal antibodies. Proc Soc Exp Biol Med Biol Med 1957; 96: 477-480.

15. Deacon WE, Freeman EM, Harris A. Fluorescent treponemal antibody test. Modification based on quantitation (FTA-200). Proc Soc Ex Biol Med 1960; 103: 827-829.

16. Deacon WE, Hunter EF. Treponemal antigens as related to identification and syphilis serology. Proc Soc Exp Biol Med 1962 ; 110: 352-356.

17. Hunter EF, Deacon WE, Meyer PE. An improved FTA test for syphilis: the absorption procedure(FTA-ABS). Public Health Rep 1964; 79: 410-412.

18. Rathlev V. Haemagglutination tests utilizing antigens from pathogenic and apathogenic *Treponema pallidum*. WHO/VDT Res 1965; 77: 65.

19. Young H. Syphilis: new diagnostic directions. Int J STD AIDS 1992; 3: 391-413.

20. Young H. Syphilis serology. Dermatol Clin 1998; 16: 691-698

21. World Health Organization. Treponemal infections. Technical reports series 674. Geneva: World Health Organization, 1982.

22. Young H, Moyes A, McMillan A, Patterson J. Enzyme immunoassay for anti-treponemal IgG: screening or confirmatory test? J Clin Pathol 1992; 45: 37-41

23. Young H, Moyes A, Ross JCD. Markers of past syphilis in HIV infection comparing with captia Syphilis G anti-treponemal IgG enzyme immunoassay with other treponemal antigen tests. Int J STD AIDS 1995; 6: 101-104.

24. Erbelding EJ, Vlahov D, Nelson TC, et al. Syphilis serology in human immunodeficiency virus infection: evidence for false-negative fluorescent treponemal testing. J Infect Dis 1997; 176: 1397-1400.

25. Byrne RE, Laska S, Bell M, Larson D, Phillips J, Todd J. Evaluation of a *Treponema pallidum* western immunoblot assay as a confirmatory test for syphilis. J Clin Microbiol 1992; 30: 115-122.

26. Fiumara NJ. Reinfection primary, secondary and late latent syphilis. The serologic response after treatment. Sex Transm Dis 1980; 7: 111-115.

27. Grimprel E, Sanchez PJ, Wendel GD, et al. Use of polymerase chain reaction and rabbit infectivity testing to detect *Treponema pallidum* in amniotic fluid. J Clin Microbiol 1991; 28: 1711-1718.

28. Noordhoek, GT, Wolters EC,. De Jonge MEJ, van Embden JDA. Detection by polymerase chain reaction of Treponema pallidum DNA in cerebrospinal fluid from neurosyphilis patients before and after antibiotic treatment. J Clin Microbiol 1991; 29: 197-198.

29. Hay PE, Clarke JR, Scrugnell RA, Taylor-Robinson D, Goldmeier D. Use of the polymerase chain reaction to detect DNA sequences specific to pathogenic treponemes in cerebrospinal fluid. FEMS Microbiol Lett 1990; 56: 233-238.

30. Musher DM. Early syphilis. In: Holmes KK, Sparling PF, Mardh P, et al Eds Sexually Transmitted Diseases, 3rd ed., New York, McGraw-Hill, 1999: 479-485.

31. Swartz MN, Healy BP, Musher DM, Late Syphilis. In: Holmes KK, Sparling PF, Mardh P et al, eds. Sexually Transmitted Diseases, 3rd ed, New York, McGraw-Hill 1999: 487-509.

32. Dawson SB, Evans A, Lawrence AG. Benign tertiary syphilis and HIV infection. AIDS 1988; 2: 315-316.

33. Gregory N, Sanchez M, Buchness MR.. The spectrum of syphilis in patients with human immunodeficiency virus infection. J Am Acad Dermatol 1990; 22: 1061-1067.

34. Musher DM. Syphilis, neurosyphilis, penicillin and AIDS. J Infect Dis 1991; 163: 1201-1206.

35. Hicks CD, Benson PM, Lupton GP, Tramont EC. Seronegative secondary syphilis in a patient infected with the human immunodeficiency virus (HIV) Kaposi sarcoma. Ann Intern Med 1987; 107: 492-495.

36. Jaffe HW, Larsen SA, Peters M, Jove DF, Lopez B, Schroeter AL. Tests for treponemal antibody in CSF. Arch Intern Med 1978; 138: 252-255.

37. Madiedo G, Ho KC, Walsh P. False positive VDRL and FTA in cerebrospinal fluid. JAMA 1980; 244: 688-691.

38. Pedersen NS, Kam-Hansen S, Link H, Mavra M. Specificity of immunoglobulins synthesized within the central nervous system in neurosyphilis. Acta Pathol Microbiol Immunol 1982; 90: 97-104.

39. Prange HW, Moskophidis M, Schipper HI, Muller F. Relationship between neurological features and intrathecal synthesis of IgG antibodies to T*reponema pallidum* in untreated and treated human neurosyphilis. J Neurol 1983; 230: 241-252.

40. Gschnait F, Schmidt BL, Luger A. Cerebrospinal fluid immunoglobulins in neurosyphilis. Br J Vener Dis 1981; 57: 238-240.

41. Tomberlin MG, Holton PD, Owens JL, Lorsen RA. Evaluation of neurosyphilis in human immunodeficiency virus-infected individuals. Clin Inf Dis 1994; 18:288-292.

42. World Health Organization 1982 Treponemal infections. Technical Report Series no 674. WHO, Geneva.

Chapter 16

Treatment of Syphilis

G Sethuraman, S Handa

Historical Perspectives[1]

Syphilis ravaged the mankind for almost 350 years after it spread in the Europe in 16th century. The prevalence rates in early twentieth century were 5-10% at autopsy and in poor socioeconomic status it reached up to 25%. It was referred to as Great Pox compared to Small Pox because of its devastating nature. The all above remind us of current AIDS scenario. The development and use of penicillin was one of the landmark breakthrough that made the treatment of Great Pox possible with one magic injection.

Until the introduction of penicillin in the year 1943, mercury and arsenic were used for the treatment of syphilis. In the beginning of twentieth century mercury was the only drug available for the treatment of syphilis. But its highly toxic nature limited its therapeutic use.

Later different forms of arsenic, Ehrlich's solution, and intravenous neoarsphenamine along with bismuth for a variable period of 9-15 months depending upon the stage of the disease, was used. Subsequently sulpharsphenamine a trivalent arsenical compound, oxophenarsine or arsphenoxide and tryparsamide have been used. Because of the serious side effects and longer duration of treatment, now a days these drugs are no longer recommended.

Bismuth has been used as a therepeutic test in patients with lesions suggestive of late syphilis and also to prevent Jarisch-Herxheimer reaction. Potassium iodide was used for many years as an adjuvant therapy especially in the gummatous lesions and also as a therepeutic test along with bismuth.

Fever, induced by mechanical means or by inoculation of infective agents such as malaria had been used in the treatment of syphilis either alone or as an adjuvant.

Penicillin was first used in the treatment of syphilis in experimental animals and in man by Mahoney, Arnold and Harris in 1943. The impure amorphous penicillin consisted of a mixture of four different penicillins called G, F, X, and K, was given at a dose of 2.4 million units every 3 hours for period of seven and half days (60 injection). Later in 1946, this treatment was proved to be ineffective due to the fact that the preparation consisted of a greater portion of penicillin K which was not effective in syphilis. It was also found that penicillin G was the most effective component against treponemes and was used at a dose of 2.4 or 4.8 million units given every two or four hours a day and night for a period of a week or more. Because of the too many injections necessitating admission and other discomfort, attempts were made to prepare long acting repository penicillins. One such preparation was calcium penicillin in arachis oil containing 4.8% of beeswax and was used at a dose of 2 ml (each ml consisted of 3,00,000 units) intramuscularly daily for a period of 8 days. A single daily injection maintained an effective level for about 24 hours. But the drug was difficult to administer and had severe reactions. The next repository preparation was the procaine penicillin, a combination of procaine and penicillin. It was used as a watery suspension in daily doses of 6,00,000 units for a period of 8-10 days. Further modification in the preparation was the suspension of procaine penicillin in arachis oil along with 2% water repellent aluminium monostearate (PAM). The advantage of this preparation was that the dose of 3,00,000 to 6,00,000 units maintained the therapeutic level of penicillin for 72 hours, which allows the patients to take the injection on alternate days.

Later, modifications and developments came with the discovery of benzathine penicillin G (dibenzyl ethylene diamine dipenicillin G), the only antibiotic formulation, which provides serum drug concentration for several weeks following a single IM injection.[2]

Treatment Guidelines

Parenteral penicillin is the treatment of choice for the treatment of all stages of syphilis. The preparations used are benzathine, aqueous procaine and aqueous crystalline penicillin.[3] Oral penicillin can also be used in the treatment but is not recommended because of reduced efficiency and lack of compliance.[1]

Mechanism of Action[1]

Penicillin at the concentration of 0.0025 units/ml kills 50% *T. pallidum* within 16 hours. The recommended concentration of penicillin in syphilis is 0.03 units/ml for a period of 7 to 10 days in early syphilis and longer time in late syphilis. Penicillin binds irreversibly to the transpeptidase enzymes of the treponemes, which are required for the biosynthesis of outer envelopes and thereby prevents closing of the gaps in the envelope lattice. This results in high osmotic pressure within the protoplasmic cylinder causing bulging of the inner membrane and bursting of the treponemes.

Treatment of Primary, Secondary and Early Latent Syphilis[3]

Recommended Regimen

- Benzathine penicillin G 2.4 million units intramuscular (IM) single dose (1.2 million units deep IM in each buttock).
- For children: Benzathine penicillin G 50,000 units/kg IM up to the adult dose of 2.4 million units in a single dose.

The treatment should be given after testing intradermal sensitivity for penicillin.

All the patients who have syphilis should be tested for HIV infection. If it is negative a repeat test should be done after 3 months especially in areas where the HIV prevalence is high. Patients with early syphilis who have features suggestive of meningitis or uveitis should be evaluated for neurosyphilis.

WHO[4] and NACO[5] recommend the following alternative regimen:

Procaine benzyl penicillin G 1.2 million IU daily

IM for 10 days. (3 vials, each having combination of 1 lakh units of benzyl penicillin G sodium and 3 lakhs units of procaine benzyl penicillin G.

Alternative Regimen for Penicillin Allergic Patients

- Doxycycline 100 mg bid orally for 2 weeks or
- Tetracycline 500 mg qid orally for 2 weeks or
- Erythromycin 500 mg qid orally for 2 weeks

The efficiency of these regimens is not well documented. Hence frequent follow up of the patients receiving these therapies is essential. The effectiveness of these therapies in HIV infected patients has not been studied. Although limited clinical studies suggest that azithromycin and ceftriaxone are effective in the treatment of syphilis, their use in the clinical practice is yet to established.[6,7]

Follow Up

Patients should be examined clinically and serologically at 6 and 12 months. There should be a four fold decrease in the non-treponemal (VDRL) titre within 6 months. Patients who have persistent symptoms or recurrence, or who have four fold increase in the VDRL titre or failure of titre to decline four fold within 6 months should be reevaluated for reinfection, treatment failure, HIV infection, or unrecognized CNS infection. All such patients should undergo a thorough neurological evaluation including CSF analysis and HIV testing. When they are retreated they should preferably be given 3 weekly doses of benzathine penicillin G 2.4 million units, unless CSF examination indicates that neurosyphilis is present.

Treatment of Late Latent Syphilis

All the patients who have latent syphilis should be evaluated for tertiary syphilis. CSF analysis is clearly indicated if any one of the following criteria is present.

- CNS or eye changes
- Evidence of active tertiary syphilis
- HIV infection
- Treatment failure
- Non treponemal titre $\geq$ 1:32

If the CSF analysis shows features of neurosyphilis then the patient should be treated for the same.

Late latent syphilis or latent syphilis of unknown duration should be treated with 3 weekly doses of benzathine penicillin G 2.4 million units IM.

Doses in Children

Three weekly injection of benzathine penicillin G at a dose of 50,000 units/kg up to the adult dose of 2.4 million units IM.

Alternate Regimen

Procaine benzylpenicillin G 1.2 million units IM daily for 20 days.

Follow Up

Quantitiative non treponemal serologic test (VDRL) should be repeated at 6, 12 and 24 months. After treatment the patient should be reevaluated for neurosyphilis if any of the following criteria is present.

- Titre increase fourfold
- An initially high titre (≥ 1:32) fails to decline at least fourfold within 12-24 months of therapy
- If the patient develops signs and symptoms of tertiary syphilis.

Alternative Regimen for Penicillin Allergic Patients

- Doxycycline 100 mg orally bid for 30 days or
- Tetracycline 500 mg orally qid for 30 days or
- Erythromycin 500 mg orally qid for 30 days.

Treament of Tertiary Syphilis (Gumma and Cardiovascular Syphilis)

Three weekly doses of benzathine penicillin G 2.4 million units IM.

Treatment of Neurosyphilis

Patients with neurosyphilis, or syphilitic eye disease in the form of neuroretinitis, optic neuritis, uveitis or any other cranial nerve palsies should have CSF examination and be treated with aqueous crystalline penicillin G 18-24 millions units per day administered as 3-4 million units IV every 4 hours or continuous infusion for 10-14 days.

Alternative Regimen

Procaine penicillin G 2.4 million units IM daily for 14 days along with probenecid 500 mg orally qid for 14 days.

Benzathine penicillin G has no role in the treatment of neurosyphilis as it does not cross the blood barrier in sufficient quantity.

Follow Up

CSF should be re-examined every 6 months until it becomes normal. CSF cell count should decrease by 6 months and CSF VDRL and protein levels by 2 years. If not, patient should be retreated.

Management of Sex Partners

The sex partners should be evaluated clinically and serologically and treated according to the following recommendations.

- Persons who were exposed within the 90 days preceding the diagnosis of primary, secondary or early latent syphilis in a sex partner might be infected even if seronegative; therefore such persons should be treated presumptively.
- Persons who were exposed >90 days before the diagnosis of primary, secondary, or early latent syphilis in a sex partner should be treated presumptively if serologic test results are not available immediately and the opportunity for follow up is uncertain.
- For purposes of partner notification and presumptive treatment of exposed sex partners, patients with syphilis of unknown duration who have high nontreponemal serologic test titres (i.e., > 1:32) can be assumed to have early syphilis.

However, serologic titres should not be used to differentiate early from late latent syphilis for the purpose of determining treatment

- Long term sex partners of patients who have latent syphilis should be evaluated clinically and serologically for syphilis and treated on the basis of the evaluation findings.

Treatment of Syphilis Among HIV Infected Patients[3]

Primary, secondary, early latent syphilis
Injection benzathine penicillin G 2.4, million units single dose IM. Some authors recommend 3 weekly doses.

Other Treatment Consideration

HIV infected persons with early syphilis are at increased risk of developing neurological complication. Hence some specialists recommend CSF examination before treatment and is treated accordingly.

Follow Up

Clinical and serological follow up are done at 3, 6, 9, 12 and 24 months. CSF examination and retreatment with 3 weekly doses of benzathine penicillin G is recommended in patients whose non-treponemal titres do not fall four fold within 6-12 months of therapy.

Late Latent Syphilis

Patients with late latent syphilis or syphilis of unknown duration should undergo CSF examination. If it is normal then 3 weekly doses of benzathine penicillin G 2.4 million units is given. If there are CSF abnormalities then they are treated as neurosyphilis.

Follow Up

Clinical and serological examination are repeated at 6, 12, 18 and 24 months after therapy. During the follow up, if clinical symptoms develop or non-treponemal titres rise fourfold, a repeat CSF examination is performed. If in 12-24 months the non-treponemal titres do not decline four fold, CSF examination is repeated and treated accordingly.

Treatment of Neurosyphilis[8]

Treatment of choice for neurosyphilis in HIV infected patients is intravenous administration of aqueous crystalline penicillin G at a dose of 18-24 million units daily for 14 days. (Given as in non HIV infected patients). If the intravenous injections can not be given then an alternative regimen of procaine penicillin G is given at a dose of 2.4 million units IM daily for 14 days along with probenecid 500 mg orally qid for 14 days. But as far as possible intravenous regimen is preferred to the IM penicillin. Some specialists recommended injection benzathine penicillin 2.4 million units IM to ensure prolonged antispirochetal activity.

Penicillin allergic patients should preferably be desensitized and given penicillin only.

Follow Up

Patients after treatment for neurosyphilis require a high index of suspicion for relapse. CSF examination should be done at 6 months interval until CSF is normal and reassessment of CSF should be undertaken when neurosyphilis is suspected.

Treatment of Syphilis During Pregnancy

Appropriate penicillin regimen should be given during pregnancy depending upon the stage. Pregnant women who are allergic to penicillin should be desensitized and treated with penicillin. No alternatives to penicillin have been proved effective for the treatment of syphilis during pregnancy. However, WHO[4] and NACO[5] recommend erythromycin as an alternative regimen in pregnant mother who are allergic to penicillin as desensitization is a very cumbersome procedure and is not feasible in most of the primary health care settings. Patients receiving erythromycin regimen should be monitored frequently and closely. Azithromycin and ceftriaxone are other potential options for penicillin allergic pregnant women, but insufficient data on efficacy limit their use.[9]

The treatment of congenital syphilis is discussed in a separate chapter.

Penicillin Allergy

Allergic reactions to penicillin may occur in 10% of patients receiving therapy. Three types of reactions can occur:

1. Penicillin Reaction

It can be either toxic or allergic.

Toxic reaction is dose related, occurring in penicillin overdose or patients with renal impairment.

Allergic reaction is immune mediated and occurs in 10% of the patients. There are divided into 4 types.

Type I	: IgE mediated - urticaria, angiodema, anaphylaxis
Type II	: Characterized by haemolytic anaemia and leucopenia
Type III	: Serum sickness
Type IV	: Delayed type reaction manifesting as maculopapular rash, toxic epidermal necrolysis, etc.

2. Procaine Reaction

Acute psychotic episode, severe anxiety, agitation, vertigo, seizures, visual and auditory hallucinations. It is thought to be due to brain microembolism secondary to inadvertent injection of crystals of procaine penicillin intravenously.

3. Jarisch-Herxheimer Reaction[1,10]

Jarisch in 1895 first described this reaction in syphilitic patients and subsequently Herxheimer in 1902 observed similar features. Since then it is known as Jarisch-Herxheimer (JH) reaction. It is also observed in other bacterial infections. The reaction occurs as "all or none phenomenon" occurring with full force if it occurs at all. Hence starting treatment with low dose of penicillin does not give any protection. It occurs most frequently (50%) with greater severity in early syphilis more so with secondary syphilis. The patients will manifest symptoms 2 to 12 hours after injection but within the first 24 hours after giving penicillin. The features in early syphilis are more like "flu like" syndrome with fever, headache, malaise, flushing and sweating, lasting for about 24 hours. The symptoms are often accompanied by local tissue reactions with temporary aggravation or flaring of primary and secondary lesions. The existing chancre may become swollen and oedematous or the patient may develop transient secondary rash. In pregnancy with early syphilis the reactions may precipitate early labour and foetal distress.

In late syphilis, the reactions are milder and occur in no more than 25% of the patients except in general paralysis of insane in which it can occur in over 50% patients. Rarely serious side effects may occur in the form of oedema of the glottis in gummatous lesions, coronary artery occlusion, cerebral thrombosis and rupture of the aneurysmal sac in cardiovascular syphilis, intensification of psychosis, epilepsy and severe attacks of lightning pain in neurosyphilis.

The exact pathogenesis of JH reaction is not known. But it has been attributed to the sudden destruction of the treponemes with the subsequent release of large amounts of antigens. The reactions are associated with an increase in circulating levels of TNF $\propto$ and interleukins.[6,8]

Treatment is supportive with fluids and NSAID. Prevention: Prednisolone at a dose of 30-40 mg given 2 days prior to the injection and continued 2-3 days afterwards, may prove to be beneficial.

Treatment of Penicillin Allergic Reactions[1]

Acute reactions: The treatment room should be well equipped with all the resuscitation measures. The patient should be given Inj. adrenaline 0.6 ml of 1:1000 solution IM along with Inj. aminophylline 250 mg in 10 ml of sterile distilled water to relieve the bronchospasm. After giving adrenaline patient may be given Inj. hydrocortisone at a dose of 250 mg followed by 1000 mg during the succeeding 24 hours.

Delayed reactions are treated with antihistamine and or steroids.

Penicillin Desensitization

Most of the time the allergic reactions occur with parenteral administration. Reactions following oral intake are rare. Re-administration of penicillin in patients who are allergic can be fatal. But in cases of syphilis in HIV infected patients, neurosyphilis and pregnancy, penicillin is the only choice even when they are allergic. Hence desensitization should be done in all such patients before administering the drug.[3]

Penicillins are low molecular weight compounds that covalenently bind to tissue carrier proteins and form drug-protein complex or haptens to become immunogenic. Ninety five percent of tissue bound penicillin is hapteneted as benzyl penicilloyl and are termed as major antigenic determinant. The remaining 5% of the molecules are termed as minor antigenic determinant which are benzylpenicillin, benzyl-penicilloate and benzylpenilloate and these are not immunologically cross reactive.

Steps of Desensitization

Step 1. Identification of Allergy Risk Patients

Most of the time, patients who experienced an allergic reaction to penicillin stop expressing penicillin specific immunoglobulin E with passage of time. It is only 10% patients who remain allergic to penicillin and are skin test positive. The first step in penicillin desensitization is to identify these high risk group. One should ask for the detailed history regarding previous penicillin hypersensitivity and also other relevant history like personal or family of atopy or allergic diathesis. A simple objective method of eliciting previous penicillin sensitization is to apply drops of procaine penicillin 300,000 units /ml to a skin scratch and to the conjunctiva. Itching, redness, oedema of the eyes within 15 minutes probably indicates sensitization. But not all patients who are allergic give a positive result. Ideally one should do skin testing with the major and minor antigenic determinants. Only the major antigenic determinant is commercially available as benzyl penicilloyl polylysine conjugate (pre-pen). For minor determinant freshly prepared penicillin G can be used as an adequate sources. Testing with only the major determinant and penicillin G identifies approximately 90-97% of the currently allergic patients. Hence extreme caution should be exercised in remaining 3-10% of patients.

Step 2. Penicillin Skin Testing

Patient should be tested in the tertiary care centre where intensive care setting is available in which treatment for anaphylaxis is undertaken. Ideally the patients should not have taken antihistamines in the recent past

The major and minor antigenic compounds of penicillin are given in Table 1.

Dilute the antigens to 100 fold for preliminary testing

Table 1.   Skin Test Reagents for Identifying Persons at Risk for Adverse Reactions to Pencillin

Major Determinant
- Benzylpenicilloyl poly-L-lysine (Pre-Pen 6x 10^{-5}M).

Minor Determinant Precursors
- Benzylpenicillin G (10^{-2} M, 3.3 mg/mL, 6,000 units/mL),
- Benzylpenicilloate (10^{-2} M, 3.3 mg/mL),
- Benzylpenilloate (or penicilloyl porpylamine) (10^{-2} M, 3.3 mg/ mL).

Positive Control
- Commercial histamine for epicutaneous skin testing (1 mg/mL).

Negative Control
- Diluent used to dissolve other reagents, usually phenol saline.

Adapted from CDC Treatment of sexually transmitted diseases 2002.

if the patient has had a life threatening reaction to penicillin or 10 fold if the patient has had another type of immediate, generalized reaction to penicillin within the preceding year.

Epicutaneous (prick) Test

Drops of reagents for skin testing are placed on the volar surface of the forearm, and the underlying epidermis is pierced with a 26 gauze needle without drawing blood. Reading is taken after 15 minutes. The test is considered positive if the diameter of the wheal is 4 mm larger than that of negative control, otherwise the test is negative. The histamine control should be positive to ensure that results are not falsely negative because of the effect of antihistamines.

Intradermal Test

If the prick test is negative then intradermal test is done. 0.02 ml antigenic solution is injected intradermally with a 26 or 27 G needle on a syringe, on the volar surface of the forearm. Reading is taken after 15 minutes. The test is said to be positive if the average wheal diameter is $\geq$ 2 mm larger than the initial wheal size and also is $\geq$ 2 mm larger than the negative control. Otherwise the test is negative.

Step 3. Desensitization

Skin test positive patients should be desensitized and it should be done orally because it is safer than parenteral. The schedule begins by administering extremely small doses of penicillin with a doubling of dose every 15 minutes. Full dose therapy should be completed and the overall time to complete the process of desensitization is approximately 4 hours. If a dose is missed then repeat the desensitization. The oral desensitization protocol is given in Table 2. After desensitization the patient can be given parenteral penicillin

The process of desensitization induces immunotolerance by administartion of very small doses of antigen. Hypersensitivity to penicillin still persist but antibodies of the IgE class bind to scanty amounts of antigen, hence the reaction is faint and remains subclinical.[11] In case of repeat administration of penicillin in the same patient is required in future, skin testing should be done again and if positive desensitization should be repeated.[12]

Table 2. Oral Desensitization Protocol for Patients With A Positive Skin Test

Pencillin V Suspension dose	Amount (units/mL)	mL	Units	Cumulative dose (units)
1	1,000	0.1	100	100
2	1,000	0.2	200	300
3	1,000	0.4	400	700
4	1,000	0.8	800	1500
5	1,000	1.6	1600	3100
6	1,000	3.2	3200	6300
7	1,000	6.4	6400	12700
8	10,000	1.2	12000	24700
9	10,000	2.4	24000	48700
10	10,000	4.8	48000	96700
11	80,000	1.0	80000	176700
12	80,000	2.0	160000	336700
13	80,000	4.0	320000	656700
14	80,000	8.0	640000	1296700

Note: Observation period: 30 minutes before parenteral administration of penicillin.
Adapted from CDC Treatment of Sexually Transmitted Diseases. 2002

References

1. King A, Nicol C, Rodin P, In: Treatment of syphilis. eds. Venereal diseases. 4th Ed. London: ELBS; 1980. p. 144-164.
2. Markowitz M. Long-acting penicillins: historical perspectives. Pediatr Infect Dis 1985; 4: 570-573.
3. Centre for Disease Control. Sexually transmitted diseases. Treatment guidelines. MMWR, 2002; 51/RR-6.
4. WHO/RHR/01.10. Guidelines for the management of sexually transmitted infection. 2001
5. Sexually transmitted infection treatment recommendations. NACO 2002.
6. Augenbraun MH. Treatment of syphilis 2001: nonpregnant adults. Clin Infect Dis 2002; 35: S187-190.
7. Pao D, Goh BT, Bingham JS. Management issues in syphilis. Drugs 2002; 62: 1447-1461.
8. Treponemal infection is HIV disease. In: Powderly WG edr. Manual of HIV therapeutics. 2nd edn. Philadelphia: Lippincott Williams & Wilkins; 2002. p. 229-238.
9. Wendel Jr GD, Sheffield JS, Hollier LM, et al. Treatment of syphilis in pregnancy and prevention of congenital syphilis. Clin Infect Dis 2002; 35: S200-209.
10. Van Voorst, Vader PC. Syphilis management and treatment. Dermatol Clin 1998; 16: 697-711.
11. Sanchez MR. Syphilis. In: Freedberg IM, Eisen AZ, Wolff K, et al, eds. Dermatology in general medicine. 5th edn. New York: McGraw-Hill; 1999. p. 2551-2581.
12. Macy E, Mellan MH, Schatz M, et al. Drug allergy. In Adelman DC, Casale TB, Correu J, eds. Manual of allergy and immunology. 4th edn. Philedelphia: Lippincott Williams & Wilkins; 2002. p. 219-241.

Chapter 17
Endemic Treponematoses

Yogesh S Marfatia

Introduction

Endemic treponematoses include non-venereally transmitted treponemal infections namely yaws, endemic syphilis and pinta. These diseases are of great public health significance because of their easy communicability and crippling, invalidating and disfiguring sequelae. It is said that syphilis goes with civilization, while endemic treponematoses start where the highway ends[1] and overcrowding as well as poor socioeconomic conditions prevail. It is postulated that all treponematoses are merely variants of a single disease, the expression of which has been modified by environmental factors, especially temperature.[2]

All these conditions are caused by subspecies of *Treponema pallidum* and hence show remarkable similarities in morphology and antigenic make up of causative organisms, as well as in immune response pattern in terms of serology by non-specific and specific tests. The difference lies in epidemiology, pathogenicity for experimental animals and clinical features of individual diseases. The general pattern of clinical stages of various treponemal diseases is remarkably similar and characterized by initial primary lesions followed by more extensive secondary manifestations and they all exhibit the phenomenon of latency.[3,4]

History

It has been postulated that *T. pallidum* originally arose from free living treponemes in mud; *T. zulezerae* still remains as a representative of this form of life. These organisms ultimately evolved into human saprophytes. Diseases then developed as natural selection ensured the optimal survival of more virulent organisms.[5]

Treponematoses are the diseases of antiquity and bones discovered in a cemetery of an ancient Greek colony in Southern Italy contain unequivocal evidence of the presence of syphilis or yaws in an era well before Columbus. Bone lesions with probable yaws have been traced down to AD 854 on the Mariana Islands in the West Pacific.[1]

Global Epidemiology

In early 1950s, there were estimated 50-150 million cases and hence WHO in collaboration with UNICEF launched Global Endemic Treponematoses Control Program in the period 1952-1964. More than 50 million cases were treated with long acting penicillin in 46 countries, reducing the overall disease prevalence by more than 95%. The control strategy subsequently was changed from a vertical program to one that was integrated into basic health services. By the end of 1970s, resurgence of endemic treponematoses had occurred in many areas.[3]

According to an estimation in 1996, the population at risk is estimated at 34 millions i.e. 5% of the total world population (mainly infants, children and to a lesser extent, adolescents and young adults). They all live in the developing countries, with 21 million living in the so called least developed countries. The regions most affected are Africa and South East Asia, with some foci in Central and South America, the Middle East and the Pacific Islands. The total number of cases estimated globally is 2.6 million and infectious cases 460,000, of which there are 400,000 cases in Africa. The number of disabled persons due to endemic treponematoses is estimated at 260,000 globally.[3]

Yaws

Nomenclature: *frambesia* (German and Dutch), *pian*

(French), *parangi* (Sinhalese), *buba* (Spanish), *bouba* (Portuguese)

Distribution: Exclusively found in the humid regions between the Tropics of Cancer and Capricorn, central and northern part of South America, the Caribbean, Africa and South East Asia.

Epidemiology

The causative organism is '*Treponema pertenue*' discovered by Castellani in 1905. The disease is commonly found in early childhood, 2-10 years of age, incidence being more in males than females. Transmission is between children or family members from moist early lesions by skin to skin contact. The entry is facilitated by excoriations, abrasions and bites. Thus most primary lesions occur over exposed parts on legs, arms, buttocks or face.[5]

Indirect transmission by the fly, *Hippelates pallipes* has been suggested.

Clinical Features

The incubation period varies from 3 to 6 weeks.

Primary Stage

The initial lesion is known by a variety of names such as primary or 'mother yaw', *frambesia, pianoma, buba madre, mannanpian*. The 'mother yaw' begins as an erythematous infiltrated papule which enlarges by extension at the periphery or by confluence with satellite nodules. The lesions then ulcerate and are covered by yellowish crust formed by exudates. The lesions are symptomless, highly infectious and vary in size from 1 to 5 cm. It may be accompanied by fever, joint pains or regional lymphadenopathy. It heals spontaneously after 3-6 months leaving atrophic and depressed scars with hypopigmented centre, sometimes surrounded by dark halo.

Secondary Stage

The secondary stage starts few weeks after the appearance of mother yaw and is characterized by:

Cutaneous lesions: It resembles the mother yaws but tends to be smaller and widespread and is called 'daughter yaws'. The lesions are frequently located adjacent to body orifices and tend to expand, ulcerate and exudate fluid rich in treponema. Occasionally peripheral extensions or coalescence of several lesions result in circinate and annular lesions resembling tinea. These are referred to as 'tinea yaws' or 'circinate yaws'.[4] Condylomatous lesions in the axillae and groins are also seen.

Palmoplantar lesions: On palmoplantar surfaces, the lesions form thick hyperkeratotic plaques which crack and fissure producing painful crab like gait (Crab yaws). Palmoplantar hyperkeratotic papules or macules, mimicking secondary syphilis are not uncommon. Papillomas arising in the nail fold cause a paronychia called 'pianic onychia'.

Bone and Joint lesions: Early bone lesions consist of painful periosteitis, polydactyleitis and fusiform swelling of metatarsals and metacarpals.

Infectious secondary lesions re-occur during ensuing 5 years and tend to be localized to axillae, perianal and circumoral areas. The disease then enters a non-infectious latent period.

Tertiary Stage (Late Yaws)

Approximately 10% of the cases develop late yaws several years after the primary infection. This stage is characterized by destructive and ulcerated cutaneous lesions, palmoplantar keratoderma, lesions of the joint, bone, gangosa and goundou.

Cutaneous lesions: Keratoderma and hyperkeratosis of palms and soles is frequently seen in late yaws. There is formation of subcutaneous nodules, which undergoes abscess formation, central necrosis and ulceration. Ulcers may become secondarily infected resulting in destruction of underlying deep structures. On healing, it may result into significant scarring, keloid formation and contractures. There is a potential risk of development of squamous cell carcinoma in the ulcerative lesions of late yaws.

Bone and Joint lesions: Osseous lesions consist of hypertrophic periosteitis, gummatous periosteitis, osteitis and osteomyelitis. Chronic osteitis of long bones such as the tibia can lead to curvature of the bone producing sabre shins. '*Goundou*' is the exostoses of the nasal bones and neighboring osseous structures producing oval thickened bony masses on either side of the nasal bridge. '*Gangosa*' (deforming rhinopharyngitis) is mutilation of the central part of face. It includes destruction of the mucosa, cartilagenous and osseous structures of nasal septum, palate and posterior aspect of pharynx.

Neurologic and Ophthalmic manifestations:

Although it is believed that yaws spares the nervous system and eyes, isolated cases of idiopathic optic atrophy and myeloneuropathies have been reported.

Attenuated Yaws

This is the mild form of the disease found in areas with low disease prevalence. It is characterized by a solitary or few lesions generally confined to skin folds. The lesions are dry and patients are less contagious. There is a great potential for missing these cases during surveillance.[4]

Differential Diagnosis

Yaws must be differentiated from venereal syphilis clinically as no serological test can distinguish the two. The skin lesions of yaws can be confused with eczema, psoriasis, keratoderma, calluses, verruca, bites and vitamin deficiencies. Leprosy, leishmaniasis, tropical ulcer, ecthyma and deep mycoses can also resemble yaws. Bone lesions can be identical to those of venereal syphilis, endemic syphilis, tuberculosis and osteomyelitis. Nasopharyngeal lesions mimic mucocutaneous leishmaniasis, rhinosporidiosis, rhinosclerosis, leprosy and tuberculosis.

Endemic Syphilis

Nomenclature: *Syphilis insontium, bejel* (Middle East), *njovera* (Zimbabwe), *siti, dichuchwa* (Botswana), *skeljevo, bishel* or *belesh* (Saudi Arabia).

Distribution

Endemic syphilis is prevalent in dry, arid climates. It occurs among primitive population; areas bordering deserts like in Middle East, Northern Nigeria, Southern Morocco, Botswana, Zimbabwe and Northern Australia.

Epidemiology

The causative organism is '*Treponema endemicum*'. The infection is prevalent in children between 2 to 15 years of age and has no sex predilection. The infection is transmitted from child to child by close skin contact, kissing and fomites such as communal drinking vessels. Direct lesion to skin contact among children and contact with saliva are additional modes of transmission. Occasionally, a previously uninfected nursing mother will have a primary lesion on or near the nipple from her infected infant. Unlike venereal syphilis, congenital transmission is rare and the mother does not have immunity against treponema. This represents reverse of Colle's law.[6]

Very few cases of venereal syphilis are seen in hyperendemic areas of endemic syphilis due to immunity in young adults with latent infection of *Treponema pallidum endemicum*. The venereal syphilis slowly emerges as the endemic disease is overcome and in this period of transition, mixed (endemic and venereal) disease will be found with considerable number of endemic syphilis cases in older age group.[6]

Clinical Features

Primary Stage

This stage is characterized by rare occurrence of small papules and ulcers on oropharyngeal mucosa and skin.

Secondary Stage

The initial lesions occur as mucous patches which are shallow, painless ulcers over the lips, tongue, tonsils, fauces and buccal mucosa. These are accompanied by regional lymphadenopathy. Split papules and condylomata lata over axillary and anogenital regions are other important secondary lesions. Non-pruritic papular eruptions and papulosquamous eruptions are also reported. Osteoperiosteitis of long bones occurs and causes nocturnal leg pain. Untreated secondary lesions last for 6-9 months.

Tertiary Stage

Gummata of nasopharynx, larynx, skin and bone develops 6 months to several years after inoculation and may progress to chronic destructive ulcers. In time they resolve leaving characteristic atrophic, depigmented scars, surrounded by hyperpigmentation. Gross mutilation with loss of skin, mucous membrane, muscle, cartilage and bone with destructive lesions of palate and nasal septum are disfiguring features of untreated disease. There is no reported evidence of neurological or cardiac involvement. However, ophthalmologic manifestations like uveitis, choroiditis, chorioretinitis and optic atrophy are encountered.

Attenuated Endemic Syphilis

In attenuated endemic syphilis, the number, severity and duration of both early and late lesions are reduced and majority of seropositive persons have latent disease. Improvement in the hygiene and wide availability of antibiotics are the most accepted reasons for attenuated disease.[7]

Differential Diagnosis

The most important and difficult disease to differentiate from endemic syphilis is venereal syphilis. Oral lesions must be differentiated from venereal syphilis, aphthosis, vitamin deficiencies and herpes. Mutilating nasopharyngeal endemic syphilis can be confused with tuberculosis, leprosy, rhinoscleroma and rhinosporidiosis.

Pinta

Pinta (Mexico) means spot or mark in Spanish, comes from the verb pintar 'to paint'.

Nomenclature: *Carate, cute* (Venezuela and Columbia), *mal del pinto, puru-puru , morados* and *azul* meaning 'the bluish ones'.

Distribution

It is found in remote areas of Mexico, Central and Northern South America and certain Islands of the Caribbean.

Epidemiology

Pinta caused by *Treponema pallidum (T.p.) carateum* is unique in having only skin manifestations and affects persons of all ages. Majority of the cases occur in children younger than 15 years and young adults are the main reservoir of infections. Mode of transmission is by repeated lesion to skin contact.

Clinical Features

Primary Stage

Seven days to 2 months after the inoculation, minute papules or erythematous macules appear over the lower extremities and other exposed areas. The lesions grow by extension to periphery or by fusion with satellite lesions forming ill defined erythematous infiltrated plaques. Infection is confined to the skin with the exception of occasional juxtaarticular nodes.

Table 1.   Comparison of Epidemiologic Features of Treponematoses

Features	Yaws	Endemic syphilis	Pinta	Venereal syphilis
Organism	*T. pallidum* subsp. *pertenue*	*T. pallidum* subsp. *endemicum*	*T. pallidum* subsp. *carateum*	*T. pallidum* subsp *pallidum*
Geographical distribution	Africa, Asia, South and Central America, Pacific Islands	North Africa, South East Asia, Arabian Peninsula	South and Central America, Mexico	Worldwide, more in developing countries
Climate	Humid, warm	Arid, warm	Semi-arid, warm	
Age group	< 15 years (Early childhood)	< 15 years (Early childhood)	1-15 years	Adulthood
Mode of transmission	Skin to skin	Household contacts, mouth to mouth or via shared drinking/eating utensils, insect vector?	Skin to skin	Sexual, transplacental

Secondary Stage

The secondary lesions, '*pintids*' appear as small, scaly papules that gradually enlarge and coalesce forming psoriasiform plaques. Initially they are red to violaceous and later become slate blue, brown gray or black. Several colours may exist within the same lesion. Primary and secondary stage lesions are highly infectious.

Tertiary Stage

Symmetric achromic lesions develop over body prominences, wrists, elbows and ankles from 3 months to 10 years after the appearance of pintids creating a mottled appearance. Cutaneous atrophy, hyperkeratosis and pigmentation may also be present. Generalized lymphadenopathy is also seen. Cardiovascular and central nervous systems are not involved and attenuated form of pinta has not been described.

Differential Diagnosis

Early pinta may be difficult to distinguish from the other treponematoses, venereal syphilis, yaws and endemic syphilis. Eczema, pityriasis alba, psoriasis, leprosy, lupus erythematosus, pellagra, tinea corporis and tinea versicolor can also mimic early pinta. The *leukoderma* of late pinta closely resembles vitiligo.

HIV and Endemic Treponematoses

The immunodeficiency due to HIV infection might lead to reactivation of latent treponemal infections. HIV infected persons are more likely to carry large number of treponemes and might disseminate pathogenic treponemes more effectively than HIV negative persons.[4]

Diagnosis

In the past, clinical diagnosis was accepted in area of high endemicity. After mass treatment campaigns, the clinical manifestations have changed and atypical attenuated disease is more commonly seen. Serologic tests for yaws, endemic syphilis and pinta are similar to those of venereal syphilis.

Table 2.   Comparison of Clinical Features of Treponematoses

Features	Yaws	Endemic syphilis	Pinta	Venereal syphilis
Primary lesions	Ulcerating and vegetating papular lesions with satellites	Eroded papules (rarely seen)	Non-ulcerating papules with psoriasiform plaques	Cutaneous ulcer (chancre)
Location	Extremities	Oral	Extremities, face	Genital, oral, anal
Secondary lesions	Papulosquamous lesions, warty nodules and palmo plantar 'crab yaws'	Florid mucocutaneous lesions (mucous patch, split papule, condylomata lata)	Pintids, (erythematous and psoriasiform scaly plaques) pigmentary changes	Mucocutaneous lesions, Condylomata lata
Tertiary lesions	Gummas, pintoid dyschromia, juxtaarticular nodes, gangosa, goundou, keratoderma	Serpiginous gummas, juxtaarticular nodes and on elbows only	Dyschromic, hypochromic, achromic polychromic patches	Granulomatous nodules, psoriasiform granulomatous plaques, gumma
Osseous	Yes	Yes	No	Yes
CVS manifestation	No	No	No	Yes
CNS manifestations	No	No	No	Yes
Congenital	No	No	No	Yes
Infectious relapses	Common	Unknown	None	~ 25%
Positive serum tests for syphilis	Yes	Yes	Yes	Yes
Response to penicillin	Excellent	Excellent	Excellent	Excellent

The RPR, VDRL, FTA-ABS, TPI and TPHA have all been used. No serologic test can distinguish yaws, endemic syphilis, pinta and venereal syphilis. Dark field microscopic examination as well as histopathologic and radiologic studies can aid in diagnosis and evaluation but are neither economical nor convenient.

Histopathology

Epidermotropism of *Treponema pallidum (T. p.) pertenue* as well as *T. p. carateum* compared with the mesodermotropism of *T. p. pallidum* is well established. Histologic criteria for differentiation of syphilis and yaws are unreliable. In contrast with venereal syphilis, the blood vessels show little or no endothelial proliferation. Late yaws resemble tertiary syphilis histopathologically. Histopathologic features of pinta vary according to different stages and those of endemic syphilis have not been well characterized.

Treatment

Penicillin was established as an effective treatment of treponematoses in the 1940s. The mass treatment campaigns of the 1950s and 1960s used procaine penicillin in 2% aluminium monostearate. The WHO recommends treating all cases and contacts over 10 years of age with 1.2 million units of benzathine penicillin G in single intramuscular injection and 0.6 million units in children younger than 10 years. Once injected, penicillin begins to kill the treponemes within minutes and the lesions become non-infectious within 18-24 hours. Alternative drugs used in patients allergic to penicillin include tetracyclines or erythromycin 500 mg PO four times daily or chloramphenicol for minimum 5 days. In children, oral erythromycin in a dose of 8 to 10 mg/kg four times a day for 15 days is the alternative regimen.

When the prevalence of cases with active lesions is above 10% of the population examined, penicillin should be given to the whole community; if between 5-10% it should be administered to patients, contacts and children of less than 5 years of age and if prevalence is less than 5% only active cases and their contacts in the same household should be treated.[1]

Control

In contrast to smallpox, it is highly unlikely that endemic treponematoses will ever be eradicated and that a treponemal vaccine may be developed in foreseeable future. In the former disorder, those afflicted develop life long immunity, remain contagious for brief periods and are usually symptomatic. However, victims of endemic treponematoses do not develop life long immunity, remain contagious for protracted periods of time and may harbour subclinical or mild disease. In mass treatment campaigns of 1950s and 1960s though the diseases were controlled, subsequently many countries failed to integrate continued active control measures into local health services. This led to gradual rebuilding and extension of treponemal reservoirs. For halting the transmission of the diseases, the mass treatment approach must be followed by periodic screening surveys of children and others at risk and by long term sero surveillance.[4]

The future may bring the emergence of plasmid-mediated antibiotic resistance among the non-venereal treponematoses. These diseases are not perceived as high priority because they are not fatal and are largely restricted to remote, poor and rural populations. The enigma whether these organisms are truly different organisms or demonstrating various clinical expressions caused by divergent environmental conditions can be settled by newer molecular techniques.

References

1. Morton RS. The treponematoses. In: Rook A, Wilkinson DS, Ebling FJG, et al, eds. Textbook of Dermatology. 6th edition. London: Blackwell; 1998. p. 1237-1275.
2. Sheila A. Lukehart. Endemic Treponematoses. In: Fauci AS, Braunwald E, Kasper DL, et al, eds. Harrison's Principles of Internal Medicine. 15th edition, New York: McGraw Hill; 2001. p. 1053-1055.
3. Meheus, A Tikhomirov E. Endemic Treponematoses. In: Holmes KK, Mardh PA, Sparling SF, et al eds. Sexually Transmitted Diseases. 3rd edition. New York: McGraw Hill; 1999. p. 511-513.
4. Koff AB, Rosen T. Nonvenereal treponematoses: yaws, endemic syphilis, and pinta. J Am Acad Dermatol 1993; 29: 519-535.
5. King A, Nicol C, Rodin P, eds. Yaws; Endemic syphilis; Bejel; Pinta. In: Venereal Diseases, 4th edition, London: Balliere Tindall; 1980. p. 333-345.
6. Willcox RR, Willcox JR. Venereological Medicine. Oxford: Oxford University Press; 1992. p. 151-160.
7. Castro LG. Nonvenereal treponematoses. J Am Acad Dermatol 1994; 31: 1075-1076.

Chater 18

Chancroid

C Balachandran, Sathish Pai B

Introduction

Ulceration of the genitalia is a common presentation of sexually transmitted diseases (STD). In developing countries especially India and Africa, chancroid and granuloma inguinale are more common, whereas in developed countries most of the cases are due to genital herpes or syphilis.[1]

Chancroid is also called as soft sore, soft chancre and ulcus molle. It is an acute infectious disease caused by a gram negative bacillus, *Haemophilus ducreyi* and is clinically characterized by one or more genital ulcers with inguinal lymphadenitis.

History

Chancroid was first described as a separate disease from syphilis in 1838 by Ricord. In 1889 Ducrey isolated the organism and described it as a short, compact streptobacillary rod.[2] The intradermal test with *H. ducreyi* was reported by Ito in 1913[3] and the work was confirmed by Reenstierna in 1923.[4]

Incidence

Although chancroid is not a problem in industrialized nations,[5] it is endemic in many developing countries.[6] In Kenya, Zambia and Zimbabwe chancroid is considered to be the most common cause of genital ulceration.[7] The disease is more prevalent in communities with low hygienic standards. Uncircumcised men are more susceptible to infection with *H. ducreyi*.[8] The male to female ratio ranges from 3:1 to 53:1.[7] The disease is transmitted from person to person mainly through heterosexual contact and is usually acquired from prostitutes.

Causative Organism

The causative organism of chancroid is the gram negative, facultative anaerobic bacillus *H. ducreyi*. Gram stain shows groups of organisms, which are often arranged in chains of two's or four's giving the typical appearance of a "school of fish or rail road track".

The biochemical and nutritional characteristics of *H. ducreyi* are;

(a) It requires haemin (X factor) for growth
(b) It reduces nitrate to nitrite
(c) It has a DNA guanosine-plus-cytosine content of 0.38 mole fraction
(d) It is oxidase positive, produces alkaline phosphatase but is catalase negative

It is a fastidious organism and culture is difficult. The organism can be easily demonstrated in the pus aspirated from an inguinal abscess, whereas open lesions on the genitalia may not reveal any *H. ducreyi* because of secondary bacterial infection.

Pathogenesis

The organism is inoculated into the tissues, possibly through a minor abrasion or trauma, which occur during the sexual intercourse. In the tissue the organism is usually present within macrophages, neutrophils and also as clumps in the interstitium. Cytotoxin produced by the organism cause cell damage, which may result in the formation of an ulcer.

Both virulent and avirulent strains of *H. ducreyi* have been demonstrated in animal and human studies. Virulent strains show greater capacity than the avirulent strain to attach to the epithelial cells. Avirulent organisms are more susceptible to antimicrobial agents.

Cinical Features

Chancroid presents as a painful ulcerative disease of the genitalia. The incubation period is usually short and ranges from 1 to 14 days,[9] with a median of 7 days between inoculation and appearance of the first skin lesion.[5]

Initially, a small inflammatory papule surrounded by erythema develops on the genitalia, which rapidly progresses to a pustule. Multiple often foul smelling ulceration quickly develops. Classically, the ulcers are painful, sharply circumscribed with ragged undermined edges (**P XIII, Fig. 52–54**). The floor of the ulcer may be covered by a yellow necrotic purulent exudate and removal of the exudate may reveal unevenly distributed very vascular granulation tissue, which may bleed on scraping or gentle manipulation. Characteristically the base of the ulcer is non-indurated.

The common sites of infection are the external or internal surface of the prepuce, the frenulum, the coronal sulcus and occasionally external urinary meatus and the shaft of the penis may be involved. Extragenital chancroid is rare.

In women, chancroid may have a more variable course than in men. Most females with ulcers are unaware of their infection and the presenting symptoms may include pain on urination or defaecation, vaginal discharge and dysparaeunia. The common sites of involvement are the fourchette, vestibule, labia, clitoris, vagina and the perianal area (**P XIII, Fig. 55**). Extragenital lesions on the breasts, fingers, thighs and in the oral cavity have been described. Female genital ulcers have been reported to heal faster than their male counterparts.[10]

The various clinical types of chancroid are the follicular chancroid, the dwarf chancroid, transient, papular chancroid, giant chancroid and the phagedenic chancroid.

Painful inguinal lymphadenitis develops in 30 to 60% of the patients within 1 to 2 weeks of the development of genital ulcers (**P XIV, Fig. 56**). This adenopathy is unilateral in most patients. The nodes become enlarged, tender and then matted together. If untreated in about 25% of patient suppuration occurs with the formation of a unilocular abscess called as bubo.[11] The overlying skin is erythematous and shiny. The buboes if untreated rupture through the skin with formation of a single sinus. The opening of the sinus may break down to form a chancroidal ulcer, which may then enlarge to form a giant ulcer. Most of the patients have genital ulcers along with the inguinal

bubo. This clinical finding along with other features may help us to differentiate it from LGV bubo. Some patients may develop buboes during antibiotic therapy while the ulcers are healing.[12] Bubo pus is usually thick, creamy and viscous. In female patients both lymphadenitis and bubo formation are less common. Scar formation, fibrosis and lymphoedema may occur in affected patients.[12]

Other complications of chancroid include phimosis, paraphimosis, urethral fistula and phagedenic ulcerations. The phagedenic ulcers are due to superadded infection with Vincent's organisms, which cause widespread necrosis of the tissue leading to the formation of large destructive ulcers.

Pseudogranuloma inguinale is a variety of chancroid that closely resembles granuloma inguinale (**P XIV, Fig. 57**).[13,14] Clinically the ulcers have the features of granuloma inguinale but on culture *H. ducreyi* is grown.

Diagnosis

Diagnosis of chancroid is basically made on clinical grounds, which has an accuracy rate of 30 to 50%.[15,16] Isolation of *H. ducreyi* from the genital ulcer or bubo is an important laboratory investigation in the diagnosis of chancroid.

Smears are taken with cotton swabs from beneath the undermined edges of ulcers and stained with Gram or Wright stain. Pleomorphic gram negative coccobaclli arranged in parallel chains of two's or four's described as "school of fish" may be demonstrated. This finding may be suggestive of chancroid, but lacks sensitivity and specificity for a definitive diagnosis.[17]

Ito-Reenstierna test is an intradermal test wherein a cutaneous reaction is produced by intradermal injection of a vaccine containing killed *H. ducreyi* in a suspension. The test is said to be positive if an inflammatory papule of 0.5 to 1 cm diameter develops at the site after 48 hrs. This diagnostic test is now obsolete.

A definitive diagnosis of *H. ducreyi* infection requires growth of the organism in culture. A special culture media is required and the recovery rates have ranged from 0 to 80%. Various culture medias used are chocolate agar enriched with 1% isovitalix, defibrinated rabbit blood and foetal bovine serum agar, which are made selective by addition of vancomycin. Cultures are incubated at 35°C in a candle jar.

Small, non-mucoid, yellow-gray, semiopaque colonies appear 2 to 4 days after inoculation. A positive culture is obtained in about 80% of patients with clinical chancroid in experienced laboratories. Anaerobes like *B.melaninogenicus*, *B.fragilis* and anaerobic cocci were isolated more frequently from ulcers of chancroid associated with fluctuant bubo suggesting that they may play a role in the development of bubo.[18] Recent developments in the diagnosis are polymerase chain reaction (PCR)[19] and indirect immunofluorescence using monoclonal antibodies.[20] Recently monoclonal antibody against haemoglobin receptor (HgbA) of outer membrane protein of *H.ducreyi* has shown a sensitivity of 100% and ability to detect 2×10^6 CFU, 8.5 ng of purified HgbA and holds promise of serodiagnosis of chancroid.[21] PCR is the most sensitive technique but is not commercially available. Multiplex test which combines PCR for *H. ducreyi*, *T. pallidum* and HSV has been developed by Roche.[22]

The Centres for Disease Control (CDC) proposes that a probable diagnosis of chancroid can be made if following are present:[21]

1. One or more painful genital ulcers.
2. Dark field examination of ulcer exudate is negative for *T. pallidum*.
3. A non-reactive serological test for syphilis performed atleast 7 days after the onset of ulcers.
4. A typical clinical presentation with findings suggestive of chancroid along with regional lymphadenopathy.
5. A negative test for herpes simplex virus (HSV).

Histopathology of Chancroid

Histopathology of the ulcer shows three distinctive zones, which is helpful in a presumptive diagnosis of chancroid in many instances. The zone at the top is narrow and consists of neutrophils, fibrin, erythrocytes and necrotic tissue. The middle zone is wide and is made up of newly formed blood vessels. The lower zone contains a dense infiltrate of plasma cells and lymphoid cells.

Management

A painful ulceration associated with tender inguinal lymphadenopathy is suggestive of chancroid, whereas the development of associated suppurative adenopathy is almost pathognomonic.[23] Successful treatment cures infection, resolves clinical symptoms and prevents further transmission of the disease to others.

The CDC recommends the following regimens

(a) Azithromycin 1gm orally in a single dose
or
(b) Ceftriaxone 250mg intramuscularly in a single dose
or
(c) Ciprofloxacin 500mg orally two times a day for 3 days.
or
(d) Erythromycin base 500mg orally four times a day for 7 days.

Earlier a combination of trimethoprim-sulfamethoxazole (TMP-SMZ) was used widely in the treatment of chancroid. But because of the development of resistance to this drug, it is no longer recommended.[24,25]

β lactam antibiotics are effective against *H.ducreyi*,[7] however plasmid mediated β lactam resistance to *H. ducreyi* have been described.[26] Many studies have demonstrated that *H. ducreyi* are capable of producing β lactamase.[7,27] So β lactamase resistant or inhibiting antibiotics are recommended in the treatment of chancroid eg. ceftriaxone.

Quinolones have shown significant activity against *H. ducreyi* in vitro.[28] A cure rate of 95–100% has been demonstrated with ciprofloxacin.[28,29]

Cordero in 1961 first used the macrolide antibiotic, erythromycin in the treatment of chancroid.[30] Erythromycin and rosaramicin (another macrolide antibiotic) have been found to be effective in the treatment of culture proved *H. ducreyi* infections.[31,32] Macrolide antibiotics are inexpensive, well tolerated and widely available. Compliance can be a problem with erythromycin as it requires multiple daily doses for 1 to 2 weeks. Recently, thiamphenicol 5.0 g orally as single dose was evaluated in a study of 1128 cases in Brazil, the treatment was successful in 99% cases.[33] Co-infection with *T. pallidum* or HSV has been demonstrated in approximately 10% of patients with chancroid which requires careful evaluation.

Management of Bubo

Fluctuant bubo should be aspirated using a wide bore needle from the non dependent part and adjacent healthy skin. Multiple aspirations were required prior to the advent of antimicrobial agents. With adequate antimicrobial treatment, a single aspiration is usually sufficient even in patients with large buboes.[34]

The antimicrobial agents have effect on genital ulcer as well as the inguinal bubo. In the presence of a bubo, the antimicrobial agents may have to be continued for a longer period till the bubo heals. Patients with inguinal lymphadenitis without suppuration usually respond without developing a bubo. Buboes less than 5cm in diameter tend[10] to resolve along with the healing of genital ulcer, whereas buboes more than 5cm resolve slowly and healing does not correspond to the resolution of genital ulcers.[10]

A randomized study has shown that careful incision and drainage is an effective and safe method for treating fluctuant bubo and avoids frequent needle re-aspiration.[35]

Treatment for Pregnant or Lactating Mothers and Children

Antimicrobial agents like erythromycin and ceftriaxone can be used during this period. Ciprofloxacin is contraindicated during pregnancy, lactation and in children and in adolescents less than 18 years of age.

The safety of azithromycin during pregnancy and lactation has not been established.

HIV Infection and Chancroid

There is a complex interaction between STD and the human immunodeficiency virus (HIV). On one hand, the natural history of STD is altered by concurrent HIV infection and on the other, the transmission and course of HIV is modified. During the last decade, enough evidence has been gathered to say that there is an increased risk of transmission of HIV in patients co-infected with a STD.

Ulcerative STD such as chancroid, primary syphilis and herpes simplex are all associated with an increased relative risk of infection. HIV sero conversion occurred more frequently in heterosexual men with genital ulcer disease (GUD) than in men without GUD.

Effect of HIV on Chancroid

   (a) Healing of the ulcer is delayed in HIV infected persons.

   (b) Treatment failures are more common.

   (c) Alteration of clinical picture. Extensive

necrotizing ulcers and multiple or multilocular buboes have been reported

Follow Up

After initiating the treatment, patients should be reviewed at day 3 and day 7. Genital ulcers are likely to improve symptomatically within 3 days and significant re-epithelialization occurs within 7 days.

References

1. Rosen T, Brown TJ. Genital ulcers evaluation and treatment. Dermatol Clin 1998; 16: 673.
2. Ducrey A. Experimentelle Untersuchunger uber den Ansteckungstoff des weichen Schankers und uber die Bubonen. Monatshr Prakt Dermatol 1989; 9: 387.
3. Ito T. Kliniche und bacteriologische studies uber Ulcus Molle und Ducreysche streptobazillen. Arch Dermatol Syph 1913; 116: 341.
4. Reenstierna J. Chancre mou experimental chez le singe et le lapin. Acta Dermatol Venereol 1921; 2: 1.
5. Ronald AR, Plummer FA. Chancroid and *Haemophilus ducreyi*. Ann Intern Med 1985; 102: 705-707.
6. Bilgeri YR, Ballard RC, Duncan MO, et al. Antimicrobial susceptibility of 103 strains of *Haemophilus ducreyi* isolated in Johannesburg. Antimicrob Agents Chemother 1982; 22: 686-688.
7. Boyd AS. Clinical efficacy of antimicrobial therapy in *Haemophilus ducreyi* infections. Arch Dermatol 1989; 125: 1399-1405.
8. Hart G. Venereal disease in a war environment: Incidence and management. Med J Aust 1975;1:808.
9. Felman YM, Nikitas JA. Sexually transmitted diseases: update on chancroid. Cutis 1983; 602: 607-608.
10. Fast MV, Nsanze H, Plummer FA, et al. Treatment of chancroid: a comparison of sulphamethoxazole and trimethoprim - sulphamethoxazole. Br J Vener Dis 1983; 59: 320-324.
11. Jones CC, Rosen T. Cultural diagnosis of chancroid. Arch Dermatol 1991; 127: 1823-1827.
12. Kraus SJ, Kaufman HW, Albritton WL, et al. Chancroid therapy: a review of cases confirmed by culture. Rev Infect Dis 1982; 4: S848-S856.
13. Rosen T, Dhir A. Chancroid, granuloma inguinale and lymphogranuloma venereum, In: Arndt KA, edr. Cutaneous medicine and surgery an integrated program in dermatology. Philadelphia: WB Saunders; 1996. p. 973-982.
14. Werman BS, Herskowitz LJ, Olansky S, et al. A clinical variant of chancroid resembling granuloma inguinale. Arch Dermatol 1983; 119: 890-894.
15. Chapel TA, Brown WJ, Jeffries C, et al. How reliable is

the morphological diagnosis of penile ulcerations? Sex Transm Dis 1977; 4: 150-152.

16. Sturm AW, Stolting GJ, Cormane RH, Zanen HC. Clinical and microbiological evaluation of 46 episodes of genital ulceration. Genitourin Med 1987; 63: 98-101.

17. Strakosch EA, Kendall HW, Craig KM, et al. Clinical and laboratory investigation of 370 cases of chancroid. J Invest Dermatol 1945; 6: 95-107.

18. Kumar B, Sharma VK, Bakaya V, Ayyagiri A. Isolation of anaerobes from clinical chancroid associated with fluctuant bubo in men. Indian J Med Res 1991; 93: 236-239.

19. Joseph AK, Rosen T. Laboratory techniques used in the diagnosis of chancroid, granuloma inguinale and lymphogranuloma venereum. Dermatol Clin 1994; 12: 1-8.

20. Karim QW, Finn GY, Easmon CSF, et al. Rapid detection of *Haemophilus ducreyi* in clinical and experimental infections using monoclonal antibody. Genitourin Med 1989; 65: 361-365.

21. Patternson K, Olsen B, Thomas C, et al. Development of a rapid immunodiagnostic test for *Haemophilus ducreyi*. J Clin Microbiol 2002; 40: 3694-3702.

22. Radchiffe K, Jushuf IA, Cowan F, et al. National guideline for the management of chancroid. Sex Transm Inf 1999; 75: S43-S45.

23. Brown TJ, Yen-Moore A, Tyring SK. An overview of sexually transmitted diseases. Part I. J Am Acad Dermatol 1999; 41: 511-532.

24. Van Dyck E, Bogaerts J, Smet H, et al. Emergence of *Haemophilus ducreyi* resistance to trimethoprim - sulfamethoxazole in Rwanda. Antimicrob Agents Chemother 1994; 38: 1647-1648.

25. Kumar B, Sharma VK, Bakaya V. Sulphaphenazole, streptomycin and sulphaphenazole combination,

trimethoprim, and erythromycin in the treatment of chancroid. Genitourin Med 1990; 66: 105-107.

26. Brunton JL, Maclean IW, Ronald AR, et al. Plasmid mediated ampicillin resistance in *H. ducreyi*. Antimicrob Agents Chemother 1979; 15: 294-299.

27. Fast MV, Nsanze H, D'costa LJ, et al. Treatment of chancroid by clavulanic acid with amoxicillin in patients with beta-lactamase positive *Haemophilus ducreyi* infection. Lancet 1982; 2: 509-511.

28. Reeves DS, Bywater MJ, Holt HA, et al. In vitro studies with ciprofloxacin: a new 4-quinolone compound. J Antimicrob chemother 1984; 13: 333-346.

29. Naamara W, Plummer FA, Greenblatt RM, et al. Treatment of chancroid with ciprofloxacin: a prospective randomised clinical trial. Am J Med 1987; 82: 317-320.

30. Cordero FA. Propionyl erythromycin ester lauryl sulphate in the treatment of treponematoses and chancroid. Antibiot Chemother 1961; 11: 764-771.

31. Carpenter JL, Back A, Gehle D, et al. Treatment of chancroid with erythromycin. Sex Transm Dis 1981; 8: 192-197.

32. Sng EH, Lim AL, Rajan VS, et al. Characteristics of *Haemophilus ducreyi* : a study. Br J Vener Dis 1982; 58: 239-242.

33. Belda Junior W, Siqueira LF, Fagundes LJ. Thiamphenicol in the treatment of chancroid. A study of 1128 cases. Rev Inst Med Trop Sao Paulo 2000; 42: 133-135.

34. Ronald AR, Albritton W. Chancroid and *Haemophilus ducreyi*. In: Holmes KK, Mardh P, Sparling PF, et al, eds. Sexually transmitted diseases. 2nd edn. New York: McGraw Hill; 1990. p. 268.

35. Ernst AA, Marvez - Vells E, Martin DH. Incision and drainage versus aspiration of fluctuant buboes in the emergency department during an epidemic of chancroid. Sex Transm Dis 1995; 22: 217-220.

Chapter 19

Donovanosis

R Ganesh

Synonyms

Granuloma venereum, Granuloma inguinale, Granuloma inguinale tropicum, Granuloma venereum genito-inguinale, Ulcerating granuloma of the pudenda, Ulcerating sclerosing granuloma, Infective granuloma, Serpiginous ulceration of the groin

Donovanosis is a chronic destructive and slowly progressive, mildly contagious disease caused by *Calymmatobacterium granulomatis* and is characterized by granulomatous ulceration affecting primarily the genitalia.

History

McLeod first described the clinical aspect of donovanosis in 1882 who called it as serpiginous ulcer of the groin. Donovan discovered the causative organism, *Calymmatobacterium granulomatis* in 1905. It was Greenblatt and his associates who described the intracellular bodies in 1937. Anderson achieved the culture of the donovanosis microorganism in 1943.[1-3] A monograph on donovanosis written by Rajam and Rangiah was published by WHO in 1954.[2]

Epidemiology

The disease is endemic in southern China, the Far East, northern Australia, Africa (west and central), and West Indies. In India donovanosis is endemic along the East Coast i.e., Orissa, Andhra Pradesh and Tamil Nadu. In USA sporadic occurrence of the disease has been reported. The disease is more prevalent among the blacks. The prevalence of the disease only in certain parts of the world may be related to the humidity and constant high temperature. Low socioeconomic conditions,

overcrowding and poor hygiene have also been implicated as probable predisposing factors. It is far less common than syphilis, chancroid and herpes. The male to female ratio is 4:1.[1,2,4,5]

Aetiology

Calymmatobacterium granulomatis otherwise known as *Klebsiella granulomatis* is a gram negative intracellular bacterium measuring 1 to 1.5 × 0.5 to 0.7μm, usually seen within the vacuoles of large mononuclear cells (histiocytes) or occasionally inside polymorphonuclear cells.[6] They reproduce in multiple foci resulting in 20 to 30 organisms occurring in a vacuole inside the host cell. The organism has a surrounding cell membrane and an overlying cell wall with a capsule in mature forms. Fimbriae (pili) like projections are seen on the cell wall.[1]

Two characteristic appearances of the organism have been described:

(i) A larger capsulated form with ovoid or bean shaped body, having well defined pinkish material surrounding a blue bacillary body with dark blue or black chromatin inclusions. These inclusions may be rounded, rod shaped and positioned centrally, peripherally or in a bipolar fashion.

(ii) The noncapsulated forms were described as minute deeply staining bodies of varying morphology-coccoid, bacillary, diplococcoid, often with a closed safety pin or telephone handle shape surrounded by a halo of unstained area. These forms are smaller; measuring 0.6 to 1μm and both may coexist in the same host cell.

Apart from the organisms, certain inclusion bodies

have been reported inside infected mononuclear cells. They may be sharply defined globular mass homogeneously staining deep pink or blue and lying away from the intact nucleus of the cell. Deeply staining spherical bodies almost filling the cell and obscuring the nucleus have also been documented. Such inclusions seem to be non-nuclear in origin, as the nucleus is intact.[2]

Pathology

The marginal epithelium often shows pronounced proliferation with irregular acanthosis and elongation of rete pegs that may simulate early epithelioma (hence called peudoepitheliomatous change). Clusters of polymorphonuclear leucocytes (PMN) forming microabscess may be seen in the epidermis.

Large mononuclear cells, 25 to 90 µm in diameter containing intracytoplasmic vacuoles filled with clusters of donovan bodies are the diagnostic hallmark of the disease. These cells are scattered diffusely throughout the dermis. Dense infiltrate of plasma cells along with scanty PMN and variable number of eosinophils is also seen. Fibrosis and oedema are seen in some of the patients. Capillaries with hypertrophy of the endothelium giving the appearance of solid cords of large pale staining cells is seen.[1,2]

Clinical Features

The incubation period is variable and it may range from 3 days to 3 months. The average incubation period is 40 to 50 days. Rajam and Rangiah have experimentally produced the lesion in a volunteer in 17 days.[2]

The disease begins as single or multiple firm papules, which erode to form well defined granulomatous ulcer. The ulcer is usually painless, beefy red in colour and bleeds easily on touch. Phimosis or lymphoedema of distal tissues is common in active phase of the disease.

The genitalia are the most common sites involved in 90% of the cases. Other sites of involvement are inguinal region in 10%, anal region in 5-10% and other sites in 1-5%. Verrucous type of disease is usually seen in perianal area. Infection of oral cavity and face has also been reported.

Lymph nodes are not usually involved in donovanosis, however in cases of secondary infections or coexisting syphilis or chancroid or rarely in malignant transformation, they can be involved. Infection spreads by direct continuity along the dermis of the skin or by autoinoculation of apposing surfaces or through fingernails. Lesions appearing in the groin may present like lymphadenopathy prior to the rupture and have been referred to as pseudo bubo (**P XIV, Fig. 58**).

Involvement of deeper parts of the vagina and cervix is usually associated with vulval lesions and occasionally it may be the primary lesion. The disease readily involves the perianal margins in the female as well as in homosexual men, but rectum is usually spared. It is hypothesized that while stratified squamous epithelium is susceptible, the columnar epithelium lining the urethra and rectum could be resistant to the disease. Rare cases of involvement of uterus and tubes, lips, gum, cheek, palate, pharynx, larynx, and neck have been reported .[5]

Rajam and Rangiah have reported liver and bone involvement besides extension of genital lesion to the trigone of the bladder in a female. Metastatic haemotogenous spread to bones, joints, lung and liver have been reported[2].

Based on the clinical and pathological features four morphological patterns are described:

- Classical granulomatous type (**P XIV, Fig. 59**)
- Hypertrophic type: shows predominantly fibrous tissue reaction throughout the dermis (**P XV, Fig. 60, 61**).
- Sclerotic or cicatricial type of granuloma: hyalinised collagenous fibrous tissue dominates the histological picture.
- Destructive necrotic (phagedenic) variety: shows extensive tissue destruction due to secondary fusobacillary infection.[2]

Morphological Variants

Classical or fleshy exuberant type is the most common presentation involving the genito inguinal region in both the sexes. The granulation tissue overflows the edges of the lesions, suggesting herniation of fleshy mass through the skin. The edge is thin and often undermined. Skin around the ulcer is slightly oedematous and infiltrated. Offensive serosanguinous discharge may be noticed. The young non-capsulated forms of the organism are found both inside and outside the mononuclear cells.

Hypertrophic type is also seen in both the sexes. The ulcer is raised above the surrounding skin and consists of pale red coarse, warty granulation tissue resulting in a buckled appearance. The edge is thickened and greyish white. There is no exudate and lesion is painless. Lesions may remain stationary for months. Capsulated intracellular organisms are seen only in the deeper parts of the lesion.

The sclerotic or cicatricial type is more common in women and is recognized by early and extensive formation of fibrous tissue. Breaking down of the scar by islands of active ulceration is a frequent occurrence. The hard fibrous tissue may result in deformities of the genitalia and demonstration of the organism is difficult.

The destructive, necrotic (phagedenic) type is often due to the superadded anaerobic infection, (fusospirillary) and is seen in chronic cases. It results in rapidly spreading necrotic inflammation with abundant foul smelling exudate. The ulcers are painful and the inflammation rapidly spreads both superficially and deeply with extensive tissue destruction. In the female, rectovaginal fistula resulting in a cloaca has been reported.

In men, partial or complete amputation of the penis has been reported. Occasionally the condition can be fatal.[1,2,5] Extragenital donovanosis is a controversial subject but several cases have been reported.[8-9]

Diagnosis

The identification of intracellular donovan bodies is the gold standard for the diagnosis. It can be demonstrated by direct microscopy of crushed tissue smear stained with Giemsa or Leishman, obtained from the active lesion (**P XV, Fig. 62**). Biopsy is less reliable and more traumatic. Serological tests using complement fixing technique and skin tests using material obtained from proved cases have not been found to be of reliable practical use. Culture using yolk sac of chick embryo,[3] and recently using human peripheral blood monocytes and HEp-2 cells had been successful but is not useful for routine use.[9] PCR technique has also been described.[10]

Recently a colorimetric detection system for *Calymmatobacterium granulomatis* has been developed.[10]

Course and Prognosis

The disease progresses very slowly and the tendency for spontaneous healing is low and recurrence in already healed areas is not uncommon. Persistent oedema of the distal tissues may result in pseudoelephantiasis,

particularly in females (15 to 20%). Subsequent excoriation and ulceration result in deformities resulting in difficulty in micturition, defaecation, sexual intercourse and delivery. Even walking may be difficult for the patient with advanced disease.[5]

Females may suffer from stenosis of urethra, vulva or anal orifice particularly in the sclerotic type. Healing may result in extensive scarring leading to infibulation of the vaginal introitus. Rectovaginal fistula has also been reported. Epidermoid carcinoma has been documented in chronic cases (0.25%). Haematogenous spread to bones and joints, particularly during pregnancy has been reported.[1,2] Adhesion of penis to scrotum, partial or total amputation or lateral or backward deformity of penis has been reported in males.

Psoas and perinephric abscess and spinal cord compression has been documented as rare complications.[12] Secondary anaemia and tuberculosis may be seen in some patients.

In oral lesions, adhesion of lip and cheek to the gum may result in microstomia (difficulty in opening the mouth), difficulty in swallowing food and nasal regurgitation. Vertical transmission is rare though lesions on the ears of infants borne to mothers with donovanosis have been documented.[13] Associated HIV infection may result in aggressive ulceration and poor tendency for healing.[14]

Differential Diagnosis

Syphilis

Primary chancre is differentiated by its classical button like indurated non-bleeding ulcer and the associated rubbery lymphadenopathy. Dark field microscopy and serology can further confirm the diagnosis.

Condyloma lata of secondary syphilis, particularly in perianal margins may mimic donovanosis, but in the later the lesions are moist with broad base and flat top and teeming with treponemes which can further be confirmed by dark field microscopy and serology.

Nodulo-ulcerative benign tertiary syphilis may sometimes confuse the clinician, especially due to absence of lympha-denopathy. The punched out appearance of the ulcer with tendency for central healing and peripheral spread besides positive serology help in making the diagnosis.

Chancroid

Chancroid is recognized by the short incubation period.

The ulcers are multiple painful with necrotic slough and an undermined edge. It is often associated with painful suppurative lymphadenopathy and demonstration of Gram negative *H. ducreyi* bacilli in their classical school of fish appearance in microscopy.

Bubo of LGV

Bubo of LGV can be confused with pseudobubo of donovanosis. Late cases of LGV with elephantiasis may show secondary ulcerations and deformities but the involvement of lymphnodes help in clinical diagnosis. Serology using microimmunofluorescence assay for chlamydia is confirmatory.

Herpes Genitalis

When associated with advanced HIV infection herpes genitalis may present with granuloma like appearance (pseudogranuloma herpeticum). Absence of donovan bodies, presence of epithelial giant cells and response to acyclovir therapy help in diagnosis.

Amoebiasis

Amoebiasis of the genitalia in homosexuals may resemble donovanosis, and is differentiated by microscopy or therapeutic trial.

Malignancy

Particularly epidermoid carcinoma may mimic donovanosis in the early stages. Classical stony induration and lymphadenopathy differentiates the disease. Biopsy is confirmatory.

Donovanosis may coexist with other sexually transmitted infections, hence routine screening for them, particularly syphilis and HIV is mandatory.

Like other genito-ulcerative diseases donovanosis can predispose to both acquiring and spread of HIV infection. Delayed response to therapy and relapse may be noticed in the presence of immune deficiency. The advent of syndromic approach to STD and increased use of condoms in HIV era may be responsible for decreasing incidence of donovanosis in recent times.

Treatment

The following antimicrobials have been used successfully in various centres:

- Streptomycin 1 g IM bid for 10 to 14 days
- Gentamycin 1 mg/kg body wt IM 8th hourly for 2 weeks
- Chloramphenicol 0.5 g orally tid
- Tetracycline 0.5 g orally qid for 2 to 3 weeks
- Erythromycin 0.5 g orally qid
- Ampicillin 0.5 g orally qid for 12 weeks
- Cotrimoxazole 2 tablets bid for 3 weeks [15]
- Azithromycin 1 g once per week for 3 weeks
- Erythromycin is the drug of choice in pregnancy and during lactation. Children borne to infected and untreated mothers must be closely monitored and a course of prophylactic antibiotics may be considered.

Recommended Regimen by WHO (2001)

Azithromycin 1g orally on day 1 and then 500 mg orally once a day
or
Doxycycline 100 mg orally bid

Alternative Regimens

Erythromycin 500 mg orally qid
or
Tetracycline 500 mg orally qid
or
Cotrimoxazole 2 tablets orally bid

Response to treatment should be noticed in a week, otherwise alternate regimen may have to be considered. WHO (2001) recommends that treatment should be continued until all lesions have completely epithelialized.

Associated HIV infection may necessitate prolonged antimicrobial therapy and more frequent review. Addition of aminoglycoside (gentamycin) to one of the oral regimens should be strongly considered. Recently trovofloxacin and ceftriaxone have been successfully used in the treatment of chronic donovanosis. [17-18]

Recommended Regimen by NACO (2002)

Doxycycline 100 mg orally bid for 14 days/ Tetracycline 500 mg orally qid for 14 days

or

Erythromycin base/stearate 500 mg orally qid for 14 days

or

Azithromycin 500 mg orally bid for 14 days.

All sex partners should be examined and treated. Epidemiological treatment is not recommended routinely.
Local hygiene is generally enough.
Surgical repair of scar tissues may not be rewarding.

Follow Up

Patients must complete the recommended course. Review is preferable monthly for first 3 months when concomitant syphilis and HIV can also be ruled out. Subsequent follow up depends on level of healing and possible relapse. Partner notification and safe sex education with condom promotion must be emphasized.

References

1. Hart G. Donovanosis. In: Holmes K, Mardh PA, Sparling FP, et al eds. Sexually Transmitted Diseases. 3rd edn. New York: McGraw-Hill; 1999. p. 393-397.
2. Rajam RV, Rangiah PN. "Donovanosis" (granuloma inguinale, granuloma venereum) WHO Monograph 1954; 24: 1-72.
3. Anderson K, De Monbreun WA, Goodpasture EW. An etiological consideration of Donovania granulomatis cultivated from granuloma inguinale (three cases) in embryonic yolk. J Exp Med 1943; 8: 25-40.
4. Goldberg J. Studies on granuloma inguinale: Some epidemiological considerations of the disease. Br J Vener Dis 1964; 40; 140-145.
5. Sehgal VN ed. Donovanosis. New Delhi: Jaypee Brothers; 1-49.
6. Carter JS, Bowden FJ, Bostain I, et al. Phylogenetic evidence of reclassification of *Calymatobacterium granulomatis* as *Klebsiella granulomatis* comb. nov. Int J Systematic Bacteriol 1999; 49: 1695-1700.
7. Rao MV, Thappa DM, Jaishankar TJ, Ratnakar C. Extragenital donovanosis of the foot. Sex Trans Infect 1998; 74: 298-299.
8. Sanders CJ. Extragenital donovanosis in patients with AIDS. Sex Trans Infect 1998; 74: 142-143.
9. Carter J, Hutton S, Sriprakash KS, et al. Culture of the causative organism of donovanosis in HEp-2 cells. J Clin Microbiol 1997; 35: 2915-2917.
10. Carter J, Bowden FJ, Sriprakash KS, Kemp DJ. Diagnostic polymerase chain reaction for donovanosis. Clin Infect Dis 1999; 28: 1168-1169.
11. Carter J, Kemp BJ. A colorimetric detection system for *Calymmatobacterium granulomatis*. Sex Transm Infect 2000; 76: 134-136.
12. Paterson DL. Disseminated donovanosis (granuloma inguinale) causing spinal cord compression; Case report and review of donovanosis involving bone. Clin Infect Dis 1998; 26: 379-383.
13. Govender D, Naidoo K, Chetty R. Granuloma Inguinale; an unusual case of otitis media and mastoiditis in children. Am J Clin Pathol 1997; 108: 510-514
14. Jamkhedkar PP, Hira SK, Shroff HJ, Lanjewar DN. Clinico epidemiologic features of granuloma inguinale in era of acquired immunodeficiency syndrome. Sex Transm Infect 1998; 25: 196-200,
15. Lal S, Garg BR. Further evidence of the efficacy of co-trimoxazole in donovanosis. Br J Vener Dis 1980; 56: 412-413.
16. Bowden FJ, Mein J, Plunkett C, et al. Pilot study of azithromycin in the treatment of genital donovanosis. Genitourin Med 1996; 72: 17-19.
17. Hsu SL, Chia JK. Trovofloxacin for the treatment of chronic granuloma inguinale. Sex Transm Infect 2001; 77: 137.
18. Merianos A, Gilles M, Chuah J. Ceftriaxone in the treatment of donovanosis in central Australia. Genitourin Med 1994; 70: 84-89.

Chapter 20

Gonorrhoea

K Venkateswaran, S Mohan

Introduction

The word *gonorrhoea* is derived from combination of gonos, '*seed*' and rhoea, '*flow*'. It was considered that gonorrhoea and syphilis are caused by the same organism till Albert Neisser identified the organism to be *Neisseria gonorrhoeae* in 1879.

Gonorrhoea is one of the commonest sexually transmitted disease. The infection primarily affects the urethra in both the sexes but it may spread to paraurethral glands, cervix, endometrium, fallopian tubes and peritoneum in females. Anorectal and oropharyngeal infection is common with persons, who practice anal or oral intercourse. In children, gonorrhoea is mostly sexually transmitted[1] and rarely through accidental inoculation. Occasionally the gonococcal infection can present as disseminated form in immunocompromised patients and it accounts for less than 3% of the cases.[2] The commercial sex workers are the main source of infection in a developing country like India. However, the incidence seems to be higher in homosexual men.[3]

Aetiology

Neisseria gonorrhoeae is a gram-negative, non-motile, non-sporing diplococci. The organism is present intracellularly in the polymorphonuclear leucocytes(PMN). Of the Neisseria species *N. gonorrhoeae*, *N. meningitidis* are pathogenic, and *N. cartarrhalis*, *N. pharyngis sicca*, *N. lactamica*, and *N. subflava* are usually non-pathogenic.

Electron microscopically gonococci are of two types: pilated and non-pilated. 'Pili' or 'fimbriae' are hair like structures seen on the entire outer surface of the organism. It is presumed that these pili are required for attachment, or invasion into the host cell, or serve as targets for host immune defenses. Auxotype AHU (arginine, hypoxanthine, uracil) requiring gonococci are of epidemiologic importance as they have resistance to killing by normal human serum, propensity for asymptomatic male urethral infection and increased likelihood of causing bacteremia.

Pathogenesis

Primary infection commonly occurs in the columnar epithelium of the urethra, para-urethral ducts and glands, cervix, conjunctiva, Bartholin's ducts, and rectum. Primary infection may also occur in the stratified squamous epithelium of the vagina in prepubertal girls (gonococcal vulvovaginatis). The female urethra often escapes infection, owing to its lining with stratified squamous epithelium with only a few scattered areas of columnar epithelium. The male urethra is lined with stratified or pseudo stratified columnar epithelium and favours penetration of gonococcus.

Penetration of the organism takes place through the intercellular spaces and organisms reach the sub epithelial connective tissue on the third and fourth day of infection. Dilated capillaries are responsible for the exudation of cells and serum. The cellular infiltrate predominantly consists of PMN with small number of lymphocytes, plasma cells and mast cells. Involvement of the epithelium is patchy with intervening areas of normal epithelium. Large numbers of PMN containing gonococci find their way into the lumen of the urethra. These together with the serum and desquamated epithelium form the profuse yellow and sometimes sanguinous discharge which is characteristic of the disease.

In the female, the cervix, urethra and Bartholin's glands are the usual sites of primary infection and one or more of these structures may be involved at the same time. The rectum is frequently the site of secondary infection in the female and is rarely the primary focus.

Clinical Features

The incubation period ranges from 1 to 14 days but majority of men develop symptoms within 2 to 5 days.[4] Anterior urethritis is the most common manifestation of gonococcal infection in men. It starts with mild irritation, scanty mucopurulent or mucoid discharge per urethra in men (**P XVI, Fig. 63**). As it progresses, within 24 hours the dischrage becomes thick, purulent and profuse with intense burning and pain during micturition[5] (**P XVI, Fig. 64**). It is associated with increased frequency and urgency. The direct contact of the discharge may give rise to balanoposthitis characterized by sharply marginated, light red erosions along with discrete pustules on the coronal sulcus and rarely pustular lesions on the fingers. In 15% of males the disease is mild or asymptomatic.[6]

Gonococcal infection accounts for 90% of the infection in females.[7,8] The primary site of infection is endocervical canal and only about 50% of infected females are symptomatic.[9] The commonest symptoms in female are moderate burning micturition, frequency and urgency. The discharge is scanty because of the short urethra in female. There may be peri-meatal erythema and oedema.

Ano-rectal Gonorrhoea

Ano-rectal gonorrhoea, may be primary or secondary. Secondary infection occurs chiefly in women and prepubertal girls with a primary genito-urinary infection and occasionally due to bursting of gonorrhoeal abscesses into the rectum. Primary infection usually results from anal intercourse but may be accidental and in many cases it has followed the insertion of contaminated thermometers or enema nozzles.

Complications in Men

These include posterior urethritis, infection of Cowper's and Tyson's glands, epididymitis, acute or chronic prostatitis, seminal vesiculitis and periurethral abscess (**P XVI, Fig. 65**). The disease may reach both diaphragmatic and bulbar portions of the glands of Cowper; either by way of the columnar lined duct, which opens on the floor of the bulb or by lymphatic route. Inflammation, often subacute throughout, may progress to abscess formation (**P XVI, Fig. 65**). A diaphragmatic abscess rarely remains localized between the two layers of the urogenital diaphragm, the pus tracking either downwards presenting as perianal, ischiorectal, or perianal abscess, or upwards to form a perirectal or peri-prostatic abscess. Chronically inflamed Cowper's glands are hard and brick-like consistency, size varying from that of a pea to hazelnut. Untreated gonorrhoea may rarely lead to water can perineum (**P XVI, Fig. 66**).

Epididymitis

Involvement of the epididymis is the most frequent complication before the introduction of the sulphonamides and penicillin, which usually follows trauma to the posterior urethra. Gonococci penetrate the columnar epithelium of the tubules of the epididymis. The only distinctive feature is the formation of multiple miliary abscesses in the subepithelial connective tissue, which rarely coalesce to form extensive abscesses. There is often an associated inflammation of the rete testis and an inflammatory hydrocele.

Acute Prostatitis

Acute inflammation of the prostatic ducts and gland with peri-glandular inflammation may cause swelling of one or both lateral lobes, which may progress to form prostatic abscess.

Infection may also spread by continuity in the columnar epithelium of the short ejaculatory ducts or by the lymphatic vessels to one or both of the seminal vesicles.

Complications in Women

Salpingitis

It is usually bilateral, may present as acute, subacute and mild form. In both the types there is tendency for the tubes to get closed to form hydrosalpinx or pyosalpinx. Acute salpingitis or pelvic inflammatory disease (PID) is the most common complication of gonorrhoea in women. They present with lower abdominal pain, dysparuenia, abnormal periods, etc. The details are discussed in chapter on PID.

Bartholin's Gland Abscess

Inflammation is commonly unilateral and remain confined to the ducts and the periglandular tissues. The orifice often has a red halo, exudes pus on pressure (**P XVII, Fig. 67**). It may develop a small indurated swelling, or a large abscess, often preceded by cystic swelling of the duct or gland.

Complications in Infants

Ophthalmia Neonatorum

Primary gonococcal infection of the conjunctiva occurs rarely in adults but is common in babies infected during birth, starting within 21 days of birth. It accounts for 5-15% of conjuctivitis in the new born. It is characterized by intense redness and swelling of the conjunctiva, associated with a profuse purulent and often blood stained discharge. The ocular conjunctiva, swollen with an inflammatory oedema, bulges over the cornea and for the same reason the upper lid may overlap the lower (**P XVII, Fig. 68**). An intense inflammatory reaction develops in the subepithelial connective tissue of the conjunctiva during the first 24 hours and gonococci can be demonstrated on the second day of the disease. Corneal ulceration is caused by manipulation, excessive inflammatory oedema of the conjunctiva and pressure under the lids which macerates the cornea.

Metastatic Complications

Disseminated Gonococcal Infection

Disseminated gonococcal infection (DGI), is the most common systemic complication of acute gonorrhoea.[2] It manifests as acute arthritis-dermatitis syndrome. The syndrome has been estimated to occur in 0.5 to 3 percent of patients with untreated gonorrhoea. DGI results from gonococcal bacteremia and is most often manifestated by acute arthritis, tenosynovitis, dermatitis or combination of these findings. The most common clinical manifestation of DGI is joint pain and skin lesions, the arthritis-dermatitis syndrome. Skin lesions present as macules, papules, pustules, petechiae, bullae, or ecchymoses. The skin lesions tend to be located on distal portions of the extremities. Approximately 30 to 40 percent of patients with DGI have overt arthritis. Any joint may be involved, although DGI most often involves wrist, metacarpophalangeal, ankle and knee joints. Iris, conjunctiva, endorcardium, pericardium, meninges and nerves are also involved. Disseminated gonococcal infection is more common in women than in men.

Gonococcal Arthritis

Gonococcal inflammation of the joints is commonly polyathritic. The joints most often involved are the knees, ankles, and small joints of the feet. It may occur at any stage of the disease and has usually an acute onset; a subacute onset is rare. There are three main type of acute joint affection in gonorrhoea: arthralgia, acute synovitis, and acute arthritis which includes serofibrinous arthritis and the purulent form. The details are discussed in a separate chapter.

Meningitis

The complication may be blood borne from primary foci. Autopsy showed patches of purulent exudates containing gonococci in the subarachnoid space, the exudates being most obvious in the frontal and parietal regions, as seen in other type of purulent meningitis.

Lab Diagnosis

The diagnosis of gonorrhoea includes microscopy and culture. VDRL and HIV serology testing should be done after getting the informed consent.

Microscopy

Specimen is collected with help of sterile cotton wool swabs. If no discharge is present, urethral or prostatic massage is performed and specimen is collected from the distal urethral meatus. In female specimen is collected from the endocervix, urethra, rectum or oropharynx. The urethral discharge is homogenously spread over the slide by rolling the swab onto a clean slide. Allow the smear to dry before it is stained. Fix the dried smear by passing the slide rapidly three to four times over a flame. The slide is stained with Gram stain and examined under oil immersion 100 x objective. The gonococci are seen as gram–negative diploccoci within PMN cells (**P XVII, Fig. 69**). The specificity of gram stain is 95-97% from culture positive male urethral discharge, 40-60% from endocervical secretion and in asymptomatic patients, the smear is mostly negative.[10]

Culture

The culture is the most specific investigation and the commonly used selective media for *N. gonorrhoeae*, are modified Thayer Martin (MTM), Chacko Nayar Medium (Trypsin digested beef extract), Martin Lewis (ML) media, and New York City (NYC) medium. The direct plating of organism has better success in growing organism. If direct plating is not available the swabs are transported to the laboratory in Stuart's medium or Amie's medium. The inoculated plates are placed in an atmosphere containing 5% CO_2 at 37°C and examined every 18-24 hours until 48-72 hours.[10] Small pinpoint colonies of 0.5 to 1mm diameter of *N. gonorrhoeae* can be seen.

The isolation rate decreases with increase in time difference between the specimen collection and inoculation, 90% within 12 hours and 100% within 6 hours of obtaining specimen and the acceptable result can be expected if the transport time is <2 days.[10] The oxidase reaction aids the search for gonococcal colonies in mixed cultures. A drop of tetra methyl-*p*-phenylene diamine hydrochloride is poured over suspected gonococcal colonies, which quickly turn pink and then dark blue.

Gonococci are fastidious organisms, it requires an enriched culture media for its growth, which also selectively supresses the normal flora. Vancomycin, colistin, trimethoprim and nystatin are added to inhibit the growth of bacterial and fungal organisms.

Monoclonal antibodies for fluorescence, co-agglutination or enzyme are highly sensitive and specific to *N. gonorrhoeae* and they have the advantage of identifying *N. gonorrhoeae* 24 hours before the conventional culture technique.[10]

ELISA technique is much less reliable in women than in men and should only be considered for use in female population with high prevalence of gonorrhoea, if culture and transport media are not available. The specificity of DNA hybridization is superior to the ELISA though the sensitivity is almost same in symptomatic females.

Serology

The complement fixation, latex agglutination immunofluorescence and anti surface pili assays, haemagglutination, radioimmunoassay, ELISA and immunoblotting can be used to detect serum antibody against *N. gonorrhoeae* but it is not useful as it can't differentiate between the present and past infection.

The acidometric method, iodometric test and chromogenic cephalosporin test are used to detect the resistance of *N. gonorrhoeae* to penicillin.[10] β lactamase, an extra cellular enzyme produced by many strains of bacteria, specifically hydrolyze amide bond with β lactam ring of penicillin analogues, rendering the antibiotic inactive. Penicillinoic acid is formed with a resulting colour change. A rapid carbohydrate utilization test, (RCUT) is used for β lactamase production by Neisseria species. The production of β lactamase from *N. gonorrhoeae* can be detected by the change in colour of the phenol red pH indicator red to yellow. The test can thus be used both for identification and testing for β lactamase production.

Treatment[11]

Uncomplicated Gonococcal Infections of the Cervix, Urethra, and Rectum

Cefixime 400 mg orally in a single dose,
or
Ceftriaxone 125 mg IM in a single dose,
or
Ciprofloxacin 500 mg orally in a single dose,
or
Ofloxacin 400 mg orally in a single dose,
or
Levofloxacin 250 mg orally in a single dose,
Plus,
If Chlamydial infection is not ruled out
Azithromycin 1 g orally in a single dose
or
Doxycycline 100 mg orally bid a day for 7 days.

Uncomplicated Gonococcal Infections of the Pharynx

Ceftriaxone 125 mg IM in a single dose
or

Ciprofloxacin 500 mg orally in a single dose
plus
If Chlamydial infection is not ruled out
Azithromycin 1 g orally in a single dose
or
Doxycycline 100 mg orally bid for 7 days.

Gonococcal Conjunctivitis

Ceftriaxone 1 g IM in a single dose.
Note: Consider lavage of the infected eye with saline solution once.

Disseminated Gonococcal Infection (DGI)

Ceftriaxone 1 g IM or IV every 24 hours.
Alternative regimens
Cefotaxime 1 g IV every 8 hours,
or
Ceftizoxime 1 g IV every 8 hours,
or
Ciprofloxacin 400 gm IV every 12 hours,
or
Ofloxacin 400 mg IV every 12 hours,
or
Levofloxacin 250 mg IV daily,
or
Spectinomycin 2 g IM every 12 hours.
All of the preceding regimens should be continued for 24-48 hours after improvement begins, at which time therapy may be switched to one of the following regimens to complete at least 1 week of antimicrobial therapy.
Cefixime 400 mg orally bid daily,
or
Ciprofloxacin 500 mg orally bid daily,
or
Ofloxacin 400 mg orally bid daily
or
Levofloxacin 500 mg orally od daily

Gonococcal Meningitis and Endocarditis

Ceftriaxone 1-2 g IV every 12 hours
Therapy for meningitis should be continued for 10-14 days; therapy for endocarditis should be continued for at least 4 weeks. Treatment of complicated DGI should be undertaken in consultation with a specialist.

Ophthalmia Neonatorum Caused by N. gonorrhoeae

Ceftriaxone 25-50 mg/kg IV or IM in a single dose, not to exceed 125 mg.
Note: Topical antibiotic therapy alone is inadequate and is unnecessary if systemic treatment is administered.

Management of Sex Partners

All sex partners of patients who have *N.gonorrhoeae* infection should be evaluated and treated for *N.gonorrhoeae* and *C.trachomatis* infections if their last sexual contact with the patient was within 60 days before onset of symptoms or diagnosis of infection in the patient.

Follow Up

Treated patients with CDC regimen need not follow up to confirm their cure but the patient with persistent symptoms may be tested for antimicrobial susceptibility and other cause and treated accordingly.

References

1. Neinstein LS, Goldenring J, Carpender S. Nonsexual transmission of sexually transmitted diseases : an jnfrequent occurrence. Paediatrics 1984; 74: 67-76.
2. Disseminated gonococcal infection. Lancet 1984; I: 832-833.
3. Hook EW, Holmes KK. Gonococcal infection. Ann Intern Med 1985; 102: 229-243.
4. Hay RJ, Adriaans BM. Bacterial infection. In: Champion RH, Burton JL, Burns DA, Breathnach SM, eds. Rook Textbook of Dermatology. Oxford: Black well Science; 1998. p. 1140-1141.
5. Gonorrhoea in males. In: King A, Nicol C, Rodin P eds. Venereal diseases. 4th edn. London: ELBS; 1980. p. 200-213.
6. Feingold DS, Peacocke M. Gonorrhoea. In. Freedberg IM, Elisen AZ, Wolff K, et al. eds. Dermatology in general medicine. 5th edn. McGraw Hill: New York ,1999: 2598-2603.
7. Thin RN, Shav EJ. Diagnosis of gonorrhoea in women. Br J Vener Dis 1979; 55: 10-13.
8. Barlow D, Phillips. Gonorrhoea in women: Diagnosis clinical and laboratory aspects. Lancet 1978; 1: 761-764.
9. Tiwari VD, Talwar S, Grewal RS. Urethritis, pelvic

inflammatory disease and Reiter's disease. In: Valia RG, Valia AR, eds. IADVL Textbook and atlas of Dermatology. 2nd ed. Mumbai: Bhalani publishing house; 2001. p. 1423-1442.

10. Gonorrhoea . In: Dyck EV, Meheus AZ, Piot P, eds.. Laboratory diagnosis of sexually transmitted diseases. Geneva: WHO; 1999. p. 1-21.

11. Centre for Disease Control. Sexually Transmitted Diseases. Treatment guidelines. MMWR 2002; 51 (RR-6) : 36-42.

Chapter 21

Chlamydia Infections and Non-Gonococcal Urethritis

Sabyasachi Majumdar, G C Saha

Urethritis

The urethra is a tube like structure in the penis that carries urine from the urinary bladder to the opening of the penis. Urethritis refers to inflammation of urethra and presents with discharge, discomfort during urination, and burning micturition or itching at the end of the urethra. But there may be no noticeable signs of infection or inflammation at all. The confirmatory test is the finding of an increased number of polymorphonuclear leukocytes (PMNL) in the urethral smear or in the sediment of the first voided urine (FVU). If the cause of the inflamed urethra is gonococcus, then the inflammation is called gonococcal urethritis. If it is some other microorganism or another cause altogether, it is called non-gonococcal urethritis or NGU. The term 'non-gonoccocal' is preferred to 'non-specific' to describe the latter type of urethritis because it has specific causes, some of which have been elucidated.[1] The reason for using the latter term is to denote multifactorial aetiology. NGU occurring soon after curative therapy of gonorrhoea is called postgonococcal urethritis (PGU).

Non-Gonococcal Urethritis (NGU)

Historical Aspects

The Bible has said much about sexual behaviour, but it contains hardly any reference to sexually transmitted diseases. It may be for this reason, a passage from Leviticus is often quoted which in the authorised version reads: "when any man hath a running issue out of his flesh, because of this issue he is unclear". The word issue meant a discharge of matter from the body. The "running issue" might have been a genital discharge.[2] Celsus (25BC—50AD) described "profusio seminis as the shedding of semen, which occurs without sexual desire or erotic dreams, and in such a way that in time, the patient is consumed by wasting". Galen[2] (130-200 A.D.) coined the word gonorrhoea (Greek gonos, semen and rhoia, to flow).

During the early middle ages, an acute purulent urethritis was reported, first in Egypt and later in Europe.[2]

In the early 19th century it was believed that urethritis was due to either a venereal infection like gonorrhoea or to a non-specific inflammation which, although it might follow sexual intercourse was not strictly "venereal" because it could follow other events. Swediaur in 1805 introduced the word blennorrhagia, which meant any inflammation of genital mucosae.[3]

NGU after Neisser (1880-1970)

For the first few years after 1879 it was believed that all cases of acute urethritis were gonococcal,[4] but the invention of Gram staining and the development of culture systems during 1880s made the laboratory diagnosis of gonorrhoea more accurate; false positive results were reduced, and research papers on NGU began to appear. Gram positive diplococci, diphtheroids and coliforms were recovered not only from men with NGU, but from their sex partners as well.[2] Another line of enquiry began with the description of an "aseptic urethritis" in which conventional microscopy and culture failed to reveal any growth of microorganisms from the works of Waelsch (1901)[5] and Glingar (1914).[6] Later on, Lindner (1910) found inclusions in the urethral cells in about 40% of NGU patients and he suggested the possibility of a "genital trachoma".[7] Sadly, these pioneering studies were not pursued and were largely forgotten until, fifty years later, the importance of chlamydia in the pathogenesis of NGU and its complications was finally realized.

The inclusion urethritis was isolated in late 1950s by incubation of the yolk sac of chick embryos.[8] In 1966, Dunlop et al[9] described the NGU in more detail. At this time, the organisms now classified as *Chlamydia trachomatis* were often called 'TRIC agents' (TRachoma, Inclusion Conjunctivitis). The mycoplasmas were later additions (*Ureaplasma urealyticum* and *Mycoplasma hominis*). From time to time, other microbes were suggested[2] *Corynebacterium vaginale*, coagulase negative staphylococci, corynebacteria and *Hemophilus equigenitalis*. Recently, however, there has been some compelling evidence regarding *M. genitalium* in NGU.[10]

Aetiology

Acute NGU

Men with acute NGU can be categorized into those with or without *Chlamydia trachomatis* infection.[11] Study reports from late 1970's and early 1980s show that 35-50% of cases of NGU were due to *Chlamydia trachomatis* infection.[12-14] More recently chlamydial NGU cases have been found to be as low as 15%,[15] possibly because of the improvement in screening and treatment programmes for *C. trachomatis* during the past decade. Therefore, the majority of cases of NGU can be classified as non-chlamydial non-gonococcal urethritis (NCNGU). The probable or proven causative organisms for acute NGU are listed in Table 1.

Chronic NCNGU

It is defined as persistent or recurrent urethritis within 6 weeks following appropriate treatment for acute NGU in a man in whom reinfection or non-adherence to antimicrobial therapy is not suspected, and in whom *C. trachomatis* is not isolated. Men with NCNGU are more likely to develop chronic urethritis.[11] Although, no identifiable urethral pathogen can be identified in almost all cases. In addition, it is not known whether the syndromes of persistent NGU (PNGU) and recurrent NGU (RNGU) have different etiologies. The microbial organisms responsible for acute NCNGU have been

Table 1. Aetiology of NGU

Chlamydia trachomatis
Ureaplasma urealyticum
Mycoplasma genitalium
Trichomonas vaginalis

Other infectious causes
    Bacterial
                Staphylococcus saprophyticus
                Haemophilus species
                Bacteriodes ureolyticus
    Yeasts
    Viral
                Herpes simplex virus
                Adenovirus
Oral flora (oral insertive sex)[11]
    Neisseria meningitidis[16-18]
    Streptococcus pneumoniae[19]
Non-infectious causes
    Pre-existing urethral stricture
    Traumatic
    Chemical & Immunological
    Neoplastic
    Foreign body e.g. catheterisation
    Kidney transplantation
    Caffine, alcohol
    Altered sexual activity

isolated in several studies.[16-19] Chronic NCNGU is one of the most frustrating problems faced by patients and clinicians in STD clinics, almost like recurrent genital herpes.

The majority of current cases of acute NGU are not caused by *C. trachomatis*, and in fact, the aetiology is not ascertained in most cases. *U. urealyticun* has been implicated as a cause with stronger evidence for an association with a first episode of acute NCNGU than with subsequent episodes. *M. genitalium* appears to be a likely urogenital pathogen, but data are conflicting. Other organisms, including *T. vaginalis* cause a minority of cases. The aetiology of chronic NCNGU is even less clear.

Biology of Chlamydia trachomatis

Chlamydia trachomatis, an important human pathogen is one of the four species within the genus Chalmydia.[20] Chlamydia belong to order *Chlamydiales*, family *Chlamydiaceae* and has four species namely *C. trachomatis*, *C. psittaci*, *C. pneumoniae* and *C. pecorum*. *C. trachomatis* causes diseases in human, *C. psittaci* in birds & lower mammals, *C. pneumoniae* in humans and *C. pecorum* in sheep, cattle and swine. *C. trachomatis* has iodine-staining inclusions and is susceptible to sulfonamides, where as other species have no iodine staining inclusions and are not susceptible to sulfonamides. *C. trachomatis* is readily differentiated from others by two simple laboratory tests, but others can only be differentiated by DNA hybridization assays and by using monoclonal antibodies. There are about 18 serovars of chlamydia of which type A, B, C, L1, L2 and L3 are important pathogens.[21]

Human diseases caused by *C. trachomatis* are recognized since antiquity and are listed in Table 2. *C. trachomatis* was first visualized in 1907 by Halberstaedter and Prowazek[21] in stained conjunctival scrapings from orang utans and was first isolated in 1930 by Hellerstrom and Wassen.

Table 2.   Human Diseases Caused by Chlamydia

Species	Serovar	Disease
C. psittaci	Many unidentified serotypes	Psittacosis
C. peumoniae	TWAR	Respiratory disease
C. trachomatis	L1, L2, L3	Lymphogranuloma venereum (LGV)
C. trachomatis	A, B, Ba, C	Hyperendemic blinding trachoma
C. trachomatis	B, D, E, F, G, H, I, J, K	Inclusion conjunctivitis (adult and newborn) NGU Others

Morphology & Composition

Chlamydia are structurally complex microorganisms. They are obligate intracellular, prokaryotic parasites of eukaryotic cells and unequivocally established as one of the etiological agents in NGU. The organism has bacterial properties (Table 3) including replication by binary fission, possession of both DNA and RNA, a discrete peptidoglycan cell wall and membranes biochemically similar to that of gram negative bacteria,[22] protein synthesis via ribosomes, and susceptibility to certain antibiotics. However, their cell walls do not contain significant quantities of muramic acid. The chlamydial cell wall consists of subunits approximately 20 nm in diameter arranged in a regular geometric pattern. The outer membrane of Chlamydia contains a Major outer membrans protein[21] which is approximately 30% of the weight of the organism and approximately 60% of the weight of the outer membrane. The size of this protein varies by serovar, with a molecular weight

Table 3.   Comparative Features of Chlamydia, Bacteria and Viruses

Feature	Chlamydia	Bacteria	Virus
Size (< 500 nm)	+	–	+
Cell Wall	+	+	–
DNA & RNA	+	+	DNA or RNA
Ribosomes	+	+	–
Metabolism	+	+	–
Energy production	–	+	–
Antibiotic inhibition	+	+	–
Obligate intracellular organisms	+	–	+

range of 38-43 kDa.[23] It appears to be a major structural protein and functions in maintenance of the structural integrity of cell wall. It is cysteine rich protein linked by disulfide bonds to itself and two other proteins.[21]

The chemical composition of the organism is approximately 35% protein and 40-50% lipid with both RNA and DNA, RNA being more in reticulate bodies. Chlamydia do not appear to be able to utilise thymidine,[24] and there is no detectable thymidine kinase.[25] Chlamydia appear to contain a number of penicillin binding proteins. The lack of muramic acid and peptidoglycan does not seem to interfere with the effects of penicillins. The inclusion bodies contain glycogen and that is why they are stained with iodine. A complex life cycle includes two distinct forms: an elementary body (EB) and a reticulate body (RB) being the infective and metabolically active states respectively. EB has a diameter of 200-300 nm, is gram negative, heat labile (inactivated by heat at 56°C, ethyl alcohol, phenol and formalin) and can be preserved at −70°C with lyophilisation. RB has a diameter of 500-1000 nm and has less disulfide bridges between MOMP and other cysteine-rich proteins in the cell wall.[21] Electron micrographs have shown regular arrangement of spikelike protuberances, which occur in only a limited area of EB.[21] EB-RB forms are specially adapted for extracellular survival, cell to cell transfer and intracellular growth.

Developmental Cycle

It is the developmental cycle of chlamydia that sets them apart from all other bacteria. The cycle comprises the following steps:

1.   Initial attachment of the EB or infectious particle to the host cell.

2. Entry into the cell.
3. Morphologic change of the EB into the RB with intracellular growth and replication.
4. Morphologic change of the RB to the EB.
5. Release of the infectious particle or EB.

Growth & Culture

As chlamydia are obligatory parasites, it is necessary to supply a living host cell to support their growth. The organism can be recovered from patients in 48-72 hours.[21] The growth of chlamydia within the cell requires that the cell receive its essential nutrients. It has been observed that the growth of chlamydia in cell culture can be regulated by the amino acid concentration in the medium. The most commonly used procedure involves treatment of the host cell with cycloheximide before or after centrifugation of the inoculum.[26] *C. psittaci* requires isoleucine, valine and phenylalanine[27] while *C. trachomatis* appears to require histidine.[28] Cyclic AMP (cAMP) inhibits chlamydial growth and the action has been shown on the RB to EB transformation.[29]

Immunology

There is little knowledge about the structure and chemical composition of chlamydial antigens. The biological role of antibodies or cell-mediated immunity (CMI) resulting from exposure to chlamydial antigens in either enhancing or protecting against disease or infection is also not yet clear. The most easily detected antigen is the chlamydial group antigen,[21] shared by all members of the genus and is responsible for the complement fixing reactions. Chlamydial EB and RB contain a lipopolysaccharide (LPS) antigenically similar to that of some gram negative bacteria and it demonstrates a positive limulus lysate test. Chlamydial LPS has two antigen sites. One is identical to that of *Acinetobacter calcoaceticus* and *Salmonella typhimurium* while the other is chlamydia specific.[21]

The sub species or serovar specific antigens are common only to selected strains within the chlamydial species. Till now, 18 serovars of *C. trachomatis* have been identified. Serovar specific monoclonal antibody (MoAb) is now available for typing purposes. The MOMP appears to contain antigens of serovar, serogroup and species specificity.[30] MoAb directed against MOMP are capable of neutralising infectivity in cell culture and are protective against toxic effects.

Immunity

Immunity induced by chlamydial infection is not well understood. It is not the single infection but multiple, often homo or heterotypic infection which will result in solid immunity to reinfection. Unfortunately, the natural infection is not readily quantifiable in terms of inoculum size and thus relative degrees of immunity may exist. However, some immunity probably develops following initial or serial infection.

There are now many in vitro studies[21] showing that immunization with purified, synthesized, or recombinant peptides can induce neutralising antibodies. Synthetic vaccines have also been developed, sometimes by artificially juxtaposing synthesized conjugates of T-helper sites with selected B-cell sites predicted to result in neutralizing antibody and finding that such antibodies are indeed generated. Chlamydia do not appear to survive well in polymorphonuclear leukocytes (PMNL). It is possible that antibody enhanced phagocytosis plays an important role in clearance of infection and in resistance to infection. Chlamydia are rapidly internalized by human PMNL and the majority are rendered non-infectious within an hour. Most of the EB are found in PMNL phagosomes where lysosomal fusion has occurred. The mechanism of killing by PMNL is not known, but both oxygen dependent and oxygen independent mechanisms may be involved, and it is also active in presence of inhibitors such as azide or cyanide.

Leukocytes play an important role in resistance to infection and in clearance of primary infection. Results of different studies[21] have suggested a defense role for both antibody and CMI responses. Both CD4+ and CD8+ T-cells have protective roles in animal models. The predominant accummulating evidence suggests that Th1-type cell responses involving CD4+ T-helper cells are likely to play an important role in protective immunity.[31,32] However, the actual mechanism is not clear, and the demonstration of cytotoxic CD8+ T-cells capable of lysing chlamydia infected cells suggests their role too.[33]

Chlamydial NGU in Adults

It has already been stated that *C. trachomatis* is the main causative organism of NGU in adults. Since the early 1970s, *C. trachomatis* has been recognized as a genital pathogen for a variety of clinical syndromes (Table 4).

Table 4. Clinical Syndromes Caused by *C. trachomatis*

	Site of infection	Clinical syndrome
Men	Urethra	NGU, PGU
	Epididymis	Epididymitis (Infertility)
	Systemic	Reiter's Syndrome
Women	Urethra	Urethritis (NGU/NSU)
	Bartholin's glands	Bartholinitis
	Cervix	Cervicitis
	Fallopian tubes	Salpingitis
		Ectopic pregnancy (spontaneous abortion)
	Uterus	Endometritis
	Liver	Perihepatitis
	Systemic	Arthritis
		Dermatitis
Both	Conjunctiva	Conjunctivitis
	Heart	Endocarditis
	Pharynx	Pharyngitis
	Inguinal lymph nodes	LGV
	Rectum	Proctitis
	Large intestine	Crohn's disease
	Systemic	Sexually acquired reactive arthritis (SARA)
Infants & Children	Conjunctiva	Conjunctivitis
		Trachoma
	Lung	Pneumonia
		Chronic lung disease
	GIT	Gastroenteritis

Epidemiology

NGU is prevalent all over the world. In STD clinics in USA, the incidence of NGU varies from 19-78%.[1] On college campuses, more than 85% of urethritis were nongonococcal. The peak age group affected is 20-24 years. In another study at Victoria, Australia,[34] it was found that patients were primarily adolescents or young adults, 66% were women; men were commonly asymptomatic. The World Health Organization (WHO) estimates that 89 million new cases of genital chlamydial infections occurred worldwide in 1995.[35] In the United States, 4-5 million cases of chlamydial infection occur annually.[36] In a study of 113 patients with NGU and 89 men with gonorrhoea, it was seen that NGU patients were more often white, better educated, more likely to be students and less likely to be unemployed, members of a higher socio economic status, older at first intercourse and had fewer sex partners.[37] However, owing to limited laboratory facilities and difficulty in diagnosis, the exact incidence of NGU in India is difficult to assess.[1]

Clinical Features

Method of Spread

There is, little doubt that this condition is spread by sexual intercourse, but clearly, this opinion is based only on epidemiological experience. However, *C. trachomatis* is often recovered from women whose sexual partners have chlamydial urethritis, but seldom from those whose partners have NCNGU.

Clinical Course

The incubation period is highly variable. Although it is considerd as 1-3 weeks, shorter and considerably longer incubation periods are also described.

The usual presentation is with low grade urethritis with scanty or moderate mucoid or mucopurulent urethral discharge and variable dysuria, but in a majority of cases the appearance of the discharge and the severity of the condition make it clinically indistinguishable from gonococcal urethritis. In a small number of cases the discharge is accompanied by haematuria and symptoms of cystitis, when it is usually called 'acute abacterial haemorrhagic cystitis'. On the other hand, subclinical urethritis tends to be common. The patient does not notice the condition but it may be found in course of routine examination or when the patient presents with complications.

Infections in Men

The prevalence of chlamydial urethral infection ranges from 3-5% of asymptomatic men seen in the general medical settings to 15-20% of all men seen in STD clinics.[38,39] Of 1221 patients screened for urethral infection in a STD clinic, 5% and 14% of homosexual and heterosexual men respectively had positive urethral cultures for *C. trachomatis*.[1] Serologic studies showed that chlamydial infection increased with age in homosexuals, but appeared relatively constant with increasing age in heterosexual and bisexual men. The incidence of chlamydial infections in men has not been well defined since in most countries, these infections either not reported or microbiologically diagnosed or being asymptomatic, escape attention.

Urethritis

Clinically it is very difficult to differentiate between

chlamydia positive and chlamydia negative NGU on the basis of signs and symptoms. Both usually present after a 7 to 21 day incubation period with dysuria and mild to moderate whitish or clear urethral discharge. Examination reveals no abnormalities other than discharge in most cases, associated adenopathy, focal urethral tenderness and meatal or penile lesions should suggest herpetic urethritis. Neither abnormal prostatic examination nor prostatic inflammation have been convincingly linked with chlamydial urethritis.[40]

Post-gonococcal urethritis (PGU) occurring in heterosexual men, like NGU frequently results from *C. trachomatis*. These patients probably acquire gonorrhoea and chlamydial infection simultaneously but because of the longer incubation period of the latter, develop a biphasic illness if the gonorrhoea is treated with an agent that does not eradicate chlamydia. This has given rise to the development of the concept of syndromic approach.

Littritis

This is inflammation of Littre's glands, which are present in the wall of the urethra. It is probably inevitable in the course of any urethral infection.

Epididymitis

It has been proposed that *C. trachomatis* causes most cases of what was previously termed idiopathic epididymitis in young, heterosexually active males. Clinically, chlamydial epididymitis presents as unilateral scrotal pain, swelling, tenderness and fever in a young male who often has associated chlamydial urethritis. The urethritis, however, may often be asymptomatic and evident only as urethral inflammation on Gram stain. Men with chlamydial epididymitis improve rapidly with tetracycline treatment, supporting the causal role of *C. trachomatis*. However, one must exclude epididymo-orchitis, testicular torsion and malignancy before treatment.

Prostatitis

It should be more accurately called prostatovesiculitis due to simultaneous involvement of seminal vesicles. Despite several studies, the role of *C. trachomatis* in causing non-bacterial prostatitis (NBP) remains unclear[40], with NBP being the most common form of prostatic inflammation (40-60% of all prostatitis).[41] Some authors[42]

point to an autoimmune aetiology and the role of urine reflux into the canaliculi of the gland causing chemical inflammation. The patient is generally asymptomatic, or may present with discomfort on passing urine and vague pain in the perineum, groins, thighs, penis, suprapubic region or back. There may also be painful ejaculation.

Proctitis

The clinical manifestations of rectal infection in infants and adult women have not been studied extensively. The clinical syndrome in homosexual men usually presents with subacute manifestations like proctocolitis and hyperplasia of intestinal and perirectal lymphoid tissue (lymphorrhoids) or late/chronic manifestations such as perirectal abscesses, ischiorectal fistula and rectal stricture or stenosis.

In men the rectal mucosa can be infected directly with chlamydia during receptive anal intercourse or by lymphatic spread from the male posterior urethra. Most *C. trachomatis* infected patients have abnormal numbers of PMNL in their rectal mucous on Gram stain and on sigmoidoscopy, those with symptoms exhibit friable rectal mucosa and mucopus. In the pre-AIDS era, *C. trachomatis* appeared to be responsible for up to 15% of proctitis seen in homosexual males.[56]

Reiter's Syndrome

Both Reiter's syndrome (urethritis, conjunctivitis, arthritis and characteristic mucocutaneous lesions) and reactive tenosynovitis or sexually acquired reactive arthritis (SARA) without the other components of Reiter's syndrome has been related to genital infection with *C. trachomatis*. Studies of untreated men with characteristic Reiter's syndrome using the micro-immunofluorescent antibody assay (micro-IF) indicate that preceding or concurrent infection with *C. trochomatis* is present in more than 80% of cases. The class I HLA-B27 haplotype appears to confer a tenfold increased risk of developing Reiter's Syndrome, and 60-70% of persons with the syndrome are HLA-B27 positive.

Infections in Women

Cervicitis

The prevalence of chlamydial infections has ranged from 3-5% in asymptomatic women to over 20%

of those attending STD clinics. The incidence of *C. trachomatis* infection in women is even less well-defined[1] than in men because the former produces no specific symptom, is rarely confirmed microbiologically and is not reported. Virtually no data on incidence is available. *C. trachomatis* causes cervicitis and is responsible for 60% of pelvic inflammatory disease (PID)[43] in Northern European countries. Genital tract infection in women is usually asymptomatic as compared to 5-10% of men attending genitourinary medicine (GUM) clinics.[44]

Although women with chlamydia isolated from the cervix are usually asymptomatic, at least one third of them generally have signs of infection on gynaecological examination. The most common presentation is a mucopurulent discharge (37%) and hypertrophic ectopy (19%).[40] The latter refers to an area of ectopy, which is oedematous, congested, and bleeds easily. The number of PMNL in cervical mucous is correlated with chlamydial infection of the cervix.[40] There appears to be a wide range of normal leukocyte values in women without cervical infection, possibly due to the influence of the menstrual cycle, contraceptive practices, sexual activity and other infections. One study[45] showed that on univariate analysis age, combined oral contraceptives and ectropian were risk factors for the laboratory detection of *C. trachomatis*. There was a reported association between the week of the menstrual cycle and the detection of *C. trachomatis*.[45] *C. trachomatis* was detected more often in the later part of the cycle, but others have found no such association.[46–48] The variation in the detection of *C. trachomatis* with the menstrual cycle could be either due to a direct hormonal effect on chlamydial replication or alternatively, an indirect effect acting through local immune factors, or a combination of both.[45]

Clinical recognition of chlamydial cervicitis depends on a high index of suspicion and a careful cervical examination. There are hardly any genital symptoms, which can specifically be correlated with chlamydial cervical infection. The clinical findings on examination suggestive of chlamydial infection include easily induced endocervical bleeding, mucopurulent endocervical discharge and oedema within an area of ectopy. The differential diagnosis of mucopurulent discharge from the endocervical canal in young, sexually active women include gonococcal endocervicitis, salpingitis, endometritis and IUCD induced inflammation. Gram stain of appropriately collected mucopurulent endocervical discharge from patients having chlamydial endocervicitis usually shows more than 30 PMNL per × 1000 field, absence of gonococci and occasional other bacteria.[40] Nearly all women with endocervical chlamydial infection have or develop antibodies to *C. trachomatis* in serum (20-30% have IgM antibody) assessed by micro-IF assay.

Urethritis

C. trachomatis can be cultured from both cervix and urethra in 50% of cases and either site alone in 25% of cases. The usual presenting complaint is dysuria, frequency and pyuria. Although urethral symptoms may develop in some women with chlamydial infection, the majority of female STD clinic patients with chlamydial urethritis do not have dysuria or frequency and even the signs of urethritis (urethral discharge, meatal erythema or oedema) are infrequent. However, the presence of mucopurulent cervicitis in a woman with dysuria and frequency should suggest the diagnosis.

Bartholinitis

C. trachomatis may produce an exudative infection of Bartholin's ducts in a way similar to gonococci. Purulent Bartholinitis may be owing to chlamydial infection, either alone or with simultaneous gonococcal infection or some anaerobic organisms viz. *Bacteroides* spp.

Endometritis

Histological evidence of endometritis, often with immunohistological and or cultural evidence of *C. trachomatis* is present in about 50% of patients suffering from chlamydial mucopurulent cervicitis and in almost all patients having chlamydial salpingitis. There may also be associated abnormal vaginal bleeding, menorrhagia and metrorrhagia. Chlamydial endometritis is characterized by infiltration of the endometrial stroma by plasma cells and infiltration of the endometrial superficial epithelium by PMNL. Besides nonpuerperal endometritis, association of intrapartum fever and late post-partum endometritis with untreated antenatal *C. trachomatis* infection has been suggested.

Salpingitis

The proportion of acute salpingitis due to *C. trachomatis* varies geographically and with the population studied. Cases of chlamydial salpingitis are usually associated with mild or absent symptoms and signs. Despite progressive tubal scarring, they result in ectopic pregnancy and infertility, thus giving rise to the term "silent salpingitis".

Perihepatitis (Fitz-Hugh-Curtis Syndrome)

Previously, perihepatitis occuring after or with salpingitis was considered a complication of gonococcal infection. But studies in the last 15 years suggest that chlamydial infection is in fact more commonly associated with perihepatitis than is *N. gonorrhoeae*.[40] Perihepatitis should be suspected in young, sexually active women who develop right upper quadrant pain, fever, nausea or vomiting. It may present as an acute abdomen, and may also mimic acute cholecystitis. A recent study has demonstrated that perihepatitis is strongly associated with extensive tubal scarring, adhesions, and inflammation observed at laparoscopy as well as with high titres of antibody to the 57-kDa chlamydial heat shock protein.

Infection in Pregnancy

Chlamydial infection in pregnancy can cause (1) spontaneous abortion, (2) neonatal conjunctivitis, (3) low birth weight (LBW) (4) prematurity and (5) preterm delivery. Postnatal infection can cause (1) neonatal conjunctivitis, (2) ophthalmia neonatorum, (3) pneumonia and (4) chronic lung or eye diseases.

Diagnosis

Many diagnostic tests for *C. trachomatis* have been available over the past decade, from antigen detection by monoclonal or polyclonal antibodies to molecular biologic methods.[11] The bedside diagnostic test, "Two glass test of urine", however, still remains an effective clue.

Cell Culture

In earlier days, cell culture had been the gold standard test for detection of *C trachomatis* over the years. Being an intracellular pathogen, *C. trachomatis* requires a cell culture system for propagation in the laboratory. However, its stringent requirements both in terms of technical expertise and specimen transport make cell culture impractical in settings in which neither a cold chain

nor a cell culture system can be maintained. Further, a carefully collected sample of columnar epithelial cells from the cervix or urethra is necessary and specimens composed purely of PMNL or mucopurulent discharge are inadequate. For culture, specimens may be collected with a cotton tipped swab (wooden sticks are not recommended as they are inhibitory to chlamydial growth). For endocervical specimens, a cytobrush may increase the culture sensitivity due to collection of more cells. Specimens must be placed in specific transport media and kept refrigerated until they are inoculated within 24 hours onto cell culture plates. Cell culture has the benefit of an excellent specificity while the sensitivity is now recognized to be less than optimal.[49] The cell line cultures used for isolation are HeLa 229 and McCoy cell lines.[50]

Owing to the inadequacies, cost and technical difficulties of cell culture, the development of non-culture tests has been a major research priority over the past 15 years. As a result, many non-culture non-invasive diagnostic tests for *C. trachomatis* are now commercially available, which can be classified as follows:

1. Antigen detection tests.
2. Nucleic acid hybridization.
3. Nucleic acid amplification.
4. Urethral lymphocyte isolation.

Antigen Detection Tests

Detection of a urethral chlamydial infection has been traditionally performed by testing urethral swabs with epithelial cells from the mucous membrane.[11] The procedure is painful and inconvenient to the patient. The recommended alernatives include antigen detection tests which use monoclonal or polyclonal antibody against chlamydial lipopolysaccharide (LPS) or MOMP,[49] as a means of detecting chlamydial EB in genital specimens. The most widely used of these assays are the direct immunofluorescence assay (DFA) and enzyme immunoassay (EIA). The DFA has a sensitivity of 80-85%, but overall sensitivity depends both on the experience of the person performing the test and on collection of an adequate specimen. The specificity of DFA is very high (>99%). EIA is one of the most commonly used tests for chlamydial diagnosis. It is evaluated on FVU or first catch urine (FCU; the first 10-30 ml of stream) for the rapid detection of chlamydia in infected symptomatic men.[11] Although EIA is easy to perform with an automatic test procedure, its sensitivity is influenced by the amount of antigen present in urine. Sensitivity of EIA generally is in the range of 60-80%.[40] In another study, it was reported that DFA and EIA have sensitivities from 64-100% with specificities from 89-100%.[51] It is a rapid test requiring less than 30 minutes from sample collection to result, does not require specialised equipment or extensive training and can be used 'on site'. Its cost is £ 2.62 (approx. Rs. 200/-) per patient. It is useful if used as an adjunct to the routine screening tests.[51,52]

Nucleic acid hybridization technique

An alternative diagnostic test to EIA for screening of *C. trachomatis* uses nucleic acid hybridization, commercially available as PAGE 2 assay by Genprobe. It detects but does not amplify chlamydial nucleic acid and results on endocervical and urethral specimens are comparable to that of DFA and the best EIAs.

Nucleic acid amplification assays

The most exciting recent development in chlamydial diagnostic procedures has been that of automated methods for the detection of amplified *C. trachomatis* DNA or RNA. The two most widely used methods are ligase chain reaction (LCR) and polymerase chain reaction (PCR), both of which can be used for cervical, urethral and urine specimens from both males and females. Although the PCR uses primers, nucleotides and the enzyme taq-polymerase, the LCR is based on the ligation of oligonucleotide probes that serve as a copy of the original target sequence and are immediately adjacent to each other.[11] The specificity of these tests has consistently been above 99%, as they can detect small amounts of chlamydial DNA.[11] Another methodology, transcription-mediated amplification assay, amplifies RNA sequences and replaces the DNA/RNA hybridization test PAGE 2 for the diagnosis of *C. trachomatis*.[11]

POLYMERASE CHAIN REACTION (PCR)

The first commercially used PCR for chlamydial diagnosis uses an endogenous 207 based plasmid target DNA sequence and has been compared to culture in a variety of clinical studies in Europe and United States, with a sensitivity of 87.1%-97.4% for FVU compared with cell culture. The test has detected upto approximately 40% more infections than urethral culture in some studies. However, in one study PCR performed on male urine specimens was significantly less sensitive than LCR, owing to PCR specific inhibitors present in fresh urine. Among females, PCR performed on FCU has demonstrated a sensitivity of 82-93%.[79] Unexpectedly, performance of PCR on endocervical specimens has been variable, with sensitivities ranging from 60-92%.

LIGASE CHAIN REACTION (LCR)

It was first described in 1989 and it can be performed on urine specimens in men and women, thus providing a non-invasive technique for chlamydial testing.[53] The sensitivity of LCR on urine range from 85.4%-96.4% in different studies depending on whether cell culture or an expanded gold standard was used for calculations.[54] Its sensitivity performed on endocervical specimens has ranged from 81-100%. In another study, the performance of LCR assay was as follows: its sensitivity was 100%, 91% and 95% respectively for cervical, vaginal and urine samples for women, when compared with DFA staining of cervical samples and 100% and 91% respectively, for urethral and urine samples for men, when compared with DFA staining of urethral smears. An EIA has only 65% sensitive for cervical samples.

The advantage of using PCR or LCR method is that these methods allow simultaneous detection of more than one STD agents.[55] The use of PCR and LCR has increased the percentage of infected people detected compared with previously used methods e.g. DIF and EIA.[53] The ability of chlamydial diagnostic tests e.g. EIA and LCR to identify positive women should be similar among the patients attending a GUM clinic and those taking part in a population screening programme; and a sensitive molecular assay e.g. LCR, should identify subjects with a low organism load in both groups.

Urethral Lymphocyte Isolation

Shahmanesh et al[56] described this method. Urethral lymphocytes were extracted from FVU of patients with NGU and gonococcal urethritis (GU) using magnetic beads coated with antibody against either the pan-T cell marker CD2 or CD4.

Urethral exudate from patients with NCNGU contains significantly less CD2+ lymphocytes (as pan-T lymphocytic marker also present on natural killer

(NK cells) compared with those in whom *C. trachomatis* was isolated. There is increasing evidence for a potential role of CD4+ and even CD8+ cells in host defence against chlamydial infection.

Serologic techniques[40]

Serologic tests have not been widely used for the diagnosis of chlamydial genital tract infection other than LGV. The major problems for this issue are as follows:

1. The baseline prevalence of antibody in populations of sexually active persons who are at the risk of *C. trachomatis* infection is high (45-65%). The high prevalence of seropositivity in culture negative, asymptomatic patients probably reflects either previous infection or persisting, chronic, asymptomatic infection not easily detectable by current culture techniques.

2. The lack of an abrupt onset of symptoms in a lot of chlamydia infected patients means that they are seen during periods when IgM antibody or rising or falling titres of IgG antibody could not be demonstrated. Thus, the serologic parameters of recently acquired infection are often absent.

3. Superficial genital tract infection e.g. urethritis and cervicitis, generally produces micro IF antibody titres in the range of 1:8 to 1:256, but rarely higher. 60% of men with NGU who were initially seronegative but later develop IgG antibody to chlamydia, have titres 1:8 to 1:32 and the rest 40% between 1:64 and 1:256. Women with salpingitis and perihepatitis have even higher titres, over 1:256 and 1:1024 respectively.

4. Cross reacting antibody developing to *Chlamydia pneumoniae* may obscure serodiagnosis.

The summary of the diagnostic criteria in different clinical syndromes in men and women are given in Tables 5 and 6.

Table 5. Diagnosis of *C. Trachomatis* in Men

Clinical syndrome	Clinical criteria	Laboratory criteria	
		Presumptive	Diagnostic
NGU	Dysuria, urethral discharge	Urethral GS* with >5 PMNL/ HPF (× 1000) Pyuria on FVU	Positive culture or nonculture tests (urethra or FVU)
Acute epididymitis	Fever, epididymal or testicular pain, evidence of NGU, epididymal tenderness or mass	As for NGU	As for NGU; Positive test on epididymal aspirate
Acute proctitis (Non-LGV stain)	Rectal pain, discharge, bleeding, abnormal anoscopy (mucopurulent discharge, pain, spontaneous or induced bleeding)	Rectal GS with >1 PMNL / HPF (× 1000)	Positive culture or direct FA (rectal)
Acute proctocolitis (LGV strain)	Severe rectal pain, discharge, hematochezia, markedly abnormal anoscopy (as above) with lesions extending to colon; fever, lymphadenopathy	Rectal GS with > 1 PMNL/ HPF (× 1000)	Positive culture or direct FA (rectal), complement fixation antibody litre

*GS = Gram Stain; PMNL = Polymorphonuclear leukocytes; NGU = Non-gonococcal urethritis, HPF = High-power Field; FA = Fluorescent antibody; FVU = First void urine; LGV = Lymphogranuloma venereum.

Approach to Management

As with any clinical complaint, one important goal of treatment is the alleviation of symptoms. However, while approaching STD, the health of the individual, the sexual partner and the community have to be considered so that the appropriate management goes beyond simply treating the infection. Management of patients with urethritis also includes the following:

1. Screening for other treatable STD.
2. Counselling and offering serologic testing for HIV.

Table 6.　Diagnosis of *C. Trachomatis* Infections in Women[40]

Clinical Syndrome	Clinical criteria	Laboratory criteria	
		Presumptive	Diagnostic
Mucopurulent cervicitis	Mucopurulent cervical discharge, cervical ectopy and oedema, spontaneous or easily induced cervical bleeding	Cervical GS★ with > 30 PMNL/HPF (× 1000) in NMW.	Positive culture or non-culture test (cervix, FVU).
Acute urethral syndrome	Dysuria–frequency syndrome in young, sexually active women, recent new sex partner, often > 7 days of symptoms.	Pyuria no bacteria.	As above
PID	Lower abdominal pain; adnexal tenderness on pelvic exam; evidence of MPC often present.	As for MPC; cervical GS positive for gonococcus. Endometritis on endometrial biopsy.	Positive culture or non-culture test (cervix, FVU, endometrium, tubal).
Perihepatitis	Right upper quadrant pain, nausea, vomiting, fever, young sexually active women; evidence of PID.	As for MPC and PID.	High titre IgM or IgG antibody to *C. trachomatis*

★GS = Gram stain; PMNL = Polymorphonuclear leukocytes; HPF = High power field; NMW = Non-menstruating women; PID = Pelvic inflammatory disease; MPC = Mucopurulent cervicitis.

3. Identifying and referring infected partners for treatment.
4. Counselling on risk behaviour reduction to prevent future STD.

In most of the industrialized world, the standard management and treatment of STD are based on laboratory diagnosis. But nowadays, the approach based on the recognition of syndromes and treatment of all prevalent curable causes (Syndromic Approach) is stressed in the developing world where resources are limited. In syndromic management, treatment of urethritis (dysuria or clinical evidence of urethral discharge) consists of antibiotic therapy directed against both *N. gonorrhoeae* and *C. trachomatis* without performing diagnostic tests. However, this approach still requires etiologic testing in sample populations to monitor local disease prevalence, as well as susceptibility testing of *N. gonorrhoeae* to monitor antibiotic resistance patterns. The current CDC STD treatment guidelines recommend identification of the etiologic agent of urethritis by testing for the presence of both gonorrhoea and chlamydia whenever possible to facilitate partner notification and public health intervention.[57] Syndromic management of urethritis in the industrialized countries is recommended only when diagnostic testing is not available. Management decisions based entirely on clinical experience e.g. belief that a mucoid appearance rather than a purulent appearance of urethral discharge makes gonorrhoea impossible, is discouraged in any setting.

The recommended therapy for NGU[58] includes the following:

Azithromycin 1 g orally in a single dose or doxycycline 100 mg bid for 7 days.

The alternative regimens are:

Erythromycin base 500 mg orally qid for 7 days, or Erythromycin ethyl succinate 800 mg qid for 7 days, or

Ofloxacin 300 mg bid for 7 days.

For recurrent and persistent urethritis, the recommended regimens are metronidazole 2g p.o, single dose plus erythromycin base 500 mg orally qid for 7 days, or

Erythromycin ethyl succinate 800 mg qid for 7 days.

The single dose directly observed therapy has a definite advantage in patients at high risk for non-compliance. But the higher cost of azithromycin (Rs. 100-370 per case) compared with doxycycline (Rs.50-90 per one week course of therapy) may limit its prescription among poor patients. While prescribing azithromycin, one must advise the individual to abstain from sex for 7 days after receiving therapy because earlier resumption of sexual activity with use of single-dose therapy is a concern and could theoretically result in transmission of an unresolved infection to sex partners.

In women with mucopurulent cervicitis the recommended regimen is azithromycin 1 g orally in a single dose, or doxycycline 100 mg bid for 7 days. The alternative regimens are

Erythromycin base 500 mg orally qid for 7 days, or
Erythromycin ethyl succinate 800 mg qid for 7 days, or
Ofloxacin 300 mg bid for 7 days, or
Levofloxacin 500mg orally for seven days.

In children who weigh less than 45 kgs erythromycin base or ethylsuccinate 50 mg/ kg/ day orally divided into four doses daily for 14 days and in children who weigh more than 45 kgs but who are less than 8 years old azithromycin 1 g orally in single dose are advised. For children who are of more than 8 years of age adult dosage is recommended.

Treatment recommendations of NACO[1]

Uncomplicated Non-gonococcal Infections (urethral, endocervical and rectal)

1. Doxycycline 100 mg bid × 7 days, or
2. Tetracycline 500 mg qid × 7 days, or
3. Erythromycin stearate 500 mg qid × 7 days, or
4. Sulfisoxasole 100 mg qid × 10 days, in order of preference.

Neonatal Non-gonococal Conjunctivitis

1. Erythromycin syrup 50 mg/kg/day in four divided doses for 2 weeks, or
2. Trimethioprim 40 mg/sulfamethoxazole 200 mg/kg/day two divided does × 2 weeks

Infantile Pneumonia

Treatment regimens are like that for conjunctivitis, for 3 weeks.

Treatment of Sexual Partners

Although not clearly demonstrated, treatment of sexual partners definitely diminishes the rate of recurrence of NGU. Thus, this treatment is essential for the patients own benefit. Infected women are considered as a huge reservoir of *C. trachomatis,* undiagnosed and untreated.

Control of increasing incidence of NGU is very difficult to achieve without attacking this reservoir.

Ureaplasma Urealyticum Infection

The most likely cause of NCNGU is *Ureaplasma urealyticum.* The incidence in normal controls increases sharply with the number of female sex partners.[59] There are at least 14 serotypes of *U. urealyticum* and it is possible that only one or several types produce urethritis. Some groups have demonstrated an association with serovars. The association between PGU and *U. urealyticum* is weak as compared to *C. trachomatis.*

Regarding antimicrobial therapy, one must remember that sulfonamides and rifampicin are active against *C. trachomatis* but not against *U. urealyticum* whereas spectinomycin and streptomycin are active against the latter but not against the former. As selective eradication of *U. urealyticum* is important, azithromycin and minocycline or a combination therapy may be another option.

Recurrent or Persistent NGU

This is a challenging situation to a venereologist, as recurrent genital herpes. Despite trials of several antimicrobials, the condition persists. After a careful history regarding compliance and sexual habits, the following guidelines[1] may prove useful:

1. Take a saline preparation of the exudate and microscopy or culture for *T. vaginalis.*
2. Check for fungus in a 10% KOH preparation.
3. Exclude urethral foreign bodies, periurethral fistulae and abscesses.
4. Rule out *N. gonorrhoeae* by repeated culture.
5. Rule out any persistent herpes simplex virus infection.
6. If tetracycline-resistant *U. urealyticum* is suspected, a course of erythromycin 500 mg qid for 1-2 weeks may be useful.
7. If the individual is negative for the *C. trachomatis* and *U. urealyticum*, an empirical course of doxycycline 100 mg daily for 4-6 weeks may be tried.
8. Rule out any prostatic infection.

Prognosis

The natural history of NGU suggests that it is a self

limiting disease even without treatment. Nowadays, the local complications are relatively uncommon as compared to the premicrobial era. Complications are similar to those seen in gonorrhoea but milder. Dissemination, however, to other sites is known. 1-2% of both *C. trachomatis* positive and negative individuals develop epididymitis and another 1-2% develop conjunctivitis.[60] The frequency of NGU patients developing Reiter's disease and SARA is also very low; however, its rate can be decreased by initiating therapy in both chlamydial NGU and NCNGU patients, even in HLA-B27-positive individuals. In certain individuals, NGU creates significant psychologic turmoil and counselling a by psychologist is needed.

Prevention

In a very simple way, prevention of NGU can be summarised as follows:

1. Prevention by the Clinician

- Early diagnosis and institution of treatment.
- Treatment of both gonococcal urethritis and NGU simultaneously.
- Contact tracing and adequate treatment of partners.
- Increasing diagnostic facilities.

2. Prevention by the Individual

- Avoidance of sexual promiscuity, and careful selection of partner.
- Use of condoms.
- Prompt treatment[61]

But the prevention of NGU does not end here. Since many chlamydial infections are asymptomatic, it is clear that effective control must involve periodic testing of individuals at risk. Contact tracing or partner notification is considered an essential element of STD control alongside medical management and health education.[62] National guidelines on the management of genital infection with *C. trachomatis* should include contact tracing as an essential part of patient care.

The cost of extensive screening may be prohibitory. Thus, development of an approach to define target populations at increased risk is needed. One such strategy is to designate the patients attending specific high prevalence clinic populations for universal testing such as STD, GUM, juvenile detention and some family planning clinics. This approach, however, fails to account for the majority of asymptomatic infections, since attendees at high prevalence clinics often do so because of symptoms or suspicion of infection. Consequently, selective screening have been developed for use in various clinical settings. Among females, young age (usually <21 years) is a critical risk factor for chlamydial infection. Other risk factors include the presence of mucopurulent cervicitis, multiple, new or symptomatic male sex partners and the lack of barrier contraceptive use.

Among asymptomatic males, risk factors for chlamydial infection have been less extensively explored and the effectiveness of screening programmes targeting males is not known. One approach has been to screen males for the presence of PMNL with the leukocyte esterase (LE) test[40] on urine in order to identify asymptomatic infected males. Such males are then tested specifically for chlamydial infections, or treated empirically.

References

1. Tiwari VD, Talwar S, Grewal RS. Urethritis Pelvic inflammatory disease and Reiter's Disease Valia RG, Valia AR, eds In. IADVL Textbook of Dermatology. 2nd Ed. Bhalani Publishing House; 2001. Mumbai: p. 1423-1452.
2. Oriel JD. The history of non-gonococcal urethritis. Genitourin Med 1996; 72: 374-378.
3. Swediaur F. Complet sur les Symptomes, les Eiffen Nature et le Traitement des Maladies Syphilique. Paris, chez 1 Auteur 1805. In: Readings in the history of gonorrhoea. Medical Life 1932; 39: 487-504.
4. Faitout P. Des urethrites non-gonocociennes, Gritta hospitaux de Paris 1896: 69-99.
5. Waelsch L. Uber nicht-goonrrhoische urethritis. Arch Dis Syph Wien 1904; 70: 103-124.
6. Glingar A. Uber Urethritis non-gonorrhoica. Berlin Wschr 1914; 64: 591-595.
7. Lindner K. Zur Atiologie der gonokokkenfreien Urethritis. Wien Klin Wochenschr 1910; 23: 283-284.
8. T'ang FF, Chang HL, Huang YT et al. Trachoma virus in chick embryo. Natl Med J China 1957; 43: 81-86.
9. Dunlop EMC, Harper IA, Garland JA, et al. Relation of TRIC agent to "non-specific genital infection". Br J Veneral Dis 1966; 41: 77-86.
10. Taylor-Robinson D. The history and role of *Mycoplasma genitalium* in sexually transmitted diseases. Genitourin Med 1995; 71: 1-8.
11. Stary A. Urethritis–Diagnosis of nongonococcal urethritis. Dermatol Clin 1998; 16: 723-726.
12. Bowie WR, Wang SP, Alexander ER, et al. Aetiology of non-gonococcal urethritis: Evidence for *Chlamydia*

trachomatis and *Ureaplasma urealyticum*. J Clin Invest 1977; 59: 735-742.

13. Bowie WR, Pollock HM, Forsyth PS, et al. Bacteriology of the urethra in normal men and women with non-gonococcal urethritis. J Clin Microbiol 1977; 6: 482-488.

14. Holmes KK, Handsfield HH, Wang SP, et al. Aetiology of non-gonococcal urethritis. N Eng J Med 1975; 292: 2299-2305.

15. Stamm WE, Hicks CB, Martin DH, et al. Azithromycin for empirical treatment of the non-gonococcal urethritis syndrome in men. JAMA 1995; 274: 545-549.

16. Conde-Glez CJ, Calderon EL. Urogenital infection due to meningococcus in men and women. Sex Transm Dis 1991; 18: 72-75.

17. Faigel HC. Meningococcal urethritis. J Adolesc Health Care 1990; 18: 72-75.

18. Wilson APR, Wolff J, Atia W. Acute urethritis due to Neisseria meningitidis group A acquired by orogenital contact. *Genitourin Med* 1989; 65: 122-123.

19. Noble RC. Colonization of the urethra with *Streptococcus pneumoniae*: a case report. Genitourin Med 1985; 57: 325-328.

20. Moulder JW. Order Chlamydiales and family Chlamydiaceae. In: Krieg NR, ed. Manual of Systematic Bacteriology. Baltimone: Williams and Wilkins; 1984. p. 729.

21. Schachter J. Biology of *Chlamydia tractomatis*. In: Holmes K.K., Mirdh PA, Spalring SF, et al. eds Sexually Transmitted Diseases. 3rd Ed. New York: McGraw-Hill; 1999. p. 391-405.

22. Matsumoto A, Manire GP. Electron microscopic observations on the fine structure of cell wall of *Chlamydia psittaci*. J Bacteriol 1970: 104-133.

23. Salari SH, Ward ME. Polypeptide composition of *Chlamydia trachomatis*. J Gen Microbiol 1981; 123: 197–207.

24. Palc SR, Crocker TT. Differences in utilization of labeled precursors for the synthesis of deoxyribonucleic acid in cell nuclei and psittacosis virus. Biochem J 1961; 78: 1.

25. Lin HS. Inhibition of thymidine-kinase activity and deoxyribonucleic acid synthesis in L cells infected with meningopneumonitis agent. J Bacteriol 1968; 96; 2054–2065.

26. Ripa KT, Mardh PA. Cultivation of *Chlamydia trachomatis* in cycloheximide-treated McCoy cells. J Clin Microbiol 1977; 6; 328–331.

27. Hatch TP. Competition between *Chlamydia psittaci* and L cells for host isoleutine pools: a limiting factor for chlamydial multiplication. Infect Immunol 1975; 12: 211–220.

28. Allan I, Pearce JH. Amino acid requirements of strains of *Chlamydia trachomatis* and C *psittaci* growing in McCoy cells: relationship with clinical syndrome and host origin. J Gen Microbiol 1983; 129: 2001–2007.

29. Ward ME, Salari H. Control mechanisms governing the infectivity of *Chlamydia trachomatis* for HeLa cells modulation by cyclic nucleotides, prostaglandins and calcium. J Gen Microbiol 1982; 128: 639–650.

30. Caldwell HD, Schacheter J. Antigenic analysis of the major outer membrane protein of Chlamydia spp. Infect Immunol 1982; 35; 1024–1031.

31. Cain TK, Rank RG, Local Th1-like responses are induced by intravaginal infection of mice with the mouse pneumonitis biovar of *Chlamydia trachomatis*. Infect Immunol 1995; 63; 1784–1789.

32. Su H, Caldwell HD. CD4+ T cells play a significant role in adoptive immunity to *Chlamydia trachomatis* infection of the mouse genital tract. Infect Immunol 1995; 63; 3302–3308.

33. Beatty PR, Stephens RS. CD8+ T lymphocytes-mediated lysis of *chlamydia*-infected L cells using an endogenous antigen pathway. J Immunol 1994; 153: 4588–4595.

34. Thompson SC, McEachern KA, Stevenson EM & Forsyth JRL. The epidemiology of notified genital *Chlamydia trachomatis* in Victoria, Australia: a survey of diagnostic providers. Int J STD & AIDS 1997; 8: 382-387.

35. World Health Organization. Sexually Transmitted Diseases. Press release WHO/1995; 64: 25.

36. Centres for Disease Control: *Chlamydia trachomatis* genital infections–United States 1995. MMWR 1997; 46: 193-198.

37. Holmes KK, Handsfield HH, Wands SP, et al, Aetiology of nongonococcal urethritis. N Eng J Med 1975; 292: 1199-1203.

38. Thelvin I, Wennstrom AM, March PA. Contact tracing in patients with genital chlamydial infections. Br J Vener Dis 1980; 56: 259-264.

39. McMillan A, SommerVille RG, Mckie PMK. Chlamydial infection in homosexual men. Frequency of isolation of *Chlamydia trachomatis* from urethra, anorectum and pharynx. Br J Vener Dis 1981; 57: 47-49.

40. Stamm WE. *Chlamydia trachomatis* infections eds. adult. In: Holmes KK, Mardh PA, Sparling SF, et al eds. Sexually Tansmitted Diseases, 3rd Ed. New York: McGraw–Hill; 1999. p. 407-422.

41. Ostaszewska I, Zdrodowska-Stefanow B, Badyda J. et al. *Chlamydia trachomatis*: probable cause of prostatitis. Int J STD & AIDS 1998; 9: 350-353.

42. Keetch DW, Humphrey P, Ratliff TL. Development at mouse modal for nonbacterial prostatitis. J Urol 1994; 10: 274-280.

43. Westrom L, Wolmer–Hanssen P. Pathogenesis of pelvic inflammatory disease. Genitourin Med 1993; 69: 9-17.

44. Taylor–Robinson D. *Chlamydia trachomatis* and sexually transmitted disease. BMJ 1993; 308: 150-151.

45. Crowley T, Horner P, Hughes A, et al. Hormonal factors and the laboratory detection of *Chlamydia trachomatis* in women: implications for screening? Int J STD & AIDS 1997; 8: 25-31.

46. Arya OP, Mallinson H, Goddard AD. Epidemiological and clinical correlates of chlamydia infection of the cervix. Br J Ven Dis 1981; 57: 118-124.

47. Tait A, Rees E, Hobson D et al. Chlamydia infection of the cervix in contacts of men with non-gonococcal urethritis. Br J Ven Dis 1979; 8: 37-45.

48. Orien JD, Johnson AL, Nayyar U et al. Infection of the uterine cervix with *Chlamydia trachomatis*. J Infect Dis 1978; 137: 443-451.

49. Stary A. Chlamydial Screening: which sample for which technique? Genitourin Med 1997; 73: 99-102.

50. Mabey D, Peeling RW. Tropical medicine series: Lymphogranuloma venereum. Sex Transm Infect 2002; 78: 90-92.

51. Woolley PD, Pumphrey J. Application of 'Clearview chlamydia' for the rapid detection of cervical chlamydial antigen. Int J STD & AIDS 1997; 8: 257-258.

52. Hirose T, Iwaswa A, Satish T, et al. Clinical study of the effectiveness of a dual amplified immuno-assay (IDEIA *PCE* chlamydia) for the diagnosis of male urethritis. Int J STD & AIDS 1998; 9: 414-417.

53. Dille BJ, Butzen CC, Birkenmeyar LG. Amplification of *Chlamydia trachomatis* DNA by ligase chain reaction. J Clin Microbiol 1993; 31: 729–731.

54. Chernesky MA, Jang D, Lee HH, et al. Diagnosis of *Chlamydia trachomatis* infection in men and women by testing first-void urine by ligase chain reaction. J Clin Microbiol 1994; 32: 2682-2685.

55. Mardh PA. Is Europe ready for STD screening?. Genitourin Med 1997; 73: 96-98.

56. Shahmanesh M, Pandit PG, Round R. Urethral lymphocyte isolation in non-gonococcal urethritis. Genitourin Med 1996; 72: 362-364.

57. Erbelding EJ, Quinn TC. Urethritis treatment. Dermatol Clin 1998; 16: 735-738.

58. Centre For Disease Control. Sexually Transmitted Diseases. Treatment guidelines MMWR 2002; 51: 31-36.

59. Mc Cormack WM, Lee YH, Zinner SH. Sexual experience and urethral colonization with grnital mycoplasma-a study in normal men. Ann Intern Med 1973; 78: 696-703.

60. Terho P. Chlamydia trachomatis in non-specific urethritis. Br J Ven Dis 1978; 54: 251-253.

61. Charke J. Contact tracing for chlamydia: date on effectiveness. Int J STD AIDS 1998; 9: 187-191.

62. Riddell LA, Sherrard J. Chlamydia tracing detection-is it doctor dependendent? Int J STD AIDS 2001; 12: 58-60.

Chapter 22

Lymphogranuloma Venereum

A K Bajaj, Rajeev Sharma

Synonyms

Climatic bubo, tropical bubo, lymphopathia venereum, lymphogranuloma inguinale, Durand-Nicholas-Favre disease

Description of lymphogranuloma venereum (LGV) dates back to 1833 when Walkee first identified the condition. It was extensively studied and described in detail by Durand, Nicolas and Favre. It was Frei, in 1925 who for the first time developed a intradermal test. *Chlamydia trachomatis* was first identified as the causative agent of LGV in 1927. The causal relationship was established by inoculating monkeys (intracerebral) by Favre and Hellerstom. The first successful drug for treating LGV was a sulphonamide. LGV was first described from India in 1902 by Caddy.[1]

Definition

Lymphogranuloma venereum (LGV) is a sexually transmitted infection affecting primarily the lymphatic system, caused by *Chlamydia trachomatis* serovars L1, L2 and L3. It is characterized by regional suppurative lymphadenopathy, which is preceded by a small transient, inconspicuous lesion at the site of inoculation, usually the genitalia.

Prevalence

LGV has a worldwide distribution and no predilection for any race, colour or religion. However, it occurs more commonly in the tropical and the subtropical regions. It is endemic in India and South-East Asia, East and West Africa, South America and the Caribbean islands.[2] Cases have been reported from Europe, North America and Australia mostly in people travelling to or living in the endemic area.[3]

Actual prevalence in India is not known. The data from STD clinics in different parts of India indicates a prevalence rate of 6%, ranging from 0.27% to 11.5%.[4-20] A higher incidence (8%) was reported from Madagascar.[21] It is a relatively uncommon sexually transmitted disease (STD). Recently there was an epidemic of LGV with HIV infection with crack cocaine use in Bahamas, where LGV was confirmed in 23 out of 47 cases of bubo by PCR and microimmuno fluorescence.[22]

Aetiological Agent

Chlamydia are gram-negative, intracellular, obligate parasites. They measure from 0.3 to 1.0μ. In their infective state they have a cell wall, contain both DNA and RNA and divide by fission. *Chlamydia* are divided into four species, *Chlamydia trachomatis, Chlamydia psittcai C. pneumoniae and C. pecorum.*[23] *C. trachomatis* has two major biovars, Trachoma (TRIC) and LGV. There are 15 serotypes and types L1, L2 and L3 cause LGV.[22] Infection occurs by a metabolically inactive form of *Chlamydia* called 'elementary bodies'. These undergo changes to form a metabolically active 'reticular body' in 6-8 hours of infection. The organisms lack the ability to synthesize high-energy compounds such as ATP. They multiply in the host cells by binary fission. After a few such fissions, the reticular body cells condense and form an elementary body. The newly formed elementary bodies burst out of the host cells. The complete cycle takes about 48-72 hours. Human beings are the sole natural hosts for *C. trachomatis*. It can be experimentally transmitted to monkeys, mice and guinea pigs. It can be readily grown in the yolk sac of developing chick embryo, HeLa 229 cell line culture, and Mc Coy tissue culture.[23,24] It is inactivated by low concentrations of formalin, phenol or ether and by heat (56°C).[1]

Transmission

LGV is a sexually transmitted infection. Rarely it can be transmitted by non-sexual contact.[23] There is no vertical transmission of the infection but infection may occur while passing through an infected birth canal.[2]

Clinical Features

The incubation period is usually around a week (3-12 days) or longer. LGV has early as well as late manifestations.[2] The clinical features can be divided into a primary stage, secondary (inguinal stage) and a tertiary stage (complications).[24]

The primary lesion is almost never noticed. The primary lesion, if present, usually last for 2-3 days. About one fourth of the patients, present with a papule, a vesicle, erosion or an ulcerated area at the site of inoculation. The site usually is the coronal sulcus of glans in men, and posterior vaginal wall in the women. The lesions may also occur on frenum, prepuce, shaft of penis, urethra and scrotum in men and fourchette, vulva and posterior lip of cervix in women. In both sexes, the lesions may have anal, rectal or oral localization according to their sexual practice. Non-specific urethritis may be a manifestation in a rare case.[27,28] Very rarely primary lesions of LGV may occur in the tonsils, nasolabial folds and submammary and umbilical regions.

Lymphangitis occurs on the dorsal aspect of the penis and soon a chord–like swelling called bubonulus makes it's appearance in men. Very often lymphangitis leads to phimosis in men and genital swelling in women. The disease then localizes in the regional lymph nodes.[1,2]

Inguinal Syndrome (Bubo)

A characteristic unilateral inflammatory swelling of the inguinal lymph nodes and their corresponding draining lymph nodes, is the most common presentation of LGV in men (**P XVIII, Fig. 70**). The involvement may be bilateral in about one third cases (**P XVIII, Fig. 71**). The interval between appearance of bubo and the time of exposure varies from 10 days to 6 months, but on an average, it takes about 10-30 days.[1,2]

Initially the supero-medial group of inguinal lymph nodes is involved in most cases but in some cases, the lateral group may also get involved. Pain accompanies a firm elastic swelling. The pain gradually increases in severity and forces the patient to walk with a limp, bending forward to control pain. The bubo then becomes fluctuant within 1 to 2 weeks The whole chain of lymph nodes in the inguino-cruro-iliac group may get involved. The lymph nodes soon become matted, the overlying skin becomes thick and dusky, and soon the bubo becomes ready to rupture.[1,2]

In about 20% of patients femoral group of lymph nodes are also involved and may be separated by the Poupart's ligament from the enlarged inguinal lymphnodes producing the **groove sign of Greenblat (P XVIII, Fig. 72)**.[2]

Constitutional symptoms often precede or follow the development of the bubo. Symptoms accompanying bubo are fever, chills, sweating, loss of appetite, joint pains and myalgia. Pain and fever are relieved once the bubo ruptures.[1,2] Suppuration occurs in majority (60-70%) of the cases while spontaneous resolution in 25-30 percent cases, while in another 5 percent cases the adenitis may persist for months. The sites of suppuration are the inguinal lymph nodes at multiple foci, giving rise to multiple sinuses. These sinuses may persist for few weeks to many months. Secondary infection is common. Healing is very slow and leaves behind contracted scars in the inguinal region. The iliac lymph nodes may rarely suppurate, but they usually undergo spontaneous resolution.[1,2]

Bilateral inguinal lymph node involvement leads to elephantiasis of the genitalia. Less than one third of the female patients with LGV develop inguinal lymphadenopathy. About one third complain of lower abdominal and back pain despite having no anorectal involvement, indicating the involvement of the deep pelvic and lumbar lymph nodes.[2]

Rarely dissemination of the organism may occur via blood stream and produce systemic disease, which may present clinically as hepatitis, pneumonitis, spondyloarthritis, endocarditis, erythema multiforme, erythema nodosum and ocular disease.[1,2] Bubonic relapse occur in about 20% of untreated cases.[2]

Genito-Ano-Rectal Syndrome

Genital involvement in LGV may be associated with hyperplastic ulcerative lesions, especially in women with LGV. Such lesions are often associated with ano-rectal involvement and this manifestation is known as genito-ano-rectal syndrome.[1] The characteristic features being proctocolitis, hyperplasia of the lymphatic tissue (lymphorrhoids), abscess formation, fistulae, stricture formation, chronic ulceration and scarring. The commonly affected sites are the rectum and the vagina.[2,25]

Anorectal involvement occurs mostly in women and homosexual men. It follows inoculation of the rectal mucosa by *Chlamydia* during peno-anal intercourse. It may also occur secondary to involvement of the posterior urethra in men, and by direct spread from vaginal secretions or by lymphatic dissemination from the cervix or posterior vaginal wall in women.[2] Perianal oedema associated with diffuse oedema of the anorectal mucosa is the only early change noticed. It may present as pruritus ani in the first few weeks. This is followed by development of multiple fissures around the anal margin. The examining finger encounters a pebbled anorectal mucosa but the elasticity of the mucosa is retained.[1]

Submucosal swellings develop as the anorectal and pararectal lymphnodes are enlarged. The rectal mucosa may have an ulcerated or granulomatous appearance on proctoscopy. The patient may have tenesmus and blood stained rectal discharge. After 3-6 months, the anorectal mucosa becomes rigid and rugose with narrowing of the lumen secondary to involvement of all layers of the bowel. Later on fully developed stricture can be felt on per rectal examination. The stricture may be annular, tubular or funnel type. There may be multiple perianal swellings and tags associated with strictures.[1]

Complications

Lymphatic obstruction leads to elephantiasis of the genitalia. The manifestation in men can be in form of (i) ram-horn penis, and (ii) saxophone penis; both being result of chronic, massive oedema of the penis.

In women, chronic oedema leads to enlargement of the vulva (elephantiasis) often referred to as 'esthiomene' (**P XVIII, Fig. 73**).[2,27] The appearance clinically may vary from swelling of one lip to giant lobulated masses hanging and obstructing the vaginal cleft. Fistulae involving the rectum and vagina, urethra and vagina, cervix and vagina or vulva may occur in women.[1] Stricture of the urethra, prostatitis, seminal vesiculitis and epididymo-orchitis may occur rarely in men.[1] Carcinoma of the rectum is known to develop in 2-5% cases of rectal stricture due to LGV.

Rare Manifestations

Papillary growths on the urinary meatus in women may lead to various urinary symptoms.[2] Uretro-genito-perineal syndrome may manifest as multiple penile, scrotal or perineal sinuses with or without urethral stenosis.[30] Generalized exanthem-papular, papulopustular, nodular, erythema nodosum and erythema multiforme have been reported.

Unilateral follicular conjunctivitis with regional lymphadenopathy may be a presenting feature after autoinoculation.[30] Rarely bilateral conjunctivitis, episcleritis, keraritis or iritis may develop during the course of LGV.[31] Extragenital LGV may lead to enlarge-

Table 1. LGV versus Chancroid Bubo

LGV Bubo	Chancroid Bubo
Genital ulcer not present	Genital ulcer present
Bubo is less painful	Bubo is painful
Constitutional symptoms present	Constitutional symptoms present
Seen in 66.7% cases	Seen in 40% cases
Bilateral in 1/3 cases	Mostly unilateral but can also be bilateral
Groove sign is positive	Groove sign may be positive
Matting of lymph nodes is present	Absent
Multilocular suppurative swelling	Unilocular suppurative swelling
Ruptures to form multiple sinuses	Ruptures to form an ulcer
Heals slowly with scarring	Heals with treatment with less scarring

ment of the axillary or cervical lymph nodes[2,32] and psoas abscess.[33]

Diagnosis

The clinical differences of LGV and chancroid bubo are given in Table 1.

The diagnosis is established after taking careful history and proper clinical examination, looking specially, for painful adenopathy.

Laboratory tests often help in establishing the clinical suspicion. Mild leukocytosis with an increase in monocytes and eosinophils is often seen in early bubo and anogenital stage of LGV. Presence of polymorphonuclear leukocytosis would indicate secondary infection in LGV buboes and abscesses.[2]

Laboratory diagnosis of LGV can be made by (i) a positive serology for *C. trachomatis*, (ii) isolation of *C. trachomatis* from infected tissue, and (iii) identification of *C. trachomatis* from infected tissue or bubo pus.

Serological Tests

Complement fixation test: It is more sensitive than Frei's test because it is the first test to become positive. It has low specificity, as it cross reacts with psittacosis and other *Chlamydia*. Low titres may persist for years. Titres greater than 1:64 are supportive of clinical diagnosis of LGV.[2]

Immunofluorescence Tests

The single L-type immunofluorescence test is more sensitive than complement fixation test but it also cross-reacts with other chlamydial antigens. Newer tests using type specific antigens can be more useful in detecting active infection.[31,32]

ELISA based tests using monoclonal antibodies are also available for LGV.[36]

Identification of *C. trachomatis* in Tissue

Presence of elementary and inclusion bodies can be demonstrated in the infected tissue or bubo pus by using special stains such as Giemsa-Romanowsky, Iodine or Macchiavello stains.[2] Immunofluorescent methods using polyclonal or monoclonal antibodies may also be used for demonstrating *C. trachomatis*.

Electron microscopy, though helpful in identifying the organism, it is not used widely in making or confirming the diagnosis.[37]
Polymerase chain reaction (PCR) method using primers of 16S ribosomal DNA can also be used to identify the organism in infected tissue or bubo pus.[37]

Histology

Histology of an infected lymph node shows multiple stellate abscesses representing areas of tissue necrosis with surrounding granulomatous infiltrate.[37]

Isolation of *C. trachomatis*

C. trachomatis can be isolated from infected tissue or bubo pus using mouse brain, yolk sac or tissue culture. Various cell lines such as McCoy, He La229, L929 treated with agents to prevent replication are used. The yield is usually poor (24-30%).[31]

Frei's Test

It was originally performed using the pus from an unruptured bubo, diluted with saline and sterilized by heating. The antigen was available commercially in the past. The test now remains one of historic interest in absence of a readily available antigen. The procedure consists of injecting 0.1 ml of the antigen into the skin on the volar aspect of a forearm and a similar amount of yolk sac or dilutent is injected on the other forearm as control. Reading is taken at 48 hours. A papule at least 6 mm in diameter indicates a positive result provided the control arm showed a papule measuring 5mm or less.[2]

The test becomes positive after the appearance of buboes. It may indicate infection with non- LGV serovars of *C. trachomatis*. The test remains positive for many years after clinical cure.[2]

Others

Barium enema is done to locate the level of stricture and to know the level of stricture and the resultant deformity. It is also used to differentiate it from carcinoma of the rectum.[2]

Lymphography, CT scan or MRI scan may be used to know the extent of lymph node involvement.[2]

Treatment

The treatment is aimed at eliminating the organism to render the patient non-infectious and prevent complications.

Centre for disease control, Atlanta, USA[38] recommends, either

(i) Doxycycline 100 mg orally bid for 3 weeks or
(ii) Erythromycin base 500 mg orally qid for 3 weeks (specially for pregnant and nursing mothers, children under 8 years of age and patients sensitive to doxycycline)

Azithromycin 1 gm orally once a week for 3 weeks is also a recommended mode of therapy though adequate trials are lacking. It is also recommended to either aspirate with a wide bore needle through normal skin or incise and drain the buboes as and when required.[38]

Other drugs used for treating LGV are:

(i) Sulphadiazine 500mg orally qid for 2-3 weeks[39]
(ii) Cotrimoxazole 2 tablets orally bid for 2 weeks.[39]
(iii) Tetracycline hydrochloride 500mg orally qid for 2-3 weeks.
(iv) Minocycline 300mg initially then 200 mg orally bid for 10 days.[40]
(v) Rifampicin 450mg orally on empty stomach o.d. for 10 days.
(vi) Azithromycin 1gm orally one dose with doxycycline 100mg bid for 7 days.[41]

The recommendations are same for HIV positive cases but they may require longer duration of treatment.[38] Sexual contacts must be treated simultaneously. Follow up must be done at every 3 months for 1 year. A surgeon or a gynecologist, depending on the merit of the case best deals with rectal strictures and fistulae surgically.

References

1. Siddappa K, Rangaiah PN. Lymphogranuloma venereum. In:Valia RG, Valia AR, eds. IADVL Textbook and colour atlas of Dermatology. 2nd edn. Mumbai: Bhalani Publishing House; 2001: p. 1466–1475.
2. Perine PL, Stamm WE. Lymphogranuloma venereum. In: Holmes KK, Sparling PF, Mardh PA, et al, eds. Sexually transmitted diseases. 3rd ed. New York: McGraw Hill; 1999. p. 423-432.
3. Abrams AJ. Lymphogranuloma venereum. JAMA 1968; 205:199.
4. Chopra A, Mittal RR, Singh P, Sharma P. Pattern of sexually transmitted diseases at Patiala. Indian J Sex Transm Dis 1990;11:43-45.
5. Bansal NK, Khare AK, Upadhay OP. Pattern of sexually transmitted diseases in and around Udaipur. Indian J Dermatol Venereol Leprol 1988; 54:90-92.
6. Nigam P, Mukhija RD. Pattern of sexually transmitted diseases at Gorakhpur. Indian J Sex Transm Dis 1986; 7:70-73.
7. Singh KG, Joshi MK, Bajaj AK. Pattern of sexually transmitted diseases in Allahabad. Indian J Sex Transm Dis 1990; 11:6-118.
8. Chaudhary SO, Bhatia KK, Bansal RK, Jain VK. Pattern of sexually transmitted diseases in Rohtak. Indian J Sex Transm Dis 1988; 9:4-7.
9. Sahib KPM, Pai GS, Pinto J, Kamath KN. Pattern of genital ulcers in and around Mangalore. Indian J Sex Transm Dis 1990; 11:52-53.
10. Arora SK, Sharma RC, Sardari Lal. Pattern of sexually transmitted diseases at Smt. Sucheta Kripalani Hospital, New Delhi. Indian J Sex Transm Dis 1984; 5:5-7.
11. Siddappa K, Jagannath Kumar V, Ravindra K. Pattern of STD's at Davangere. Indian J Sex Transm Dis 1990; 11 :39- 42.
12. Garg BR, Baruah MC, Sait MA. Pattern of sexually transmitted diseases at JIPMER, Pondicherry. Indian J Sex Transm Dis 1985; 6:41-43.
13. Kapur TR. Pattern of sexually transmitted diseases in India. Indian J Dermatol Venereol Leprol 1982; 48:23-24.
14. Vora NS, Dave IN, Mukhopadyay AK, et al. A profile of sexually transmitted diseases at Apex ESIS Hospital, Ahmedabad. Indian J Sex Transm Dis 1994; 15:36-38.
15. Rajanarayan, Kar HK, Gautam RK, et al. Pattern of sexually transmitted diseases in a major hospital of Delhi. Indian J Sex Transm Dis 1996; 17:76-78.
16. Khanna N, Pandhi RK, Lakhanpal S. Changing trends in sexually transmitted di:;eases: A hospital based study from Delhi. Indian J Sex Transm Dis 1996; 17:79-81.
17. Jaiswal AK, Bhushan B. Pattern of sexually transmitted diseases in North Eastern India. Indian J Sex Transm Dis 1994; 15:19-20.
18. Arora PN, Romasastry CV, Chatterjee RG. Changing pattern of sexually transmitted diseases in Indian armed forces: Retrospective study from 1961 to 1990. J Sex Transm Dis 1993; 14:34-37.
19. Reddy BSN, Garg BR, Rao MV. An appraisal of trends in sexually transmitted diseases. Indian J Sex Transm Dis 1993; 14:1-4.
20. Rege VL, Shukla P. Profile of genital sores in Goa. Indian J Sex Transm Dis 1993; 14:10-14.
21. Behets FM, Andriamadana J, Randrianasolo D, et al. Chancroid, primary syphilis, genital herpes and lymphogranuloma venereum in Antananarivo, Madagascar. J Infect Dis 1999; 180:1382-1385.
22. Bauwens JE, Orlander H, Gomez MP, et al. Epidemic

lymphogranuloma venerum during epidemics of crack cocaine use and HIV infection in Bahamas. Sex Transm Dis 2002; 29:253-259.

23. Schachter I, Caldwell KD. Chlamydiae. Ann Rev Microbiol 1980; 34:285-309.

24. Schachter I, Osoba AO. Lymphogranuloma venereum. Br Med Bull 1983; 39: 151.

25. Burgoyne RA. Lymphogranuloma venereum. Prim Care 1990; 17:153-157.

26. Faro S. Lymphogranuloma venereum, chancroid, granuloma venereale. Obstet Gynaec Clin North Am 1989; 16: 517-530.

27. Ghinsberg RC, Firsteter-Gilburd E, Mates A, et al. Rectal lymphogranuloma venereum in a bisexual patient. Microbiologica 1991; 14:161.

28. Watson DJ, Parker AI, Macleod TI. Lymphogranuloma venereum of the tonsil. J Laryngols, Otol 1990; 104:331.

29. Gupta S, Gupta U, Gupta DK. A gigantic esthiomene. Indian J Sex Transm Dis 1997; 18:75-76.

30. Coutts WE. Lymphogranuloma venereum: a general review. Bull WHO 1950; 2:545.

31. Kamprneir RH, Smith OW, Larsen RM. Human chlamydial infection. Am J Med Sci 1939; 198:516.

32. Heaton ND; Yates-Bell A. Thirty-year follow-up of lymphogranuloma venereum. Br J Urol 1992; 70:693-694.

33. Speers D.Lymphogranuloma venereum presenting with psoas abscess. Aust NZ J Med 1999; 29:563-564.

34. Van Dyck E, Piot P. Laboratory techniques in the investigation of chancroid, lymphogranuloma venereum and donovanosis, Genitourin Med 1992; 68:130-133.

35. Joseph AK, Rosen T. Laboratory techniques used in the diagnosis of chancroid, granuloma inguinale and lymphogranuloma venereum. Dermatol Clin 1994; 12: 1-7.

36. Mittal A, Sachdeva KG. Monoclonal antibody for the diagnosis of lymphogranuloma venereum: a preliminary report. Br J Biomed Sci 1993; 50:3-7.

37. Hadfield TL, Lamy Y, Wear Dl. Demonstration of *Chlamydia trachomatis* in inguinal lymphadenitis of lymphogranuloma venereum: a light microscopy, electron microscopy and polymerase chain reaction study. Modern Pathology 1995; 8:924-929.

38. Czelusta A, Yen-Moore A, Van der Straten M, Carrasco D, Tyring SK. An overview of sexually transmitted diseases. Part III. Sexually transmitted diseases in HIV-infected patients. J Am Acad Dermatol. 2000; 43:409-432.

39. Expert Group Recommendations on National Sexually Transmitted Diseases Control Programme. New Delhi: DGHS, Govt. of India, Sept. 26-28, 1991; 23.

40. Sowmini CN, et al. Minocycline in the treatment of lymphogranuloma venereum. J Am Vener Dis Assoc 1976; 2:19.

41. Levine WC, Berg AO, Johnson RE, et al. Development of sexually transmitted diseases treatment guidelines 1993. Sex Transm Dis 1994; 21(Suppl.2):S96-S101.

Chapter 23

Bacterial Vaginosis

Devinder M Thappa

Synonyms

Haemophilus vaginalis vaginitis; *Gardnerella vaginalis* vaginitis; Anaerobic vaginosis; Vaginal bacteriosis

Bacterial vaginosis (BV) is a common cause of abnormal vaginal discharge in women of reproductive age.[1] It is a polymicrobial syndrome involving the replacement of the normal vaginal lactobacilli by a variety of anaerobic bacteria and mycoplasmas.[2] Little is known about the incubation period of BV, but recurrences are common.[1] The importance of BV with respect to women's health is emphasized by the association between BV and pelvic inflammatory diseases (PID), adverse outcome of pregnancy, postpartum endometritis, and cuff cellulitis.[3]

Historical Aspects

Gardner and Dukes first described the syndrome as "Haemophilus vaginalis vaginitis" in 1955. They concluded that it was a sexually transmitted disease (STD) as the isolated aetiological agent, *H. vaginalis* (now renamed *Gardnerella vaginalis*), was found in the male contacts of the female cases.[4] However, Leopold had previously described a Gram negative non-motile rod isolated from men and women with symptoms characteristic of BV and it is now known that *G. vaginalis* occurs in up to 50% of women without BV.[5] Further research has implicated a wide range of other microorganisms, including Prevotella spp, *Mycoplasma hominis* and Mobiluncus spp in the syndrome.[2]

Epidemiology

The incidence of BV varies according to the population studied and the geographic location, with recorded prevalence ranging from 4% in university students to 33% in GUM clinics.[1] BV was the most common infection (26%) among the 319 women with vaginal discharge attending a reproductive health clinic in New Delhi, India. At least one STD was detected in 21.9% of women. The prevalence of *Chlamydia trachomatis* infection was 12.2%, trichomoniasis 10% and syphilis 2.2%.[6] In another study from New Delhi, BV was seen in 50% of symptomatic cases with vaginitis (out of 544 cases) and 21.8% of asymptomatic women (out of 258 cases) based on the clinical criteria and Gram's stain.[7] Bacterial vaginosis significantly correlated with increasing years since marriage, lower socio-economic status and a parity of more than two, but not with age, stage of menstrual cycle and hours since last intercourse. In a report from Chennai[8], 150 symptomatic and 50 asymptomatic women in second trimester of pregnancy in the age group of 20-30 years were screened for bacterial vaginosis by Gram stained smear of vaginal discharge utilizing the scoring system of Nugent et al. They found that 38.5% of symptomatic and 16% of asymptomatic women had BV. In our institute at Pondicherry in a group of 100 women with abnormal vaginal discharge, 16% of them were found to have BV by Amsel's criteria and it was the commonest cause of abnormal vaginal discharge (unpublished data). The prevalence of bacterial vaginosis was 37.5% among the 80 randomly selected married women from Mumbai, based on Gram's stain and Amsel's criteria.[9] In a study of hundred women with vaginal discharge at Patiala, BV was seen in 48%, candidosis in 26% and trichomoniasis in 13% of the cases.[10]

Aetiopathogenesis

The vagina is a dynamic ecosystem that is sterile at

birth and becomes colonized within a few days with a predominantly Gram positive flora consisting of anaerobic bacteria, staphylococci, streptococci, and diphtheroids.[11] The vaginal pH in premenarchal females is near neutral (pH 7.0). At the time of puberty, under the influence of estrogen, the vaginal epithelium increases to about 25 cells thick with increased glycogen levels, the predominant flora changes to lactobacilli and vaginal pH decreases to less than 4.5 due to production of lactic acid. This low pH is maintained until menopause, when vaginal pH rises above 6.0. In BV, this symbiotic relationship is broken in one or more places and lead to overgrowth of bacteria associated with BV.

BV represents a complex change in vaginal flora, characterized by the replacement of hydrogen peroxide producing lactobacilli with concentration of *G. vaginalis*, Mobiluncus species, *Mycoplasma hominis*, anaerobic gram-negative rods belonging to the genera Prevotella, Porphyromonas, and Bacteroides and Peptostreptococcus species.[12] *G. vaginalis* metabolically produces amino acids, which act as substrate for the production of volatile amines by anaerobic bacteria. The amines in turn raise the vaginal pH favouring the continued growth of *G. vaginalis* over lactobacilli.[11] Another proposed theory for the pathophysiology of BV states that the overgrowth of anaerobic microorganisms is accompanied by the production of proteolytic enzymes that act on vaginal peptides to release several biologic products including polyamines, which volatilize in the accompanying alkaline environment to elaborate foul smelling trimethylamine.[12] Polyamines act to facilitate the transudation of vaginal fluid and exfoliation of epithelial cells, creating a copious discharge. It is thought that amines produced by the microbial flora, perhaps by microbial decarboxylases, account for the characteristic abnormal fishy odor produced when vaginal fluid is mixed with 10 percent KOH.[13] This so called "Whiff test" is thought to be owing to volatilization of aromatic amines, including putrescine, cadaverine, and trimethylamine at alkaline pH. Mobiluncus is known to produce trimethylamine, but other microbial sources of the amines are still unknown. Clue cells are formed when *G. vaginalis* present in high numbers, and adhere in the presence of an elevated pH to exfoliated epithelial cells.

Synergistic relations between different BV associated organisms have now been demonstrated. The prevalence of *M. hominis* and *G. vaginalis* are known to increase following an increased prevalence of various anaerobes.[14]

The stimulation of *G. vaginalis* growth has been observed with the production of amino acids by anaerobes and ammonia by *Prevotella bivia*.

Risk Factors

BV is related to sexual activity, though it is hard to confirm that its development is entirely determined by those variables. It could be a marker of specific sexual practices or may be related to changing biological mechanisms that mean a woman's susceptibility increases with age.[1] The risk of BV is greatest among black Caribbean women. Those with a history of a bacterial STD (gonorrhoea or *Chlamydia trachomatis*) are at a greater risk of BV.[1] Previous studies have reported that the prevalence of BV also increases with the number of lifetime sexual partners and is more common in those with a lower age of first intercourse.[15]

BV is more prevalent in lesbians. In a report from London, 33% of lesbians were infected compared with 13% of heterosexuals.[16] Lesbians usually have lower rates of STD and this fact together with studies that have found BV in virgins indicate that specific practices and not sexual intercourse with an infected partner predisposes to BV.

Clinical Features

BV is the commonest cause of vaginal discharge occurring in women attending the gynaecological clinics in our country.[9] Patients often present with a malodorous vaginal discharge although many are asymptomatic. BV and "other non-sexually transmitted conditions" exhibit an age profile in direct contrast with the known STD. Both showed prevalence peaking in the over 30's when one would expect lower rates of sexual partner change than in younger adults.[1] Non-viscous homogenous, white non-inflammatory discharge that smoothly coats the vaginal walls, often visible on the labia and fourchette with characteristic odour are the features of BV.[13] The vaginal mucosa and vulva appear normal and because of this lack of inflammation it has been called as vaginosis instead of vaginitis. The majority of women with BV note a foul odor in the genital area immediately following intercourse when alkalinization of the vaginal secretions by semen occurs, leading to volatilization of polyamines.[11]

Diagnosis

Bacterial vaginosis can be diagnosed by the use of clinical or Gram-stain criteria.[17] Amsel et al[18] proposed a set of practical diagnostic criteria for the clinical diagnosis of BV that is now often accepted as the "gold standard." Diagnosis requires three or more of the following clinical/diagnostic features:

- Excessive homogeneous uniformly adherent vaginal discharge
- Elevated vaginal pH > 4.5
- Positive amine test (Whiff test)
- Clue cells (20%)

The pH of vaginal secretions should be determined by using a strip of narrow range pH paper (about 4.0 to 5.5), which may be applied to the withdrawn speculum or directly inserted into the vagina.[11] The odour of vaginal secretions should be tested by smelling the withdrawn speculum. Normal vaginal secretions do not have an unpleasant odour. If this test is negative, a more sensitive procedure for detecting the amines is performed by adding a few drops of 10% KOH to a few drops of vaginal secretions and immediate smelling ("whiffing") of the specimen for the transient "dead fish" odour that is characteristic of BV. Menses, semen or douching may affect the pH and a weakly positive whiff test may be produced by menstrual blood or semen. Wet mount of vaginal secretions should be done to look for 'clue cells', epithelial cells covered with *G. vaginalis* that Gardner and Dukes called "clues" to the diagnosis of BV (**P XIX, Fig. 74**).

Detection of clue cells (Fig. 1) is the most useful single procedure for diagnosis of BV.[13] Gram's staining of vaginal secretions is even more reliable than wet mount, with a sensitivity of 93 percent and specificity of 70 percent, but it is underused.[12] Determination of pH and amine odour can significantly enhance the accuracy of diagnosis of BV. Vaginal pH has the greatest sensitivity of the four clinical signs, but the lowest specificity. Cultures for *G. vaginalis* have little utility for the diagnosis of BV and as "test for cure".[13]

BV is diagnosed conventionally when at least three of four composite criteria are fulfilled. This, however is laborious. Alternatively, Gram's staining of the smear have been shown to be a simple, inexpensive, sensitive, specific, and reproducible way to diagnose BV.[19] Spiegel et al[20] defined criteria that made it easy to diagnose BV by scoring Gram-stained vaginal secretion smears, and this procedure was refined by Nugent et al (Table

1).[21] Nugent Gram stained criteria for diagnosis of BV has the sensitivity of 86 to 89% and specificity of 94 to 96% compared to the Amsel criteria.[13]

Table 1. Scoring System of Gram-Stained Smears (Nugent et al)

Bacterial morphological type	Score				
	None	1+	2+	3+	4+
Lactobacilli (large Gram positive bacilli)	4	3	2	1	0
Small Gram negative/ Gram variable rods	0	1	2	3	4
Curved Gram negative bacilli (Mobiluncus)	0	1	2	3	4

Interpretation
<1/oil immersion field — 1+
1-5/oil immersion field — 2+
6-30/oil immersion field — 3+
>30/oil immersion field — 4+

Score: 0-3 Normal; 4-6 Intermediate (test to be repeated later); 7-10 Bacterial vaginosis

Several other alternative methods have also been used to develop easy, inexpensive and reproducible diagnostic methods such as the rapid nucleic acid hybridization test, proline aminopeptidase activity and the amine test.[3] Laboratory diagnosis by gas liquid chromatographic identification of fatty acids is useful as a research tool.[11] A ratio of the succinate to lactate peaks of more than 0.4 is highly predictive of BV.

Differential Diagnosis

The three major causes of vaginitis (bacterial vaginosis, trichomoniasis and candida vaginitis) and their differentiating features are shown in the Table 2.[12, 22] Other possible differential diagnosis includes ulcerative vaginitis due to *Staphylococcus aureus*, vaginal ulceration associated with the use of vaginal tampons or cervical caps or spermicide, infections associated with other intravaginal foreign bodies, postmenstrual atrophic vaginitis, allergic or chemical reactions and contact dermatitis.

HIV and Bacterial Vaginosis

An understanding is emerging of how BV might enhance

Table 2.   Differential Diagnoses of Bacterial Vaginosis

Profile	Normal vaginal discharge	Candidal vulvovaginitis	Trichomonal vaginitis	Bacterial vaginosis
Aetiology	Lactobacillus predominant	Candida spp. and other yeasts	*Trichomonas vaginalis*	Associated with *G. vaginalis*; anaerobic bacteria, and *Mycoplasma hominis*
Symptoms	None	Vulval pruritus and/or irritation; external dysuria, increased vaginal discharge	Profuse discharge, often malodourous; external dysuria and genital irritation often present	Malodourous, increased discharge (commonly present at the introitus)
Discharge				
Amount	Variable; usually scant	Scant to moderate	Profuse	Moderate to profuse
Colour	Clear or white	White	White, yellow or green	White or gray
Consistency	Nonhomogenous, flocculant	Clumped, "Cheesy" adherent exudative plaques	Homogenous, watery, often frothy	Homogenous, uniformly coating vaginal walls
pH	Usually <4.5	<4.5	Usually >5.0	Usually >4.5
Amine odour with 10% KOH	None	None	Usually present	Present
Associated inflammatory signs	None	Erythema, oedema and/or erosions of vagina or external genitalia; vulval dermatitis common	Erythema of vaginal mucosa, introitus; occasional cervical petechiae; vulval dermatitis	None
Microscopy of discharge	Normal epithelial cells; lactobacilli predominate	Leukocytes, epithelial cells; yeast, mycelia, pseudomycelia seen	Leukocytes; motile trichomonads seen	Clue cells; rare leukocytes; lactobacilli outnumbered by mixed flora

the susceptibility to HIV infection.[23] Lactobacilli produce hydrogen peroxide, which is toxic to a number of microorganisms, including HIV. BV is characterized by the absence of lactobacilli and thus an elevated pH. A low vaginal pH may inhibit CD4 lymphocyte activation and therefore decrease HIV target cells in the vagina; conversely, an elevated pH may make the vagina more conducive to HIV survival and adherence. BV has also been shown to increase intravaginal levels of interleukin-10, which increases susceptibility of macrophages to HIV.

Complications

Women with BV have fivefold increased risk of late miscarriage or preterm delivery.[19] Studies are underway to determine whether intervention can prevent a woman with BV having a late miscarriage and preterm delivery.

Other reported complications in pregnancy are low birth weight, premature rupture of membranes (PROM), chorioamnionitis and amniotic fluid infection. Causal relations have also been established between BV and postpartum endometritis, vaginal cuff cellulitis (occurs when vaginal bacteria contaminate the operative field during a hysterectomy), post abortion and spontaneous PID.[13]

The Association Between BV and Other Genital Tract Infections

The association between BV and other genital tract infections may reflect biological interactions in the vaginal microflora rather than common risk factors for their acquisition.[1] Those presenting with BV are more likely to have a concurrent infection with gonorrhoea, but less likely to be diagnosed with a protozoal, viral, or

Table 3. Treatment of Bacterial Vaginosis

WHO (2001)[25]	CDC (2002)[17]	NACO (2002)[26]
Metronidazole 500 mg PO bd 7 days	Metronidazole 500 mg PO bd for 7 days	Only symptomatic women to be treated
Or 2 gm PO single dose (in pregnancy, Metronidazole can be used in 2nd and 3rd trimester)	Or Metronidazole gel 0.75%, one full applicator intravaginally, OD × 5 days.	Metronidazole 400 mg PO bd for 7 days
Or Clindamycin 300 mg bd for 7 days alternative	Or Clindamycin cream 2% one full applicator intravaginally at bed time × 7 days	Or metronidazole 2 gm PO single dose
Metronidazole 2 gm PO single dose	Alternatives	Alternatives
or Clindamycin vaginal cream (2%) 5 gm at bed time for 7 days	Metronidazole 2 gm PO single dose	Cream and pessaries
or	Or Clindamycin 300 mg PO bd for 7 days	
Metronidazole gel (0.75%) 5 gm bd 5 days	Or Clindamycin ovules 100 g intra vaginally OD at bed time × 3 days	
or		
Clindamycin 300 mg (bd) for 7 days		

fungal infection. An inhibitory effect of the bacterial amines, putrescine and cadaverine on the cell division and germ tube formation of *Candida albicans* has recently been reported. [24]

Routine treatment of sex partners is not recommended, since likelihood of relapse or recurrence is not affected by her sex partner treatment. Asymptomatic women with BV may be offered treatment if requested.

Pregnant Women

BV during pregnancy is associated with adverse pregnancy outcomes, including PROM, preterm labour, preterm birth, and postpartum endometritis.[17] The results of several investigations indicate that treatment of pregnant women who have BV and who are at high risk for preterm delivery (i.e., those who previously delivered a premature infant) may reduce the risk for prematurity. All symptomatic pregnant women should be tested and treated. Metronidazole 250 mg orally three times a day for 7 days or Clindamycin 300 mg orally twice a day for 7 days is the recommended treatment.

Currently, pregnant women with asymptomatic bacterial vaginosis are not routinely screened or treated for this syndrome.[27] As the treatment of BV in asymptomatic pregnant women at high risk for preterm delivery with a recommended regimen has reduced preterm delivery in three of four randomized controlled trials, some specialists recommend the screening and treatment of these women.[17]

Treatment

The treatment of bacterial vaginosis as recommended by CDC, WHO and NACO is summarised in Table 3.

Recurrence

After therapy, approximately 30 percent of patients with initial response have a recurrence of symptoms within three months.[12] The reasons are unclear; they include reinfection, but recurrences more likely reflect vaginal relapse caused by failure to eradicate the offending organisms or to re-establish the normal protective vaginal flora dominated by lactobacillus. Optimal treatment for recurrent BV is unknown. Options include re-treatment with metronidazole or clindamycin and local therapy with clotrimazole. If an intrauterine device is present, its removal should be considered.[22]

Partner Treatment

Treatment of the male sex partner has not been beneficial in preventing the recurrence of BV.[17]

HIV Infection

Patients who are co-infected with HIV and BV may receive the same treatment regimen as those who are HIV-negative.[17]

Prevention

It is difficult to define useful approaches for the prevention of this condition in the scenario of poorly understood host factors and agents involved. Since BV is associated with sexual activity, abstinence may represent the most effective means to prevent its occurrence.[13]

References

1. Morris MC, Rogers PA, Kinghorn GR. Is bacterial vaginosis a sexually transmitted infection? Sex Transm Infect 2001; 77: 63-68.

2. Krohn M, Hillier S, Eschenbach D. Comparison of methods for diagnosing bacterial vaginosis among pregnant women. J Clin Microbiol 1989; 27: 1266–1271.

3. Wolrath H, Forsum U, Larsson PG, Boren H. Analysis of bacterial vaginosis-related amines in vaginal fluid by gas chromatography and mass spectrometry. J Clin Microbiol 2001; 39: 4026-4031.

4. Gardner H, Dukes C. *Haemophilus vaginalis* vaginitis: a newly defined specific infection previously classified "non-specific vaginitis". Am J Obstet Gynecol 1955; 69: 962-976.

5. Leopold S. Heretofore undescribed organism isolated from the genitourinary system. US Armed Forces Med J 1953; 4: 263-266.

6. Vishwanath S, Talwar V, Prasad R, Coyaji K, Elias CJ, de Zoysa I. Syndromic management of vaginal discharge among women in a reproductive health clinic in India. Sex Transm Inf 2000; 76: 303-306.

7. Bhalla P, Kaushika A. Epidemiological and microbiological correlates of bacterial vaginosis. Indian J Dermatol Venereol Leprol 1994; 60: 8-14.

8. Mathew R, Kalyani J, Bibi R, Mallika M. Prevalence of bacterial vaginosis in antenatal women. Indian J Pathol Microbiol 2001; 44: 113-116.

9. Saharan SP, Surve C, Raut V, Bhattacharya M. Diagnosis and prevalence of bacterial vaginosis. J Postgrad Med 1993; 39: 72-73.

10. Chopra A, Mittal RR, Kanta S, Kaur R. Vaginitis and vaginal flora –Study of 100 cases. Indian J Sex Transm Dis 1993; 14: 52-54.

11. Schmid GP, Arko RJ. Vaginitis. In: Morse SA, Moreland AA, Thompson SE, eds. Slide Atlas of Sexually Transmitted Diseases. New York: Gower Medical Publishing; 1992. p. 1-8.

12. Sobel JD. Vaginitis. New Engl J Med 1997; 337: 1896-1902.

13. Hilliers S, Holmes KK. Bacterial vaginosis. In: Holmes KK, Mardh PA, Sparling PF, et al eds. Sexually Transmitted Diseases. 3rd edn. New York: McGraw-Hill; 1999: p. 563-586.

14. Pybus V, Onderdonk AB. Microbial interactions in the vaginal ecosystem, with emphasis on the pathogenesis of bacterial vaginosis. Microbes Infect 1999; 1: 285–292.

15. Larsson P, Platz-Christensen J, Sundstrom E. Is bacterial vaginosis a sexually transmitted disease? Int J STD AIDS 1991; 2: 362–364.

16. Bump R, Buesching W. Bacterial vaginosis in virginal and sexually active adolescent females: evidence against exclusive sexual transmission. Am J Obstet Gynecol 1988;158: 935–939.

17. Centre For Disease Control. Sexually transmitted diseases: Treatment guidelines 2002. MMWR 2002; 51 (No.RR-6): 42-44.

18. Amsel R, Totten P, Spiegel CA, Chen KC, Eschenbach D, Holmes KK. Non-specific vaginitis: diagnostic techniques and microbial and epidemiologic associations. Am J Med 1983; 74: 14–22.

19. Hay PE, Lamont R, Taylor-Robinson D, Morgan DJ, Ison C, Pearson J. Abnormal bacterial colonization of the genital tract and subsequent preterm delivery and late miscarriage. BMJ 1994; 308: 295–298.

20. Spiegel CA, Amsel R, Holmes KK. Diagnosis of bacterial vaginosis by direct Gram stain of vaginal fluid. J Clin Microbiol 1983; 18: 170-177.

21. Nugent RP, Krohn MA, Hillier SL. Reliability of diagnosing bacterial vaginosis is improved by a standardized method of Gram stain interpretation. J Clin Microbiol 1991; 29: 297-301.

22. Celum CL, Wilch E, Fennell C, Stamm WE. The Practitioner's Handbook for the Management of Sexually Transmitted Diseases, revised second edition, Seattle, WA: Health Sciences Centre for Educational Resources, University of Washington: 1998; p. 31-34, p. 76-77.

23. Schmid GP, Markowitz LE, Joesoef R, Kouman E. Bacterial vaginosis and HIV infection. Sex Transm Inf 2000; 76: 3–4.

24. Rodrigues AG, Mardh PA, Pina-Vaz C, Martinez-de-Oliveira J, d-Fonseca AF. Is the lack of concurrence of bacterial vaginosis and vaginal candidosis explained by the presence of bacterial amines? Am J Obstet Gynecol 1999; 181: 367-370.

25. Guidelines for the management of sexually transmitted infections. WHO/HIV/AIDS 2001.01 WHO/RHR/01.10.

26. Guidelines for treatment of sexually transmitted diseases NACO (2002).

27. Hillier SL, Nugent R, Eschenbach D, et al. Association between bacterial vaginosis and preterm delivery of a low birth weight infant. N Engl J Med 1995; 333: 1737–1742.

Chapter 24

Herpes Genitalis

Joseph A Sundharam

Genital herpes simplex virus infections are now one of the commonest sexually transmitted diseases (STD) afflicting both men and women. The incidence has increased manifold in the last two decades and has assumed major public health significance especially because of association with HIV infection. The reasons for its increase are: the decrease in the treatable bacterial STD, the high recurrence rates and asymptomatic recurrences with transmission in the absence of symptoms. The morbidity of the illness is due to the high recurrence rates, the severity of the primary infections, and the high mortality and morbidity in neonates is of great concern to both patients and health care workers.

Aetiology[1]

Herpes genitalis is caused by a DNA virus, herpes virus hominis. There are two types—type 1 and type 2. The predominant type isolated from the genital area is type 2, although in a third of the cases, type 1 may be isolated.

Herpes simplex virus (HSV) is characterized by persistence in the sensory nerve ganglia after primary infection (latency). During this period of latency, the virus cannot be detected by the host defence mechanisms. Following various triggers, the virus may be reactivated, travel peripherally to the skin and mucous membranes, and replicate to cause recurrent disease. Virus shedding may occur even without lesions (asymptomatic shedding); however, the number of virus particles shed is considerably less than from active lesions (up to a 1000 times less).

Thus, although the characteristic clinical feature of HSV infections is the recurrent vesicular eruption, the disease is best understood as a chronic persistent infection of the sensory ganglia with varying unpredictable degrees of epithelial expression (asymptomatic or symptomatic recurrences).

Structure

The herpes simplex virus is composed of four basic components

- The core—which consist of a linear double stranded DNA coding for over 70 different polypeptides.
- The capsid—a 20 sided (icosahedral) protein shell which protects the DNA core. The capsid is composed of 162 structural units known as capsomeres.
- The tegument—an amorphous proteinaceous material which covers the capsid
- The envelope—a lipid membrane derived from the host-cell nuclear membrane. The envelope contains 11 glycoproteins which are the major target of the humoral and cellular immune response.

Epidemiology

Spread occurs through direct contact with infected secretions. The incubation period varies from 5 to 14 days. All patients with HSV infections are potentially contagious, whether or not lesions are visible. Transmission often occurs in the absence of lesions because of asymptomatic shedding.

The epidemiology of type 1 and type 2 infections differ. In developing countries, the majority of the adult population is infected in childhood by the type 1 virus; in the developed countries the proportion is lower.[2] Type 2 virus infection is typically post pubertal. There is a paucity of Indian studies; in the US, approximately 25% of the population is seropositive to HSV type 2. Orogenital contact may lead to transmission of type 1 virus to the genitalia and up to a third of genital HSV infections are caused by the type 1 virus.

The prevalence of genital herpes has increased markedly between the 1960's and 1990's. These increases have been seen not only in STD clinics in India, but also all over the world and 6 to 10 fold increases have been reported from centres in the UK and USA.[3]

One recent study published from Sweden[4] challenges the traditional view that HSV 2 infections remain confined below the waist, while HSV 1 tends to cause infections on the upper half of the body. In this study, cultures from lesions at all sites were taken over a four year period. While among 631 orofacial isolates, 96% were HSV 1, of 3085 anogenital isolates, 29% were HSV 1 and the rest (71%) were HSV 2. On the fingers and hands, 46% of 69 isolates were HSV 2, while at other sites (such as the foot and abdomen), 40% of 95 isolates were HSV 2. It seems, therefore, that except for the orofacial region, both viral types are capable of, and well adapted to infecting other body regions.

Both humoral and cell mediated immune responses follow primary infection. These, however, do not fully prevent either the recurrences or reinfection. Infection with HSV of a different type produces a first episode nonprimary infection. This is usually milder. The importance of the immune system is demonstrated by herpes in immunodeficient individuals such as patients on immunosuppressive or cytotoxic drugs following organ transplantation or malignancy, and in patients with AIDS. In such patients, herpes virus infections follow a prolonged and atypical course.

The importance of the immune system is also demonstrated by neonatal transmission of the disease. In maternal primary infection at the time of delivery, transmission occurs in 50% of neonates and is often severe and fatal. However, transmission to the neonate is less frequent and serious morbidity is rare in nonprimary, first episode or recurrent genital infection during pregnancy or at delivery since maternal antibodies protect the foetus.

Transmission and Viral Shedding[1,5]

Infection with the herpes simplex virus follows contact with infected secretions through oral to oral, oral to genital or genital to genital contact. Some factors influencing the transmission of HSV are listed in Table 1.

Table 1.   Factors Influencing HSV Transmission

- Gender
- Previous infection with HSV
- Frequency of recurrence
- Presence of active lesions at intercourse
- Use of barrier contraceptives
- Use of HSV suppressive therapy in the partner with herpes

In couples where one partner has a history of herpes, serologic tests show that in 25% of these couples, both partners are seropositive, suggesting that infection had already been transmitted. In the couples who were serologically discordant for HSV antibodies, the mean rate of transmission was 12% per year.[6]

Pathology

The herpes simplex virus infects the epidermal cell. Oedema of the cytoplasm produces the characteristic "ballooning degeneration". Giant cells formed from epidermal keratinocytes containing 2 to 15 nuclei, and intranuclear inclusions can also be seen.

Vesicles in the epidermis are formed by coalescence of intercellular oedema as well as degeneration of epidermal cells. Polymorphonuclear leukocytes infiltrate the dermis and subsequently the epidermis.

Clinical Manifestations[1]

The severity and frequency of clinical manifestations (Table 2) may be influenced by a number of viral and host factors. Viral factors include the viral type (type 1 or type 2), while host factors include the immune status of the host and prior exposure to autologous or heterologous virus type.

Table 2.   Classification of Herpes Virus Infections

- First episode

  True primary—in a seronegative individual
  Nonprimary—first episode in a previously infected individual

- Recurrent

The first time that a nonimmune person develops herpes is known as a primary infection. The first episode of herpes in an immune person (i.e., infected by another virus type) is termed a nonprimary first episode. Recurrences may follow first episode infections in a proportion of individuals. The first episode of infection is usually more severe and more frequently associated with systemic symptoms. However, the acquisition of infection in many individuals may go unnoticed and without any associated signs or symptoms, and in one study almost half of seroconversions of HSV 2 infections were asymptomatic.[7]

Only fifty percent of patients who present with their first episode of genital herpes have a true primary infection with either HSV 1 or 2. In the remainder, there is serological evidence of earlier infection, usually with HSV 1. About a fourth of patients presenting with their first episode of clinical HSV infection have serological evidence of previous HSV 2 infection, in these cases, this is not a primary infection, but probably a recurrence in an individual with an asymptomatic first episode.

The incidence of genital HSV 1 infections is rising with up to a third of true primary infections being caused by HSV 1. Prior nongenital HSV 1 infection protects against acquisition of genital HSV 1 infection, but protection against genital HSV 2 infection is incomplete. However, prior HSV 1 infection reduces the severity of first episode genital herpes.

Primary Genital Herpes

In primary genital herpes, systemic symptoms (fever, headache, myalgias and malaise) are prominent and prolonged. The disease is more severe in women and systemic symptoms are experienced by more than three fourths of women, but less than half the men. Symptoms are maximal in the first few days after onset of lesions. Painful ulcers are present in almost all patients and may last up to 2 weeks. The severity of local symptoms is similar with both types of HSV infection. Urethral and vaginal discharge and local lymphadenopathy are common but suppurative lymphadenopathy does not occur.

The lesions start as grouped vesicles but rapidly become pustular and ulcerate (**P XIX, Fig. 75**). At presentation, large coalescent areas of ulceration, often with polycyclic margins are usually present (**P XIX, Fig. 76**). New lesions continue to form in the first 8

to 10 days and complete re-epithelization may take as long as three weeks or more. Viral shedding usually continues for the first two weeks. Scarring is uncommon.

Systemic signs and symptoms are uncommon in patients with first episode nonprimary genital HSV 2 infections.

Cervicitis is commonly (upto 90%) associated in first episode HSV 2 infections in women and it is often ulcerative or necrotic. However, an examination of the cervix is usually not performed in the presence of painful vulval lesions. Proctitis caused by the herpes simplex virus is more commonly seen in homosexual men, and is the most common cause of nongonococcal proctitis. It is frequently severe and associated with severe systemic symptoms. It is usually limited to the lower third of the rectum. Anorectal infections may be occasionally seen in women and may be related to recurrences in the sacral ganglion rather than anal intercourse. Pharyngeal infection is often associated. In 20% of patients it may be the presenting complaint and may be associated with orogenital exposure. Autoinoculation during the course of primary gingivostomatitis to the genitalia sometimes occurs in children.

Complications of First Episode Genital Herpes

CNS involvement: Aseptic meningitis, transverse myelitis and sacral radiculopathy have been reported. HSV may be isolated from the CSF. Pleocytosis in the CSF may occur. Autonomic dysfunction (urinary retention, constipation, perineal hyperaesthesia or anaesthesia) may also be seen in the more severe cases.

Extragenital lesions: Extragenital lesions are frequent on the thigh, buttock or groin, but occasionally on the hand or eye. They are more common in women and with primary HSV 1 infection (25%) as compared to primary HSV 2 infection (9%) and usually appear in the second week. Autoinoculation, rather than viremic spread is probably the mode of spread.

Disseminated infection: This is rare, viremic spread occurs early, and it is associated with more severe disease. Disseminated infection is often associated with aseptic meningitis, hepatitis or pneumonitis. Pregnancy, immunosuppression, atopic eczema may predispose to disseminated infection.

Secondary infection: Bacterial superinfection manifesting as cellulitis and secondary pyoderma is not uncommon. Fungal vaginitis may be associated and usually emerges in the second week.

Recurrent Genital Herpes

Recurrences generally follow first episodes of infection, but in many cases the first episode may be asymptomatic or so mild as to remain unrecognized. Recurrent episodes are milder, lasting only 5 to 7 days. Over 90% of patients with recurrent disease have prodromal symptoms varying from a mild tingling sensation to shooting pains from an hour to up to 5 days prior to the appearance of the lesions. In a fifth of episodes there may be only prodromal symptoms without appearance of lesions.

Recurrent genital herpes is milder in men as compared to women, and is usually confined to one side. The duration of viral shedding is usually about 3 to 4 days and healing is usually complete by 7 to 10 days. However, even in the same patient there may be considerable variation in severity between episodes. The same strain of virus may have markedly different patterns of reactivation between persons and even in the same individual. The intervals between recurrence and duration of consecutive episodes are unpredictable.

Recurrences may not always be "typical" with grouped vesicles leading to crusting in a few days. In one study,[31] a third of the women in whom HSV was isolated, only linear superficial fissures or erosions were seen which were initially thought to be traumatic or monilial in origin.

Rate of Recurrences

After the primary episode, patients with HSV 2 infections have more frequent recurrences and earlier recurrences than those with HSV 1. The time to first recurrence after primary infection was about 10 months for HSV 1 infection but only about 6 weeks for HSV 2 infection.[8] Patients with more severe and prolonged first episode disease (> 5 weeks) have more frequent recurrences than those without. Genital herpes caused by HSV 2 may recur up to six times more frequently than that caused by HSV 1. During the first year, after a symptomatic episode of primary genital herpes caused by HSV type 2, almost 90% have at least 1 recurrence, 38% have more than six and 20% may have more than 10 recurrences. Recurrences are more common in men. The number of recurrences varies from 4 to 5 per year.

The frequency of recurrences shows a declining trend over the initial years of infection at the rate of about 1 recurrence per year. However, this is variable and up to a fourth of these patients may actually show an increase in the number of recurrences in the fifth year.[9]

In contrast to HSV 2, only 60% of patients with HSV 1 will have a recurrence in the first year of follow up. Rates of recurrence are also low at about 1 recurrence per year and less than 5% of patients with HSV 1 average more than 4 recurrences, that too mostly in the first year.

Asymptomatic Shedding

Although HSV infections are frequent, less than 20% of patients are aware that they are infected. Among HIV negative homosexual men, asymptomatic shedding from anogenital sites occurs on an average 2.2% of days sampled (range 1-24%).[10,11] Thus the majority of HSV seropositive individuals are unaware of their infection and yet are capable of shedding the virus and hence of transmitting the infection. Complicating this is the fact that over half of the men who were HSV 2 seropositive in the above study were also HSV 1 seropositive and shed the virus from the oral cavity on about 2% of the days.

Asymptomatic viral shedding is responsible for at least 70% of viral transmission.

Genital Herpes Complicating Pregnancy[12]

There are no studies addressing the seroprevalence of HSV type 2 infections in Indian women and one has to rely on figures from studies in other countries. In the US, approximately 25% of women in the reproductive age group are infected with the HSV 2 virus, more blacks (55%) being seropositive as compared to whites (19%). In studies from antenatal clinics, HSV 2 seroprevalence rates vary from less than 10% (UK, Japan, Italy and Spain) to intermediate (11 to 30%) reported from Australia, Finland, France and Sweden to high (more than 30%) in USA and Brazil.[13] Most of these patients are unaware of the fact and only a fourth of infected women report signs and symptoms suggestive of recurrent herpes.

It is important to classify genital herpes in pregnancy accurately based on typing of the genital isolate and serotyping the patient with type-specific serologic assays as the incidence and severity of neonatal infection depend on this.

First Episode Genital Herpes in Pregnancy

Genital herpes is acquired for the first time during

pregnancy in 2-3% of the pregnant women. Among seronegative pregnant women who have seronegative partners, the rate of transmission (acquisition) of herpes is 13% by the end of pregnancy. Most of these cases of herpes acquired during pregnancy are asymptomatic, and since in most cases seroconversion has occurred by the time of labour, the foetus is not in any danger. However, in patients acquiring infection late in pregnancy in which HSV seroconversion has not been completed by the time of labour, there is a 40% risk of transmission of herpes to the newborns.

Recurrent Genital Herpes in Pregnancy

The progressive decline in the immune competence that occurs during pregnancy results in an increase in the frequency, duration and severity of symptomatic recurrences as pregnancy progresses. During and around the time of labour, approximately 2% of seropositive women suffer a symptomatic recurrence, with another 2% having a culture positive asymptomatic shedding, and about 20% showing PCR positive tests.

Symptomatic recurrences during advancing gestation may be atypical and more severe, sometimes even resembling first episode disease. To complicate matters, some seropositive women who have been earlier asymptomatic, may experience a first-ever recurrence in advanced pregnancy. In one study of 29 women who presented with what appeared clinically to be primary genital herpes in the latter half of pregnancy, it was determined serologically that only 4 (14%) of these were actually true first episode disease and all the remaining were HSV seropositive and experiencing a first ever recurrence.[14] It is important, in view of both social implications as well as implications to the newborn that type specific serology should be determined as well as culture and typing of the viral strain isolated from the genitalia – antibodies to the same viral type isolated from the genitalia would indicate that the infection most likely antedated the pregnancy.

Transmission During Pregnancy and Delivery

Despite the frequency of genital herpes infection in women, the transmission of genital herpes to neonates is relatively rare, and is estimated to be less than 3%. The risk increases more than ten fold if a woman acquires genital HSV in the third trimester and delivers prior to the development of antibodies. Currently

available data suggest that the risk of transmission to the infant from a mother with primary HSV infection of either type is 50%, while in a first episode (nonprimary) HSV 2 infection in a woman with a past HSV 1 infection is 20%. In recurrent HSV 2 the risk of neonatal transmission is less than 1%.[1]

Neonatal Herpes

Neonatal herpes is a serious and frequently fatal disease and is of major concern to patient with genital herpes. This is the most serious complication of genital herpes occurring during pregnancy. The prevalence varies with the prevalence rate of maternal infection and reported rates range from up to 50 per 100,000 live births in the US to 6/100,000 in Sweden, 8/100,000 in Australia and 3/100,000 in the UK.[13]

Eighty percent of the infants in whom neonatal herpes develops have mothers who report no history of exposure to HSV and are asymptomatic at delivery. Some 25% of infants who contract herpes at delivery will develop disseminated herpetic infection, which has a high mortality (>40%) despite antiviral therapy. Congenital infection is rare and can occur through transplacental transmission of the virus. It may lead to spontaneous abortion, prematurity and a host of other abnormalities.

Only 5% of infants with neonatal HSV are born with the disease (suggesting *in utero* transmission), with most infections being acquired during labour or delivery. It is estimated that about two-thirds of these infections are caused by asymptomatic first episode genital herpes.

HSV type 1 is more easily transmitted to the newborn as compared to HSV 2. However, neonatal HSV 2 infections are more serious, with frequent dissemination to the CNS and fatal outcome, as compared to HSV 1 infections which are usually limited to the skin, eyes and mucous membranes.

The diagnosis of neonatal herpes is often overlooked early on and made late in the course of the disease. This may happen because lesions in the mother may be absent (asymptomatic) or not recognized or hidden (e.g., on the cervix), or the fact that the long incubation period (5 to 21 days) allows the mother to take home a healthy looking newborn that sickens at home. Further, the initial manifestations are non-specific (irritability, lethargy, poor feeding) and skin lesions are present only in a minority of infants.

Most cases of neonatal herpes cannot be anticipated

and hence are not preventable even with the best of antenatal and obstetric care. It has been estimated that even if every patient entering pregnancy with symptomatic recurrent genital herpes was delivered by a caesarean section, only a minority of cases of neonatal herpes would be prevented.

Unrecognized HSV 2 Infection

In a large survey in the US, only 9% of HSV 2 infected persons reported a history of genital herpes. Of individuals with genital HSV infection, approximately 20% have symptomatic disease that they recognize as genital herpes, another 60% have symptoms that they attribute to genital herpes only after being taught about the manifestation of infection, and the remaining 20% lack any sign or symptom of genital herpes.[15]

Herpes Genitalis in Patients with Concomitant HIV Infection[16]

Current seroprevalence studies suggest that HSV is the most common opportunistic infection occurring among HIV infected adults. In developed countries, up to 90% of men who have sex with men, and 40–60% of injection-drug users have antibodies to HSV-1, HSV-2 or both, while studies from Africa suggest that most (up to 90%) persons infected with HIV are co-infected with HSV-2.[17] It is probable that the genital ulcers of HSV facilitate the transmission of HIV.

Atypical presentations are common in patients with AIDS. These include deep progressive infection, disseminated infections, and prolonged viral shedding (Table 3)

Table 3. Atypical Presentations of Herpes Genitalis in Patients with AIDS

- Deep progressive ulceration
- Haemorrhagic and ecthyma-like lesions
- Hyperkeratotic verrucous lesions resembling condylomata
- Pseudotumour of the tongue
- Esophagitis, hepatitis, pneumonitis or life threatening disseminated infections associated with viremia
- Continuous and prolonged viral shedding

Differential Diagnosis

Many clinicians are under the impression that genital herpes has a characteristic appearance, comprising of easy to recognize blisters or ulcers. However, these so-called 'typical' signs and symptoms of herpes are in clinical practice not the commonest sign of herpes genitalis, and recurrent episodes of viral shedding may be associated with a wide variety of non-specific signs and symptoms such as erythema, small fissures, excoriated skin and burning or itching which frequently fail to be recognized as herpes. It should be emphasized also, that owing to the distribution of sacral sensory nerves, recurrences may occur anywhere below the waist; particularly common sites are on the buttocks, lower back, thighs and around the anus.

All ulcerative conditions of the genitalia, sexually transmitted or otherwise, must be suspected to be herpetic and appropriate tests must be performed.

Laboratory Tests

The diagnosis of herpes genitalis is usually made clinically in typical cases. It is important to realize however, that the sensitivity of clinical diagnosis is low—in one recent study, the sensitivity was only 39%, while the specificity was 96%.[7] However, in view of the fact that herpes may masquerade as a number of genital diseases with ulceration such as syphilis or chancroid, or even as non-specific lesions such as erosions or fissures, and in a proportion of cases may be asymptomatic, laboratory tests are frequently called upon to resolve the issue. As a thumb rule, all genital lesions regardless of appearance must be evaluated for herpes.

Laboratory tests available for the diagnosis of herpes virus infection include

- Tzanck smear
- Histopathology
- Viral culture
- Serology

Tzanck Smear

A smear taken from the base of a vesicle or erosion and stained with Giemsa stain may show multinucleate giant cells (**P XIX, Fig. 77**). This test is not sensitive and may be negative in later lesions. Specimens cannot be taken from dry lesions or crusts. Varicella-zoster virus infections may show a similar picture, although the clinical picture usually is distinctive enough to avoid confusion. Also, the Tzanck smear does not distinguish between HSV 1 and 2 infections.

Immunofluorescence staining of a Tzanck smear increases the sensitivity and specificity of the Tzanck test, but is not available in most laboratories.

Histopathology

Genital lesions are rarely biopsied. However, the presence of balloon cells and multinucleate giant cells will confirm the diagnosis of herpes. Histopathology is occasionally necessary in chronic herpes virus infections in HIV infected individuals wherein the morphology and clinical course are atypical. Again, as in the case of the Tzanck smear, the presence of giant cells does not distinguish between type 1 and 2 herpes simplex virus infections, nor does it exclude varicella zoster virus infections.

Viral Culture

This is the definitive means for diagnosis of herpes. The technique is demanding. The material for culture is collected with special (Dacron) swabs, placed in a viral transport medium which is then refrigerated and transported to the laboratory. Refrigeration is necessary, as otherwise negative results may occur. In the laboratory, the swabs are inoculated into either human diploid fibroblast cultures or green monkey kidney (GMK) cell cultures. The virus grows rapidly, and cytopathic effects are visible within a few days, although the cultures are observed for two weeks if there is no growth. Virus cultures are generally not available in most laboratories.

Cultures are usually positive in primary or first episode infections, but may be negative in up to 50% of patients with recurrent infections. Cultures are also frequently negative from dry erosions or crusts.

Serology[15,18]

These tests detect antibodies to the herpes simplex virus in the blood and include

- Enzyme linked immunosorbent assay (ELISA)
- Complement fixation test (CFT)
- Western Blot

Both ELISA and CFT detect circulating antibodies and are over 90% sensitive but the specificity is low (50%). Serologic testing may be useful to distinguish true primary HSV infections in which there is only increased IgM from first episode nonprimary infections (increased IgG with or without increased IgM). The Western Blot is another serologic technique which distinguishes between HSV 1 and HSV2 with high sensitivity and specificity (> 99%).

Earlier tests were misleading, inaccurate and had low sensitivity and specificity. The current generation of tests based on enzyme immunoassays are highly sensitive and specific and use type specific glycoproteins gG1 and gG2 from HSV 1 and HSV 2 respectively. Kits have been developed for office use with results within hours. The Pockit tests can detect HSV 2 antibodies within 15 days on an average although response times vary from 3 to 102 days (within 4 weeks in over 80% of episodes) Because of the wide variation in seroconversion, negative results should be repeated after 3 months for confirmation.

Unfortunately, the serological tests being performed at most commercial laboratories in India still utilize the older generation ELISA tests.

Management[19]

When seeing a new patient with suspected genital herpes, the clinician should establish a working diagnosis and a swab should be taken for confirmation if possible. Coexisting STD should be looked for, and appropriate screening tests should be performed. The importance of evaluating the sexual partners should be discussed with the patient.

The patient with herpes should be counseled and should receive a comprehensive diagnostic evaluation, information and ongoing support. Patients confronted with a diagnosis of herpes genitalis frequently report feelings of depression, isolation, loss of self esteem, and a fear of rejection and discovery; although these tend to subside over time, many patients report that these feelings never totally disappear even after many years. Although effective antiviral drugs are now available, cure of the infection is not possible, and therefore strategies to avoid contracting and transmitting infection are important and should be discussed. A professional, but non-judgemental and non-patronizing approach is essential to maintain a rapport with the patient.

Drugs available for use in herpes simplex virus infections are given in Table 4. Immunomodulators and vaccines are still in their infancy, while many drugs and modalities of treatment used in the past have now been shown to be ineffective (a few of the more popular ones are listed)

Table 4. Drugs Used for the Treatment of HSV Infections

Drugs currently in use	Vaccines and Immunomodulators	Ineffective drugs used in the past
Acyclovir	**To reduce recurrences**	Vidarabine
Valacyclovir	Imiquimod	Idoxuridine
Famciclovir	Resiquimod	Ether
Cidofovir	Vaccines	Chloroform
Trifluridine		Povidone iodine
Foscarnet	**For prevention of acquisition**	Photodynamic dyes
		BCG vaccine
	Vaccines	Nonoxynol-9

There are currently three drugs approved for the treatment of herpes genitalis – acyclovir, famciclovir and valacyclovir. Of these, only acyclovir is available in India and famciclovir has recently been launched. They are nucleoside analogues and prevent replication of herpes simplex virus by interfering with the formation of viral DNA. They are active only in herpes virus infected cells, making them extremely safe and well tolerated. Acyclovir's only drawback is poor bio-availability, less than a fifth of each dose is absorbed. Famciclovir is the oral prodrug of penciclovir, which has a similar, but not identical mechanism of action to acyclovir. Famciclovir is well absorbed orally, making twice daily oral therapy possible. Valacyclovir is metabolized to acyclovir in vivo, and has the same mechanism of action as acyclovir. Valacyclovir is almost completely absorbed orally and so lower doses and less frequent dosing is possible.

Drugs less commonly used, usually only in special circumstances such as acyclovir resistance, include foscarnet, cidofovir and trifluridine. Foscarnet is a viral DNA polymerase inhibitor; it has potent antiviral activity, but its insolubility precludes oral formulations. Intravenously, it is used in doses of 40 mg/kg every eight hours, but is toxic to the kidney and may produce hyperphosphatemia. It has been shown to be efficacious in acyclovir resistant recurrent HSV infections as a 0.3% and 0.1% cream.

Cidofovir is an acyclic nucleoside phosphonate which is phosphorylated only by cellular enzymes and hence is active against thymidine kinase deficient acyclovir resistant HSV strains. Intravenous cidofovir is effective, but is toxic to the kidney. Topical cidofovir, as a 0.3 and 1% gel formulation has been shown to help healing of non healing skin lesions of HSV in AIDS patients; however, almost one fourth of the treated patients had mild to moderate local side effects.

Trifluridine is a topical antiviral (since it is toxic when given internally). Interferon a may potentiate its antiviral effect. It could become a useful alternative in acyclovir resistant HSV infections.

Drug Regimens

Available antivirals may be used in different ways including:

- Symptomatic management using only applications designed to reduce symptoms and improve healing
- Episodic (intermittent) therapy: to abort or reduce the duration of the episodes
- Continuous antiviral therapy – suppressive therapy to prevent recurrences

In 'episodic' treatment, oral antiviral therapy is used intermittently by the patient whenever a recurrence is experienced. In 'suppressive' (preventive) treatment the patient takes antiviral therapy continuously to prevent recurrences. While episodic therapy may only decrease the duration of lesions by one to one and a half days, some patients may find this effect clinically significant. Suppressive therapy generally reduces the number of recurrences, and virus shedding) by 85-90 percent.

Dosage schedules used to treat initial and recurrent episodes of herpes genitalis are given in Table 5. The probability of recurrences should be discussed with the patient after an initial episode and the decision to use episodic or suppressive treatment should be evolved in consultation with the patient. The potential benefits of antiviral therapy should be discussed with all patients. As many patients are unaware of the options available to them, the responsibility lies with the clinician to provide patients with sufficient information to enable them to participate fully in management decisions. Once the patient is fully informed about the options available, the patient and clinician together should agree upon a management strategy.

Patients who have four or less recurrences per year are best managed with episodic therapy. Patients managed by episodic antiviral therapy can start therapy themselves each time they detect the first signs of a recurrence. Self initiation allows each recurrence to be treated more expeditiously than if a physician had to be consulted. Education directed at recognition of early signs and symptoms, including the prodrome, is very important. Allowing patients to self initiate treatment

Table 5. Treatment of Herpes Genitalis

Initial episodes	Acyclovir	200 mg 5 times daily for 7-10 days★ or 400 mg thrice daily for 7-10 days
	Valacyclovir	1 g twice daily for 7-10 days★
	Famcyclovir	250 mg twice daily for 7-10 days
Recurrent episodes#	Acyclovir	200 mg 5 times daily for 5 days★ or 400 mg thrice daily for 5 days or 800 mg twice daily for 5 days
	Famciclovir	125 mg twice daily for 5 days
	Valacyclovir	500 mg twice daily for 3-5 days 1 g once daily for 5 days

★every 4 waking hours # commence in prodromal period or at symptom onset
Adapted from CDC 2002.Guidelines for treatment of sexually transmitted diseases. MMWR 2002; 51 (No.RR-6) 12-17).

without having to go back to the physician also returns control of the infection to the patient.

Based on the fact that viral shedding (and by inference, viral replication) is generally halted within 48 hours, some workers have studied shorter courses of antiviral drugs for episodic treatment of recurrent genital HSV type 2 infections including

- A 2-day course of acyclovir 800 mg thrice daily[20]
- A 3-day course of valacyclovir twice daily[21]

Both these regimens have been shown to be as effective as the recommended 5-day course. In the case of valacyclovir the shorter course results in a 40% reduction in dose, and thus the cost.

None of the currently available antivirals offers any greater clinical benefit as compared to the other. Although less frequent dosing may be an advantage, cost considerations and availability may favour acyclovir.

Suppressive therapy should be considered for patients with severe, frequent or distressing recurrences (Table 6)

In the original benchmark study[22] of suppressive therapy with acyclovir (400 mg twice daily), 20% of patients remained recurrence free for the entire period

Table 6. Indications for Suppressive Therapy in Patients with Recurrent Genital Herpes

Severe recurrences
Frequent recurrences (>6 per year)
Distressing recurrences
Severe associated prodromes
To decrease risk of transmission★
Psychological and psychosexual problems linked to infection
Immunocompromised patients

★may decrease asymptomatic viral shedding and thus transmission

of 5 years. In the multicentre trial of 1100 patients with over 12 episodes of herpes genitalis per year, in the first year of treatment the recurrence rate was only 1.7 during the first year and 0.8 in the fifth year. There were no serious side effects, nor was there any cumulative toxicity. Some patients required higher doses up to 800 mg twice daily.

Table 7. Suppressive Therapy

Immunocompetent patients	Acyclovir	400 mg twice daily
	Famciclovir	250 mg twice daily
	Valacyclovir	500 mg once daily (<10 recurrences per year) 1000 mg once daily(> 10 recurrences per year)
Immunocompromised patients	Acyclovir	400 - 800 mg twice daily to five times daily (more frequent doses if repeated breakthrough recurrences)
	Famciclovir	250 mg twice daily, revise upwards if breakthrough recurrences★
	Valaciclovir	500 mg twice daily

★CDC 2002 treatment guidelines recommend 500 mg twice daily

Immunomodulation

Resiquimod an immune response modifier is a potential treatment option for genital herpes. Unlike nucleoside analogues, immune response modifiers have no direct antiviral activity. Resiquimod stimulates the innate immune response to produce cytokines such as tumour necrosis factor α, interleukin 12 and interferon γ as well as the antigen-presenting cells (APC) present in the skin. Once HSV in neurons has reactivated and translocated to cells in the skin, it can be recognized by skin-based APC stimulated by resiquimod. Thus resiquimod stimulates the development of Th1 acquired, cell mediated immune response against HSV infected cells thereby preventing HSV recurrences. Results from a Phase II clinical trial[23] of resiquimod (0.01 or 0.05% gel for 4 to 9 doses) as a treatment for genital herpes in patients have been promising, with a tripling of time to recurrences from 57 days to 169 days in the resiquimod treated patients.

Management of Herpes Genitalis in Pregnancy[1,12]

Herpes virus infections prior to labour have no effect on pregnancy outcome. Antiviral chemotherapy is indicated only for the treatment of maternal disease and should be restricted only to treat the more severe infections – whether recurrent or first episode.

There are no data with the use of either valacyclovir or famciclovir in pregnancy, but published literature suggests that acyclovir is safe and well tolerated even during the first trimester. Acyclovir is readily transferred to the amniotic fluid with an amniotic fluid to serum concentration of 5:1. At term the maternal serum to cord blood ratio is approximately 1.15:1.

Management of HSV Infections at Labour

It has been suggested by some workers in the past that all women with symptomatic genital herpes should be delivered by caesarean section. As discussed earlier, however:

1. Most neonates who develop herpes have mothers who either have no past history of herpes and have no active lesions at the time of delivery
2. Most of symptomatic lesions at term are recurrent HSV 2 which usually does not lead to infection of neonates.
3. Most neonatal herpes is a consequence of asymptomatic 1st episodes and caesarean section for all symptomatic lesions at term will prove ineffective in preventing neonatal HSV infection
4. HSV 1 infections during pregnancy and at term are rare but more easily transmissible to the neonate.

Since acyclovir is safe, two studies have been conducted using suppressive acyclovir treatment at term in pregnant women, and it was shown to be effective in suppressing symptomatic recurrences at term. However this strategy is not advocated for routine use for prevention of HSV neonatal infections.

Recommendations for the management of HSV infections in pregnancy[12]

1. HSV type specific serology should be determined at the first prenatal visit when all routine pregnancy blood tests are obtained to:

   - Detect HSV seronegative as well as HSV 1 seropositive women—these are the women who are at risk for acquisition of genital herpes late in pregnancy. At a subsequent visit, the partners of these women can be tested to identify serologically discordant couples. These women are liable to acquire genital herpes and if this occurs at the time of labour transmission of the herpes virus to the newborn may occur. These couples should be counselled regarding methods to prevent the women from acquiring genital herpes, including abstinence, use of condoms, and suppressive antiviral therapy for the male throughout the pregnancy.

   - Identify those women who are already infected by HSV 2 at their initial prenatal visit—these patients who have a high rate of symptomatic shedding at labour and it would be prudent to avoid invasive obstetric procedures including foetal monitoring, with scalp electrodes, rupture of the foetal membranes, forceps and vacuum extractors. A patient who is known to be HSV 2 seropositive during pregnancy and has recurrent lesions at the time of delivery may be delivered vaginally (since the child had passive immunity, and HSV 2 does not infect the neonate that easily). However lesions of HSV 1 on the vulva, or women with active lesions who have not yet seroconverted should be delivered by caesarean section.

   - Since nearly two thirds of the patients are asymptomatic, routine serologic testing of pregnant women will identify a large number of seropositive women who are unaware of their disease. They can be counselled regarding their infection, recognition of recurrences and methods of avoiding transmission to their sexual partner.

2. Women presenting for the first time with genital lesions in pregnancy should have viral cultures and typing obtained from lesions on the cervix and type specific HSV serology determined for reasons mentioned earlier

3. Routine antepartum and intrapartum HSV cultures of pregnant women known to have HSV infection are now not recommended. Such cultures do not predict newborns who will acquire neonatal herpes.

4. Although known to be effective in suppressing recurrent herpes, acyclovir suppressive therapy is presently not recommended for pregnant women who are known to suffer from recurrent herpes.

5. In women with active genital lesions of herpes at the time of labour:

   • In the absence of prior information on the serologic profile of the patient or if appropriate tests (such as the more accurate type specific serologic tests) are unavailable, the presence of active genital lesions of herpes at the time of labour should be taken as primary infection and a caesarean section would be prudent. There is evidence that the risks of vaginal delivery for the foetus are small and must be set against risks to the mother of caesarean section.

   • However, if such lesions are known to be recurrent, or if they are distant from the genitalia (buttock) the lesions can be covered with an occlusive dressing and a vaginal delivery can be allowed.

   • The mother should be treated with appropriate antiviral drugs, and the babies should be carefully followed up in the first three weeks for signs of neonatal herpes infection.

It should be pointed out that these recommendations revolve around the identification of HSV infection by culture and serology, and serotyping of the infection in the pregnant woman, and her spouse. These are not available in most developing countries and the costs and benefits of identifying susceptible women by means of type specific antibody testing have not been fully evaluated.

A simpler strategy could involve asking all women at their first antenatal visit if they or their partner have ever had genital herpes. Female partners of men with genital herpes, but without a history of genital herpes, should be strongly advised not to have sex at the time of lesional recurrence. The regular use of condoms throughout pregnancy may diminish the risk of acquisition. Pregnant women should be advised of the risk of acquiring HSV 1 as a result of oro-genital contact.

All women, not just those with a history of genital herpes should undergo careful vulval inspection at the onset of labour to look for clinical signs of herpes infection. Mothers, staff, and other relatives/friends with active oral lesions should be advised about the risk of postnatal transmission.[24]

Management of Genital Herpes in HIV-Infected Patients[16]

The management of genital herpes in human immunodeficiency virus (HIV) infected (HIV positive) patients differs from that in individuals not infected with HIV (HIV negative) for three reasons. Firstly, recurrent herpes simplex virus (HSV) genital infection in HIV positive patients tends to be persistent rather than self-limiting as in HIV negative individuals. This is particularly true in cases where the CD4 positive cell count falls below 100×10^6 cells/l. Secondly, HSV infection increases the replication and possibly the transmission of HIV infection. Finally, HIV immunosuppression increases the likelihood that antiviral therapy will lead to the emergence of drug-resistant mutants and with it, the associated failure of therapy.

Management of Primary and Initial Genital Herpes HIV-infected Patients

Initial genital herpes infection in HIV negative patients may be severe and prolonged but resolves spontaneously. In HIV infected patients, primary genital herpes may not resolve spontaneously but rather cause progressive, severe, multifocal and coalescing mucocutaneous anogenital lesions. Conventionally used doses of acyclovir, valacyclovir or famciclovir frequently effective in primary and initial genital herpes but higher doses of acyclovir (400 mg three to five times daily) have been recommended for HIV infected patients with severe genital infection and continuation of treatment until all lesions have crusted or re-epithelized This will generally exceed the 5–10-day duration of treatment that is recommended for HIV negative patients.[25]

Management of Recurrent Genital Herpes in HIV Infected Patients

Genital herpes disease in HIV-infected patients may recur more frequently than in HIV negative patients, especially those with a CD4 positive cell count of <50 × 10^6 cells/l, and cause extensive, severe anogenital ulceration that does not resolve spontaneously. Managing recurrent genital herpes in HIV infected patients requires close attention both to the treatment of the HIV infection itself and to the recurring HSV infection. Highly active antiretroviral therapy (HAART) has been shown to reduce the risk of retinitis due to reactivation of another herpes virus, cytomegalovirus (CMV), by 83% and extrapolating these results, optimizing the control of HIV disease is of fundamental importance for the management of genital herpes in these individuals.[16]

Episodic Therapy for Recurrent Genital Herpes in HIV Infected Individuals

Collectively, the available data support the choice of acyclovir 200–400 mg five times daily, famciclovir 500 mg twice daily or valacyclovir 1 g twice daily for 5–7 days for episodic treatment of recurrent genital herpes in HIV positive individuals.[16] Whereas 3 days' treatment of recurrent genital herpes can be as effective as 5 days' therapy in HIV-negative adults,[20] the appropriate duration of therapy in HIV infected adults appears to be at least 5–10 days (Table 8).

Table 8.   CDC Recommended Regimens for Episodic Infection in Persons Infected with HIV[30]

Acyclovir	400 mg orally three times a day for 5–10 days 200 mg five times a day for 5–10 days,
Famciclovir	500 mg orally twice a day for 5–10 days
Valacyclovir	1.0 g orally twice a day for 5–10 days

Suppressive Therapy of Recurrent Genital Herpes in HIV Infected Individuals

In addition to the indications for suppressive antiviral therapy of recurrent genital herpes discussed in non-HIV infected individuals earlier, recurrent disease that is either slow to respond to treatment or has a marked adverse psychological impact may be added. HIV infected patients with recurrent genital herpes lesions should initially be treated with one of the regimens for episodic therapy to achieve lesion resolution, after which a suppressive regimen as for HIV negative individuals can be initiated. Until optimal drug regimens are defined, available data indicate that valacyclovir 500 mg twice daily should be the preferred regimen for suppressive therapy of recurrent genital herpes in HIV infected individuals. Breakthrough recurrences may occur, but if frequent may necessitate an upward revision of the dose or assessment for resistance to the drug.

Management of Acyclovir-resistant Infection

Acyclovir-resistant strains of HSV were first reported over 20 years back, but are only now assuming significance with the epidemic of AIDS. Drug resistance appears to be uncommon in the immunocompetent population but more common in HIV-infected patients with prevalence rates of 4 to 7%. Acyclovir-resistance is most commonly due to a mutation in the gene encoding HSV thymidine kinase (TK), resulting in TK that either possesses reduced affinity for acyclovir or is not synthesized (TK–). Moreover, as famciclovir and ganciclovir are also subject to the same initial phosphorylation activation step mediated by TK, acyclovir resistance also extends to famciclovir and ganciclovir. Acyclovir-resistance may also be due to a mutation in the HSV DNA polymerase that results in a reduced affinity for acyclovir-triphosphate. Infection caused by isolates with altered TK or reduced affinity of HSV DNA polymerase should theoretically respond to higher doses of acyclovir and indeed, successful treatment of a patient with acyclovir-resistant HSV that had a TK with altered affinity, using intravenous acyclovir 1.5–2.0 mg/kg per hour for 6 weeks has been reported.

Long-term management of genital herpes in patients with resistant disease is unsatisfactory. Although both foscarnet and adenine arabinoside, show in vitro activity against acyclovir-resistant HSV, a controlled clinical trial demonstrated healing of mucocutaneous lesions due to acyclovir-resistant HSV only in recipients of foscarnet 120 mg/kg per day for an average of 14 days but not in those treated with adenine arabinoside 15 mg/kg per day intravenously; the latter was also associated with significant toxicity (neurotoxicity). Unfortunately, recurrences, mostly with acyclovir resistant virus occurred a median of 14 days after foscarnet was stopped in most of the treated patients.

Topical trifluridine alone or in combination with interferon-alpha, cidofovir gel and foscarnet 1% cream have been reported to have clinical utility for the treatment of acyclovir-resistant HSV genital ulcers.

The Role of Antiherpes Drugs in the Management of HIV and HSV Co-infection[17]

HSV infection increases HIV replication, and possibly the transmission of HIV infection, raising the possibility of a role for antiherpes drug therapy in controlling HIV disease and reducing HIV transmission. Epidemiological observations suggest that HSV-2 infection facilitates HIV transmission. HSV is a potent stimulator of HIV replication in co-infected CD4-positive cells in vitro. A survival benefit of treatment with acyclovir, 3200–4800 mg per day, has been demonstrated by a meta-analysis of eight randomized trials in patients with HIV and herpes virus infections.[17] The advantage was seen specifically in studies in which the incidence of HSV and varicella zoster virus (VZV) clinical disease was high, with >25 cases per 100 patient years. Acyclovir decreased HSV and VZV but not CMV infections as well as reducing mortality. These data suggest an important pathogenetic interaction between HIV and the herpes viruses, HSV and VZV. Controlled prospective studies with optimal HAART co-therapy are needed to confirm this and to justify chronic administration of antiherpesvirus drugs to control HIV infection and its transmission.

Prevention of Transmission of Genital Herpes

The only methods currently available for preventing transmission of genital herpes infections are male and female condoms. There have been no studies evaluating the efficacy of female condoms in preventing the transmission of herpes simplex virus infections. In one recent large study of over 500 serodiscordant couples enrolled in a candidate HSV 2 vaccine trial where participants were followed for 18 months participants using condoms were less likely to acquire HSV 2.[26] The efficacy of condoms was especially marked among women. Unfortunately, condoms are not acceptable to all users and the male condom does not provide coverage

of all susceptible surfaces. Altering sexual behaviours represents a cost-effective and safe measure that may significantly reduce new infections. Consistent and correct use of latex condoms appears to protect women from HSV 2 infection, and should be emphasized in pregnant women at risk of HSV 2 to prevent neonatal herpes.[27]

HSV vaccines are still in development. There are currently over nine types of live attenuated as well as inactive vaccines under evaluation. Although vaccines may not offer absolute protection, it is possible that they might ameliorate the disease or reduce recurrences. However, recent trials of some of the vaccines have not been very encouraging showing only minimal protection.[28]

Table 7. Potential Methods of Preventing Transmission of Genital Herpes

Condoms
Vaccines
Microbicides
Monoclonal antibodies

Another approach is the use of topical microbicides. These have been investigated in the prevention of other STD and have been found to be useful. Among the first such topical agents to be used was nonoxylenol-9. A variety of novel microbicides are in various stages of development[29] and these include sulphated polymer based inhibitors, acid buffers and surfactants. Sulphated polymer based inhibitors interfere with transmission by binding to pathogens and/or target cells and preventing the pathogen from attaching to its target. Acid buffers are designed to maintain the natural vaginal acidity in the presence of the alkalinizing effects of semen, thereby inactivating acid sensitive pathogens. Surfactants solubilize membranes and viral envelopes.

In contrast to the topical microbicides which are non-specific, monoclonal antibodies are highly specific. Monoclonal antibodies have been shown in experimental studies to protect against other sexually transmitted infections such as *Candida albicans*, *Chlamydia trachomatis* and *human papilloma virus* among others.

Monoclonal antibodies can also be used for preventing vertical transmission (neonatal herpes).[29] Microbicidal agents such as vaginally applied chlorhexidine have been used in the past to prevent neonatal transmission of HSV, HIV and other sexually transmitted infections. Based on the fact that antibodies prevent vertical transmission of hepatitis B and varicella zoster and also that maternal antibodies to HSV are associated with low transmission to infants by infected women systemically delivered anti HSV monoclonals given to women at risk for neonatal transmission, have been suggested as an alternative to or in conjunction with suppressive acyclovir therapy. Systemically delivered HSV specific antibodies have been shown to protect neonatal mice and guinea pigs from mucosal challenge, even when given 2 days after viral challenge and to prevent oral transmission of infection in a neonatal macaque model.

References

1. Corey L and Wald A. Genital herpes. In: Holmes KK, Mardh PA, Sparling PF, et al. eds. Sexually Transmitted Diseases. 3rd Edition. New York: McGraw-Hill; 1999. p. 285-312.

2. Xu F, Schillinger JA, Sternberg MR, et al. Seroprevalence and coinfection with herpes simplex virus type 1 and type 2 in the United States, 1988-1994. J Infect Dis 2002; 185: 1019-24.

3. Kumar B, Sahoo B, Gupta S, Jain R. Rising incidence of genital herpes over two decades in a sexually transmitted disease clinic in North India. J Dermatol 2002; 29: 74-78.

4. Lowhagen GB, Tunback P, Bergstrom T. Proportion of herpes simplex virus (HSV) Type 1 and Type 2 among genital and extragenital isolates. Acta Derm Venereol 2002; 82: 118-120.

5. Wald A. Herpes: Transmission and viral shedding. Dermatol Clin 1998; 16: 795-7.

6. Mertz G, Coombs R, Ashley R, et al. Transmission of genital herpes in couples with one symptomatic and one asymptomatic partner: a prospective study. J Infect Dis 1988. 157; 1169-1177.

7. Langenberg AGM, Corey L, Ashley RL, et al. A prospective study of new infections with herpes simplex virus type 1 and type 2. N Engl J Med 1999; 341: 1432-8.

8. Wald A, Zeh J, Selke S, et al. Reactivation of genital herpes simplex virus type 2 infection in asymptomatic seropositive persons. N Engl J Med 2000; 342: 844-850.

9. Benedetti JK, Zeh J, Corey LK. Clinical reactivation of genital herpes simplex virus infection decreases in frequency over time. Ann Intern Med 1999; 131: 14-20.

10. Krone MR, Wald A, Tabet SR, et al. Herpes simplex virus Type 2 shedding in human immunodeficiency virus-negative men who have sex with men: frequency, patterns, and risk factors. Clin Infect Dis 2000; 30: 261-267.

11. Stanberry RL. Editorial Response: Asymptomatic Herpes Simplex virus shedding and Russian roulette. Clin Infect Dis 2000; 30: 268-269.

12. Brown ZA. Genital herpes complicating pregnancy. Dermatol Clin 1998; 16: 805-809.

13. Mindel A, Taylor J, Tideman RL, et al. Neonatal herpes prevention: a minor public health problem in some communities. Sex Transm Inf 2000; 76: 287-291.

14. Hensleigh P, Andrews W, Brown Z, et al. Genital herpes during pregnancy: inability to distinguish primary and recurrent infections clinically. Obstet Gynecol 1997; 89: 891-895.

15. Ashly RL. Genital herpes: Type specific antibodies for diagnosis and management. Dermatol Clin 1998; 16: 789-793.

16. Aoki FY. Management of genital herpes in HIV-infected Patients. HERPES 2001; 8: 41-45.

17. Schacker T. The role of HSV in the transmission and progression of HIV. HERPES 2001; 8: 46-49.

18. Goldman BD. Herpes serology for the dermatologist. Arch Dermatol 2000; 136: 1158-1161.

19. Barton SE. Herpes management and prophylaxis. Dermatol Clin 1998; 16: 799-803.

20. Wald A, Carrell D, Remington M, et al. Two day regimen of acyclovir for treatment of recurrent genital herpes simplex virus type 2 infection. Clin Infect Dis 2002; 34: 944-948.

21. Leone PA, Trottier S, Miller JM. Valacyclovir for episodic treatment of genital herpes: a shorter 3-day treatment course compared with 5-day treatment. Clin Infect Dis 2002; 34: 958-962.

22. Goldberg LH, Kaufman R, Kurtz TO, et al. Long-term suppression of recurrent genital herpes with acyclovir: a 5-year benchmark. Arch Dermatol 1993; 129: 582-587.

23. Spruance SL, Tyring SK, Smith MH, Meng TC. Application of a topically applied immune response modifier, resiquimod gel, to modify the recurrence rate of recurrent genital herpes: a pilot study. J Infect Dis 2001; 184: 196-200.

24. National guidelines for the management of genital herpes. Sex Transm Infect 1999; 75 (Suppl 1): S24-28

25. Drew WL, Stempien MJ, Kheraj M, Erlich KS. Management of herpes virus infections (cytomegalovirus, herpes simplex virus and varicella-zoster virus). In: Sande MA, Volberding PA, eds). The Medical Management of AIDS. 6th edn. Philadelphia: WB Saunders; 1999. p 444.

26. Wald A, Langenberg AG, Link K, et al. Effect of condoms on reducing the transmission of herpes simplex virus type 2 from men to women. JAMA 2001; 285: 3100-3106.

27. Casper C, Wald A. Condom Use and the prevention of Genital Herpes Acquisition. HERPES 2002; 9: 10-14.

28. Stanberry LR, Cunningham AL, Mindel A, et al. Prospects for control of herpes simplex virus disease through immunization. Clin Infect Dis 2000; 30: 549-566.

29. Larry Zeitlin, Kevin J Whaley. Microbicides for preventing transmission of genital herpes. HERPES 2002; 9: 4-9.

Chapter 25

Anogenital Warts

N Usman

Definition

Wart is a viral infection caused by human papilloma virus (HPV). It can affect both the skin and mucosa. Anogenital warts refer to the infection of the anal and genital mucosa and its adjoining area. Many authors use the term "Anogenital Warts" synonymously with "Condylomata acuminata", although the later is described with a characteristic histology.[1]

Prevalence

Prevalence of genital HPV infection and distribution of specific HPV types appears to be similar in different regions of the world. Current evidence suggests that over 50% of sexually active adults have been infected with one or more HPV types. In United States estimated prevalence among men and women between 15-49 years of age with genital warts is 1.4 million and 19 million have subclinical infections.[2] In Britain and Ireland 80000 new cases of anogenital warts are reported yearly.[3] The prevalence of genital warts in India have been reported to be 5.1% to 25.2% of STD patients. [4-6] In a report by Arora et al, the incidence of anogenital warts had increased from 7.2% to 8.8% among the HIV infected patients over a period of five-years.[7]

Aetiology

The causative agent of anogenital warts is HPV, which is a naked, double stranded DNA virus. There are at present more than 100 different genotypes. Of these forty-five genotypes have been found to infect the genital epithelium.

HPV belongs to the family Papovaviridae along with polyoma virus. They are non-enveloped and are composed of 72 pentameric capsomers forming the outer coat. This coat consists of major and minor capsid proteins and these are arranged on a skewed icosahedral lattice. The capsids are approximately 60 nm in diameter. The genome consists of circular double stranded DNA, which encodes for overlapping genes and a single control region. The genes are distributed into early (E_1-E_7) and late (L_1 and L_2) regions. The early genes encode for proteins that are involved with regulation of viral DNA replication and transcription, whereas the late region encodes as L_1 and L_2 for major and minor capsid protiens, respectively. Early genes (E_6, E_7) are involved in oncogenic transformation in high-risk HPV types.[8,9]

HPV are epitheliotropic, and their replication depends on the presence of differentiating squamous epithelium. Viral DNA but not structural (capsid) protein can be detected in the lower layer of the epithelium. Capsid protein and infectious virus are found in the superficial differentiated cell layers. The different types of HPV cannot be differentiated serologically like other virus groups, because of the lack of antigen available to produce antibodies for testing, and these viruses cannot be grown in vitro. So far no HPV type has been shown to transform cells in vitro. The use of raft culture system, which forms a stratified squamous epithelium, has now produced limited amounts of infectious HPV.

Several types of HPV can co-exist in the same wart. The common types of genital HPV and their associations are shown in Table 1.[10]

Transmission of the Virus

Genital HPV infections are transmitted primarily through sexual contact. The infectivity of HPV between sexual

Table 1. HPV Types and Clinical Disease

Clinical diseases	HPV types (frequent)	HPV types (less frequent)
Condylomata acuminata	6, 11	1-5, 10, 16, 18, 30, 31, 33, 35, 39-45, 51-59, 70, 83
Cervical intraepithelial neoplasia (CIN/CIL)		
Low-grade	6, 11	16, 18, 26, 27, 30, 31, 33-35, 40, 42-45, 51-58, 61, 62, 67-69, 71-74, 82
High-grade	16, 18	6, 11, 31, 33, 35, 39, 42, 44, 45, 51, 52, 56, 58, 59, 61, 64, 66, 68, 82
Bowenoid papulosis	16	34, 39, 40, 42, 45
Cervical cancer	16, 18	31, 33, 35, 39, 45, 51, 52, 56, 58, 59, 66
Giant condyloma of Buschke and Lowenstein and other verrucous carcinomas	6, 11	57, 72, 73
Oral/laryngeal papilloma (Recurrent respiratory papillomatosis)	6, 11	2, 16, 30, 32, 40, 57
In HIV patients	7, 72, 73	

partners is estimated to be 60%. During the sexual act micro-abrasions occur in male and female genitalia and anus in homosexuals. It is believed that these micro-abrasions permit the transfer of HPV virions from the epithelial cells of the infected partner to the basal layer of recipient. It is thought, but not proven that moisture and abrasions of the epithelial surface enhance HPV transmission. Transfer by fomites, is not a known factor in transmission of genital HPV. Digital transmission has been reported. Perinatal transmission has been observed in infants born to women with genital warts during pregnancy. These infants developed laryngeal papillomas and congenital condylomas. This type of transmission is rare.[2]

Immunology of Warts [2]

Inability to propagate HPV in the laboratory has hampered investigation of the immunology of warts. Both cell-mediated immunity (CMI) and humoral response have been demonstrated in patients with genital warts

Humoral Immunity

Almedia *et al*[11] showed "one way cross reactivity" between cutaneous and anogenital warts. The cutaneous warts are auto-inoculable on to the genital mucosa, where as the genital warts are not able to produce any lesion on the glabrous skin. The aetiological difference

between cutaneous and genital warts is also seen in their serological behaviour. The serum from patients with cutaneous wart interacts with antigen from cutaneous as well as anogenital warts, whereas the serum from patients with anogenital warts interacts with the antigen of anogenital wart only.

Various studies have shown that human sera have antibodies that react to HPV proteins. The earlier studies used HPV expressing fusion proteins or synthetic peptides and used antibody assays that recognized only linear epitopes. Thus the heterogeneity of the virus particles were not taken into account. Almedia[12] analyzed the sera of 42 patients with warts and only half of these patients had demonstrable antibody. No particular correlation between presence of antibody, types and duration of the lesions had emerged, though recurrence did seem to be associated with lack of antibody. HPV capsids are the new generation of antigen targets. These antigen targets have defined specificity, which are obtained from recombinant vaccinia virus or baculovirus expressing L_1 and L_1 plus L_2. Using capsids in an ELISA, type specific antibodies to L_1 protein had been detected, and these antibodies strongly correlate with history of HPV-associated disease. Experimentally infected animals generated similar antibodies that have been shown to be neutralizing. It has been also noted that the tempo for developing serum anticapsid antibodies is slow. The median time to seroconversion is approximately one year and antibodies persist for decades.[2] Though circulating antibodies are detected in patients with warts, they do not help in the elimination of the lesion or in the prevention of recurrences.

In patients with regressing warts, IgM (100%), IgG (97%) and IgA (80%) classes of antibodies to HPV antigens were detected. In 83% of these patients, IgM class of antibodies to virus-infected cells was also seen. Only 12% of the patients with non-regressing warts showed antibodies (IgM) to the infected cells. Pyrhonen[13] showed that when complement-fixing (CF) antibodies (IgG) were present, the cure rate was high. In 75% of such patients cure was observed during first 2 months. The cure rate was high in those with CF antibodies and warts of short duration (less than one year). In contrast, absence of CF antibodies correlated with slow healing process. Increase in the circulating antibodies has been demonstrated in regressing warts. Whether this increase in antibodies is the result of the regression of the wart or it is responsible for the regression of the warts, is not known.

Cell Mediated Immunity

Increase in the CMI has been shown to be effective both in elimination and in the prevention of recurrence of warts. Evidence for the involvement of CMI in wart regression has come from observations that patients with immunodeficiency have an increased incidence of warts. It was noted that those patients with a predominantly cell mediated defect or a mixed antibody and cell-mediated defect were susceptible, in contrast to those with only antibody defects. A study on the immunocompetence of wart patients revealed a relative deficiency of cell mediated immunity which appeared to be related to the duration of infection,[14] thus confirming the observations of Brodersen, Genner and Brothagen that children with warts showed reduced tuberculin reactivity when compared to unaffected controls. In addition to the observation, that a marked dermal infiltrate of mononuclear cells present around spontaneously resolving warts, suggests the role for CMI in wart regression.

The lack of detectable local immunological response may be due to the fact that (i) the virus producing cells are away from the basement membrane as far as the immune response is concerned (ii) inadequate production of viral particles and viral antigens. This is supported by the smaller number of mature particles seen in genital warts either by immunoperoxidase staining or electron microscopic studies and (iii) the infected cells may exhibit insufficient histocompatibility antigen display on their surface as seen with other virus induced tumours.

The primary infected cells in a wart are not recognized by the immune system because of the local inhibitory effect of these cells. This is evidenced by the absence of Langerhans cells and T cells in the epidermis surrounding the wart in comparison to the normal epidermis. The antigen of HPV is situated in the granular layer of epidermis, therefore exposure of the antigen to the immune system is hampered and thus, there is delay in development of CMI against warts. Regression of warts due to increase in CMI in wart patients was demonstrated by Viac et al.[15] Cytotoxic T lymphocytic response seems to play an important role in the elimination of warts.[2] Although neutralizing antibodies may be useful in preventing infection, the cell–mediated immune response is likely to be important in controlling reactivation and regression of infection.[16]

Clinical Features

HPV after entry may remain dormant without producing any lesions[16] or may produce symptomatic or asymptomatic lesions.

Symptomatic

The lesions appear after the incubation period of 1-8 months with an average of three months. Rarely they may resolve after some time without any treatment. Anogenital warts may be single or multiple. In men genital warts most commonly appear first on the inner lining of the prepuce (subpreputial region) and the frenulum followed by the glans, coronal sulcus, urinary meatus, penile shaft, and the scrotum. In women, the common sites involved are posterior part of the introitus, labia, perineum and perianal area. Lesions can also be seen intravaginally or in the cervix, but these areas are affected more commonly in subclinical infections. The lesions are verrucous papules or pedunculated lesions. Some times they coalesce to form verrucous plaques or cauliflower like growths. Generally the lesions are pink and painless. Depending upon the clinical appearance warts can be classified as, condylomata acuminata, papular wart, keratotic wart, and flat topped papular warts.

1. Condylomata Acuminata

The lesions are pedunculated masses (cauliflower like)

with fissures and irregular surface (**P XX, Fig. 78–80**). The colour of the lesion varies from red to pink or white with characteristic warty digitations. Such lesions are usually seen in the moist partially keratinized epithelium.[2]

2. Papular Wart

These are non-pedunculated, hemispherical masses or dome shaped, 1-4 mm in diameter and are located on fully keratinized epithelium.[2]

3. Verruca Vulgaris Type or Keratotic

These are firm papular lesions with slightly rough horny surface with no pedicle; size ranging from few millimeters to few centimeters in diameter (**P XX, Fig. 81**). They are usually seen on dry areas like shaft of penis, outer aspect of prepuce, labia majora, and perineum.[2]

Sessile warts are tiny lesions with no horny surface. They are usually detected on fully keratinized epithelium.

4. Flat-topped Papules

These appear macular to slightly raised. They are detected on either partially or fully keratinized epithelium.[2]

5. Bowenoid Papulosis

A variant form of papular wart characterized by hyperpigmented dome shaped, smooth and flat-topped papules, the size of which is around 7 mm in diameter (**P XXI, Fig. 82, 83**). Histologically it shows high grade squamous intraepithelial neoplasia, and is positive for HPV 16 DNA. In men, it appears on the shaft or glans penis and in women around the labia majora and minora, inguinal folds and perianal region.[2] Recurrence rates of 20% have been reported. Recently HPV 16/11,16/18, 31/33/51 has been demonstrated in Bowenoid papulosis by in situ DNA hybridization technique.[17] The viral typing and clinical variation of anogenital lesions have no correlation. The clinical presentation at the anogenital region is dependent on the anatomical site of occurrence, abundance of moisture, concomitant infections and immune status of the patient.

Subclinical HPV Infections

Subclinical HPV infections, together with latent infections are probably the most likely outcome after exposure to HPV. They present with symptoms such as burning, fissuring and dyspareunia in some patients. Only these patients should be offered treatment. Predominantly, subclinical infections are asymptomatic. Aceto-white test with 3-5% acetic acid has been described to detect the same, but with variable specificity and this procedure is commonly not recommended.[9]

Diagnosis

Diagnosis of warts in the anogenital region is based on the history of the exposure, clinical appearance, epidemiological proof of the warts in the sexual contact and the histological appearance. The most sensitive method for detection of HPV DNA is PCR. This technique is able to detect latent infection, but has little benefit in routine diagnosis and management of condyloma and is primarily used as a research tool. Gel electrophoresis and restriction endonuclease cleavage are other methods employed in the detection of viral warts.[18]

Histopathological Features

Gross et al[19] studied warts of different clinical types and correlated them histologically and virologically. The histological characteristics of the 'classical' protuberant growth-type of condyloma acuminatum in the anogenital region are:

1. Mainly parakeratotic hyperkeratosis of varying degree
2. Moderate granulomatosis
3. Pronounced acanthosis and sometimes marked papillomatosis
4. Marked perinuclear vacuolization with marginal nuclei of sickle form, partially intranuclear oedema and basophilic inclusions in the malphigian and granular layer
5. Increase in the mitotic activity in the basal layers.
6. Koilocytes, which are mature squamous cells with a large, clear perinuclear zone, scattered throughout the outer cell layers. The nuclei of koilocytes may be enlarged and hyperchromatic and double nuclei are often seen. Ultrastructural studies show virus in some of the cell nuclei. Although koilocytes are thought to represent a specific cytopathic effect of HPV, koilocytic features often subtle, and other cellular changes

may mimic koilocytic changes. Thus, detection of koilocytes is not a sensitive or reliable predictor of cervical HPV infection.[4]

7. Viral antigen can be demonstrated in the nuclei of cells in the stratum granulosum by peroxidase-antiperoxidase test, indirect immunofluorescence and indirect immuno-alkaline phosphatase reaction.

The variations occurring in histopathology of plane warts versus genital wart is that, plane wart would reveal basket weave orthokeratosis, while hyperkeratosis would be demonstrated by genital wart.

Differential Diagnosis

Genital warts are to be differentiated clinically from the other verrucous lesions of the genitalia, like condyloma lata of syphilis, non-venereal treponematosis, hypertrophic verrucous type of granuloma inguinale, tuberculosis verrucosa cutis, skin tags and malignancy. Small warts are most often confused with pearly penile papules, others being herpes progenitalis, molluscum contagiosum and hirsutoid pappillomas, Fordyce's spots, urethral curuncle, capillary angioma, lichen planus, foreign body granuloma, schwannoma[20] and focal dermal hypoplasia (Goltz syndrome)[21]. The complication of lymphogranuloma venereum and filariasis (due to lymphatic obstruction) may mimic genital warts. Benign tumours like neurofibroma, lipoma and certain cysts are other genital conditions to be considered in the differential diagnosis of genital warts. Normal physiological glands like Tyson's may look like early warts. In multiparous women, mucous tags due to trauma may give misleading appearance of vaginal warts. Around the anus, prolapsed & sentinel piles and anal tags are the important clinical entities to be excluded. In unhygienic persons, dry smegma may appear like warts and hence cleaning the sub-preputial region is emphasized before the examination of warts in the male genitalia.

Treatment Modalities for Anogenital Warts[22]

The preference of patient, the available resources, and the experience of the health care provider should guide treatment of genital wart. No definite evidence suggests that any of the available treatment is superior to others.

The treatment modality should be changed if a patient has not improved substantially after three provider-administered treatments or if the warts have not cleared after 6 treatments.

(a) Extragenital/Periananl warts

Recommended regimens

Patients applied	Imiquimod 5% cream Podofilox 0.5% solution/gel
Provider administered	Cryosurgery with liquid nitrogen/(Cryoprobe repeat applications every 1-2 weeks.) or Podophyllin resin (10-25%) or Trichloro acetic acid (TCA)/ Bichloro acetic acid (BCA) 80-90%. Small amounts are applied on warts till frosting develops. or Surgical removal (Tangential scissor excision, tangential shave excision, curretage or electro-surgery)
Alternative regimens	CO_2 laser or Intralesional interferon

(b) Cervical Warts

(Management of exophytic cervical wart should include consultation with specialist, and should rule out high grade squamous intra epithelial lesions (SIL).

(c) Vaginal Warts

Recommended regimen
Cryosurgery with liquid nitrogen
Cryoprobe not recommended due to risk of vaginal perforation and fistula formation.
or
TCA / BCA (80-90%)

(d) Urethral Meatal Warts

Recommended regimen	Cryosurgery with liquid nitrogen or Podophyllin 10-25%

(e) Anal Warts

(Rectal mucosal involvement should be managed with consultation of a specialist).

Recommended regimen	Cryosurgery with liquid nitrogen or TCA/BCA (80-90%) or Surgical removal

(f) Oral Warts

Cryosurgery with liquid nitrogen (Recommended regimen) or Surgical removal

Podophyllin was introduced in the treatment of warts in 1942. It is a complex resinous material containing podophyllotoxin, alphapeltatum and betapeltatum, obtained from American plant *Podophyllum peltatum* and *P. emodi*, an Indian plant, grows in Himalayas (May apple or mandrake).[23] Podophyllin inhibits mitosis and causes swelling and necrosis of cells. It is used as dry powder or by making solutions with mineral oil, linseed oil, rectified sprit, liquid paraffin, propylene glycol; and tincture of benzoin 20% to 50% is the usual form used worldwide. Podophyllin is contraindicated in pregnancy. It may produce foetal deaths and abortions. Systemic absorption of podophyllin can rarely result in renal toxicity, neuropathy, coma, hepatotoxicity, granulocytopenia and thrombocytopenia. Prolonged use of podophyllin is not to be advocated for the fear of its oncogenic potential. Podophyllin is applied to the warts by clinicians using cotton tipped swab once or twice a week for upto six weeks. Applications are limited to less than 0.5 ml or 10 cm² per treatment session. One to 4 hours after application, it is completely washed off. After 6 sittings if the warts persists, other treatment modalities need to be considered.

Podofilox is 0.5% solution or gel purified from podophyllin. Podofilox has stable shelf life, does not need to be washed off after application and less likely to cause systemic toxicity. The solution or gel is applied with cotton swab or finger respectively, over the condylomas (also on normal appearing skin between the lesions) twice daily for three days, followed by 4 days of no therapy. Such treatment is given for a total of 4 cycles. The total area of treatment should not exceed 10cm² and total volume should not exceed 0.5ml. The initial application is by health care provider to demonstrate proper application and subsequently by patients themselves.

Imiquimod is a new immune response modifier for local application that induces the release of cytokines including interferon gamma, tumour necrosis factor, and certain interleukins by peripheral mononuclear blood cells and lymphocytes. There is no direct antiviral activity. 5% cream is applied to warts with fingers three times per week (every other night) upto sixteen weeks. The area is washed with mild soap and water 6 to 10 hours after application.[24] The most commonly reported side effect is local irritation.

Imiquimod and podofilox have not been approved for treatment of perianal, rectal, urethral, vaginal, or cervical warts. Safety in pregnancy has not been established for both the agents.[2]

Cryotherapy is a very useful for treatment of warts. It is particularly suitable for internal warts, especially meatal and does not require anaesthesia. The cryoprobe, which depends on a supply of nitrous oxide, is manufactured with number of probes with different sizes (including a cervical cone that may also be used for treating cervical erosions). The tip of a suitable probe or the surface of wart should be sparingly covered swith KY jelly before freezing. Two short freeze-thaw cycles are probably just as effective as a single one minute freeze, which is time consuming when multiple warts are present.

Liquid nitrogen is applied by pressing cotton wool swabs on orange sticks dipped in liquid nitrogen on the warts and holding for a minute; adherence to the warts is better if before use the cotton wool tips are teased to make the ends ragged before application.[9]

All patients are offered a follow up evaluation at 3 months after treatment. Women with genital warts or whose husband has genital warts should be counselled about the need for regular cytologic screening.

The comparative efficacy of different modalities of therapy is given in Table 2.[25]

Table 2. Clearance and Recurrence Rates with Different Treatment Modalities for Genital Warts

Treatment	Clearance Rates (%)		Recurrence Rates
	End of Treatment	3 Months or More	
Cryotherapy	63–88	63–92	0–39
Electrocatutery	93–94	78–91	24
Interferon			
Intralesional	19–62	36–62	0–33
Systemic	7–15	18–21	0–23
Topical	6–90	33	6
Laser therapy	27–89	39–86	<7–45
LEEP	<=90	——	——
Podophyllin★	32–79	22–73	11–65
Podophyllotoxin (Podofilox)	42–88	34–77	10–91
Surgical/scissors excision	89–93	36	0–29
Trichloroacetic acid	50–81	70	36
5-fluorouracil	10–71	37	10–13

★Studies using more than one treatment strength have been grouped together.
LEEP = loop electrocautery excision procedure.

Complications

Warts may resist most of the treatment modalities and persist for as long as ten years and cause embarrassment to the patient. They may increase in number and size. In men urethral meatal lesion may cause obstruction to the flow of urine. These types of warts after cauterization are liable to produce meatal stenosis. In women larger warts may cause cervical dystocia. Ulcerations, secondary infection and haemorrhage are the other complications of anogenital warts. Giant condyloma described by Buschke and Lowenstein is histologically benign (intact basal layer) and clinically manifest as large, foul smelling, cauliflower like masses, locally invasive, destructive and nonmetastasizing lesions. They are usually positive for HPV6 DNA. Malignant transformation of genital warts has also been reported. A constant problem of warts for both patients and clinician are their recurrences.[4]

Anogenital Warts and Pregnancy

Warts flourish in pregnancy and there is increase in both size and number. This may be due to the influence of increased hormone level, vascularity and immune deficiency, which are seen in pregnancy. Larger warts may cause dystocia. Even without treatment warts may resolve after delivery. The newborn may pick up infection during labour. Cryotherapy and TCA are ideal for warts in pregnant women. Larger warts can be surgically excised. Podophyllin, podofilox, imiquimod are not advocated in pregnancy. Some clinicians prefer elective caesarian section to prevent transmission of the infection to the neonate.[4]

Anogenital Warts in Children

The mode of infection in children is uncertain. Infants can acquire warts from maternal genital condyloma, at the time of delivery with resulting genital or laryngeal disease. Laryngeal papillomatosis occurs predominantly in infants and young children. There may be an increased risk of laryngeal papillomas in children whose mothers have had genital warts at the time of delivery, but the processes involved in their pathogenesis are unknown. There have been several reports, of condyloma acuminata in young children, which may be the result of sexual abuse. It is believed that infection may also occur through close non-sexual contact within a family.[2,27]

Anogenital Warts and HIV

Before the acquired immunodeficiency syndrome (AIDS) epidemic, it was well documented that immunosuppressed patients were at increased risk for the benign and malignant manifestations of HPV infection. Iatrogenic immunosuppresion such as that of transplantation patients, confers an increased risk for HPV associated neoplasms. The risks of carcinoma in situ of the cervix, vulva, and anus are estimated to be from 14 fold to 100 fold higher in renal transplantation patients than in normal women.

The HPV types detected in immunosuppressed patients have been found to be similar to those associated with warts in immunocompetent persons. Although at least one investigator found a selective increase of high-risk HPV types among transplantation patients, another investigator reported "nononcogenic" HPV viruses, such as HPV types 6 and 11 associated with cancers in immunosuppressed patients. A few studies suggested that intraepithelial neoplasia develops into cancer at an accelerated rate and that the natural history of cancers is altered by immunosuppression. Given such data, it was expected that similar changes would be seen in the natural history of HPV infection among those with HIV induced immunosuppression. It was reported that the incidence of venereal warts was 8.2 compared with 0.8 per 100 person years of follow up for HIV 1 seropositive and HIV 1 seronegative women, respectively. Studies examining HIV infected women in the United States, Europe, East Africa and West Africa found genital HPV DNA in 8% to more than 50% of HIV seronegative women and 37% to 78% HIV seropositive women[28]. Smaller studies have reported that 26% to 60% of HIV seropositive men and 15% to 29% seronegative men have anal HPV DNA. Among women in whom cervical HPV DNA was detected, HIV seropositive women were more likely to harbour high risk HPV types 16 and 18 than were HIV seronegative women. Cervical cancer is now considered as AIDS defining illness in women.[28] Increasing HIV induced immunosuppression, as measured by CD4+ counts correlates with increased likelihood of detecting HPV DNA in men and women. It was found low CD4+ counts ($200/cm^3$) to be a risk factor for detection of anal HPV DNA. HIV infection and immunosuppression play an important role in modulating the natural history of HPV infection.[29] HIV infection influences local immunity by altering HPV transcription and by systemic immunodeficiency.[30]

Mechanisms of Interactions Between HIV and HPV

Alterations in the natural history of HPV infection and of HPV related neoplasia among HIV seropositive individuals are probably the result of general or local HIV induced immune system dysfunction. It is possible, for example that control of HPV is impaired when large numbers of lymphocytes or Langerhans' cells in

the area are infected with HIV. Some small studies found that among HIV seronegative women, those with squamuos intraepithelial lesions (SIL) had fewer Langerhans' cells than those without SIL and that HIV seropositive women with cervical SIL had even fewer Langerhans' cells than HIV seronegative women with SIL. It is also possible that HIV acts directly on HPV. In vitro studies have shown that intracellular HIV 1 tat m RNA can transactivate HPV type 16, E6 and E7, a step that is important in development of squamous cell neoplasias. In vitro studies have also shown that extracellular HIV 1 tat protein can enter HPV infected cells and upregulate HPV type 16 E6 and E7. The HIV 1 tat protein enhances E2 dependent HPV type 16 transcription. It is possible that extracellular tat migrates from Langerhans' cells or other HIV infected mononuclear cells that abut HPV infected epithelial cells and upregulates HPV. However, although several in vitro studies suggests that HIV could enter and establish infection in epithelial cells, the mechanisms remain controversial.[28]

Anogenital Warts and Malignancy

Role of the HPV in the aetiology of anogenital cancers has been firmly established based on large number of molecular and epidemiological studies. Predictions of the role of HPV in neoplasia induced by experimental studies, which are consistent with the natural history of cervical cancers. The genital HPV have been grouped in to high and low risk types based on the potential of the infected cells to progress to carcinoma. HPV types 16, 18, 31, 33, 35, 39, 45, 51, 52, 54, 56, 66, 68 are associated with cancers.[31]

Vaccine

Prophylactic Vaccine

Several human phase I trials have established the safety and immunogenicity of candidate prophylactic vaccines. All these preparations are based on virus like particles (VLP), which are recombinant versions of the major capsid protein (L1) of the relevant HPV types. The individual L1 molecules self assemble into empty viral capsids that assume correct information and induce type specific neutralizing antibodies. The VLP lack nucleic acids and are thus incapable of replication and are noninfectious.

In models using animals and their corresponding papillomaviruses, vaccines based on VLP have been protective. In humans, phase I trials have shown that neutralizing antibodies are present in sufficient titre in genital secretions to block infection in model system. Thus large scale trials are being mounted to determine clinical efficacy in phase III trials. Phase III studies are planned for HPV 16 VLP vaccine developed through the National Cancer Institute. HPV 16 is the most common HPV type associated with cervical cancer and dysplasia. The outcome studied in this placebo controlled trial will be on HPV 16 induced SIL (squamous intraepithelial lesion) with a planned 4 year follow up. Another planned phase III study is of a quadrivalent VLP based preparation. This preparation contains VLP from HPV types 6,11,16 &18. HPV types 6 and 11 are the most common types associated with condyloma acuminata, and types 16 and 18 are the most common types associated with cervical cancer.

Therapeutic Vaccines

Although production of neutralizing antibody may eventually prove to be sufficient to prevent disease; antibodies alone will not suffice to alter the course of established disease. A variety of strategies are being tested to produce a cellular immune response that is thought to be necessary to eliminate an established intracellular viral infection. The strategies that have proven immunogenic are the use of DNA based vaccines and the use of VLP that have proteins other than the L1 protein included in the vaccine. Some of the preparations are now in phase II and III trials in patients with established pre-existent cervical, vulvar, or anal intraepithelial neoplasia due to target HPV types, mainly HPV 16. Outcomes measured in the study lesion are stabilization, and progression or regression.

References

1. Oriel JD. Genital Papilloma Virus Infections; clinical manifestations. In: Morten RS, Haris JRW, eds. Recent advances in sexually transmitted diseases. New York: Churchill Livingstone; 1988. p. 127-145.

2. Koutsky LA, Kiviat NB. Genital human papilloma virus. In: Holmes KK, Sparling PF, Mardh PR, et al. eds. Sexually transmitted Diseases. 3rd Edn. New York: McGraw Hill; 1999. p. 347-359.

3. Maw RD. Genital Warts – approaching rational treatments. Indian J Sex Trans Dis 1999; 20: 30-32.

4. Kura MM, Hira S, Kohli M, et al. High occurrence of HBV among STD clinic attendees in Bombay, India. Int J STD AIDS 1998; 9: 1101-1103.

5. Chopra A, Dhalival RS, Chopra D. Pattern and changing trend of STD at Patiala. Indian J Sex Transm Dis 1999; 20: 22-25.

6. Aggarwal K, Jain VK, Brahma D. Trends of STD at Rohtak. Indian J Sex Transm Dis 2002; 23: 19-21.

7. Arora R, Rawal RC, Bilimoria FE. Changing Pattern of STD and HIV prevalence among them at five year interval. Indian J Sex Transm Dis 2002; 23: 22-25.

8. Brentjens MH, Yeung-Yue KA, Lee PC, Tyring SK. Human papilloma virus: a review. Dermatol Clin 2002; 20: 315-331.

9. Saunders NA, Frazen IH. Simplifying the molecular mechanisms of human papilloma virus. Dermatol Clin 1998; 16: 823-827.

10. Nebesio Cl, Mirowski GW, Chuang TY. Human papilloma virus: Clinical significance and malignant potential. Int J Dermatol 2001; 40: 373-379.

11. Almedia JD, Oriel JD, Stannard LM. Characterization of the virus found in Human genital warts. Micro bios 1969; 3: 225-232.

12. Almedia JD, Goffe AP. Antibody to wart virus in human sera demonstrated by electron microscopy and precipitin tests. Lancet 1965; 2: 1205-1207.

13. Pyrhonen S. Johansson E. Regression of warts. An immunological study. Lancet 1975; 1(7907): 592-596.

14. Morison WL. Viral warts, herpes simplex and herpes zoster in patients with secondary immune deficiencies and neoplasms. Br J Dermatol 1975; 92: 625-630.

15. Viac J, Thivolet J, Chardonnet Y. Specific immunity in patients suffering from recurring warts before and after repetitive intradermal tests with human papilloma virus. Br J Dermatol 1977; 97: 365-370.

16. Bunny MH. Viral warts: a new look at old problem. Br Med J 1986; 293: 1045-1046.

17. Salvatore P, Irina P, Amina V. The presence of HPV types 6/11, 6/18, 31/33/ 51 in Bowenoid papulosis demonstrated by DNA in situ Hybridization. Int J STD AIDS 2000; 11: 823-824.

18. Strand A, Rylander E. Human papilloma virus sub clinical and atypical manifestation. Dermatol Clin 1998; 16: 817-822.

19. Gross G, Pfister H, Hagedorm M, Gissman L. Correlation between human papilloma virus (HPV) type and histology of warts. J Invest Dermatol 1982; 78: 160-164.

20. Ghaly AF, Orange GV. Not every penile lump is a wart! Schwannoma of the penis. Int J STD AID 2000; 11: 199-200.

21. Singh S, Singh A, Gupta S, Thappa D. Perianal papillomas in focal dermal hypoplasia (Goltz Syndrome) mimicking Condyloma acuminata. Indian J Sex Trans Dis 2000; 21: 87-89.

22. Centre For Disease Control. Sexually transmitted diseases.

Treatment guidelines 2002. MMWR 2002; 51 (No. RR-6): 53-57.

23. Bhargava RK, Joshi R. Viral STD In: Valia RG, Valia AR, Eds. IADVL textbook and atlas of Dermatology. Mumbai: Bhalani publishing house, 2001. p. 1476-1491.

24. Mohany CO, Law C, Gollnick HPM, Marini M. New patient applied therapy for ano genital wart is rated favourably by patients. Int J STD and AIDS 2001; 12: 565-570.

25. Beutner KR, Wiley DJ. Recurrent external genital warts: A literature review. Papillomavirus Report 1997; 8: 69-74.

26. Willcox RR, Willcox JR. In: Pocket consultant – venereology, Maruzen Asian Edition. London: Grant MCln Tyre Ltd, 1981. p. 264-268.

27. Usman. N, Shakir FH, Gajendiran K. Anal condylomata acuminata in eleven months old Infant. Indian J Sex Transm Dis 1985; 6: 61-62.

28. Kiviat MB. Human papilloma virus and hepatitis viral infections in human immuno deficiency virus infected persons. In: Devita Jr VT, Hellman S, Rosenberg SA, Curran J, Essex M,. Fauci AS, Es. AIDS Aetiology, Diagnosis, Treatment and prevention. New York: Lippincott – Raven: 1997. p. 281-291.

29. Ahdieh L, Klein RS, Burk R, et al. Prevalence, incidence and type-specific persistance of human papilloma virus in human immuno deficiency virus (HIV)-positive and HIV- negative women. J Infect Dis 2001; 184: 682-690.

30. Aramy I, Typing SK. Systemic immuno suppression by HIV infection influences HPV Transcription and this local Immuno responses in condyloma acuminatum. Int J STD and AIDS 1988; 9: 268-271.

31. Galloway DA. Biology of Genital human papilloma virus, In: Holmes KK, Sparling PF, Mardh PA, et al, Eds. Sexually Transmitted Diseases. 3rd New York: Mc Graw – Hill; 1999. p. 335–346.

Chapter 26

Balanoposthitis

PN Arora, S Arora

Definition

Balanitis is defined as inflammation of the glans penis and posthitis is inflammation of mucous surface of the prepuce. It may occur individually or in combination i.e. balanoposthitis.

Incidence

The overall incidence of balanoposthitis reported is less than 2 percent.[1] However in the recent years, the incidence has gone up to 20 percent.[2]

Aetiology

Balanoposthitis is a disease confined to uncircumcised males. The warm, humid and relatively anaerobic environment of the preputial sac predisposes to the growth of aerobic and anaerobic organisms. Balanitis alone is far less seen in circumcised males. Balanoposthitis occurring for the first time in elderly males is highly suggestive of diabetes mellitus[3] whereas in younger age group it commonly results from sexually transmitted diseases. The various predisposing and etiological factors are given below.

Predisposing Factors

(a) Poor personal hygiene
(b) Long prepuce
(c) Congenital or acquired phimosis
(d) Failure to dry the glans and prepuce after a bath
(e) Hot and humid climate

Systemic diseases like diabetes mellitus[3], candidiasis,

Reiter's disease, Crohn's disease[4], ulcerative colitis[5], HIV infection and other diseases or drugs leading to immunosuppression also predispose to balanoposthitis.

Classification of Balanoposthitis[6]

Infections

1. Fungal

    (a) *Candida albicans* (commonest cause of infective balanoposthitis[7,8])
    (b) *Pityrosporum orbiculare*[9]

2. Anaerobic Organisms (recorded in 76% of cases[10])

    (a) Diphtheria
    (b) Diphtheroids
    (c) Fusospirochetes

3. Spirochaetal

    Treponema pallidum

4. Viral

    (a) Herpes simplex[11]
    (b) Human papilloma virus (HPV)

5. Mycobacterial

    (a) *Mycobacterium tuberculosis*[12]
    (b) *Mycobacterium leprae*[13]

6. Aerobic Organisms[14]

    (a) *Gardnerella vaginalis*

(b)   Group B streptococcus
(c)   *Staphylococcus aureus*
(d)   *Calymmatobacterium granulomatis*
(e)   Mycoplasma
(f)   Pseudomonas
(g)   Gonococci
(h)   *Haemophilus ducreyi*
(i)   Chlamydia

7. Protozoal

(a)   *Trichomonas vaginalis*[15]
(b)   *Entamoeba histolytica*

8. Parasitic

(a)   Scabies
(b)   Pediculosis
(c)   Creeping eruptions[16]

Irritants

(a)   Smegma
(b)   Perfumed soaps
(c)   Retention of soaps or detergents in preputial sac
(d)   Persistent moisture
(e)   Contraceptives
(f)   Irritation from infected urine and faeces
(g)   Irritants from vaginal secretions
(h)   Podophyllin
(i)   Vaginal spermicides
(j)   Spermicidal lubricants
(k)   Condoms

Trauma

(a)   Postcoital or post masturbation trauma
(b)   Sharp cuts inflicted by pubic hair
(c)   Laceration of prepuce by fasteners
(d)   Frictional trauma
(e)   Teeth bites
(f)   Pin pricks
(g)   Excoriations
(h)   Self inflicted

Fixed Drug Eruptions

(a)   Sulfonamides
(b)   Barbiturates

(c)   Tetracycline
(d)   Carbamazepine
(e)   Salicylates
(f)   Oxyphenbutazone
(g)   Dapsone
(h)   Griseofulvin[17]
(i)   Chlordiazepoxide
(j)   Phenolphthalein
(k)   Morphine
(l)   Codeine
(m)   Quinine
(n)   Phenacetin
(o)   Erythromycin
(p)   Metronidazole[18]

Premalignant Conditions

(a)   Erythroplasia of Queyrat (Bowen's disease of glans penis)
(b)   Leukoplakia
(c)   Extramammary Paget's disease.

Malignant Diseases

(a)   Squamous cell carcinoma
(b)   Basal cell carcinoma
(c)   Basisquamous or metastatic basal cell carcinoma
(d)   Melanoma

Cutaneous and Mucocutaneous Disorders

(a)   Pemphigus (**P XXI, Fig. 84**)
(b)   Dermatitis herpetiformis
(c)   Erythema multiforme
(d)   Stevens' Johnson syndrome
(e)   Toxic epidermal necrolysis
(f)   Lichen planus
(g)   Psoriasis
(h)   Behcet's disease
(i)   Aphthae
(j)   Porokeratosis of Mibelli
(k)   Herpes zoster
(l)   Varicella

Miscellaneous

(a)   Circinate balanitis
(b)   Zoon's balanitis

(c) Balanitis xerotica obliterans and lichen sclerosus et atrophicus

(d) Pseudoepitheliomatous micaceous and keratotic balanitis of Civatte

Clinical Manifestations

Balanoposthitis is a spectral disorder varying from an insignificant localized lesion to gangrenous ulceration. There is invariably overlap of clinical presentation of one disease and manifestation of others. It is important to rule out the underlying diseases or to investigate the basic etiopathogenic factors.

The natural course of the disease is that of the predisposing factors and the etiological factors mentioned above leading to the inflammation with or without break in the continuity of the surface of the glans or undersurface of the prepuce. This is followed by preputial oedema, phimosis, and copious, thick, offensive subpreputial discharge accompanied with pain, pruritus, feeling of pricking or of insect crawling or sense of stretching of the affected parts, meatal inflammation and burning micturition. Occasionally painful lymphadenopathy develops if left untreated and may progress to extensive ulceration, perforation of prepuce and even sloughing gangrenous ulceration (phagaedena) of the glans an or prepuce, particularly when infected with fusospirochetes. The progress of the disease is arrested as the symptomatic treatment is started and the underlying cause is dealt with.

Manifestations of balanoposthitis irrespective of aetiology are much more severe when associated with HIV infection, particularly so in the advanced stage.[19,20]

The clinical manifestations of different etiological factors leading to balanoposthitis are described under respective headings in different chapters. However, distinctive features of some of the conditions deserve special mention.

Candidal Balanoposthitis

It is the commonest type. Two types of clinical patterns have been described. The first one is due to the presence of *C. albicans* and manifests as small papules or fragile papulopustules on the glans or in the coronal sulcus which break open and leave behind superficial erythematous erosion having a collarette of whitish scales or a thrush like membrane. It may also present as longitudinal fissures on the undersurface of the prepuce. Preputial oedema leads to phimosis and anaerobic infection with offensive purulent curdy discharge from the preputial sac. The second type is due to the hypersensitivity reaction to *C. albicans* and present with transient erythema and burning, shortly following intercourse wih partners having candidal vaginitis. Healing in these cases may be rapid with topical application of corticosteroids rather than with antifungals.[7,8,21,22]

Anaerobic Balanoposthitis

It is thought to be caused by non-sporing anaerobic bacteria. It presents as erosive balanoposthitis, ulceration and as foul smelling discharge. In a study of 104 patients with above signs, 29 of the culture positive infections were due to mixed anaerobes and 8 due to single anaerobes. A rapid response to treatment with metronidazole also confirmed the anaerobic cause of the infection.[23]

Non-Syphilitic Spirochaetal Balanoposthitis

It has been described from many tropical countries including from India.[24,25] Clinically it is characterized by the presence of an extensive tender ulceration of the glans accompanied by a foul smelling purulent discharge. The foul smelling discharge is often due to the associated anaerobic infection. It is caused by *T. refrigens, T. phagedenis, T. balanitidis* and *T. vincenti*. These organisms have characteristic *eel* like movements and few coils on DGI. Treatment with penicillin and metronidazole may prevent the progression to phagedenic complications (**P XXI, Fig. 85**).

Herpetic Balanoposthitis

Genital herpes presents as grouped small circular erosions lasting for less than a week in recurrent genital herpes but for more than three weeks in a primary infection. Necrotizing balanitis has been described with primary HSV infection.[26,27]

Balanoposthitis due to HPV Infection

HPV infection may present as balanoposthitis. A careful examination and penoscopy with acetowhite test may be needed.[28] High power magnification can illustrate warty balanitis or balanoposthitis.

Trichomonal Balanoposthitis

It is distinguished by invariably accompanying history of urethritis and associated vaginitis in sexual partner. The discharge is copious, mucopurulent, greenish, frothy and has a fishy odour.[29]

Gonococcal Balanoposthitis

It follows sexual exposure with an infected partner. Clinical features include pain, burning, urgency and frequency of micturition; thick, creamy, greenish yellow purulent urethral discharge. Demonstration of intracellular diplococci on Gram's stain and culture of gonococci and biochemical tests confirm the diagnosis.[30]

Behçet's Syndrome

It is a chronic relapsing disease of unknown cause and usually starts with oral ulcers followed by genital lesions, which may be followed by scarring. Fibrosis may be seen under magnification. Occasionally eye lesions may precede cutaneous lesions. Recurrent arthritis and other systemic features may occur.[31]

Penile Psoriasis

It manifests as bright red colour of variable severity covered with white silvery scales in circumcised patients. Moist erythematous plaques without scaling occur in uncircumcised males. It usually has an annular or circular morphology with psoriatic lesions elsewhere.

Circinate Balanitis

In uncircumcised men, it presents as classical painless, serpiginous geographic dermatitis of the glans penis, whereas in circumcised men, it manifests as hyperkeratotic papules.[32] Other features of Reiter's disease are invariably associated and discussed in the respective chapter.

Bowen's Disease

Bowen's disease of glans may be confused with psoriasis but is gradually progressive in size whereas psoriasis is variable in its course. Histopathology is characteristic.

Balanitis Xerotica Obliterans (Lichen Sclerosus et Atrophicus)

It is characterized by a chronic inflammation followed by atrophic sclerosis, depigmentation, induration, urethral stricture and phimosis.[33]

Zoon's Balanitis

Chronic benign circumscribed plasma cell balanoposthitis of Zoon is usually seen in middle aged or elderly patients. Classically it presents as shiny red velvety patches often with characteristic 'cayenne pepper' stippling due to hemosiderin. The lesion is usually solitary, asymptomatic or mildly pruritic. Erosive and vegetative types have also been described. Aetiology is unknown. Usual sites are glans penis and/or inner surface of the prepuce. The characteristic histopathological features include a thin epidermis showing 'lozenge' keratinocytes, occasional dyskeratotic cells and mild spongiosis with dermal lichenoid infiltrate.[34]

Pseudoepitheliomatous Micaceous and Keratotic Balanitis of Civatte (PMKB)

It was first described by Lortat-Jacob and Civatte in 1961. Clinically it presents as crusty hyperkeratotic plaques on the penis. The term micaceous refers to the white scaly appearance of the lesion. The lesions tend to progress slowly and recur locally. Some authors suggest that it is a premalignant condition or locally aggressive low-grade malignancy, which has been associated with the development of a verrucous carcinoma.[35,36] Histologically, PMKB reveals hyperplastic epidermis with massive hyperkeratosis and elongated rete ridges, at times surrounded by dense polymorphonuclear infiltrate. Few atypical cells and mitoses may also be seen.

Balanoposthitis Associated with Leukemia

Rarely ulcerative balanoposthitis has been described as initial presentation of acute promyelocytic leukemia.[37]

Balanoposthitis and Circumcision

The presence of prepuce predisposes to collection of microorganisms that contribute to inflammation presenting as balanoposthitis. In a study of 305 patients, all cases of Zoon's balanitis, Bowenoid papulosis, and nonspecific balanoposthitis were observed in uncircumcised males. Lichen sclerosus et atrophicus was diagnosed in only 1 circumcised patient. Most patients with psoriasis (72%), lichen planus (69%) and seborrheic eczema (72%) were seen in uncircumcised males.[38]

Complications

- (a) Recurrence
- (b) Chronicity
- (c) Relapse
- (d) Re-infection from the sexual partner
- (e) Phimosis
- (f) Paraphimosis
- (g) Balanitis xerotica obliterans
- (h) Depigmentation of glans or prepuce
- (i) Hyperpigmentation of the affected parts
- (j) Preputial adhesions
- (k) Perforation of prepuce
- (l) Gangrene (phagaedena)
- (m) Scarring
- (n) Meatitis
- (o) Meatal stricture
- (p) Carcinoma of penis in long standing cases.

Diagnosis

The clinical diagnosis of balanitis, posthitis or balanoposthitis is not difficult by the presence of signs of inflammation of the affected part. Subpreputial wash followed by naked eye examination of urine for haze will clinically differentiate it from urethritis. The importance of comprehensive and detailed history cannot be overemphasized for etiological diagnosis. A thorough examination of the glans penis, coronal sulcus, urethral meatus, undersurface of the prepuce and frenulum must be done to establish a clinical diagnosis. Prepuce if present must be examined and retractility should be assessed. Dorsal slit may be mandatory where retraction of prepuce is not possible. Laboratory tests like complete blood count, urine examination for glucose, subpreputial

discharge in normal saline for *T. vaginalis,* KOH preparation for *C. albicans,* dark ground microscopy, Gram's or Giemsa staining and culture for aerobes and anaerobes particularly for mixed infections, blood for VDRL, HIV, patch testing (for condom and contraceptive allergic tests), skin biopsy for histopathological tests and other relevant investigations like examination of vaginal secretions of sexual partners, particularly when trichomonal vaginitis is suspected, may be required to establish the etiological diagnosis. The diagnostic criteria of genital ulcer diseases, premalignant and malignant conditions and other disorders involving the cutaneous and mucocutaneous regions are discussed in the respective chapters.

Treatment

The general treatment of balanoposthitis irrespective of aetiology remains almost the same, depending on the stage of the disease. Subpreputial wash or irrigation, when the prepuce cannot be retracted, with normal saline or 1:10000 potassium permanganate solution, 1% boric acid solution, 0.6% magnesium sulphate solution or 1% lead acetate solution for 15-20 minutes thrice daily for fifteen minutes each after voiding urine, helps in reducing the inflammation.

Specific treatment depends on the aetiology and is discussed in the relevant chapters. Aggressive treatment is warranted when balanoposthitis is associated with HIV infection.

Preventive treatment in the form of (a) Personal hygiene, (b) Circumcision for phimosis (congenital or acquired), chronic circumscribed balanitis of Zoon, and recurrent relapsing chronic persistent, intractable balanoposthitis, (c) Examination of sexual partner for candidal, trichomonal, or other STD induced balanoposthitis whenever indicated. (d) Management of systemic diseases, if any.

Topical corticosteroids have been used with variable efficacy in treatment of balanoposthitis due to psoriasis, lichen planus, fixed drug eruption, plasma cell balanitis and allergic contact dermatitis.

For treatment of PMKB, topical application of 5% 5-FU has been used with encouraging results, but definitive therapy is Moh's microsurgery.

Surgical treatment e.g. meatoplasty, meatotomy, repair of perforation, dorsal slit or circumcision may be required for complications of balanoposthitis after the medicinal treatment is over.

Post treatment surveillance is essential for a variable period depending on the aetiological cause.

References

1. Arora PN, Chaterjee RG. Changing patterns of sexually transmitted diseases (thirty years retrospective study), Indian J Sex Transm Dis 1993; 14: 24-37.

2. Rajnarayan, Kar HK, Gautam RK, et al. Pattern of Sexually Transmitted Diseases in a Major Hospital in Delhi. Indian J of Sex Transm Dis 1996; 17: 76-78.

3. Waugh MA, Evans EGV, Nayyar KE, Fong R. Clotrimazole (Castren) in the treatment of candidal balanitis in men. Br J Venereal Dis 1978; 54: 184-186.

4. Wijesurenda CS, Singh G, Manuel ARG, Morris JA. Balanoposthitis-An unusual feature of Crohn's disease. Int J STD AIDS 1993; 4: 184.

5. Lytde PH. Ulcerative colitis and balanoposthitis. Int J STD AIDS 1994; 5: 72-73

6. Waugh MA. Balanitis. Dermatol Clin 1998; 16: 757-762.

7. Oriel JD, Partridge BM, Denny MJ, et al. Genital yeast infection. Br Med J 1972; 4: 761.

8. Sharma VK, Kumar B, Ayyagiri A, et al. Microbial flora in balanoposthitis: study of 100 cases. Indian J Sex Transm Dis 1990; 11: 19-22.

9. Smith EL. Pityriasis versicolor of the penis. Br J Vener Dis 1978; 54: 441.

10. Masfari AN, Kinghorn GR, Duerden BI. Anaerobes in genitourinary infection in men. Br J Vener Dis 1983; 59: 255-9.

11. Chakraborty AK, Dutta AK, Herpetic balanoposthitis. Indian J Dermatol 1981; 26: 15-23.

12. Pavithran K, papulonecrotic tuberculids, on the glans penis. Indian J Dermatol Venereol Leprol 1982; 48: 42-44.

13. Chaudhury DS, Chaudhury M. A case report of gangrenous balanitis in progressive reaction in leprosy. Lepr Rev 1966; 37: 225-6.

14. Bhargava RK, Thin RNT. Subpreputial carriage of aerobic micro organisms and balanoposthitis. Br J Vener Dis 1983; 59: 131-133.

15. Dal S, Barua MC, Padiyar NV. Ulcerative Balanoposthitis due to Trichomonas vaginalis. Indian J Sex Transm Dis 1982; 3: 72-74.

16. Pavithran K, creeping eruptions on the genitals. Indian J Sex Transm Dis 1990; 11: 33-34.

17. Arora PN, Aggrawal SK. Drug eruptions. Indian J Dermatology 1989: 34: 75-80.

18. Arora SK. Metronidazole causing Fixed drug eruptions. Indian J Dermatol Venereol Leprol. 2002; 68: 108-109.

19. Franca I, Mansinho K, Claro C, Baptista AP, Nunes JM, Champalimaud J. Isolated hyperplastic balanitis. Int Conf AIDS. 1994: Aug 7-12; 10: 183.

20. Potekayev N, Yurin O, Potekayev S, Pokrovsky VV. Chancriform pyodermia as an indicator for HIV-infection. Int Conf AIDS 1992: Jul 19-24; 8: 124.

21. Martin AG, Kobayashi GS. Yeast infections; candidiasis, pityriasis (Tinea) versicolor. In: Freedberg IM, Eisen AZ, Wolf K, et al, eds. Dermatology in general medicine. 5th Ed. New York: Mc Graw-Hill; 1999: p. 2358-2371.

22. Kumar B, Sharma VK, Malhothra S, Talwar P. Balano posthitis. Contribution of women. Indian Sex Transm Dis 1991; 21: 66-68.

23. Cree GE, Willis AT, Phillips KD, Brazier JS. Anaerobic balanophosthitis. Br Med J (Clin Res Ed) 1982; 284: 859-860.

24. Piot P, Duncan M, Dyck EV, Ballare RC. Ulcerative balanoposthitis associated with non-syphilitic spirochete infection. Genitourin Med. 1986; 62: 44-46.

25. Chakraborthy AK. Clinico pathological study of balanoposthitis in male. Indian J of Dermatol. 1982; 27: 105-108.

26. Peutherer JF, Smith IW, Robertson DHH. Necrotizing balanitis due to a generalized primary infection with herpes simplex virus type 2. Br J Vener Dis J 1979; 55: 48-51.

27. Powers RD, Rein MF, Hayden FG. Necrotizing balanitis due to herpes simplex type 1. JAMA 1982; 248: 215-216.

28. Wikstrom A, Van Krogh G, Hedblad MA, Syrjanen S. Papilloma virus associated balanoposthitis. Genitourin Med 1994; 70: 175-181.

29. Michalowski R. Balano posthites à Trichomonas. A propos de 16 observations. Ann Dermatol Venereol 1981; 108; 731-738.

30. Landergren G. Gonorrhoeal ulcer of the penis; report of a case. Acta Derm Venereol 1961; 41: 320-323.

31. Jorizzo JL. Behçet's syndrome. Arch Dermatol 1986; 122B: 556-558.

32. Rice PA, Handsfield HH. Arthritis associated with sexually transmitted diseases. In: Holmes K, Mardh PA, Sparling PF, et al eds. Sexually transmitted diseases. 3rd Ed. New York: Mc Graw Hill; 1999: p. 921-935.

33. Stühmer A. Balanitis xerotica obliterans (post-operationem) und ihre beizhunger zur "Kraurosis glandis et praeputii penis". Arch Dermatol Syph 1928; 156: 613-623.

34. Souteyrand P, Wong G, MacDonald DM. Zoon's balanitis (balanitis circumscripta plasmacellularis). Br J Dermatol 1981; 105: 195-199.

35. Read SI, Abell E. Pseudoepitheliomatous, keratotic balanitis. Arch Dermatol 1981; 117: 435-437.

36. Beljaards RC, VanDijk E, Hausman R. Is pseudoepitheliomatous, micaceous and keratotic balanitis synonymous with verrucous carcinoma? Br J Dermatol 1987; 117: 641-646.

37. Steinbach F, Essbach U, Florschutz A, Gruss A, Allhoff EP. Ulcerative balanoposthitis as initial manifestation of acute promyelocytic leukemia. J Urol 1998; 160: 1430-1431.

38. Mallon E, Hawkins D, Dinneen M, Francics N, Fearfield L, Newson R, Bunker C. Circumcision and genital dermatoses. Arch Dermatol 2001; 737: 503-504.

Chapter 27

Miscellaneous Sexually Transmitted Diseases

Dinesh C Govil, Vinod K Sharma

Introduction

A large number of infections besides the traditional sexually transmitted diseases (STD) are now recognized as being sexually transmitted. Their role in the causation of STD is undisputed since several studies have shown that they are present in significant proportion of patients in association with the traditional STD. Moreover, the causative organisms are isolated with equal frequency in both the sex partners. They are described under miscellaneous STD (Table.1).

Table 1. Miscellaneous Sexually Transmitted Diseases

Viral Infections
    Molluscum contagiosum
    Hepatitis A,B,C and D
    Cytomegalovirus
    Epstein Barr virus
Parasitic Infestations
    Scabies
    Phthirus pubis
Bacterial Infections
    Ureaplasma and Mycoplasma
    Bacterial vaginosis
    Enteric Pathogens
Protozoal and Fungal Infections
    Trichomoniasis
    Candidiasis

Viral Infections

Molluscum Contagiosum[1-7]

Molluscum contagiosum is a common cutaneous disease caused by a pox virus- Molluscum contagiosum virus (MCV).

Epidemiology

The molluscum contagiosum infection is commonly seen in school going children. Molluscum contagiosum in adults over the genital areas is sexually transmitted. Transmission occurs through close skin to skin contact with infected person or fomites. Since 1991, there is a progressive increase in patients with molluscum contagiosum localized to the genital area. Lesions on the genitalia and perianal skin of children are not uncommon but sexual abuse should be ruled out in such cases.

Aetiology

MCV is a brick shaped approximately $300 \times 200 \times 100$ nm sized virus, with a biconcave viral core enclosed by an inner membrane and an outer envelope. MCV cannot be grown in tissue culture or egg yolk. However it has been shown to produce typical changes on human keratinocytes culture in immuno-incompetent mice. Two types of MCV have been recognized by DNA endonuclease restriction techniques: MCV-1 and MCV-2. Majority of the infections (76-97%) is caused by MCV type-1.

Clinical Features

Incubation period of molluscum contagiosum is 2 to 3 months though the range varies from 2 weeks to 6 months. The onset is gradual and most patients are asymptomatic. Some may complain of itching or tenderness. The lesions are skin coloured or pearly white papules, size 3 to 5 mm in diameter. Papules are firm, dome-shaped and umblicated with a central pore from which cheesy material can be expressed (**P XXII, Fig. 86**). Rarely some lesions become very large reaching upto 1 to 2 cm or larger in size and are called as giant molluscum contagiosum.

In adults the lesions most often occur on the thighs, inguinal region, buttock, lower abdominal wall, external genitalia and perianal region especially mucosal surfaces. In contrast, in children the lesions are usually distributed on exposed areas of the limbs, face and neck. However, 10 to 50% of children may have lesions on the genital area.

MCV is a common cutaneous pathogen in HIV infection. MCV tends to appear when CD-4 cell count is below 200/mm^3 and the severity of infection tends to parallel with the stage of HIV disease with a prevalence of 5 to 18 % among the HIV infected patients. The distribution of lesions of molluscum contagiosum in HIV infected individuals is usually over the face, neck and trunk rather than the genitalia. The lesions may be in hundreds and of larger size ranging from 1 cm to 5 - 10 cm. These may be follicular. Mucosal lesions are seen when the CD 4 cell count is less than 50/mm^3.

Diagnosis

The diagnosis of molluscum contagiosum is often clinical. In less typical cases the differential diagnosis includes – plane warts, vaccinia, eruptive xanthomas, syringoma, lichen planus, histiocytosis and when large and solitary, pyogenic granuloma, acanthoma or an epithelioma and disseminated cryptococcosis especially in HIV infected individuals.

Direct microscopic examination of unstained curetted lesion crushed on a slide establishes diagnosis. Thin smears of the expressed cheesy core material stained with Wright, Giemsa or Gram stain demonstrates the pathognomic enlarged epithelial cells with cytoplasmic molluscum bodies. Diagnosis is confirmed by histopathologic examination. Typically brightly eosinophilic cytoplasmic inclusion bodies -"molluscum bodies" otherwise known as Henderson-Paterson bodies can be demonstrated in lower epidermis.

Antibodies were demonstrated in both HIV positive and negative persons and there was no correlation with number of lesions and duration. Other methods of detection include electron microscopy, detection of MCV antigen by fluorescent antibody techniques or using dot blot hybridization technique to demonstrate MCV DNA.

Treatment

The disease is self limiting and may clear spontaneously. However, to prevent auto inoculation and spread to others, therapy is needed.

The simplest and most widely used technique is expression of contents of papules with forceps followed by cauterization of base of the lesion with electrodessication or a chemical agent such as silver nitrate, trichloroacetic acid or iodine. Cryotherapy is effective. Destruction by laser may also be considered.

For tiny lesions, which may be difficult to curette, topical preparations can be used to produce an inflammatory response. These preparations are 10 – 20% phenol, tretinoin, 5% imiquimod cream, 5% potassium hydroxide, cantharidin and 0.5% podophyllotoxin cream. A course of oral cimetidine has been found to be effective. Interferon alpha has been used to treat molluscum contagiosum in immunodeficiency. In HIV patients HAART may lead to regression of lesions. The antiviral agent cidofovir has been shown to be effective (used either IV or 1 – 3% ointment topically). It should be considered for treatment of extensive molluscum contagiosum in HIV disease.

Viral hepatitis[8–10]

Both Hepatitis A virus (HAV) and Hepatitis B virus (HBV) can be transmitted sexually. Hepatitis C virus (HCV) is predominantly a blood borne infection although less efficient, occupational, perinatal and sexual exposure also can result in the transmission of HCV.[19] Hepatitis delta virus may also be transmitted sexually.

Hepatitis A

HAV is an RNA containing picornavirus, known to cause only acute and not chronic hepatic disease. It is a non-enveloped virus and the size is 27 nm. It is heat, acid and ether resistant. There are four polypeptide capsids VP1 – VP4 in HAV. The virus is inactivated by boiling for 1 minute, by contact with formaldehyde, chlorine and by ultraviolet light.

Prevalence

HAV is most commonly transmitted by faecal-oral route. Hepatitis A, like other enteric infections can be transmitted during sexual activity especially involving oroanal or digital-rectal intercourse. Inapparent fecal contamination is commonly present during sexual intercourse. Measures like condom use to prevent other STD do not protect from HAV. HAV transmission through sexual activity may play a major role in the developed countries with good public health system. In developing countries with inadequate sanitary and water system, water borne infection is so prevalent that sexual mode of transmission becomes insignificant. Outbreaks of hepatitis A have occurred among homosexual men. Some studies have associated the various risk factors like having a greater number of sex partners, frequent oral-anal contact, insertive anal intercourse or serologic evidences of other STD with HAV. Parenteral spread can occur in intravenous drug users,haemophiliacs using contaminated factorVIII and other recipients of blood products.

HAV replicates in the hepatocytes and appears in bile. It is shed in high concentration in faeces from 2 weeks before to 1 week after the onset of illness.Viraemia roughly parallels shedding of virus in faeces and can persist for several weeks after the onset of symptoms.

Clinical Features

The incubation period from the time of exposure to the onset of symptoms is approximately 4 weeks (range 15 – 50 days). It starts with a prodromal illness which will last for about 2 weeks, followed by icteric hepatitis that lasts for a few weeks, sometimes longer than 3 months.There is no prolonged carrier state and infection with HAV produces immunity and hence symptomatic reinfections rarely occur. Chronic infections usually do not occur.

Antibodies to HAV (anti HAV) can be detected concurrent with the clinical onset of hepatitis. The early antibody response is predominantly IgM and persists for several months. Anti HAV IgG appears shortly after the appearance of symptoms and during convalescence, and may remain detectable lifelong.

Diagnosis

A specific diagnosis of viral hepatitis-A requires the demonstration of IgM anti HAV, which is virtually present in the serum of all patients. Rheumatoid factor may be falsely positive. Absence of anti-HAV IgM is strong evidence against current infection with HAV. Anti-HAV IgG persists for life and is not useful for acute illness.Tests can also be positive after hepatitis-A vaccination.

Treatment

Patients with hepatitis-A infection usually require only supportive care. Patient developing dehydration due to nausea and vomiting or patients with signs and symptoms of acute liver failure may require hospitalization.

Prevention

Both passive vaccination with immunoglobulin (IG) and active vaccination with formalin inactivated cell-cultured-derived HAV are available. HAVRIX[R] contains inactivated Hepatitis A virus HM 175 strain. It is not recommended for children under 2 years.Adults (older than 18 years) should receive two 1.0 ml injections containing 1440 enzyme linked immunoassay units (ELU) 6 to 12 months apart. Children aged 2 to 18 years should receive 0.5-ml injections containing 360 ELU at 0,6,12 months or two 0.5-ml injections containing 72 ELU, 6 to 12 months apart. Another vaccine manufactured by Merck is also available for prevention.

A combined hepatitis-A and B vaccine has been developed for adults.When administered at 0, 1 and 6 months schedule, the vaccine has equivalent efficacy to that of the monovalent vaccines.

Immunoglobulin (IG) when administered before or within 2 weeks of exposure is 80 to 90 percent effective in protecting against Hepatitis A. Previously unvaccinated persons exposed to patients with HAV (e.g. through household or sexual contact or sharing needle with a person who has hepatitis A) should be administered a single dose of IG (0.02 ml/kg) as soon as possible, but not more than 2 weeks after exposure. Hepatitis A vaccine can be administered simultaneously at different sites. Adverse drug reactions to IG are minimal and occur in about 1 % of all recipients.

Hepatitis B[11–15]

HBV is a double stranded DNA virus in the Hepadnaviridae family. It has been cultivated on different cell lines. The HBV genome has four genes: pol, env, precore and X that encode for viral DNA polymerase, envelope protein, pre-core protein (which is processed to viral capsids) and protein X respectively. HBV has three antigens – HbsAg and HBcAg & HBeAg present in the surface envelope and in the core protein of virus respectively. They are also produced by infected hepatocytes. HBcAg is obtained on vigorous disruption of the virus core.

Presence of HBsAg in blood is diagnostic of HBV infection. The core antigen HBcAg is not seen in blood and is detected in hepatocytes. Estimation of HBeAg, which is also present in the core of the virus, is useful to assess the infectivity of the patient, especially in long-term carriers.

Prevalence

In the United States an estimated 18,000 persons were infected with HBV in 1998, and about 5,000 deaths occurred from HBV related cirrhosis or hepatocellular carcinoma. An estimated 1.25 million, chronically infected people serve as reservoir for HBV infection. Hepatitis B infection is endemic in many parts of South Asia including India.

HBV is a hepatotropic, found in the highest concentration in blood and in lower concentration in other body fluids (e.g. semen, vaginal secretion and wound exudates). The major route of transmission is percutaneous. At present as a result of screening of the blood and blood products for HBV, transmission by blood transfusion is very rare. The other routes are sexual contact and perinatal transmission especially in endemic countries. Both homosexual and heterosexual exposure may transmit HBV. Sexual transmission can be prevented by use of condom. Health care providers and patients receiving haemodialysis are also at increased risk of acquiring infection.

Various Indian studies have shown high prevalence of HBV antigens among STD patients. High (59%) serological prevalence of HBV was observed among male homosexuals. The most common risk factors for heterosexual transmission include multiple sex partners, unprotected sexual act or a recent history of STD. Changes in sexual practices to prevent HIV infection have resulted in lower risk for HBV. HBV infection is more prevalent among HIV infected population.

Clinical Features

The incubation period from the time of exposure to the onset of symptoms is 6 weeks to 6 months. It may be shorter with large inoculum and parenteral exposures and may be prolonged by administration of globulin preparations. HBV infection may be self limited or chronic. In adults 50% have silent infection resulting in permanent and solid immunity. The remaining develop symptomatic, acute HBV infections and about 1% of these cases result in acute liver failure and death.

Approximately 15 to 20 % of patients develop a transient serum sickness like illness during the prodromal or early acute stage of hepatitis B. Acute hepatitis B infection has clinical picture similar to that of HAV infection. About 90 to 95% of the acutely infected adults recover without any sequelae and about 2 to 6% develop chronic infection. Risk for chronicity is associated with age at infection. About 90% of infected neonates and 60% of infected children develop chronic infection in contrast to 2 to 6% of adults. Approximately 5% of persons with HBV infection become chronic carrier of which two-thirds have a benign form of the disease, and one-third of chronic HBsAg carriers develop chronic active hepatitis, which can be either "replicative" with virus production or "non-replicative". The "replicative" chronic HBV infections is defined by the presence of detectable HbeAg, has worse prognosis and a increased risk of developing cirrhosis and or hepatocellular carcinoma. The risk of death due to cirrhosis and or hepatocellular carcinoma is 15% to 20% among persons with chronic HBV infection.

Diagnosis

The diagnosis of acute or chronic HBV infection cannot be made on clinical grounds but requires serologic testing. Almost 90 percent of individuals with acute hepatitis B have HBsAg detectable in the serum when presenting to clinician for the first time. The remaining 10 percent HbsAg negative individuals will have antiHBc uniformly present in the sera while antiHbs may be found in some. HbsAg is detectable several weeks after infection and its appearance coincides with the onset of clinical infection. The presence of IgM antibody to hepatitis B core antigen (IgM anti-Hbc) is specific and diagnostic of acute HBV infection. It persists for 6 to 24 months. Antibody to HbsAg (anti-Hbs) is produced following a resolved infection and is the only HBV antibody marker present following immunization. The presence of Hbs Ag with a negative test for IgM anti-HBc is indicative of chronic HBV infection. The presence of anti-Hbc may indicate acute, resolved or chronic infection. Diagnosis of hepatitis B is confirmed and prognosis is assessed by liver histopathology.

Treatment

Laboratory testing should be used to confirm suspected acute or chronic HBV infection. In acute hepatitis, recovery occurs in 99% of the previously healthy adults. No specific treatment is available for persons with acute HBV infection. Anti viral agents (IFN alpha or lamivudine) are available for chronic HBV infection. Interferon alpha is administered by subcutaneous or intramuscular injection at a dose of 5,000,000 units daily for a period of 16 weeks. The patient must be monitored carefully during the treatment for side effects, like flu-like symptoms, depression, rashes and abnormal blood counts.

Prevention

Two products are available for hepatitis B prevention; hepatitis B immunoglobulin (HBIG) and hepatitis B vaccine.

HBIG is indicated for post exposure prophylaxis in the following situations: sexual contact of previously unvaccinated person with a patient who has active hepatitis B or who developed hepatitis B, or sexual contact with an HBV carrier (blood test positive for HbsAg) and household contacts. HBIG should be administered within 14 days after the most recent sexual contact. Passive immunization with HBIG provides temporary protection. Simultaneous administration of HBIG and hepatitis B vaccine should be considered.

For perinatal exposure of infants born to HbsAg positive mothers, a single dose of HBIG 0.5 ml should be administered in the thigh immediately after birth followed by the complete course of recombinant Hepatitis B vaccine within 12 hours of life. For persons with direct percutaneous inoculation or transmucosal exposure to HbsAg positive blood or body fluids, a single dose of HBIG 0.06 ml/kg should be administered as soon after exposure as possible followed by the complete course of recombinant hepatitis B vaccine within 1 week.

Pre-exposure Immunization

Pre-exposure immunization is recommended for all persons who attend the STD clinics and have not been previously vaccinated, including pregnant women with STD. Hepatitis B vaccination is offered to all persons who have not been vaccinated, universally to neonates, persons with a history of STD, persons who have had multiple sex partners, those who have had sex with injection drug user, active male homosexuals, household contacts, drug sharing partners of person with chronic HBV infection and persons on haemodialysis, receiving blood products or occupational exposure to blood products.

There are two recombinant hepatitis B vaccines available: Recombivax-HB containing 10μgm of HbsAg, Engerix-B containing 20μgm of HbsAg.

Schedule of Vaccination

Three intramuscular (deltoid, not gluteal) doses at 0,1 & 6 months

Dosage of Vaccine

Engerix-B
    10μgm in children under 10 years
    20μgm for immunocompetent children older than 10 years and adults
    40μgm for dialysis patients and immunocomprised patients

Recombinant Vax-HB
    2.5μgm for children less than 11 years of age of HbsAg negative mothers
    5 μgm for infants of HbsAg positive mothers and for children and adolescents 11 to 19 years of age
    10 μgm for immunocompetent adults
    40 μgm for dialysis and other immunosuppressed patients

HIV infection can impair the response to hepatitis B vaccine. Therefore, vaccinated HIV infected person should be tested for anti-HbsAg, 1 to 2 months after the third dose. Re-vaccination with three additional doses should be considered for those who do not respond to initial vaccination.

Safe sexual practices, rigorous screening of blood and blood products can lead to reduced transmission of HBV infection.

Hepatitis D Virus Infection (HDV)

It is a unique RNA virus that is replication defective, causing infection only when it is encapsulated by HbsAg.

It is fully dependent on the genetic information provided by the hepatitis B virus for its multiplication. It has the same the sources and modes of transmission as that of HBV and can be sexually transmitted. HDV infection occurs in two forms:

1. Acute co-infection develops after exposure to the serum containing both HBV and HDV. It results in hepatitis ranging from mild to fulminant hepatitis. Fulminant hepatitis occurs more frequently with co-infection than with HBV alone.
2. Super infection of a chronic HBV carrier with a new inoculum of HDV and it results in either one of the following clinical situation:

    a. Mild HBV may become fulminant hepatitis
    b. Acute severe hepatitis
    c. Chronic progressive disease leading to cirrhosis (80%)

IgM anti HDV is the most reliable indicator of recent HDV infection along with markers of acute /chronic HB infection. HDV antigen and HDV RNA can also be detected.

Hepatitis C virus Infection

Hepatitis C virus previously called as "non A, non B" hepatitis is a single stranded RNA virus, in the family flaviviridae. In most of the cases (> 90%) it is transmitted by blood transfusion. The other percutaneous route is self-injection. Sexual (unprotected vaginal sex) and perinatal transmission are very rare (5%). It can occur only when the level of viremia is very high in the source or when the source of infection is co-infected with HIV. Heterosexual spread of HCV has been reported from Thailand, Argentina and Egypt. However reports from Malaysia, Jamaica and Tanzania did not show significant evidence for the heterosexual spread. These studies suggest that sexual transmission may occur in resource poor countries but at a lower rate compared with other modes of transmission. Homosexual spread of HCV infection has also been reported from European countries and USA.

Clinical Features

The average incubation period is 150 days. Acute infection is largely asymptomatic (80%). Only 20% of patients develop icteric hepatitis. Fulminant hepatitis may occur with hepatitis A super infection. Chronic infection develops in about 80% of the patients (mostly asymptomatic). Symptomatic chronic infection with cirrhosis develops only in about 20% after 20 years. Coinfection with HIV may accelerate the natural course of the disease resulting in progressive liver disease, which is the major cause of morbidity and mortality. Hepatitis C infection in AIDS patients may increase the risk of hepatotoxicity due to HAART.

Diagnosis & Treatment

Detection of IgG anti HCV antibody by screening test- ELISA and RIBA test is confirmatory for both acute & chronic infections. The test will become positive 3 months after exposure to HCV but sometimes after 9 months. PCR assay can also be used to detect viral proteins. Treatment with combination of IFN (3 million units subcutaneously three times weekly) and ribavirin 800-100 mg PO daily is safe in both HIV infected and non infected patients.

Cytomegalovirus Infections[19–25]

Cytomegalovirus (CMV) belongs to Herpesviridae family and is termed as Betaherpes-viridae. CMV is a double stranded DNA virus consisting of icosahedral capsids, surrounded by an outer envelope of lipid bilayer. It is the largest member of herpes virus family and the size is 150-200 nm. The structure is like that of other herpes viruses. Of all the herpes viruses described to date, infection with CMV arguably is the most important cause of morbidity and mortality. CMV infections occur worldwide and are usually inapparent. Primary infection is followed by life long carriage of this virus with intermittent shedding in various secretions. The shedding may increase in conditions of immuno-suppression by diseases or by therapy and in pregnancy.

In clinical specimens, one of the classic hallmark of CMV infection is the cytomegalic inclusion cells, first described by Ribbert in 1904. These cells are markedly enlarged with large purple intranuclear inclusions surrounded by a clear halo and smaller basophilic cytoplasmic inclusions producing "owl's eye" appearance.

Prevalence

Poor personal hygiene and communal living facilitates the spread of infection. Virus is present in saliva, urine, semen, breast milk, blood, transplanted donor organs and cervical and vaginal secretions and may be acquired from these sources. In adulthood, sexual activity is the most important route of CMV transmission. Kissing may transfer CMV from toddlers to adults. CMV may also be transmitted by blood transfusion and solid organ transplant.

The prevalence of CMV infection in the adult population ranges from 40% in Europe to 100% in Africa and Far East. The age at which an individual acquires CMV depends greatly on geographic location, socio-economic status, cultural factors and child rearing practices. Acquisition of CMV in the newborn period is common – either transplacental or perinatal. More than 50% infants become infected with CMV infected breast milk. Others, not infected in infancy may acquire CMV in day care centres.

Clinical Features

Congenital CMV disease may be symptomatic or asymptomatic. In the most severe forms it leads to hepatosplenomegaly, jaundice and purpura. Most infants die within two months and survivors usually (90%) suffer from some neurological damage. Purple or red papules or nodules develop in the skin because of erythropoietic tissue collection in the dermis and lasts for 4 to 6 weeks. Asymptomatic congenital CMV may cause sensorineural hearing loss in 15 to 20% of the cases.

Typical CMV mononucleosis is a disease of young adults. There is fever and lymphocytosis. The lymphadenopathy and splenomegaly may not be striking. Transfusion acquired CMV disease presents as CMV mononucleosis. The incubation period is 20 to 60 days. CMV infection in the immunocompromised patients can be severe and even be fatal. Infection may occur because of reactivation of latent viral infection or may be newly acquired. Viral dissemination leads to multiple organ system involvement with pneumonitis, hepatitis, gastro-intestinal ulceration, retinitis and super infection with other opportunistic pathogens. Neurological complications include encephalitis, myelitis and myeloradiculitis when the peripheral nerve roots are infiltrated with lymphocytes in AIDS.

CMV produces a necrotic, rapidly progressing retinitis with characteristic white perivascular infiltrates with haemorrhage (bush-fire retinitis). It was the most common cause of blindness in adult patients with AIDS before the advent of highly active anti-retroviral therapy (HAART) for HIV infection. It occurs in 90% of the affected individual. In contrast to adults CMV associated retinitis in children is rare. CMV retinitis is less common in transplant patients also.

In AIDS, CMV also causes erosive oesophagitis with symptoms similar to those caused by Candida and HSV. Colonic infection can result in diarrhoea. True CMV pneumonia may occur.

Diagnosis

Virus culture from throat washings, urine, bronchoalveolar lavage fluid, cervico-vaginal secretions, CSF, blood or biopsy material is carried out in human embryo fibroblast, and the cell culture is monitored for the development of the characteristic CMV associated cytopathic effect. It takes 5 to 28 days to produce cytopathic effect. Looking for CMV early antigen after 24 to 48 hours of culture (shell-vial assay) can make the diagnosis earlier. A positive blood culture is almost always diagnostic. Urine and saliva may be positive due to routine viral shedding. Newer diagnostic tools like PCR and direct detection of CMV antigenemia are useful rapid methods with greater sensitivity and can be used to monitor CMV disease in immuno-compromised host. Demonstration of CMV antibody is diagnostic of primary CMV infection. Congenital CMV may be diagnosed by virus isolation or the presence of CMV IgM antibody within 3 weeks of birth.

Treatment

CMV infection in a normal host rarely requires treatment. However, in life threatening situations such as AIDS or other immunocompromised situations, therapy is often required. Three antiviral therapies – gancyclovir (GCV), cidofovir (HP MPC) and foscarnet (PFA) are approved by US FDA for prophylaxis or therapy of CMV infection. The latter two are more toxic. Treatment should be monitored by experienced physician.

Prevention

Vaccines are under trial. Until the goal of a CMV vaccine is realized, educating women of child-bearing age about the risk of CMV and modes of prevention are the only control strategies available.

Epstein-Barr Virus Infection[26–28]

Epstein-Barr virus (EBV) is a DNA virus and is named

after Tony Epstein and Yvonne Barr who first described the virus in patients with Burkitt's lymphoma. It is a gamma virus a, member of Herpesviridae family. Icosahedral nucleocapsids and the viral envelope surround the viral genome. Following primary infection EBV establishes life long latency in the B-lymphocytes in the host.

Prevalence

EBV spreads by close contact especially kissing and can be sexually transmitted. During the dormant state of the virus there is a periodic activation and shedding of viruses in the oropharyngeal secretions. Transmission of the virus through air or blood does not usually occur. However transmission by blood transfusion and bone marrow transplantation has been described. The infection occurs worldwide and is the most common in early childhood with a second peak during late adolescence. Usually the infections in children are asymptomatic. But with poor hygiene and socioeconomic status, the infection in children may be symptomatic.

Pathogenesis

The virus is transmitted by saliva and infects the epithelium of the oral cavity. The B-lymphocytes are the target cells and they become infected after contact with the epithelial cells. The virus is attached to the EBV receptors CD21 present on the surface of the B cells and also epithelial cells and is internalized by cell. Inside the cell the viral DNA forms a loop of DNA and enters the cell nucleus. The viral DNA is then integrated into the host DNA. The viral proteins are expressed with the formation of new virus. EBV remains latent in few cells in the throat and in the B cells. They persist in the form of an episome. Six viral genes termed EBNA 1-6 are expressed and they transform the B cell into an immortal continuous dividing cells.

Clinical Features

Primary Syndromes
    Infectious mononucleosis
    Chronic EBV infection
    X linked lymphoproliferative syndromes
Reactivation Syndromes
    Lympho proliferative disorders in immunocompromised patients

Burkitt's lymphoma
Nasopharyngeal carcinoma
Oral hairy leucoplakia
Hodgkins lymphoma

Infectious Mononucleosis (IM)

The incubation period is 4 to 7 weeks. Clinically it is characterized by a prodrome of fatigue, malaise and myalgia which will last for about 1-2 weeks and is followed by fever, pharyngitis and generalized lymphadenopathy. The cutaneous manifestations are morbilliform rash, sometimes erythema nodosum and erythema multiforme. Other features are splenomegaly, hepatomegaly, abnormal liver function test and atypical lymphocytosis in the peripheral blood. Usually the disease is self-limiting but sometimes the convalescence may be prolonged.

Complications are neurological (meningitis, encephalitis, Guillaine Barre syndrome, acute transverse myelitis and peripheral neuritis), autoimmune haemolytic anaemia, splenic rupture, upper airway obstruction and bacterial super infections.

Chronic EBV infections

Chronic EBV infections are very rare and patients have an illness lasting for more than 6 months with marked increase in the EBV antibody titre. There is usually systemic involvement in the form of hepatomegaly, lymphadenopathy, pneumonitis, uveitis and neurologic disease.

Lymphoproliferative Disorders

It has been described in immunosupressed patients (both congenital and acquired immunodeficiency). There is a polyclonal proliferation of EBV transformed B cells in the lymph nodes and multiple organs.

X linked Lymphoproliferative Syndrome (Duncan's Syndrome)

It is a rare disorder of young boys who have a normal response to childhood infection but develop fatal lymphoproliferative disorders after infection. Most of the patients die of severe IM. The other complications are hypogammaglobulinemia, malignant B cell lymphoma, aplastic anaemia and agranulocytosis.

The other diseases, which are associated with EBV, are OHL, Burkitt's lymphoma, nasopharyngeal lymphoma, Hodgkin's lymphoma and leiomyosarcoma.

Oral Hairy Leucoplakia (OHL)

OHL is a white corrugated lesion normally seen along the lateral borders of the tonque on both sides. It may extend over to the ventral surface or the adjacent buccal mucosa. It usually occurs in HIV infected individuals with the CD4 count of <300 mm^3 and occasionally in organ transplant patients. Most often it is confused with oral candidiasis in which the whitish lesions can easily be removed with a spatula. OHL is not a premalignant lesion. Histologically OHL shows hyper keratosis, parakeratosis, acanthosis and large vacuolated cells in the prickle layer. The specific diagnosis depends on the demonstration of EBV in the sample by electron microscopy, in situ hybridization, immunohistochemical staining or PCR.

Diagnosis

Paul-Bunnel test (Heterophil test) is positive in 70-80% of patients acute IM. Heterophil antibodies agglutinate sheep or horse erythrocytes but do not react with EBV antigens directly. Heterophil antibody titre of 1: 40 is highly diagnostic of acute IM. EBV specific IgM antibody to viral capsid antigens (VCA) is also very useful in the diagnosis of IM. IgG antibody to VCA is elevated in the past infection and it persists for life. Anitbodies to early antigens (EA) are seen either as diffuse pattern in the nucleus and the cytoplasm of the affected cell (EA-D) or as a restrictive pattern in the cytoplasm (EA-R). EA-D antibodies are elevated in acute illness and also in nasopharyngeal carcinoma or chronic active EBV infection. Elevated EA-R antibodies are often seen with Burkitt's lymphoma or chronic active EBV infection. IgA antibodies to EBV antigens may be useful for the diagnosis of nasopharyngeal carcinoma. EBV DNA, RNA or proteins can be detected in tissues from patients with OHL or other malignancies. PCR technique can also be used in viral detection.

Treatment

Treatment of IM is usually symptomatic. A short course of steroids may be useful in severe disease. Patients with severe pharyngitis are treated with appropriate antibiotics. For the treatment of OHL, oral acyclovir (400-800mg five times a day) or topical tretinoin or podophyllin may be used. Therapy for EBV lymphoproliferative disorders is directed towards the reduction of immunosuppressive medication. Newer therapies that are being tried interferon-alpha or infusion of donor T cells or EBV specific cytotoxic T cells.

Parasitic Infestations

Scabies[29–34]

Scabies is one of the first diseases with a known cause. The itch mite *Sarcoptes scabiei var-hominis* was first described in 1687. Scabies affects all races and socioeconomic classes. Both sexes are affected equally although earlier studies have described a male preponderance.

Transmission of scabies occurs through close physical contact e.g. during playtime in young children, sharing of bed or prolonged handholding. Transmission may also occur through fomites like bed linen, towels, though it is less likely. *Sarcoptes scabiei* mite cannot survive for more than 1 to 2 days away from the skin of host. Transmission of scabies during sexual contact particularly in sexually active young adults is not uncommon. Patients with scabies attending Genito-urinary medicine (GUM) clinic had comparable number of STD, as were seen in other GUM clinic population. The diagnosis of scabies in the sexually active age group particularly when genital lesions are present should prompt a search for co-existing STD especially gonorrhoea and syphilis.

Clinically, the following features suggest diagnosis of scabies in a patient.

1. Types of lesions: papules, nodules, vesicles, pustules, ulcers, secondary eczematization, excoriation and infection
2. Distribution – in finger web space, hands, wrist, elbows, anterior axillary folds, areola in female, abdomen, genitals and buttocks.
3. Burrow, especially when present in finger web space or penis is pathognomonic (**P XXII, Fig. 87**).
4. Severe pruritus with nocturnal exacerbations.
5. Presence or history of scabies or pruritus in family members.

Besides the classical sites, erythema and scaling may

occur on face, neck, scalp, and trunk and may generalize. Nails may become dystrophic. The disease occurs in mentally retarded or physically debilitated persons or those who are immunologically deficient. Desai observed that half of the patients had evidence of malnutrition, the other half had other underlying diseases like lepromatous leprosy, pulmonary tuberculosis, carcinoma, mongolism and pemphigus vulgaris.

The presence of HIV disease in patients may modify scabies. Crusted Norwegian scabies or hyperkeratotic plantar plaques may develop. Norwegian scabies is highly contagious with large number of mites in the exfoliating scales. Itching is minimal or absent. The number of mite may be in millions. Large warty crusts form on the hands, feet, palms and soles. They are hyperkeratotic with fissures. Patients undergoing immunosuppressive therapy or with immunosuppression can also develop crusted scabies with bizarre lesions.

Scabies incognito is seen in those patients whose symptoms and signs are modified with topical or systemic use of corticosteroids. There are unusual clinical manifestations, atypical distribution and usually extensive involvement.

Diagnosis is most often clinical. But absolute diagnosis is made with the identification of mite with skin scrapings or other techniques. A burrow is gently scraped off with a blunt scalpel, care is taken to include the blind end. The scraped material is placed on a microscopic slide and a drop of 10 -20 % potassium hydroxide or mineral oil (xylol) is added. Finding of mites, eggs or fragments of egg shells or faeces (scybala) on examination confirm the diagnosis. Concentration techniques for high yields have been described.

Skin biopsy may also reveal section of mite or pellets of faeces. Epidermal shave biopsy may also help in the demonstration of mite.

Treatment

General: For successful treatment, it is essential that the patient applies antiscabetic medicines properly. Detailed instructions should be given to the patients explaining the treatment regimen and warning against excessive use. They should be explained that following effective therapy, the itching may persist for a few days but will usually resolve within 2 weeks. The medicine is applied to the entire body below neck after a good scrub bath with soap and water and after drying the skin preferably at night. After the contact period of 12 hours (next day morning) the patient should take a bath and change the bed linen. Disinfection of clothing and bedding, other than by ordinary laundering is not required. All members of the family and close physical contacts should be treated, whether having evidence of scabies or not; the symptom free incubation period may be 1 to 2 months.

Different antiscabetic preparations available are:

1. 5% permethrin is the drug of choice because it has excellent activity and low toxicity. Clinical trials show that 5% permethrin is as effective as lindane and more effective than crotamiton with toxic effects 40 times lower than 1% lindane.
2. Gamma benzenehexachloride (GBHC) – A single 6 hour application of 1% lindane effectively treats scabies. Some clinicians use a second application after one week.
3. 10% crotamiton cream, applied for 24 hours on five consecutive days.
4. Oral ivermectin, which interrupts GABA – induced neurotransmission, has shown good effect as a single dose ($200\mu g/kg$). It has recently been introduced in India.
5. A preliminary open study of 0.8% ivermectin lotion has also shown good results.

Scabies not responding to conventional treatment may be presenting feature of HIV infections. Crusted scabies is treated with permethrin followed by lindane and sulfur if necessary. Pretreatment with keratolytics may be useful.

Pediculosis pubis[29, 35,36]

Pediculosis pubis is an infestation of hair bearing area, most commonly pubic region and is sexually transmitted. The incidence of infestation is related to promiscuity and poor hygiene. The disease occurs throughout the world. Many of the patients infested with *P. pubis* had other sexually transmitted diseases. The population with the highest incidence of pubic lice is similar to that of gonorrhoea and syphilis. Pediculosis pubis is rare in persons older than 35 years.

The Organism

The pubic or 'crab louse' – *Phthirus pubis* has squat body. The female pubic louse is 1 mm in length, the male is slightly smaller. It has 3 pairs of legs. The first set of legs terminate in slender claws, while the second and third pair of legs have well developed claws, perfectly adapted for grasping the hair. They move upto 10 cm a day. The legs are light brown in colour cemented to the hair of host. Eggs are laid in batches of 20 or 30 and hatch in a week time. Development of adult, since the laying of eggs, takes 22 to 27 days. *Pthirus pubis* is a strict human parasite, but infestation among dogs has also been reported.

Clinical Features

The commonest site is the pubic region. However in hairy individuals, the thighs, trunk, perianal area and occasionally the axilla, beard and moustache may get involved (**P XXII, Fig. 88**). Meinking and Taplin observed involvement of sites other than pubic areas in 60% of their study group of homeless population. Infestation of the eye lashes and scalp hair occurs mainly in children. It is not indicative of sexual abuse though this may occasionally be the case. Children may acquire infection from infected parents or shared beds or other fomites.

Patients who have pediculosis pubis usually seek medical attention because of pruritus or because they notice lice or nits on their pubic hair. Itching occurs mainly in the evening and night. A complete body examination is important in all patients. Excoriation may lead to secondary pyoderma and eczematization. Blue-grey macules (maculae caeruleae) are occasionally seen on the skin of lower abdomen and upper thighs (**P XXII, Fig. 89**). Their exact pathogenesis is unknown, probably they develop as a response to altered blood pigment or a reaction to the louse's saliva. These persist for several days.

Munoz-Perez and colleagues reported pediculosis pubis in 26% among 1161 HIV 1 positive patients over a period of 38 months. Infestation may be severe with extensive colonization in HIV positive individuals.

Diagnosis

A careful history and examination for lice or nits confirms the diagnosis. Lice are observed as yellowish brown specks clinging closely to the base of hair. Nits on the hair are cemented at an oblique angle. The diagnosis of pediculosis pubis should initiate search for other STD.

Treatment

Permethrin 1%, GBHC 1% or pyrethrins with piperonyl butoxide are recommended. Permethrin 1% rinse or pyrethrins with piperonyl butoxide is applied to the affected areas and washed after 10 minutes. GBHC 1% lotion or shampoo is applied to affected area and washed after 4 minutes. GBHC is not recommended for pregnant or lactating women and for children under 2 years.

Permethrin, GBHC or Pyrethrins should not be applied to the eyes. Pediculosis of the eyelashes should be treated by applying occlusive ophthalmic ointment to the eyelid margins twice a day for 10 days. The remaining nits may be removed mechanically with forceps. Application of freshly prepared 10-20 percent flourescein eye drops is also said to be effective.

Pediculosis pubis patient with HIV should receive the same treatment regimens. Bedding and clothing should be decontaminated.

Follow Up

Patients should be evaluated after 7 to 10 days if the symptoms persist. A second application of same or alternative pediculicide is given if lice are or nits are observed at the hair skin junction.

Management of Sexual Partners

Sexual partners of the patient within the last month should be treated. The patient should avoid sexual contact with their sex partner(s) until patients and partners have been treated and re-evaluated to rule out persistent disease.

Genital mycoplasmas[37–41]

Mycoplasmas belonging to class named Mollicutes (mollis, soft; cutis, skin, in Latin) are the smallest free-living organisms. They are widespread in nature as parasites of humans, mammals, reptiles, fish, arthropods and plants. Mycoplasmas are distinguished phenotypically from other bacteria by their minute size and total lack of a cell wall. The primary habitats of human mycoplasmas are the mucous surfaces of the respiratory and urogenital tracts, the eyes, alimentary canal and joints. Frequently isolated organisms from the urogenital tract are mycoplasma and the ureaplasma. There are eight genera, five namely mycoplasma, ureaplasma, acholeoplasma, anaeroplasma and astreoleplasma, which collectively form 120 species.

Infections with pathogenic mycoplasmas are rarely

of the fulminant type, but follow a chronic course. Several virulence factors have been associated to mycoplasmas. The mildly toxic byproducts of mycoplasma metabolism, such as hydorgen peroxide and superoxide radicals, have been incriminated as causing oxidative damage to host cell membranes. Most mycoplasmas adhere to the epithelial linings of the respiratory or urogenital tract, so they may be considered surface parasites. While mycoplasmas such as *M. penetrans* and *M.genitalium* appear to enter the cells through their specialized tip structure, other mycoplasmas internalize, such as *M. fermentans* and *M. hominis*, have no tip structures. Data indicate that pathogenic mycoplasmas reside and replicate intracellulary over extended periods in human cells. Intracellular location may protect mycoplasmas against the effects of the host immune system and antibiotics.

The clinical picture of mycoplasma infections in humans and animals is more suggestive of damage due to host immune and inflammatory responses rather than to direct toxic effects by mycoplasma cell components. Non-specific immunomodulatory effects may contribute to their pathogenic properties, enabling them to evade or suppress their host defense mechanisms and establish a chronic, persistent infection.

Epidemiology

Several mycoplasma species (16 in total) have been isolated from humans. *M. genitalium, M. spermatophilum*

and *M. penetrans*, the genital tract is the main site of colonization. Some of them are considered as not having pathogenic potential (*M. primatum, M. spermatophilum*). The most recently discovered, *M. penetrans*, has been isolated from the urine of HIV 1 positive homosexual men.

In adults, colonization following puberty occurs primarily as a result of sexual contact, colonization increases in relation to the number of sexual partners for both *Mycoplasma hominis (M. hominis)* and Ureaplasma urealyticum (*U. urealyticum*). A recent case control study (men and their female partners) revealed that for *M. genitalium* couples had concordant status, pertaining to the sexual transmission of *M. genitalium* and it was concluded that it behaves in a similar way as *C. trachomatis*. The various clinical syndromes that are associated with genital mycoplasmas are given in Table 2. The list includes both causal role and association effect on different clinical syndromes of genital mycoplasma.

Non-gonoccocal Urethritis

NGU is the most common STD syndrome that occurs in men. Collected data support that *M. hominis* on its own is not a cause of NGU, and it has been found more frequently in men who did not have NGU than those who did.

U. urealyticum have been isolated from 0-56% of healthy men, and from *5.6-42%* of men with urethritis. Results of an experiment suggest that *U. urealyticum*

Table 2.   Clinical Syndromes and Genital Mycoplasma

Clinical Syndromes	Mycoplamsa
Non gonococcal urethritis	*U. urealyticum* (20-40%)
	M. genitalium (24-26%)
Nongonococcal nonchlamydial urethritis (acute)	*U. urealyticum* (26-50%)
	M. genitalium (12-19%)
Nongonococcal nonchlamydial urethritis (chronic)	*U.urealyticum* (12-19%), *M.hominis* (4%), *M. genitalium* (1%)
Prostatitis	*U. urealyticum* (13-47%), *M.hominis* (10-12%), *M. genitalium* (4%)
Epididymitis	*U.urealyticum* , *M. hominis*, ? *M. genitalium*
Reiter's disease	? *M. genitalium*
Bacterial vaginosis	*M. hominis, U. urealyticum*
Pelvic inflammatory disease	*M. hominis*
Post partum/ post abortal fever	*M. hominis*
Urinary calculi	*U .urealyticum*
Pyelonephritis and urinary tract infection	*M .hominis*, ? *U. urealyticum*
Involuntary infertility	?*U. urealyticum*
Habitual spontaneous abortions and still birth	?*Mycoplasmas*
Low birth weight	? *M. hominis* , ?*U. urealyticum*

may cause disease the first time it gains access to the urethra but subsequent invasion result in colonization without disease. This finding may explain the frequent isolation of ureaplasmas from the urethras of healthy men.

M. genitalium prevalence amongst urethritis patients varies from 8% amongst urology patients to 29% amongst STD patients. The prevalence amongst asymptomatic patients varies from 0% (again amongst urology patients) to 9% amongst STD patients. Men with NGU tend to harbour *C. trachomatis* or *M. genitalium* separately rather than together. *M. gentalium* was found more often in *C. trachomatis*-negative NGU (NCNGU) patients than in those with chlamydial urethritis. In a recent study from Sweden, involving 51 men with urethritis, no co-infection with *M. genitalium* and *C. trachomatis* was detected. According to these studies *M genitalium* could be considered an important cause of NGU, constituting 13-45% of *C. trachomatis*-negative NGU cases.

The association of *M. genitalium* with persistent or recurrent urethritis (PRU) is also noted by some authors. *M. genitalium* was detected in 19-27% of men with PRU, suggestive of the aetiological role. *M. gentialium* patients were more likely to have had a previous urethrits in comparison to other patients with non-chlamydial NGU. This could indicate that *M. genitalium* urethritis may have a tendency to recur. There is recent evidence showing that *M. genitalium*-related PRU is more likely associated with persistent or recurrent infection rather than with immunologically mediated inflammation.

M. genitalium has been associated with chronic 'abacterial' prostatitis. In one study, 135 patients with chronic abacterial prostatitis underwent transperineal prostatic biopsies to detect microorganisms by PCR, 10 (8%) harboured a STD pathogen in their prostate (*M. genitalium* was detected in 4%).

Bacterial Vaginosis

Genital mycoplasmas are amongst the major aetiological agents currently believed to be part of a synergisitc mixture in bacterial vaginosis (BV), but the particular organism in this mixture essential for the developing and maintence of the condition is not known.

A number of works have shown *M. hominis* to be asociated with BV in pregnant women and in non-pregnant women. *M. hominis* has been reported in 58-76% of women with BV and from significantly fewer patients with a normal vaginal examination. The connection between *U. urealyticum* and BV is less obvious: *U. urealyticum* is isolated from a high percentage of patients (62-92%) who have a diagnosis of BV, higher apparently than that from control patients.

In a study of role of male partner in the lower genitourinary tract infection of females, 93 consecutive patients in the reproductive age group with symptoms of vaginal discharge along with their sexual partners were evaluated microbiologically. The predominant pathogen isolated was *Ureaplasma urealyticum* seen in 43.01% of females and 24.7% of males.

Cervicitis

The controversial role of gential mycoplasmas is particularly true for cervicitis. *M. hominis* and *U. urealyticum* seem not be have a role in the aetiology of mucopurulent cervicts. There are much fewer studies published on *M. genitalium* infections on women than in men. The connection of *M. genitalium* with cervicits has been suggested. The prevalence of *M. genitalium* is significantly greater in *C. trachomatis*- negative women with genital infections (cervicits, adnexitis) than in asymptomatic pregnant women.

The other manifestitations have been enumerated in the above table, and detailed discussions regarding PID and prostatitis have been given in separate chapters.

Diagnosis

In men the diagnosis, is made by collecting and testing the urethral swab or the first void urine sample, and in women high vaginal smear or endocervical swabs. The collected swabs are to be immediately instilled in the transport media and the swab is not allowed to dry. The culture is done on a beef heart infusion broth (PPLO broth) with 10% fresh yeast extract, 20% horse serum. The culture colonies on the media would look like classical 'fried egg' appearance and the size (200-300 μ) in case of *M. hominis* and smaller (10-30μ) without the fried egg appearance in case of ureaplasma. Commercial kits for detection of *M. hominis* and ureaplasma are available. DNA probes for detection of mycoplasma and ureaplasma have been developed, but they are not beneficial as compared to culture methods. Serological tests have also been described, and in combination with identification of the organism it can enhance the specificity of the diagnosis.

Treatment

Treatment of choice for both genital mycoplasma and ureaplasma infection is tetracycline. The others, which can be used, are macrolides and fluoroquinolones. Tetracyclines are active against many strains of *M.hominis*. In resistant cases clindamycin should be good alternative. Around 10% of ureaplasma exhibit resistance for tetracyclines and 40% cross resistance with erythromycin. *M.genitalium* associated acute and chronic NGU can effectively treated with a five day course of azithromycin.[4]

Enteric Bacterial Pathogens[42–47]

Enteric infections traditionally have not been viewed as sexually transmitted diseases. The sexual practices that predispose to acquisition of these infections are anilingus (rimming or active oral-anal sex) and faecal-oral contact occurring indirectly when oral-genital sex (fellatio) following anal genital intercourse. These practices are more common among homosexuals than heterosexuals.

The bacterial pathogens that are sexually transmitted are salmonella, shigella, campylobacter species and *Helicobacter pylori (H. pylori)*. All these infections have become sexually transmitted because only a small inoculum that is needed to cause the disease (shigella 10-100 organisms, campylobacter 500 organisms).

Shigellosis

Shigellosis is caused by Shigella species of enteric bacteria, which are non-motile, short, gram negative rods that ferment lactose slowly or not at all. Fifty serotypes have been grouped into four serogroups A-D. Several population based incidence studies have demonstrated disproportionately higher rates in homosexuals.

The usual incubation period is 1-7 days. Clinically it presents as bacillary dysentery characterized by bloody mucoid stool accompanied with abdominal pain, tenesmus and fever. *Shigella dysentriae* type I cause the most severe infection. Cutaneous shigellosis, in the form of furuncle over the penis had been reported in a 22-year-old homosexual. Other manifestations are haemolytic uraemic syndrome. Diagnosis is made by culture, by taking direct rectal stool swab and plated on Hektoen and or MacConkey agar. Further biochemical and serological identification are unnecessary for routine purposes, but may be useful for outbreak investigations.

Treatment is by newer fluoroquinolons, ciprofloxacin 500mg bid for up to 3 days or trimethoprim sulfamethoxazole bid for 3 days. (TMP 160 mg and SMX 800mg). Other drugs are nalidixic acid 1g qid for 5 days and pivemecillinam 400mg qid for 5 days. Due to wide spread development of resistance, selection of antibiotics should be based on regional antibiotic sensitivity. An oral live attenuated *Shigella flexneri* hybrid vaccine has been used in field trials but its efficacy could not be assessed because of the low incidence of cases in the study population.

Salmonellosis

They belong to the family Enterobacteriaceae. They are anaerobic facultative, gram negative rods, do not ferment lactose or sucrose, but they are motile and always produce H_2S. They have four serogroups A-D, 75-80% of infections are caused by only 10 sterotypes.

The clinical manifestations that are produced by salmonella are acute gastroenteritis, enteric fever, septicemia and focal invasive infections. Salmonella diarrhoea is generally watery, containing mucous and very occasionally blood. Endoscopic examination would reveal colonic mucosal oedema, hyperaemia, friability and petechial hemorrhages. Salmonella septicemia is a well described entity in a HIV infected hosts and recurrent salmonella septicemia has become a CDC surveillence definition of AIDS-defining illness. Focal central nervous system involvement in HIV/AIDS patients has been reported. The usual incubation period is 1-7 days. Chronic carrier state is described in adult population. Diagnosis is by stool culture using a highly selective media. (Potassium tellurite, Wilson Blair). No antimicrobial therapy is advised in gastroenteritis with non-bloody, non-mucoid diarrhoeal stool and mild to moderate dehydration. On the contrary, patients has bloody or mucoid stools, severe illness, severe dehydration requires hospitalization. The first line of treatment is ciprofloxacin 500 mg BID for 3-5 days. Alternative regimens include aminopencillins, ceftriaxone or cefotaxime.

Campylobacter Enteritis

This infection is caused by *Campylobacter jejuni* and campylobacter like organisms (CLO). They are small, curved motile, gram negative rods microaerophilic and non-fermenting. They are isolated from 4-8% of patients with acute diarrhoea.[3] Sexual transmission of these organisms has been documented in animals and humans. The atypical form CLO are more frequently isolated from homosexual men with or without intestinal symptoms, and rarely from heterosexual men and women. In a study CLO were recovered from the stool of 26 of 158 symptomatic homosexual men, 6 of 75 asymptomatic homosexual men and 0 of 150 heterosexual men and women. Two of there CLO are identified as *C. cinaedi* and *C. fennelliae*.

Clinical manifestation runs a broad range from that compatible with mild viral gastroenteritis to severe diarrhoea with blood and pus. In around 10% of patients, abdominal pain and tenderness persists, or recurrent fever or diarrhoea occurs. Otherwise they resolve within 2-3 days. Proctocolitis is evident by endoscopic examination, associated with anal discharge, pain and fever. Faecal leucocytosis is usually present and the diagnosis is confirmed by isolating the organisms from the stool by culture on selective media with microaerophilic atmosphere. For CLO, PCR amplification of 23s rDNA sequences has been used to identify these isolates. Benefit from using antibiotics is not clear, especially if the start of treatment is delayed. Erythromycin 500mg qid for 1 week has been recommended for severe symptoms.

Helicobacter Pylori

A recent review of literature, has reported that Helicobacter infection could be transmitted sexually via oral-anal intercourse. Sexual practices where there is contact with faeces may be an important risk factor for the transmission of *H.pylori,* clinically characterized by chronic gastritis.

Candidiasis[48–52]

Syn.: Candidosis; Moniliasis; Thrush.
Candidiasis is an infection caused by the yeast *Candida albicans,* or occasionally by other species of candida like *C.glabrata, C.parapsilosis, C.tropicalis, C.guilliermondi, C.kefy* and *C.krusei.*

Aetiology

C. albicans is an oval yeast 2-6 × 3-9 μm in size which can produce budding cells, hyphae and psuedohyphae. There are over 100 species. Hyphae are usually produced during the process of tissue invasion, though yeasts without hyphae may also occur during the phase of tissue invasion. *C.albicans* is a common commensal of gastrointestinal tract. Candida yeasts are found in the mouth and gut in around 50% of the population and colonize the vagina in up to 20% of asymptomatic females. They are rarely isolated from the healthy skin.

The candidal infection often develops from the commensal reservoir with the exception of genital candidiasis which is often sexually acquired and oral candidiasis in infants. Certain factors appear to favour the presence of organism and to produce a clinical condition where it had been carried as a commensal. These include pregnancy, glycosuria and the administration of broad spectrum antibiotics, cortico steroids and other immunosuppressive drugs. In HIV positive population, oral candida carrier rates are generally high.

Clinical Features

Candida can cause superficial infections of skin and mucous membranes. Systemic infections are more serious with involvement of internal organs including septicemia, endocarditis and meningitis. In this chapter we will be describing only the genital candidiasis. Among 100 consecutive cases of candidiasis at Mumbai, 30% had vulvovaginitis.

Candidiasis in the Males

Asymptomatic colonization of the glans penis occurs both in circumcised and uncircumcised males although the uncircumcised are more likely to develop symptoms, since the internal milieu of preputial sac often favours the growth of microorganisms. Sexual contact of a patient of candidal balanitis may have either abundant vaginal candida carriage or frank vulvovaginitis. Singhi et al isolated *C.albicans* in 21% of patients with balanoposthitis. The organism was more commonly isolated from married than unmarried individuals. Pathogenic staphylococci were seen in 25% of *C.albicans* positive cases. Sharma and colleague also isolated *C.albicans* among 23% of patients with balanoposthitis, though staphylococci were more commonly isolated in their study.

In the mildest cases of candidal balanitis transient tiny papules develop on the glans penis, a few hours after intercourse evolve into white pustules or vesicles that rupture causing erosions. There may be mild soreness or irritation. Later a red glazed surface of the glans, a slightly scaling edge and eroded satellite pustules develop which is hallmark of candidal balanoposthitis (**P XXIII, Fig. 90**). In long standing chronic cases, maceration, fissuring or ulceration of the prepuce may occur with or without phimosis. Anaerobic bacterial infection may cause a foul smelling, subpreputial purulent discharge. Involvement of the penile shaft, scrotal skin and the groins coexists often in hot weather. Diabetes mellitus is frequently associated with candidal balanoposthitis. Florid persistent lesions spreading beyond the genitalia are more likely to be associated with glycosuria.

The differential diagnoses include balanoposthitis due to other causes–trichomonal, bacterial, allergic, psoriasis, lichen planus, etc.

Candidiasis in Females

Many women with candidiasis are asymptomatic or have minimal symptoms. Typical symptoms of vulvo vaginal candidiasis (VVC) include pruritus and vaginal discharge. Other symptoms are vaginal soreness, vulvar burning, dyspareunia and external dysuria. None of these symptoms is specific for VVC. On examination, there is typical dusky red erythema of vaginal mucous membrane and vulval skin with oedema associated with curdy whitish discharge, fissures and erosions. The discharge is typically thick creamy white or 'cheese like'. Generally the pH of the discharge is below 5. The rash may extend to the perineum and groins. The perianal area is often affected. Subcorneal pustules at the periphery may develop in extensive cases. Clinical manifestations of VVC are aggravated during pregnancy.

Vaginal mucosa becomes glazed and atrophic in recurrent chronic VVC.

VVC has been classified into the following 2 types based on the clinical presentation, microbiology, host factors and response to therapy.

1. Uncomplicated VVC
   Sporadic or infrequent VVC, or
   Mild to moderate vulvovaginal Candidiasis, or
   Likely to be *C. albicans*, or
   VVC in nonimmuno compromised women.
2. Complicated VVC
   Recurrent VVC, or

Severe VVC, or
Non-*C. albicans* Candidiasis, or
Women with uncontrolled diabetes, debilitation or immuno-suppression or those who are pregnant.
Approximately 10 to 20 percent of women will have complicated VVC, suggesting diagnostic and therapeutic considerations.

Diagnosis

Diagnosis of VVC depends upon the demonstration of the yeast by simple microscopic examination of vaginal secretions in 10% KOH or by Gram staining. A wet mount or saline preparation should routinely be done not only to identify yeast cells and mycelia, but also to exclude the presence of "clue cells" and motile trichomonads. The visualization of psuedohyphae strengthens the diagnosis. Vaginal secretion culture on Sabouraud's agar should be performed in the presence of negative microscopic findings. Fifty percent of patients with culture positive symptomatic VVC, have negative microscopic findings. A positive culture also does not always indicate that the yeast is responsible for the vaginal symptoms.

Treatment

The general principles include that all local topical preparations should be applied to all involved skin and mucosal surfaces. Any predisposing factor like diabetes mellitus, or HIV infection should be treated. Most women with uncomplicated VVC have no precipitating factor. VVC can occur concomitantly with other STD and the latter has to be investigated and treated. The various treatment guidelines are given in Appendix II.

Treatment of Complicated VVC

Recurrent VVC (RVVC) is defined as four or more episodes of symptomatic VVC each year and affects less than 5% of women. Clinical diagnosis should be confirmed by culture, which also helps to identify unusual species including *Candida glabrata*. Each individual episode of RVVC responds to short duration of initial therapy. A longer duration 7-14 days of topical therapy or a repeat dose of oral fluconazole 150 mg at 3 days is recommended to achieve mycological remission before initiating a maintenance antifungal regimen.

Maintenance therapy with antifungals agents include clotrimazole (500 mg) vaginal suppository once weekly, ketoconazole 100 mg once daily, fluconazole (100-150 mg) once weekly and itraconazole 400 mg once monthly or 100 mg once daily). All maintenance regimens should be continued for 6 months. Recurrence may occur in 30% to 40% women on cessation of maintenance therapy.

During pregnancy only topical azoles should be used. Therapy for VVC should not differ in HIV infected women. Recurring vulvo-vaginal candidiasis is not on indication to test for HIV.

References.

1. Mittal RR, Jha A. Molluscum contagiosum venereum. Indian J Sex Transm Dis 2000; 21: 84-86.

2. Schwartz JJ, Myskowski PL. Molluscum contagiosum in patients with HIV infection: a review of twenty seven patients. J Am Acad Dermatol 1992; 27: 583-588.

3. Konya J, Thompson CH. Molluscum contagiousm virus: antibody responses in persons with clinical lesions and seroepidemiology in representative Australian population. J Infect Dis 1999; 179: 701-704.

4. Meadows KP, Trying SK, Pavia AT, Rallis TM. Resolution of recalcitrant molluscum contagiosum virus lesions in human immunodeficiency virus infected patients treated with cidofovir. Arch Dermatol 1997; 133: 987-990.

5. Sharma AK. Cimetidine therapy for multiple molluscum contagiosum lesions. Dermatology 1998; 197: 194-195.

6. Hourihane J, Hodges E, Smith J, Keefe M, Jones A, Connett G. Interferon alpha treatment of molluscum contagiosum in immunodeficiency. Arch Dis Child 1999; 80: 77-79.

7. Cattelan AM, Sasset L, Corti L, et al. A complete remission of recalcitrant molluscum contagiosum in an AIDS patient following highly active antiretroviral therapy (HAART). J Infect Dis 1999; 38: 58-60.

8. Diegstag JL. Sexual and perinatal transmission of hepatitis C. Hepatology 1997; 26(Suppl.): 566-570.

9. Centres for Disease Control. Hepatitis-A among homosexual men – United States, Canada & Australia. MMWR 1992; 41: 155.

10. Dienstag JL, Isselbacher KJ. Acute viral hepatitis. In : Fauci As, Braunwald E, Isselbacher KJ, eds. Harrison's Principles of Internal Medicine. 15th edn. New York: McGraw Hill; 2001. p. 1677-1692.

11. Centres for Disease Control and Prevention. Sexually Transmitted Treatment Guidelines 2002. MMWR 2002; 51 (No.RR-6): 59-65

12. William J, Shanmugasundaraj A. Prevalence of hepatitis B among male homosexuals. Indian J Sex Transm Dis 1989; 10: 6-9.

13. Mahendra AK, Bhargav RK, Agarwal US et al. Hepatitis B virus marker in high risk group STD patients. Indian J Sex Transm Dis 1988; 9: 32-34.

14. Singh V, Kumar B, Bhasin DK, et al. Prevalence of hepatitis B virus and delta infection in patients with sexually transmitted disease in North India. Indian J Sex Transm Dis; 1994; 15: 13-15.

15. Puoti M, Airoldi M, Bruno R, et al. Hepatitis B virus co-infection in human immunodeficiency virus-infected subjects. AIDS Rev; 2002; 4: 27-35.

16. Brook MG. Sexually acquired hepatitis. Sex Transm Infect 2002; 78: 235-240

17. Crawford JM. The liver and the Biliary Tract. In: Cotran R, Kumar V, Collins T, eds. Robins Pathologic Basis of Diseases. 6th edn. Philadelphia: W.B. Saunders Company; 1999. p. 861-862

18. Powderly WG. Gastrointestinal aspects. In: Manual of HIV Therapeutics. 2nd edn. New York: Lippincott Williams & Wilkins; 123-129.

19. Hirsch, Martin S. Cytomegalo virus and human herpes virus 6, 7 and 8. In : Braunwald E, Fauci AS, Kasper DL, et al, eds. Harrisons Principles of Internal Medicine. 15th ed. New York: MacGraw Hill; 2001. p.1111-1114.

20. Lesher JL, Cytomegalovirus infections and the skin. J Am Acad Dermatol 1988; 18 : 1333-1338.

21. Betts RF. Syndromes of cytomegalovirus infections. Adv Intern Med 1980; 26: 447-466.

22. Sohn YM, Oh MK, Balcarek KB, et al. Cytomegalo virus infection in sexually active adolescents. J Infect Dis, 1991; 163: 460-463.

23. Said G. Peripheral neurological manifestations of infection by the human immunodedficiency virus. Rev Pract (France) 1992; 42: 173-178.

24. Puy-Montburn J, Ganansia R, Lemarchand N, Delichenault P, Denis J. Anal ulceration due to cytomegalovirus in patients with AIDS; Report of six cases. Dis Colon Rectum 1990; 33: 1041.

25. Pariser RJ. Histologically specific skin lesions in disseminated cytomegalo-virus infection. J Am Acad Dermatol 1983; 9: 173-178.

26. Strauss JH, Strauss EG. Viruses whoose life cycle use reverse transcriptase. In : Viruses and Human Diseases. New York: Academic Press. p. 246-250

27. Cohen JI. Ebstein Barr virus infections including Infectious Mononucleosis. In: Fauci As, Braunwald E, Isselbacher KJ, eds. Harrison's Principles of Internal Medicine. 15th edn. New York: McGraw Hill; 2001. p. 1089-1091.

28. Cohen JI. Ebstein Barr virus infections. In: Freedberg Im, Eisen AZ, Wolff K, eds. Fitzpatrick's Dermatology in General Medicine. New York: McGraw Hill; 1999.p. 2458-2462.

29. Burns DA. Diseases caused by arthropods and other noxious animals. In : Champion RH, Burton JL, Burns DA and Brathnach SM, eds. Text Book of Dermatology. 6th ed. Oxford: Blackwell Science ; 1998. p. 1423-1481.

30. Guggisberg D, de Viragh PA, Constantin C, Panizzon RG. Norwegian scabies in a patient with acquired immunodeficiency syndrome. Dermatology 1998; 197: 306-8.

31. David N, Rajamanoharan S, Tang A. Are sexually transmitted infections associated with scabies. Int J STD AIDS 2002; 13: 168-170.

32. Bitman LM, Rabinowitz AD. Hyperkeratotic plantar plaque in an HIV-positive patient. Crusted scabies, localized to the soles. Arch. Dermatol 1998; 134(8): 1019,ʻ1022-3.

33. Desai SC. Scabies – A mighty persistent pestering puzzle despite pesticides. Indian J Dermatol Venereol Leprol 1987; 127-133.

34. Redkar VE, Redkar SV. Epidemiological features of human immunodeficiency virus infections in western India. J Assoc Phys India 1999; 47: 261-262.

35. Imandeh NG. Prevalence of Pthirus pubis among sex workers in urban Jos, Nigeria . Appl parasitol 1993; 34: 275-277.

36. Meinking TL, Taplin D. Advances in Pediculosis, scabies and other mite infestations. Adv Dermatol 1990; 5: 131-150.

37. Uuskula A, Kohl PK. Genital mycoplasmas, including *Mycoplasma genitalium,* as sexually transmitted agents. Int J STD AIDS 2002; 13: 79-83.

38. Taylor-Robinson D, Ainsworth JG, McCormack WM. Genital mycoplasma. In: Holmes KK, Mardh P-A, Sparling PF, et al. eds. Sexually Traansmitted Diseases. 3rd edn. New York. Mc Graw Hill; 1999.p 533-548

39. Sahoo B, Bhandari H, Sharma M, Malhotra S, Sawhney H, Kumar B. Role of the male partner in the lower genitourinary tract infection of female. Indian J Med Res 2000; 112:9-14.

40. Schwartz MA, Hootan TM. Aetiology of non chlamydial non gonococcal urethritis. Dermatol Clin 1998; 16: 727-733.

41. Taylor-Robinson D. *Mycoplasma genitalium* - an up-date. Int J STD AIDS 2002; 13: 145-151.

42. Judson FN. Sexually transmitted viral hepatitis and enteric pathogens. Urol Clin North Am 1984; 11: 177-185.

43. Eslick GD. Sexual transmission of *Helicobacter pylori* via oral-anal intercourse. Int J STD AIDS 2002; 13: 7-11.

44. Quinn TC. Clinical approach to intestinal infections in homosexual men. Med Clin North Am 1986; 3: 611-634.

45. Thorpe CM, Keusch GT. Enteric bacterial pathogens: shigella, salmonella, campylobacter. In: Holmes KK, Mardh PA, Sparling PF, eds. Sexually transmitted diseases. 3rd edn. New York: Mc-Graw Hill; 1999. p-549-562.

46. Sack DA. Acute infectious diarrhoea. In: Rakel RE, Bope ET, eds. Conn's Current therapy. 54 edn. Philadelphia. W.B Saunders: 2002. P.12-18.

47. Sobel J, Swerdlow DL. Salmonellosis. In: Acute infectious diarrhoea. In: Rakel RE, Bope ET, eds. Conn's Current therapy. 54 edn. Philadelphia. W.B Saunders: 2002. P.163-166.

48. Gough DM, Warnock DW, Turner, et al. Candidosis of genital tract in non-pregnant women. Eur J Obstet Gynecol Reprod Biol 1985; 19: 237-46.

49. Bhargava RK, Singhi NK, Mangal HN, Garg SP. Balanoposthitis, diabetes and micro-organisms. Indian J Sex Transm Dis 1987; 8: 19-21.

50. Singhi NK, Bhargava RK, Mangal HN, et al . Micro-organism and balanoposthitis. Indian J Sex Transm Dis 1986; 7: 75-80.

51. Sharma VK, Kumar B, Ayyagiri A, Talwar P. Microbial flora in balanoposthitis : a study of 100 cases. Indian J Sex Transm Dis 1990; 11: 19-22.

52. Centre for Disease Control and Prevention. Sexually transmitted disease treatment Guidelines 2002. MMWR, 2002; 51 : (No RR6) 45-48.

Chapter 28

Trichomoniasis and Other Protozoal Diseases

Vinod K Sharma, Trilokraj Tejasvi

Introduction

An increasing number of diseases are currently being recognized as sexually transmitted. Bacterial and viral diseases comprise the vast majority of sexually transmitted diseases (STD), however several protozoa, nematodes and arthropod are also included in this group. It was recognized by the 1960s that enteric protozoan infections may be related to sexual behaviour, and today there is increasing concern that several protozoan infestations may be sexually transmitted.

The protozoa can be classified into major and minor protozoa and according to their primary infection site into intestinal, urogenital tract and blood and tissue protozoa. The current chapter discusses the former two groups, which are sexually transmitted. The other important protozoan infections like toxoplasmosis and *Pneumocystis carinii* (now considered as a fungus) pneumonia are opportunistic infections and are covered in chapter 7.

The major and minor pathogenic protozoa implicated

Table 1.   Major and Minor Pathogenic Protozoa[1]

	Species	Disease
Major protozoa		
Intestinal tract	*Entamoeba histolytica*	Amoebiasis
	Giardia lamblia	Giardiasis
	Cryptosporidium parvum	Cryptosporidiosis
Urogenital tract	*Trichomonas vaginalis*	Trichomoniasis
Minor protozoa		
Intestinal tract	*Balantidium coli*	Dysentery
	Isospora belli	Isosporiasis
	Enterocytozoon bienusi	Microsporidiosis
	Septata intestinalis	Microsporidiosis
	Cyclospora cayetanensis	Cyclosporiasis

Table 2.   Morphological Features of Major Protozoa[2]

Protozoan	Size (μ)	Motility	Nucleus	Others
T. vaginalis				
Trophozoite	7-23	'jerky rapid'	1	Presence of undulating membrane.
Cyst	No cyst stage			
G. Lamblia				
Trophozoite	10-20	'Falling leaf'	2('owl eyed')	Sucking disc prominent on the ventral side
Cyst	8-19	–	4	
E. histolytica				
Trophozoite	12-60	Progressive, directional,	One	RBCs in cytoplasm
Cyst	10-20	rapid	Mature-4 Immature 1-2	diagnostic of *E histoytica*

in STD are listed in Table 1 and important morphological features of major protozoa (except cryptosporidium, which is discussed under coccidian, later in the chapter.) are outlined in Table 2

The other classification is (1) Protozoa for which the principal route of transmission is sexual intercourse i.e. trichomoniasis, (2) Those for which the primary route of transmission is non-sexual but for which male homosexual activity and much less commonly heterosexual activity are thought to be associated with disease transmission (amoebiasis, giardiasis, etc.).

Trichomoniasis

Trichomoniasis is caused by *Trichomonas vaginalis* (T.

vaginalis), a protozoan belonging to the order trichomonads. Three species are found in humans: *T. vaginalis* is a parasite of the genitourinary tract, while *T. tenax* and *Pentatrichomonas hominis* are nonpathogenic trichomonads that are found in the oral cavity and large intestine respectively. Donne in 1936 first described the species from a freshly made vaginal discharge smear. [3]

Biology[3]

The shape and size of *T. vaginalis* vary depending on the vaginal microenvironment or culture conditions. It is 15 mm in length, and fusiform in shape and has a characteristic erratic, twitching motility. It has four anterior flagella that originate from the anterior kinetosomal complex, and a fifth flagellum attached to the undulating membrane, that arises from the kinetosomal complex and extends till half the length of organism (Fig. 1).

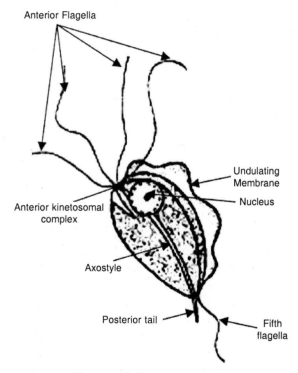

Fig. 1   *Trichomonas Vaginalis*

The other components are anterior nucleus with 5 chromosomes, golgi complex, parabasal apparatus and axostyle which runs along to form the tail or projection posteriorly. Three rows of large chromatin granules are arranged parallel to the axostyle which are hydrogenosomes. Reproduction is by mitotic division

and longitudinal fission, which occurs every 8-12 hours under optimal conditions. They are present in 2 forms: the smaller form which is more virulent, and the larger form, which is more dormant. The latter are found in asympto-matic infection, while the former in symptomatic disease.

Prevalence

The organism is responsible for approximately one-fourth of all cases of clinically evident vaginal infection. The prevalence ranges from 2-5% in middle class women, 56% in women attending sexually transmitted disease clinics; 50% of them are asymptomatic, while 30% develop symptoms within a period of 6 months of follow up. [4] A study of women with vaginal discharge at STD clinic in Mumbai, reported a prevalence of 5.9% with trichomoniasis, and a significant association between sexual habits and prevalence of gonorrhoea, trichomoniasis and HIV was observed.[5] The prevalence of trichomoniasis varies from 5.7 to 60.6% in different parts of India (Table 3).

Table 3.   The Prevalence of Trichomoniasis in Women in India[6–10]

Number studied	Place (year)	Prevalence (%)
92	Meerut 1990	60.6
350	Chandigarh 1991	9.4
100	Patiala 1993	13
142	Port Blair 1994	8.4
74	Calcutta 1994	11.1
8900	Mumbai 1991-1999	5.7

In men the prevalence has ranged from 0% in asymptomatic men at low risk to 58% among adolescents at high risk for STD. [3] In a study from Tanzania, a community of rural men with urethritis was studied, where the most prevalent pathogen was *T. vaginalis* (11%) and 50% of these men were asymptomatic.[11] In another study, 13% of men attending the STD clinic had trichomoniasis, and men older than 30 years had a higher prevalence of *T. vaginalis* infection.[12] In one Indian study, the prevalence of trichomonas infection was 6.6% in men with STD.[9] Co-infection with other organisms like *Ureaplasma urealyticum* and or *Mycoplasma hominis* in over 90%, *Gardnerella vaginalis* in about 90%, *Neisseria gonorrhoeae* in 30%, yeasts in 15% and *C. trachomatis* in about 15% has been reported.[3]

Risk factors for acquiring trichomoniasis were studied among African-American women living in low socio economic areas, in which it was observed that use of marijuana, older sex partners, non-steady partners and history of delinquency contributed to risk for acquiring infection. All of these were modifiable behavioural risks.[13]

Transmission[2]

T. vaginalis is almost exclusively transmitted by sexual intercourse. The organisms are isolated from vagina, cervix, urethra, bladder, Bartholin glands and Skene glands in females, whereas in males, organisms have been isolated from the anterior urethra, external genitalia, prostate, epididymis and semen. Rarely, transmission by contaminated fomites has been reported. *T. vaginalis* survives upto 45 minutes on toilet seats, wash clothes, clothing and bath water.

Perinatal transmission occurs to 2-17% of female children of infected mothers.[14] Reports have also documented *T. vaginalis* as a cause of neonatal pneumonia.[15]

Pathogenesis[3]

Due to lack of animal models, very little information is available on the pathogenesis of trichomoniasis. Studies have implied that various virulence-associated characteristics are important for infection with *T. vaginalis*. The presence and absence of complement and iron also play a role in pathogenesis. The findings of different studies suggest that cyto-adherence, which ultimately leads to cytotoxicity, which is a dynamic and complex process involving a cascade of reactions may be responsible for *T. vaginalis* infection. It was also observed in one study that molecular mimicry of one of the adhesion molecules with malic enzyme could be responsible for evasion of host immune defenses by the parasite.

Clinical Manifestations

T. vaginalis commonly infects the vaginal epithelium. Other sites affected are the urethra, Bartholin glands and Skene glands and rarely endocervix. In men, it most commonly involves the urethra, others being epididymis and prostate. Infection of extragenital sites like fallopian tubes, perinephric abscess, meningitis and perianal ulcers has also been reported.[3]

Manifestations in Women

The incubation period for *T. vaginalis* infection has been reported to be between 4-28 days. About 50% of women are asymptomatic, but about 30% of this group develop symptoms when they are observed for 6 months.[4]

In symptomatic women, most studies showed that vaginal secretions were usually copious, homogenous, malodourous with a pH of 4.5, and a yellow-green colour. Gardner and Dukes described the colour of discharge as gray in 46% of cases, yellow-green in 36% cases and yellow in 10%.[4] Punctate mucosal haemorrhages with ulcerations over the cervix are referred as colpitis macularis, flea-bitten or strawberry cervix, and is better visualized on colposcopy. The positivity of this finding on naked eye examination is only 2.5%, as compared to 52% on colposcopy. In another study, it was observed that vaginal fluid from women with colpitis macularis had a mean of 18 *T. vaginalis* / 400 × microscopic field to that of 7 *T. vaginalis* / 400 × microscopic field in women without colpitis macularis.[3]

Twelve percent of patients complained of abdominal pain, which could reflect the presence of severe vaginitis, regional lymphadenopathy, endometritis or salpingitis. Rarely postmenstrual and post-coital spotting are observed.[8] An overview of signs, symptoms and clinical findings in women is given in Table 4.

Reproductive complications include increased risk of HIV infection, premature rupture of membranes (PROM) and preterm birth. The prevalence of trichomoniasis in pregnant women ranges from 12 to 27%.[16] In one study from India, a high infection rate was found in women of higher parity. The risk of PROM was found to be almost 2.5 times that in uninfected pregnant women, but there was no association with preterm labour and IUGR.[17] A large multicenrtic study, which included multivariate analysis to correct the potential confounding variables, revealed a correlation between *T. vaginalis* and PROM and low birth weight. In the puerperal period, *T. vaginalis* was associated with a risk of febrile mortality. There was also an association between postabortal infection and trichomonas colonization.[18]

Clinical Manifestations in Men

The most common manifestation of *T. vaginalis* infection in men is urethral discharge, or symptoms of urethritis. They may also complain of dysuria, urgency, and post-

Table 4.   Symptoms, Signs and Clinical Findings in Women with Trichomoniasis[14]

Symptoms	%	Signs	%	Findings	%
None	9-56	None	15	pH>4.5	66-91
Discharge		Diffuse vulval erythema	10-37	Positive whiff test	~50
Malodourous	50-75	Excessive discharge	50-75	Wet mount:	
Pruritus	23-82	Yellow, green	5-42	Excess PMNs	~75
Dypareunia	10-50	Frothy	8-50	Motile trichomonas	40-80
Dysuria	30-50	Vaginal wall inflammation	20-75	Fluorescent antibody	80-90
Lower abdominal pain	5-12	Strawberry cervix:		Acridine orange	50-90
		Naked eye	1-2	Giemsa	50-90
		Colposcopy	45-90	Papanicolau	56-70
				Culture	95-97

coital burning. They also may have asymptomatic urethritis. *T. vaginalis* has been reported to cause 1-17% of cases of nonchlamydial nongonococcal urethritis (NCNGU). The urethral discharge in *T. vaginalis* infection is less profuse and purulent compared to that of gonococcal or chlamydial urethritis.[19] In one large study of 447 men attending an STD clinic it was observed that the majority of the patients had symptoms of urethritis, and both spontaneous resolution (33%) and prolonged asymptomatic carrier states were observed.[3]

The other less known presentations are: balanoposthitis, inflammation of external genitalia, urethral stricture, epididymitis and infertility. Though many studies, indicate that the second most common manifestation of *T. vaginalis* infection is prostatitis, definitive evidence is still lacking. A study on aetiology of chronic prostatitis reported that second commonest cause of chronic prostatitis was *T. vaginalis* (52/276 patients), next only to *C. trachomatis*.[20]

Diagnosis

Diagnosis based solely on clinical signs and symptoms is unreliable, and it has to be confirmed by laboratory investigations.

Direct Microscopic Examination [3]

Making a wet mount of vaginal discharge and examination of urine in males can be used in making the diagnosis in clinical practice. The detailed methodology for these is described in chapter 12. The sensitivity of detection ranges from 42-92% depending on the experience and expertise of the examiner. Various staining methods have been described, which include

Gram's, Giemsa, Papanicolaou, PAS, acridine orange, fluorescein, neutral red and peroxidase stains. Routine Papanicoloau stained smears have demonstrated *T. vaginalis* on cytological examination in asymptomatic women.

Culture

Culture is the 'Gold standard' for diagnosis of trichomoniasis. It is especially of significant use when the organism load is low, especially in asymptomatic women and men with chronic disease. Various media have been used to detect trichomonas, such as Diamond (tripticase, yeast and maltose), modified Diamond, Kupfurberg, Lash, NIH and Feinberg-Whettington media. In one study, it was found that with Diamond and modified Diamond media, detection rate was 90-97% compared to other media.[3] In another study, which compared broth culture to that with modified Columbia agar, showed that the latter was more sensitive (98.5%) than broth (92.1%).[21] The yield on culture usually takes 3-7 days. Culture systems like InPouch TV®, which allows direct inoculation, transport and culture are commercially available, and results are obtained earlier than the routine culture.[2]

Immunological and Molecular Methods

Various serological assays with good sensitivities have been described, but they are less specific than culture and sometimes even wet mount. Other detection methods are antigen-detection immunoassay using monoclonal antibody and nucleic acid based tests, PCR. In an observational study of 337 women with a new PCR test for *T. vaginalis*, it was found that the sensitivities of wet preparation and culture were 52% and 78% respectively, compared to that of the PCR which was

84% sensitive and 94% specific on the same specimens. It was concluded that women with high risk and asymptomatic infection would be benefited with this PCR.[22] In another study, 5' nuclease assay for detection of *T. vaginalis* DNA from female genital specimens showed that sensitivity and specificity were 97.8% and 97.4% respectively, compared to those of broth culture. It was also reported to have advantage of detection, among large clinical samples in a short time compared to culture.[23] In a study, for improved detection of DNA amplification of *T. vaginalis* in males, prevalence of trichomoniasis was estimated by culture and PCR analysis of urine and urethral swab specimens. The prevalence estimated was 5% by culture and 17% by the PCR. Urine specimens yielded more positive specimens than urethral swabs. The sensitivity of the PCR analysis of the urine specimens in comparison to that of culture was 100%.[24]

Treatment[25]

Recommended Regimen
Metronidazole : 2g orally in a single dose.
Alternative Regimen
Metronidazole : 500 mg twice a day for 7 days.
The nitroimidazoles comprise the only class of drugs useful for the oral or parenteral therapy of trichomoniasis. Of these, only metronidazole is readily available and approved by the FDA for the treatment of trichomoniasis. In randomized clinical trials, the recommended metronidazole regimens have resulted in cure rates of approximately 90%-95%; ensuring treatment of sex partners might increase the success rate. Treatment of patients and sex partners results in relief of symptoms, microbiologic cure, and reduction of transmission.

Follow Up

Follow up is unnecessary for men and women who become asymptomatic after treatment or who are initially asymptomatic. Certain strains of *T. vaginalis* can have diminished susceptibility to metronidazole; however, infections caused by most of these organisms respond to higher doses of metronidazole. If treatment failure occurs with either regimen, the patient should be retreated with metronidazole 500 mg twice a day for 7 days. If treatment failure occurs again, the patient should be treated with a single, 2 g dose of metronidazole once a day for 3-5 days.

Patients with laboratory documented infection who do not respond to the 3-5 day treatment regimen and who have not been reinfected should be managed in consultation with a specialist; evaluation of such cases should ideally include determination of the susceptibility of *T. vaginalis* to metronidazole.

Management of Sex Partners

Sex partners of patients with *T. vaginalis* should be treated. Patients should be instructed to avoid sex until they and their sex partners are cured i.e., when therapy has been completed and patient and the partner(s) are asymptomatic (in the absence of a microbiologic test of cure).

Special Considerations

Allergy, Intolerance and Adverse Reactions

Patients with an immediate-type allergy to metronidazole can be managed by desensitization. Topical therapy with drugs other than nitroimidazoles can be attempted, but cure rates are low ($\leq$50%).

Pregnancy

Vaginal trichomoniasis has been associated with adverse pregnancy outcomes, particularly PROM, preterm delivery, and low birthweight. Data have not indicated that treating asymptomatic trichomoniasis during pregnancy lessens the risk of adverse outcome. Women who are symptomatic with trichomoniasis should be treated to ameliorate symptoms.

Women may be treated with 2g of metronidazole in a single dose. Multiple studies and meta-analyzes have not demonstrated a consistent association between metronidazole use during pregnancy and teratogenic or mutagenic effects in the infants.

HIV positive patients should receive the same treatment regimen as those who are HIV-negative.

Other Therapies

Active immunization against trichomoniasis is done in Europe. Other therapies which have proved useful are metronidazole gel, clotrimazole pessary, nonoxynol-9 and povidine iodine douches.

Metronidazole resistant vaginal trichomoniasis may

be treated with high doses of tinidazole both oral and vaginal tablets with 92% cure rate. Furazolidone and sulphimidazole are effective in vitro against metronidazole resistant *T. vaginalis.* [26] Another in vitro study showed that the combination of dipyridamole and allopurinol could be useful in treatment of trichomonaisis, and also against other parasites which use de novo purine synthesis for their metabolism. [27]

Intestinal Protozoal Infections

Intestinal infections with a wide variety of pathogens now occur as sexually transmitted diseases, and as opportunistic infection in HIV/AIDS population. Protozoa are important enteric pathogens in patients with HIV infection. The spectrum of disease associated with each of these infections depends on a variety of factors which include immunological competence of the individual, the pathogenicity of the microbe and the duration of infection.

Epidemiology

The intestinal protozoal infections are now well recognized in especially risk group population like homosexuals, HIV/AIDS and bisexuals. The first published observation was in 1968 that giardiasis and amoebiasis could be sexually transmitted.[28] The initial studies concentrated on homosexual populations. The comparative studies of the prevalence of intestinal protozoal infection among the homosexual and heterosexual populations were done, where the prevalence of *E.histolytica* was 20%, *G. lamblia* 3%, *E.coli* 20%, *Endolimax nana* 24%, *E.hartmanii* 14% other nonpathogenic amoebae 8% in homosexuals compared to other group (heterosexuals), *E.histolytica* 0%, *G.lamblia* 2%, *E.nana* 5% and other amoebae 9%.[29] Various studies have put prevalence of *E.histolytica* 21-32% and giardiasis at 12-18% among homosexual populations.[29-31] In another study which examined the prevalence of enteric protozoal infection and their associations between the gender, sexual preference and practices in 180 consecutive patients at STD clinic, 19.6%, 3.9% and 23.5% of homosexuals were infested with *E.histolytica, G.lamblia* and other non-pathogenic entamoeba respectively, whereas bisexuals were infected with 2.1%, (*E.histolytica*) 4.2% (*G.lamblia*) and 10.4% (non-pathogenic entamoeba), and heterosexuals had no *E.histolytica* or

G.lamblia infection and 9.4% had non-pathogenic entamoeba in their stools. Homosexuality and oral anal sex were the most important risk factors.[32] In an another study in homosexual men with or without gastrointestinal symptoms, *E.histolytica* was observed in 29% of symptomatic men and in 25% of asymptomatic men; *G. lamblia* was found in 14% symptomatic and 4% asymptomatic men. On the whole, the initial studies which were done in homosexual population showed that there was definite association between sexual practices and higher prevalence of *E. histolytica* and *G. lamblia* infection.

With HIV/AIDS population increasing, various other exotic protozoal infections have become common. These are referred as new or emerging protozoal infections. In a recent study in Africa where aetiology of acute, persistent and dysenteric diarrhoea was evaluated, *E.histolytica* was found in both HIV positive and HIV negative individuals, where as microsporidium species and *Blastocystis hominis* were found only in HIV positive patients. [33] In an another study from Africa, among 50 AIDS patients, 57% had a variety of intestinal protozoa; isosporiasis was detected in 7 and cryptosporidiosis in 2 patients. [34] In another comparative study between HIV positive and negative individuals *Cryptosporidium parvum* was found exclusively in HIV positive patients where as *G.lamblia* was found in both the groups. [35]

In the current scenario of HIV/AIDS, the opportunistic protozoal infections have outnumbered the major protozoal infections. Various studies have documented prevalence of new or emerging protozoal infections: cryptosporidiosis (7.2-30%), isosporiasis (1.2-12%), cyclosporiasis (11.1%), microsporidiosis (9-20%), blastocystosis (10-51%) and nonpathogenic entamoeba (16-25%). These parasitic infections were either found exclusively or in majority of HIV/AIDS patients compared to that of infection caused by *E.histolytica* and *G.lamblia* which were of prevalence 0-25% and 2.2-6.2% respectively. [34,36-38] Recent studies from North India on prevalence of intestinal pathogens in HIV positive patients have been reported and are given in Table 5.

Transmission of Intestinal Protozoal Infection[16]

Transmission of giardiasis, amoebiasis, cryptosporidiosis and other coccidian intestinal protozoa infections is primarily by the faecal-oral route. Drinking faecal

Table 5. Prevalence of Protozoal Infections in HIV Positive Patients[39,40]

	Lucknow (n=26)	Chandigarh (n=120)
E.histolytica	11.5%	1.6%
G.lamblia	3.8%	8.3%
Cryptosporidium	11%	10.8%
B. hominis	8%	3.3%
Isospora belli	31%	2.5%
Cyclospora	–	3.3%
Enterocytozoon	–	2.5%

contaminated water and having sexual contact with an infected individual appear to be the most frequent causes of infection.

It has been estimated that 500-1000 cysts of *G. lamblia* and 2000-4000 cysts of *E. histolytica* can infect an individual. The primary infectious form is the mature quadrinucleate cyst. In most parts of the world, the usual source of infectious material is faecal contaminated water. Food handlers, flies or cockroaches, and poor hygiene in institutionalized individuals can also spread this disease.

E. histolytica is the most common intestinal parasite seen in gay communities throughout the world, with an average prevalence of 25% noted for this group of individuals. High risk behaviour found in this group that would easily predispose individuals to infection includes analingus (anal-oral contact) or fellatio (oral-genital contact) after anal-genital intercourse. Digital anal manipulation or poor hygiene after anal intercourse can easily result in generalized faecal contamination and subsequent infection. It is believed that direct rectal inoculation of trophozoites can occur, but this is thought to be an uncommon method of transmission. It has been shown that cleaning of the anus prior to intercourse does reduce the prevalence of infection, but sharing cleansing equipment among groups of individuals can, in fact, promote infection. It appears that the rate of amoebiasis in homosexual men has decreased during the last 5 years. This decrease may be because of safe sex practices that have been adopted in an attempt to decrease the incidence of AIDS in the gay community.

Despite the high prevalence of *E. histolytica* among homosexual men, it has been well documented that relatively few cases of invasive amoebiasis have occurred in this group. In addition, amoebiasis has only rarely been reported as a cause of morbidity in patients with AIDS. Analyzes has shown that the isolates of *E. histolytica* taken from several populations of homosexuals in the

United States and Europe almost always belong to nonpathogenic zymodemes. This apparently is not the case in Japan, where 15% of gays in large cities appear to have pathogenic organisms on the basis of serologic studies.

Heterosexual transmission of *E. histolytica* has also been described. Women can develop genital disease due to poor perineal hygiene. Heterosexuals practising anal intercourse or oral-genital sex in a manner similar to homosexuals can also be infected through the faecal-oral route.

Transmission of *Giardia lamblia* by sexual contact is almost exclusively seen in male homosexuals. Sexual behaviour that is responsible for the transmission of this organism is similar to at responsible for the spread of amoebiasis. There have been rare reports of proctitis and vaginitis caused by *Giardia lamblia*, which indicate the possibility of direct trophozoite transfer as an initiating factor in the development of infection.

It has been proposed that because of the compromised gut immunity in patients of HIV/AIDS, infection with the coccidian intracellular parasites like cryptosporidium, isospora have increased.

Giardiasis

Giardiasis is the human infection caused by the flagellated protozoan *Giardia lamblia*. Loeuwenhoek described the organism in 1679 and in 1859, Lambl re-described it. In 1915, Stiles renamed it *in Giardia lamblia*. The prevalence of *G.lamblia* is 2.9% general population,[41] and in homosexuals it is as high as 12 -18%.[30] A study among the HIV positive patients attending the AIDS clinic, reported a prevalence of 55% and giardiasis was associated significantly with penoanal sex. [42]

Biology[41]

G. lamblia is a flagellated protozoan belonging to the phyllum sarcomastigophora. It has two distinct life forms, the trophozoite and the cyst. The trophozoite stage is responsible for colonization in man. It is pear shaped and of length 10-20μ (average 14μ), 6-15μ wide and 1-3μ thick with an ovoid sucking disk occupying the anterior ventral surface.

The dorsal surface provides an area for diffusion of nutrients as the adults line the upper jejunal sections of the small intestine. The sucking disk appears to be a rigid structure connected to the exterior by a canal containing flagella. It is hypothesized that the beating

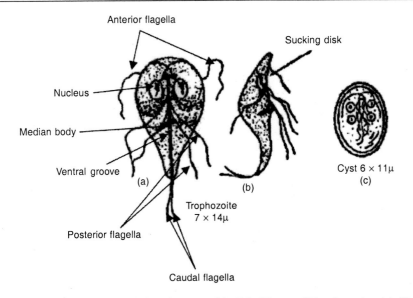

Fig. 2   *Giardia Lamblia* (a) Trophozoite (b) Side View of Trophozoite (c) Cyst

of the flagella produces a negative pressure in the concavity of the ventral surface causing its attachment to the microvilli of the small intestine. Eight large flagella are present in four symmetric pairs, and there are two distinct nuclei responsible for the characteristic "monkey-face" appearance on light microscopy (Fig. 2). *G. lamblia* multiplies by binary fission; therefore, as long as host nutrition and immediate environmental conditions are satisfactory, the parasite can maintain itself within the host indefinitely.

It is generally believed that the trophozoite stage interferes with the integrity of the brush border of the upper small intestine. The exact mechanism has not been defined, but it has been proposed that it may obstruct absorption by direct microvillous attachment and associated factors, such as fungal or bacterial overgrowth, or the production of an enterotoxin by *Giardia lamblia* itself. In fact, it is a combination of all factors responsible for the pathologic activity.

The cyst state is responsible for the environmental contamination and transmission of this parasite. The cysts are oval, 8 to 14μ long (average 12μ) and 6 to 10μ wide. Four nuclei are present, usually positioned near one end of the cyst. Once passed in faeces, the cysts survive best in wet, cool conditions. They are capable of surviving standard concentrations of chlorine used routinely for water purification systems. Oral contact with the cysts through contaminated water food, hands, or other body contact then reintroduces the cysts into the human host. Once ingested, the cysts apparently need the acidic environment of the stomach to signal excystation. The excystation is completed in the alkaline environment of the upper duodenum where a mature cyst releases a four-nucleated trophozoite. Once the trophozoite has established itself, it can multiply by binary fission every 5 hours, thus rapidly establishing its presence in great numbers. From ingestion to the appearance of symptoms it takes approximately 21 days but may as short as 3 days (range 3 to 41 days).

Clinical Features[41]

The most characteristic early phase of giardiasis is an acute diarrhoeal illness of brief duration. The diarrhoea usually lasts 2–3 days. The infection can be acute or chronic. In acute giardiasis, the manifestations are diarrhoea (95%), fatigue (93%), abdominal pain (74%), foul stool (77%), bloating (71%), weight loss (65%), nausea (60%), greasy stool (56%), flatulence (56%), anorexia (60%), frothy stool (48%), vomiting (23%), fever (19%), belching (26%) and constipation (9%).

The chronic phase of giardiasis is characterized by recurrent bouts of diarrhoea over 2–3 years, and flatulence (94%), upper abdominal pain (84%), epigastric gnawing (75%), nervousness (72%), weight loss (53%), constipation (47%), diarrhoea (41%), anorexia (38%), dizziness (34%), pruritus ani (28%), mucous in stool (25%), palpitation (22%), irregular fever (22%), urticaria (19%), nausea (16%), blood in stool (6%) and vomiting (6%).

Diagnosis[28]

Identifying the characteristic cyst or trophozoite of the parasite can establish the diagnosis of giardiasis. This is accomplished by obtaining appropriate samples of stool or duodenal fluid. The fresh stool is concentrated by flotation in 33% zinc sulfate or by formalin ether sedimentation. The concentrate is then stained with 1% potassium iodide. On microscopy, motile trophozoites are looked for. The sensitivity is better with active diarrhoea and is specific in experienced hands, but finding trophozoites does not prove disease causation. Microscopy of duodenal aspirate or jejunal biopsy or imprint is used, where the sensitivity is 34-98% and approaches 100% by latter method.

Serological tests like IFA using patients cysts / trophozoites have 89% sensitivity in symptomatic patients and 71-100% specificity. Immunodiffusion with sonicated cysts and IFA (with cultured trophozoites) have 91-97% sensitivity and 85-100% specificity, while ELISA (cultured trophozoites) has sensitivity of 87% and specificity of 88%.

Treatment[28]

Various antibiotics have been used for treatment of giardiasis. They include acridine derivatives like quinacrine 100mg tid for 5-7 days with 63-100% cure rates. Metronidazole 250-750mg tid for 3-10 days has been used with cure rates of 56-95%. Highest cure rate (95%) is obtained with metronidazole 750mg tid for 3-10 days. Tinadazole 2g single dose or 125 mg bid for 7 days yields cure rates of 93-97%. Furazolidone at 100mg tid for 7 days has 72-92% cure rates.

Amoebiasis

Amoebiasis is caused by the protozoan *Entamoeba histolytica*. Timothy Richard Lewis first described amoebae in human stools in 1869. In 1893, Quincke and Roos first described amoebic cysts. In 1903 Fritz Schandinn named the parasite *Entamoeba histolytica*. [28]

The majority of cases occur in tropical countries, the prevalence ranging from 15 to 40%; published reports place the prevalence of *E. histolytica* in homosexual men at 7-30%.[16] In patients with AIDS, *E. histolytica* is rare, but still should be considered as a cause of diarrhoea in addition to cryptosporidiosis and isosporiasis.

Biology[16]

E. histolytica is a protozoan. Of the seven species that make up the genus entamoeba, it is the only known human pathogen. *E. histolytica* primarily exists in two forms, trophozoites and cysts. The trophozoite, motile by means of its pseudopodia, is approximately 25 to 50μm in diameter. It has a single nucleus with a distinct, central nucleolus, its cytoplasm consists of a clear, outer ectoplasm and a more central, finely granular endoplasm (Fig. 3). The organism multiples by simple binary fission within the intestinal lumen. Unless diarrhoea is present, trophozoites become rounded and develop into cysts within the intestinal lumen before being excreted in the stool. In becoming cysts, trophozoites go through a precyst and a cyst maturation process. Trophozoites can no longer encyst after stool evacuation from the host. They are fragile and do not survive long outside the host.

Mature cysts are spherical, approximately 12μm in

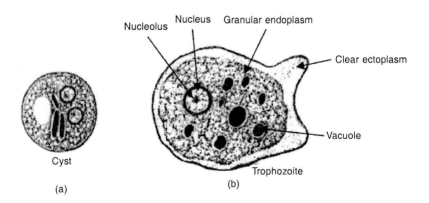

Fig. 3 *Entamoeba Histolytica* (a) Immature Binucleate Cyst (b) Trophozoite

diameter, and generally contain 4 nuclei. When a susceptible host ingests a mature cyst, its wall degenerates in the small intestine, releasing a single amoeba, which divides into eight uninucleated amoebae. These amoebae migrate to the large intestine and develop into trophozoites, which then encyst and complete the life cycle. Mature cysts can survive upto 3 months in water. They are destroyed by hypercholorination or iodination of drinking water, temperatures higher than 55°C, and prolonged exposure to carbolic acid or warm vinegar.

Pathology[16]

It is apparent that not all *E. histolytica* infections result in clinical disease exhibited by signs or symptoms of tissue invasion. It is proposed that there are distinct pathogenic and nonpathogenic strains or zymodeme groups of *E. histolytica* based on the electrophoretic motility of 4 of its basic enzymes, and certain zymodemes appear capable of causing invasive amoebiasis. It is estimated that only 10% of individuals with asymptomatic infection will have isolates that belong to a zymodeme predictive of invasive disease.

On the other hand others think that all *E. histolytica* are capable of invasion, but pathogenicity is the result of a complex interaction between host bacterial flora and the organism. Mirelman has recently demonstrated that an isolate of *E. histolytica*, obtained from an asymptomatic patient and thought to be nonpathogenic, could become pathogenic after contact with bacteria from a patient with invasive amoebiasis. [43]

E. histolytica causes local tissue injury by several biochemical mechanisms. Virulent strains are often resistant to both leukocytes and lysis by complement. Diets high in protein and low in iron restrict the growth of trophozoites and may help protect against invasive disease.

Clinical Presentation[16]

The incubation period from ingestion of mature cysts until infection is evident, ranges from days to months, but averages 2 to 4 weeks. Infected individuals can be totally asymptomatic, have symptoms primarily related to the gastrointestinal tract, or have extraintestinal manifestations of amoebiasis. The majority of patients, 50 to 90%, are believed to be asymptomatic. In one study of homosexual men infected with *E. histolytica*, 50 to 60% had mild gastrointestinal symptoms, but

symptoms were also present in a similar percentage of uninfected controls. Gastrointestinal symptoms may be mild or severe in intensity.

Individuals with nondysenteric colitis may complain of intermittent diarrhoea or constipation, mild abdominal cramping, flatulence and fat intolerance. These symptoms may begin insidiously and fatigue may also be a common complaint. Physical examination at this stage may be fairly unremarkable except for colon tympani and mild tenderness over the caecal area.

Some patients may exhibit signs and symptoms of severe amoebic dysentery. Dysenteric amoebiasis, rarely seen in homosexual men, presents with the passage of large numbers of watery stools containing clearly visible blood or mucous. In 50% of cases, the onset of illness is sudden, and fever, severe abdominal cramps, and tenesmus occur. On examination, there is usually generalized abdominal tenderness and signs of dehydration. Tender hepatomegaly occurs in 25% of cases and is due to a toxin released from infected colonic mucosa. A palpable mass and tenderness in the right lower quadrant can result from excessive production of granulation tissue in the caecum or rectosigmoid. This mass is known as an amoeboma. Although amoebomas occur very infrequently, they have been known to cause death.

Amoebic liver abscess is seen in fewer than 10% of patients infected with pathogenic *E. histolytica*, and its presence in homosexual men is extremely rare. In approximately 20% of cases, a history of prior amoebiasis is obtained. Patients initially present most (80%) of the time, with acute onset of fever and continuous, right, upper quadrant pain, temperature higher than 39°C (102.2°F), pallor and tender hepatomegaly. Intercostal and subcostal tenderness is present in 80% of patients and is a useful finding in suggesting the possibility of this diagnosis. If detected and treated early, the fatality rate for hepatic amoebic abscess is less than 1%; however, if rupture into the thoracic cavity occurs, the mortality rate increases to 6 to 30%.

Amoebic involvement of the penis or cervix typically results in ulceration and significant tissue destruction. Clinically, these lesions closely resemble squamous cell carcinoma. Penile amoebiasis has been described in both homosexual and heterosexual men.

Diagnosis[28]

A diagnosis of amoebiasis should be strongly considered

in male patients with diarrhoeal symptoms who are homosexuals. Demonstrating either the cyst or trophozoite of *E.histolytica* in stool generally makes a definitive diagnosis of intestinal amoebiasis. Three stool specimens, or one purged specimen should be examined for maximum yield. Differentiation of *Entamoeba* species requires permanent stains (trichrome or iron hematoxylin) after fixation with 10% formalin. The stool examination is positive in 90% cases of invasive amoebic colitis. If stool is negative, proctoscopy followed by colonoscopy may be required.

In vitro cultivation of the organisms may be carried out by numerous culture media including the liver extract, egg infusion media or alcohol egg extract of Nelson. Both cysts and trophozoites can be cultured. Zymodeme determination using starch gel electrophoresis of in vitro cultivates can be utilized to differentiate entamoebas.

Serology[28]

Serological techniques are quite sensitive in detection of patients with amoebic liver abscess and invasive colitis. One hundred percent positivity can be obtained by using ELISA in liver abscess and cellulose acetate membrane precipitation in rectocolitis. The other serological methods used for the diagnosis are indirect agglutination, indirect immunofluorescence, agar gel diffusion, complement fixation, immunoelectrophoresis. Latex agglutination and thin layer immunoassay demonstrates positivity of 1-52%, 55-100%, 83-100% in cyst passers, rectocolitis and liver abscess respectively.

Treatment[28]

Appropriate drug therapy of ameobiasis must take into account, the drug distribution and sites of amoebicidal activity. For cyst passers, diloxanide furoate 500mg tid for 10 days has 87-96% cure rate, diiodohydroxyquin followed by tetracycline 650mg tid for 20 days has 95% cure rate, and paramomycin 300mg/kg/day for 5-10 days has 80-90% cure rate. In invasive colitis, metronidazole 750mg tid for 5-10 days or 2.4g qd for 2-3 days has more than 90% cure rate. Tetracycline and dihidroemetine 250mg qd for 14 days and 1-1.5mg/kg/day IM for 7 days have 80-90% cure rates. In cases of liver abscess, metronidazole 750mg for 5-10 days or 2.4 g qd for 1-2 days has 99% cure rate.

Cryptosporidiasis

Cryptosporidia are tiny (4-5μ) protozoan parasites that primarily inhabit the microvillous region of epithelial cells. Tyzzer in 1907 described the organism. However the first instance of symptomatic human disease was recorded in 1976. With recognition of AIDS, multiple cases of cryptosporidium enteritis have been identified in immunocompromised homosexual men. In a study the prevalence of cryptosporidiasis in AIDS patients was reported to be 8.3%.[44] In an Indian study, cryptosporodium oocysts were detected in 46.7% of 75 immunocompromised patients which included both cancer and AIDS patients.[45] Salient features of all the coccidian protozoa and microsporidia are given in Table 6.

Biology[28]

The primary mammalian species causing diarrhoeal disease is *Cryptosporidium parvum*. They belong to the coccidian family. The estimated ID50 for humans is 132 oocytes. The life cycle of cryptosporidium is excystation of oocyte to trophozoite in the intestinal mucosa, then the trophozoite, transformed to type 1

Table 6. Salient Features of Coccidian Protozoan and Microsporidia[46]

Features	C. parvum	C. cayetanensis	I. belli	Microsporidium
Size (μ)	4-6	8-10	20-30	1-4
No. of sporocyst/oocyst	0	2	2	10-12 coils
No. of sporozoite/sporocyst	4/oocyst	2	4	-
Sporulation time after excretion	0*	7-14 days	24-48 hours	-
Stain(modified acid fast)	Yes	Variable, light pink- red	Yes (whole cyst stains pink)	Chromotope stains (bright pinkish red)

* already sporulated.

meront, which develops into a merozoite. The merozoite can become a trophozoite again or becomes a type 2 meront, the type 2 meront divides itself into macro and microgamont and after fertilization of the micro with macrogamont an immature cyst is formed, which finally becomes a mature oocyst. The oocyst sporulate *in situ* and either release sporozoites for autoinfection or pass from the body in the faeces.

The mechanism by which cryptosporidium causes diarrhoea has not been elucidated. It brings about non-inflammatory diarrhoea. Ultrastructural studies show the intestinal mucosa is intact but the microvilli are displaced at the sites of attachment to the parasite and the enterocyte may be elongated at this attachment. The type of diarrhoea caused by cryptosporidiasis is both secretory and malabsorptive.

Mode of Transmission

Since oocysts are infectious when passed in faeces, person to person transmission takes place in day-care centres, or household contacts in immunocompetent patients. In homosexuals and occasionally in heterosexuals oral-anal intercourse and fellatio after anal intercourse are common modes of transmission.

Clinical Manifestation [28]

Asymptomatic infections can occur in both immunocompetent and immunocompromised hosts. The incubation period is usually 3-14 days. In the immunocompetent host the clinical features are febrile symptoms, malaise, anorexia, vomiting, abdominal pain and cramps. Blood and pus do not occur in the stool. Diarrhoea may last as long as 4 months, but usually subsides within 6-12 days.

In immunocompromised hosts, especially in AIDS, diarrhoea can be chronic, persistent and profuse. Stool volume ranges from 1-25L/d. Weight loss, wasting, and abdominal pain may be severe. Biliary tract involvement can manifest as mid epigastric or upper quadrant pain.

Diagnosis

Faecal examination for oocytes is done by modified acid fast stain of diarrhoeal stool after sugar floation technique. In addition, the diagnosis can be established from histologic examination of jejunal biopsy or rectal mucosa for oocytes.

A direct immunofluorescent antibody stain is sensitive and specific and may require less time. ELISA for cryptosporidial antigen in stool with 83-95% sensitivity has been developed, and ELISA for IgM or IgG antibodies to cryptosporidium with 90% positivity rate has been described. [28] In a recent study, immuno-chromatographic dip-strip test for cryptosporidium oocysts in stool showed 92% sensitivity and 100% specificity. [47]

Treatment

To date, no chemotherapeutic agent is effective for cryptosporidiosis. In immunocompetent hosts, treatment is not recommended because the disease is self-limited. Although in limited studies spiromycin,[16] paromomycin (500-750mg qid) have shown modest benefit. Adequate fluid and electrolyte balance and supportive therapy are necessary. [48]

Emerging Protozoal Infections

The emerging protozoal infections are isosporiasis, cyclosporiasis, microsporidiasis and blastocystis infection. These protozoal infections have become prevalent as they cause opportunistic infections in HIV/AIDS patients.

Isosporiasis

It is caused by *Isospora belli*, another coccidian parasite frequently seen in homosexual men with enteritis. It is most commonly acquired by consumption of oocysts after which the parasite, invades the intestinal epithelial cells. In immunocompetent individuals it causes self-limited disease. But in immunocompromised individuals especially in AIDS, infection is not self-limited. The reported prevalence of isosporiasis in AIDS patients is 9.7%.[44] *I.belli* infection is indistinguishable from cryptosporidiasis. Eosinophilia which was not found in other enteric protozoal infections has been documented. *I belli* infect the entire intestine and produce severe intestinal disease. Symptoms include diarrhoea, nausea, steatorrhoea, headache and weight loss. Disease may persist for months to years. Deaths from fulminant infections have been reported. [46]

The diagnosis is usually made by detection of the large oocysts (25μ) in stool by modified acid fast staining. Sampling of duodenal contents by aspiration, string test or small bowel biopsy may help if the stool microscopy is negative.

In contrast to cryptosporidiosis, isosporiasis responds to trimethoprim sulfamethoxazole (160/800mg) qid for 10 days and then bid for 3 weeks. Other alternatives include pyrimethamine (50-75mg/day)[48] and in another report a combination of pyrimethamine and sulfadiazine for 8 weeks resulted in complete clinical and parasitological cure.[49] For prophylaxis refer to appendix VI.

Cyclosporiasis

The protozoan is another coccidian species, which is present globally, *Cyclospora cayetanensis* has been reported from the United States, Asia, Africa, Latin America and Europe. It is usually water-borne, but is also transmitted among homosexuals, and enteric infection is more common in HIV positive individuals. In a study of 450 HIV patients with diarrhoea with prevalence of, cryptosporidiosis 30%, *Isospora belli* 12%, cyclospora species 11%, *G. lamblia* 13% and *E. histolytica* 1%. The cyclospora infection studied in this group had clinical manifestations indistinguishable from cryptosporidiosis or isosporiasis. In all these patients disease manifested with profuse diarrhoea.[50] In a study from Mumbai, India, 50% of HIV patients in the study group had mixed protozoal infections and 6.6% had cyclospora species exclusively out of 334 faecal specimens.[51] The disease is characterized by non bloody profuse diarrhoea and concomitant weight loss, anorexia, bloating, abdominal cramping, malaise and fatigue. Symptoms tend to be more severe in patients of AIDS, and may persist as long as 70 days.[46]

Diagnosis is made by detection of spherical 8-10μ oocyst in stool. These refractile oocystes are acid fast variable and are fluorescent when viewed under ultraviolet light microscopy.

Cyclosporiasis is effectively treated with trimethoprim sulfamethoxazole (160/180mg bid for 7 days).[48] The study, quoted above, found 48% recurrence after 1 week of TMP / SMZ, and retreating with TMP/SMZ tid for 1 week resulted in cure.[50] But patients with HIV however experience relapses and may require long-term suppressive maintenance therapy.

Microsporidiosis[48]

These are obligate intracellular spore-forming protozoa. It has been detected recently as a human disease-causing protozoan especially in AIDS population. Currently six genera have been recognized to cause human disease: encephalitozoon, pleistophora, nosema, vittaforma, septata and enterocytozoon.

Microsporidiosis is most common among patients with AIDS. In these patients; *Enterocytozoon bieneusi* and *Encephalitozoon intestinalis* are increasingly recognized as causes of chronic diarrhoea and wasting. These infections are found in 10-40% of patients with chronic diarrhoea. The other manifestation described with microsporidiasis are AIDS cholangiopathy, acalculous cholecystitis, pneumonitis, chronic sinusitis, myositis, keratoconjuntivitis, nephritis, hepatitis and encephalitis.[46]

Microsporidia are small, gram positive with mature spores 0.5-2μ × 1-4μ. Diagnosis requires electron microscopy, although intracellular spores can be identified on routine microscopy with H&E, Giemsa and tissue Gram's stain. For the diagnosis of intestinal microsporidiosis, chromotrope 2 R-based staining and Uvitex 2B or calcofluor fluorescent staining reveal spores in faeces or duodenal aspirates. For enteric infection of *E.bieneusi* and *E. intestinalis* in HIV infected patients, therapy with albendazole may be efficacious[48]

Blastocystosis

It is caused by *Blastocystis hominis,* another protozoan, which is classified as an indeterminate form, and was initially considered nonpathogenic. Recently a study on protozoan infection on intestinal permeability using 99m technetium (99mTc labeled DTPA) assay showed that *B hominis* is also pathogenic.[52] Various studies have shown high rate of prevalence among HIV/AIDS population ranging from 10-51%.[34,36-38] They have two-forms trophozoite and cystic form. The cyst is considered infectious. They are nonmotile, 5-30μ, spherical, with 2-4 nuclei, and the cell contains a large vacuole with a thin rim of cytoplasm.[53]

They cause both asymptomatic and symptomatic infections. The spectrum of illness includes watery diarrhoea, abdominal pain, perianal pruritus and excessive flatulence.[53] Diagnosis is based on finding the cyst like stage in the stool with special stains. Indirect fluorescent antibody assay (IFA) has been found to be strongly positive in chronic infection as well as in 70% of asymptomatic patients.[54]

Blastocystosis can be treated with metronidazole and iodoquinol.[48] A study of 18 patients with blastocystosis treated with metronidazole 2g/day for 5 days showed complete clearance in 11and recurrence and relapse in 7 patients.[55]

The Impact of AIDS on Enteric Infection

Following the recognition of endemic enteric infections among homosexual men, cases of AIDS were reported in New York City, Los Angeles and San Francisco. AIDS which is characterized by an underlying cellular immune deficiency, has frequent multiple opportunistic infections and malignancies. The disease is primarily seen among homosexual men (73% of the total cases), and gastrointestinal complaints are often evident among homosexual men with AIDS. It is unclear what relation these enteric infections have with the development of AIDS, but besides the coincidence of these two epidemics and the frequent identification of these infections in patients with AIDS, case-control studies on AIDS in homosexual men have demonstrated that faecal exposure during sex and treatment for enteric parasites were significant variables for developing AIDS.

In one limited study, promiscuity, and anal intercourse were major risk factors for infection with HIV. One hypothesis relating these two syndromes includes production of a suppressor substance from *E.histolytica*, which results in alteration of the immune response, rendering a patient more susceptible to HIV which may be acquired during anal intercourse. An alternative hypothesis suggests that multiple intestinal infections, which are commonly seen in the homosexual men, result in an altered immunologic status, including activated T and B cells that are more permissive than nonactivated cells for HIV infection. In this latter hypothesis, frequent exposures to enteric infections among homosexual men would produce a more "susceptible" immunosuppressed state for HIV infection. Obviously, more research is required to explore these possible relations between multiple enteric infections and AIDS in homosexual men.

References

1. Levinson W, Jawetz E. Intestinal and Urogenital protozoa. In: Levinson W, Jawetz E, eds. Medical microbiology and immunology. 6th edn. New York: Lange Mc-Graw Hill; 2002: p. 298-304.

2. Leber AL, Novak SM. Intestinal and urogenital amoebae, flagellates and ciliates. In : Murray PR, JoBaron E, Pfaller MA, Tenover FC, Yolken RH, eds. Manual of clinical microbiology. 7th edn. Washington DC: ASM Press; 1999. p. 1391-1403

3. Kreiger JN, Alderete JF. *Trichomonas vaginalis* and Trichomoniasis. In: Holmes KK, Mardh P-A, Sparling PF, et al eds. Sexually Transmitted Diseases. 3rd edn. New York: Mc- Graw Hill 1999. p. 587-604.

4. Sweet RL, Gibbs RS. Infective vulvovaginitis. In: Sweet RL, Gibbs RS, eds. Infectious disease of the female genital tract. 4th edn. Philadelphia: Lippincott Williams and Wilkins; 2002. p. 337-354.

5. Divekar AA, Gogate AS, Shivkar LK, Gogate S, Badhwar VR. Disease prevalence in women attending the STD clinic in Mumbai, India. Int J STD AIDS 2000; 11: 45-48.

6. Kumar P, Sharma NK, Sharma U, Sharma RP, Iduani R, Agrawal AK. Trichomoniasis and candidasis in consorts of female with vaginal discharge. Indian J Sex Transm Dis 1990; 11: 54-56.

7. Sokhey C, Dhar K, Vaishnavi C, Ganguly NK, Kumar B. Isolation of pathogens from clinically suspected vaginitis. Indian J Sex Transm Dis 1991; 12: 59-62.

8. Chopra A, Mittal RR, Kanta S, Kaur R. Vaginitis and vaginal flora - study of 100 cases. Indian J Sex Transm Dis 1993; 14: 52-54.

9. Sharma PK. A profile of sexually transmitted diseases in Port Blair. Indian J Sex Transm Dis 1994; 15: 21-22.

10. Gogte A. Reproductive tract infections in women of child bearing age from Dharavi slums, Mumbai. Indian J Sex Transm Dis 1999; 20: 11-15.

11. Watson- Jones D, Mugeye K, Mayaud P, et al. High prevalence of trichomoniasis in rural men in Mwanza, Tanzania: results from a population based study. Sex Transm Infect 2000; 76: 355-362.

12. Joyner JL, Douglas JM Jr, Ragsdale S, Foster M, Judson FN. Comparative prevalence of *Trichomonas vaginalis* among men attending a sexually transmitted diseases clinic. Sex Transm Dis 2000; 27: 241-242.

13. Crosby R, DiClemente RJ, Wingood GM, et al. Predictors of infection with *Trichomonas vaginalis*: a prospective study of low income African- American adolescent females. Sex Transm Infect 2002; 78: 360-364.

14. Heine P, Mc Gregor JA. *Trichomonas vaginalis*: A reemerging pathogen. Clin Obstet Gynecol 1993; 36: 137-144.

15. McLaren L, Davis L, Healy G, James G. Isolation of *Trichomonas vaginalis* from the respiratory tract of infants with respiratory diseases. Paediatrics 1983; 71: 888-890.

16. Levine GI. Sexually transmitted parasitic diseases. Prim care 1991; 18: 101-128.

17. Mathai E, Muthaiah A, Mathai M, Jasper P. Prevalence and effects of trichomoniasis in pregnancy. Natl Med J India 1998; 11: 151.

18. Carey JC, Yaffe SJ, Catz C. The vaginal infections and prematurity study: an overview. Clin Obstet Gynecol 1993; 36: 809-820.

19. Schwartz MA, Hootar TM. Aetiology of non gonococcal nonchlamydial urethritis. Dermatol Clin 1998; 16: 727-733.

20. Skerk V, Schonwald S, Krhen I, et al. Aetiology of chronic prostatitis. Int J Antimicrob Agents 2002; 19: 471-474.

21. Stary A, Kuchinka-Koch A, Teodorwicz L. Detection of *Trichomonas vaginalis* on Modified Columbia agar in the routine laboratory. J Clin Microbiol 2002; 40: 3277-3280.

22. Wendel KA, Erbelding EJ, Gaydos CA, Rompalo AM. *Trichomonas vaginalis* polymerase chain reaction compared with standard diagnostic and therapeutic protocols for detection and treatment of vaginal trichomoniasis. Clin Infect Dis 2002; 35: 576-580.

23. Jordan JA, Lowery D, Trucco M. TaqMan-based detection of *Trichomonas vaginalis* DNA from female genital specimens. J Clin Microbiol 2001; 39: 3819-3822.

24. Schwebke JR, Lawing LF. Improved Detection by DNA Amplification of *Trichomanas vaginalis* in Males. J Clin Microbiol 2002; 40: 3681-3683.

25. Centre for Disease Control. Sexually transmitted Diseases Treatment Guidelines, MMWR 2002; 51: 44-45.

26. Sobel JD, Nyirjesy P, Brown W. Tinidazole therapy for metronidazole-resistant vaginal trichomoniasis. Clin Infect Dis 2001; 33: 1341-1346.

27. Afifi MA, el-Wakil HS, Abdel-Ghaffer MM. A novel chemotherapeutic combination for *Trichomonas vaginalis* targeting purine salvage pathways of the parasite. J Egypt Soc Parasitol 2001; 30: 735-746.

28. Guerrant RL, Sears CL, Ravdin JI. Intestinal protozoa: *Giardia lamblia, Entameoba histolytica,* cryptosporidiosis and new and emerging protozoal infection. In: Holmes KK, Mardh PA, Sparling PF, et al, eds. Sexually Transmitted Diseases. 3 edn. New York: Mc Graw Hill; 1999. p. 605-627.

29. Ortega HB, Borchardt KA, Hamilton R, Ortega P, Mahood J. Enteric pathogenic protozoa in homosexual men from San Fancisco. Sex Transm Dis 1984; 11: 59-63.

30. William DC, Shookhoff HB, Felman YM, DeRamos SW. High rates of enteric protozoal infections in selected homosexual men attending a venereal disease clinic. Sex Transm Dis 1978; 5: 155-157.

31. Law CL, Walker J, Qassim MH. Factors associated with the detection of *Entameoba histolytica* in homosexual men. Int J STD AIDS 1991; 2: 346-350.

32. Phillips SC, Mildvan D, William DC, Gelb AM, White MC. Sexual transmission of enteric protozoa and helminths in a venereal-disease-clinic population. N Engl J Med 1981; 305: 603-606.

33. Germani Y, Minssart P, Vohito M, et al. Etiologies of acute, persistent and dysenteric diarrhoea in adults in Bangui, Central African Republic, in relation to human immunodeficiency virus serostatus. Am J Trop Med Hyg 1998; 59: 1008-1014.

34. Hunter G, Bagshawe AF, Baboo KS, Luke R, Prociv P. Intestinal parasites in Zambian patients with AIDS. Trans R Soc Trop Med Hyg 1992; 86: 543-545.

35. Gomez Morales MA, Atzori C, Ludovisi A, et al. Opportunistic and non-opportunistic parasites in HIV-positive and negative patients with diarrhoea in Tanzania. Trop Med Parasitol 1995; 46: 109-114.

36. Mendez OC, Szmulewicz G, Menghi C, et al. Comparison of intestinal parasite infestation indexes among HIV positive and negative populations. Medicina 1994; 54: 307-310.

37. Manatsathit S, Tansupasawasdikul S, Wanachiwanawin D, et al. Causes of chronic diarrhoea in patients with AIDS in Thailand: a prospective clinical and micro-biological study. J Gastroenterol 1996; 31: 533-537.

38. Brandonisio O, Maggi P, Panaro MA, et al. Intestinal protozoa in HIV-infected patients in Apulia, South Italy. Epidemiol Infect 1999; 123: 457-462.

39. Prasad KN, Nag VL, Dhole TN, Ayyagari A. Identification of enteric pathogens in HIV-positive patients with diarrhoea in northern India. J Health Popul Nutr 2000; 18: 23-26.

40. Mohandas, Sehgal R, Sud A, Malla N. Prevalence of intestinal parasitic pathogens in HIV-positive individuals in Northern India. Jpn J Infect Dis 2002; 55: 83-84.

41. Jones JE. Giardiasis. Prim Care 1991; 18: 43-52.

42. Esfandiari A, Jordan WC, Brown CP. Prevalence of enteric parasitic infection among HIV-infected attendees of an inner city AIDS clinic. Cell Mol Biol 1995; 41: S19-S23.

43. Mirelman D. Effect of culture condition and bacterial associate on the zymodemes of *Entameoba histolytica*. Parasitol Today 1987; 3: 37-43.

44. Dieng T, Ndir O, Diallo S, Coll-Seck AM, Dieng Y. Prevalence of Cryptosporidium species and *Isospora belli* in patients with acquired immunodeficiency syndrome (AIDS) in Dakar (Senegal). Dakar Med 1994; 39: 121-124.

45. Ballal M, Prabhu T, Chandran A, Shivananda PG. Cryptosporidium and *Isospora belli* diarrhoea in immunocompromised hosts. Indian J Cancer 1999; 36: 38-42.

46. Ortega YR. Cryptosporidium, cyclospora and isospora. In : Murray PR, JoBaron E, Pfaller MA, Tenover FC, Yolken RH, eds. Manual of clinical microbiology. 7th edn. Washington DC: ASM Press; 1999. p . 1406-1412.

47. Llorente MT, Clavel A, Varea M, et al. Evaluation of an immunochromatographic dip-strip test for the detection of cryptosporidium oocysts in stool specimens. Eur J Clin Microbiol Infect Dis 2002; 21: 624 625.

48. Weller PF. Protozoal intestinal infection and trichomoniasis. In: Braunwald E, Fauci AS, Kasper DZ, et al, eds. Harrison's Principles of Internal

Medicine. 15 edn. New York: Mc-Graw Hill; 2001. p. 1227-1230.

49. Ebrahimzadeh A, Bottone EJ. Persistent diarrhoea caused by *Isospora belli* : therapeutic response to pyremethamine and sulfadiazine. Diagn Microbiol Infect Dis 1996; 26: 87-89.

50. Pape JW, Verdier RI, Boncy M, Boncy J, Johnson WD Jr. Cyclospora infection in adults infected with HIV. Clinical manifestations, treatment, and prophylaxis. Ann Intern Med 1994; 121: 654-657.

51. Deodhar L, Maniar JK, Saple DG. Cyclospora infection in acquired immunodeficiency syndrome. J Assoc Physicians India 2000; 48: 404-406.

52. Dagci H, Ustun S, Taner MS, Ersoz G, Karcasu F, Budak S. Protozoon and intestinal permeability. Acta Trop 2002; 81: 1-5.

53. Weber R, Canning EV. Microsporidia. In : Murray PR, JoBaron E, Pfaller MA, Tenover FC, Yolken RH, eds. Manual of clinical microbiology. 7th edn. Washington DC: ASM Press; 1999. p. 1413-1420.

54. Kaneda Y, Horiki N, Cheng X Tachibana H, Tsutsumi Y. Serologic response to *Blastocystis hominis* infection in asymptomatic individuals. Tokai J Exp Clin Med 2000; 25: 51-56.

55. Garavelli PL. The therapy of blastocystosis. J Chemother 1991; 3: 245-246.

Chapter 29

Pelvic Inflammatory Disease

Jaswinder Kalra, Sarala Gopalan

Definition

Pelvic inflammatory disease (PID) as described by the Centres for Disease Control and Prevention (CDC) is a spectrum of upper genital tract inflammatory disorder including a combination of endometritis, salpingitis, tubo-ovarian abscess and pelvic peritonitis with salpingitis being the most important component of the spectrum.[1] Acute PID, in general, refers to an infection involving the upper genital tract that is caused by the upward spread of microorganisms from lower genital tract. Chronic PID is a term used to refer to the sequelae of the acute process. PID is one of the most frequent and important infections seen in non-pregnant reproductive age women and is associated with major clinical and public health problems. In women, an increase in the prevalence of sexually transmitted diseases (STD) is associated with an increase in prevalence of acute PID and its sequelae.[2]

Prevalence

The incidence and prevalence of acute PID is very difficult to determine precisely as it is not a reportable disease in most areas and the wide spectrum of its clinical presentation and lack of accurate clinical diagnostic criteria. In addition, it has been estimated that up to two-thirds of cases of PID go unrecognized.[3] Westrom and Eschenbach noted that the incidence of PID is influenced by multiple factors, including prevalence of STD, demography, economics, health care characteristics of a population, sexual attitudes, douching, smoking and drug habits and contraceptive practices.

In a community based study in rural areas of Haryana, 61% of women of reproductive age had reported symptoms of reproductive tract infection with 41% of those who had pelvic examination, evidence of PID in

the form of cervical discharge and other signs like pelvic or lower abdominal tenderness.[4] In a study of 798 women screened in Shahjahanpur (Uttar Pradesh), 272 (34%) were symptomatic for reproductive tract infection (RTI), 54% women with vaginal discharge were found to have PID.[5] Awareness regarding the cause of RTI is very poor and none of the women in Karachi, Pakistan considered vaginal discharge as a symptom of STD.[6] In developed countries, various sources such as patient surveys, hospital discharge rates, private physician office visits, emergency room visits and retrospective self reporting have been used to calculate incidences of PID. There was an increase in the incidence of acute PID in 1970s and 1980s, as a result of STD epidemic and widespread use of intrauterine contraceptive device (IUD).[7-11] Since the peak in early 1980s, the hospitalisation rates for acute PID declined with the office visits rates remaining relatively unchanged.[11] According to the CDC report, there was a 57% decline in the number of hospitalised cases of PID from 1981 to 1996. In addition to this, with change to less expensive ambulatory treatment, there was a significant decrease in the direct medical costs for PID and its sequelae. This decline in the number of PID cases in USA was attributed to a parallel decrease in the incidence of gonorrhoea and a significant decline in the use of intrauterine devices as a method of contraception. An apparent decline in the incidence of PID was also attributed to more patients being shifted to ambulatory treatment to cut down the costs of health care by Health Maintenance Organizations.

Recently, increasing attention has been focussed on what is discussed as 'silent' or 'atypical' PID, a term used for the condition in which women with documented infertility secondary to tubal scarring and adhesions provided no past history of PID despite the fact that scarring suggested that pelvic infection had occurred in an asymptomatic or unrecognized form.[13] Such an unrecognized PID is probably as common, if not more common than clinically apparent disease.

Risk Factors

Knowledge of risk factors is required in order to prevent the significant economic impact and sequelae of PID and this has been emphasized by the CDC and others.[14,15]

Besides demographic and social indicators, important roles of sexual behaviours, contraceptive practice, health care behaviour have been stressed.[14-17]

Demographic Factors

(i) Age

Age is an important risk marker for PID and is inversely related to PID rates.[8,14] Adolescent girls are at significant risk of developing acute salpingitis. In a report by Westrom[8], nearly 70% of women with acute salpingitis were younger than 25 years, 33% experienced their first infection before the age of 19 and 75% were nulliparous. The risk of developing acute PID in the sexualy active 15 year old age group was 1:8, falling to 1:80 in women 24 years or older.[8,18] It has been suggested that the adolescent population is at greater risk because this population has a high prevalence of STD, has multiple sexual partners, tends not to use contraceptives which also protect against development of PID and in addition in this age group estrogen dominance with the resulting cervical ectopy provides a better target for attachment of microorganisms. Socioeconomic factors such as low level of education, unemployment and low income may be indirectly related to prevalence of STD and sexual and health behaviour.[15] No studies have compared PID rates in urban and rural population.

(ii) Sexually Transmitted Diseases

There is a strong correlation between exposure to STD organisms and PID, with gonorrhoea, chlamydial infection and bacterial vaginosis (BV) being the most important risk factors. In an analysis of risk factors associated with PID of differing microbial etiologies among 589 hospitalised patients with PID, Jossens et al[19] reported that an STD organism was present in

65% of PID cases and *N. gonorhoeae* and *C. trachomatis* were recovered from 55% and 22% of the patients respectively. Eschenbach et al[7] reported that a history of prior uncomplicated cervical gonococcal infection was present more often among patients with acute PID compared with controls.

(iii) Sexual Behaviour

Several aspects of sexual behaviour have been proposed to be associated with an increased risk of PID. These include multiple sex partners, high frequency of sexual intercourse and early age at first sexual intercourse. In a recent case control study of PID risk factors, identified more than one sex partner in the previous 30 days as a significant risk factor, whereas lifetime number of partners was not associated with an increased risk for PID. Coitus during menstruation has also been suggested as a risk factor for PID.[20]

(iv) Contraceptive Use

Use of different contraceptive methods has a major impact on the risk of acquiring STD, PID and their sequelae.[2,14,15,21] Non users of contraceptives are at increased risk for PID.[20] Barrier methods, mechanical and chemical, decrease the risk of STD and PID. Condoms when used appropriately are highly effective in decreasing the risk of acquiring and transmitting STD organisms associated with PID[22,26] and are associated with decreased risk of tubal factor infertility and ectopic pregnancy.[24,25] It has been suggested that vaginal spermicides decrease the risk of acquiring STD and consequently may decrease the risk of PID.[26]

The IUD is an additional predisposing factor for PID with most studies reporting an increased risk of PID and its sequelae from 2 to 9 fold. The World Health Organization has reported that in the most objective studies comparing IUD use with no contraceptive use, the increase in PID is in the range of 15 to 26 times.[27] Among different IUD, Dalkon Shield users had a maximum (13 fold) risk, with Copper T and Copper 7 having a 4 fold risk. Fairley[28] reported an increased risk of PID in the first 1 to 3 months after insertion of the device and this was related to the introduction of microorganisms into the uterus with insertion.

However, an increased risk of PID was not demonstrated with increased duration of use of IUD. Recently results from the PID evaluation and Clinical

Health (PEACH) study comparing contraceptive use in 290 women with histologic endometritis with 253 without it, demonstrated that IUD users had an increased risk of PID with an odds ratio of 13.1 (95% CI, 1.6-109.3).[29]

In contrast, most studies have demonstrated that oral contraceptives reduce the risk for symptomatic and clinically apparent acute PID by 40 to 60%.[30,31] Changes in cervical mucous, preventing ascent of vaginal and cervical microorganisms into the upper genital tract or modification of the immune response are believed to decrease the risk of PID in the pill users.

(v) Health Care Behaviour

Health care seeking behaviour influences the risk of PID.[14] Early detection and effective treatment of STD and PID in women and their partners decreases the risk of PID and its sequelae.[15]

(vi) Douching

An increased incidence of acute PID associated with history of vaginal douching has been demonstrated in several studies[20,32,33] with the risk significantly related to frequency of douching. Douching was found to be independently related to PID even after adjusting for age, marital status, lifetime partners, STD history and age at first intercourse[32]. Some case control studies have also demonstrated that vaginal douching is associated with increased incidence of ectopic pregnancy, a major sequelae of PID.[35,36]

(vii) Other Risk Factors

Cigarette smoking,[37,38] substance abuse[39] and menstruation[40] are additional factors implicated as risk factors for PID.

Aetiology

PID is a polymicrobial infection and is caused by ascent of microorganisms from the lower genital tract. The STD agents *Chlamydia trachomatis*, *Neisseria gonorrhoeae*, genital mycoplasmas, the facultative anaerobic and aerobic bacteria present in the normal endogeneous flora of the vagina and cervix are the microorganisms most frequently isolated from the upper genital tract of women with PID.[14,19,41-48] Although most proven cases of PID

are associated with *N. gonorrhoeae* or *C. trachomatis* in 30% of cases, only anaerobic and facultative bacteria are isolated such as Bacteroides species, Peptostreptococcus species, *Gardnerella vaginalis*, *Escherichia coli*, *Haemophilus influenzae* and aerobic streptococci.[19,49] Many of the non STD organisms are similar to those found associated with BV.[50,51]

Neisseria Gonorrhoeae

Gonococcus as the causative agent is implicated in 33% to 81% of the cases of acute PID when endocervical cultures are used to make a diagnosis.[44,52,53,54] When specimens are obtained from the abdominal cavity or fallopian tubes, *N. gonorrhoeae* is recovered in 18% compared to 39% from endocervix of total patients and 43% of patients with *N. gonorrhoeae* isolated from the cervix.[55] Generally, the proportion of acute PID associated with *N. gonorrhoeae* depends upon the endemic rates of gonorrhoea infection in a population. Recently, the PEACH study, a large prospective study of acute PID in United States, reported isolation of *N. gonorrhoeae* in only 4% of 274 patients where diagnosis was confirmed by histologic endometritis.[56]

Chlamydia Trachomatis

C. trachomatis is now well established to be the major aetiologic agent in acute PID. The incidence of the isolation rates of *C. trachomatis* in cases of PID depends upon several factors such as the patient population studied (mild disease or severe disease in admitted patients), cultures obtained from biopsy/needle aspiration or from peritoneal fluid or tubal exudate. The isolation rates therefore vary from 10% to 47% in the endocervix and 2% to 51% from upper genital and peritoneal cavity.[57] A 4 fold rise in levels of serum antibody to *C. trachomatis* has been seen in 19 to 62% of cases of acute PID.[57] It has been suggested that patients with milder form of PID are more likely to have *C. trachomatis* as the causative agent.[58] The two major sequelae of PID, tubal infertility and ectopic pregnancy have been found to be associated with prior chlamydial infection.[35,59-63] Recently subclinical PID was demonstrated by endometrial biopsy in 27% of women with lower genital tract infections with *Chlamydia trachomatis*.[64]

Genital Tract Mycoplasmas

The genital tract mycoplasmas such as *Mycoplasma hominis*,

Ureaplasma urealyticum and *Mycoplasma genitalium* have been suggested as potential pathogens in the aetiology of acute salpingitis.[65,66] However, their role remains controversial as some studies have shown no difference between the rates of isolation from the cervices of these patients and sexually active control patients.[44] The frequency of isolation of the mycoplasmas is low from the peritoneal cavity or fallopian tubes of patients with salpingitis (2 to 20%).[44,67] It has been suggested that mycoplasmas may be commensals rather than pathogens in PID[68] and on the other hand, failure to recover mycoplasmas from fallopian tubes in PID cases may be due to the reason that these organisms cause parametritis rather than acute salpingitis.[69] More recently another genital tract mycoplasma, *M. genitalium* has attracted attention as a causative agent for PID in animal models although its role in acute PID in women remains undetermined.[70,71]

Anaerobic and Facultative Bacteria

Nongonococcal and nonchlamydial bacteria such as bacteroides species, peptostreptococcus species, *Gardnerella vaginalis*, *Escherichia coli*, aerobic streptococci and coagulase negative staphylococci are the predominant isolates found in acute PID cases (upto 70%) in addition to *N. gonorrhoeae* and *C. trachomatis*.[20] In nearly one third of hospitalised cases of PID, these anaerobic and aerobic bacteria were found to be the only isolates recovered from upper genital tract.[19] Many of these nongonococcal, nonchlamydial microogranisms have been implicated in BV and several investigators have demonstrated an association between BV and PID.[46,47,51,62-74] Bukusi et al have observed that women with PID who are infected with human immunodeficiency virus (HIV) are more likely to have BV than HIV 1 seronegative women whereas *N. gonorrhoeae* and *C. trachomatis* infections were more common in the HIV 1 seronegative group.[48] In another study coagulase negative staphylococcus, coagulase positive staphylococci and *E.coli* were isolated in acute PID.[75]

Pathogenesis

Intracanalicular spread of microorganism from endocervix and vagina to the endometrium and fallopian tubes must occur for PID to develop.[3,14,49,76] CDC has listed 4 factors that might contribute to the ascent of bacteria from the lower genital tract and that might be associated with the pathogenesis of PID. These include uterine instrumentation, hormonal changes during menstruation leading to loss in the mechanical barrier of the cervical mucosa, retrograde menstruation and potential virulence factors of microorganisms associated with the development of PID.

An additional condition that might facilitate the ascending infection is damage to the normal clearance mechanism by the ciliated epithelial cells in the endometrium and fallopian tube.[49] Cervical ectopy occuring more frequently in adolescents and young women results in a larger area for attachment to microorganisms.[76] In chlamydial PID tubal scarring is thought to be due to an immune mediated delayed hypersensitivity type reaction, possibly involving heat shock proteins.[77]

Clinical Features and Diagnosis

Acute PID can present with a broad spectrum of manifestations that include unrecognized subclinical infection to overt infection which may be mild to severe. The most effective strategy for establishing an early accurate diagnosis of PID has not yet been identified. The specificity of any single clinical or laboratory diagnostic finding is low as no symptom or sign is pathognomonic of acute PID.[3] Nearly two-thirds of patients with post PID sequelae report no history of infection[61,78] and on the other hand one third of patients presenting with abdominal or pelvic pain suggestive of PID are found to have other conditions such as appendicitis or ectopic pregnancy or no disease at all.[3,79,80]

Silent PID

Many women with PID demonstrate vague or subtle symptoms that are not diagnosed as PID suggesting a concept of 'silent' PID.[3,13,14] Such patients in retrospective studies of post PID sequelae do not give any history of having been diagnosed or treated for PID.[13] Many studies have demonstrated the presence of inflammation or microorganisms in the endometrium and fallopian tubes of women with no symptoms of overt acute PID.[81-83] *C. trachomatis* has been recovered from endometrium by culture in 25% of infertile women and in 15% of infected women from fallopian tubes with no clinical or laparoscopic evidence of PID.[83,84] Chlamydial infection is known to persist in the tubes and endometrium in the absence of symptoms after treatment of acute PID.[85] Although the concept that ascending infection in the absence of clinical signs and symptoms can result in damage to the tubal function is widely accepted, it has been suggested recently by Wolner-Hanssen,[86] that these women with 'silent' or subclinical infection have had symptoms that were unrecognized as being associated with PID with nearly 60% of women with tubal occlusion with no history of PID had sought treatment for symptoms like abdominal pain.

Overt PID

Clinically apparent PID can present with mild to severe symptoms. The classical presentation includes symptoms and signs such as lower abdominal pain, purulent cervical discharge, cervical motion tenderness, adnexal tenderness, fever and leukocytosis. In mild to moderate cases, patient's general condition is good.[3] The onset of symptoms with gonococcal and chlamydial PID is often at the end of or just after menstruation.[92]

Severe disease is seen only in 5 to 10% of overt PID cases[3] and its clinical presentation is more characteristic with fever, chills, nausea and vomiting, abdominal guarding and rebound tenderness suggestive of peritonitis. The white blood cell count, ESR and the C-reactive proteins are raised in most of the cases. However, the accuracy of clinical diagnosis is questionable as only 65% of women with presumed clinical diagnosis of PID could be confirmed on laparoscopic visualisation with 23% having normal pelvic findings and 12% having other pelvic pathology such as appendicitis, endometriosis, ruptured ovarian cyst and ectopic pregnancy.[87] Recent studies have suggested a higher accuracy (80-90%) of clinical diagnosis of acute PID.[47,88] However, the overlap between the visually normal and the acute salpingitis group is so large that it precludes reliance on the clinical factors to differentiate the individual patient with acute salpingitis from the patient with normal pelvis.[87] In an analysis of the prevalence of clinical or laboratory findings in women with laparoscopic confirmation of PID according to aetiologic agent, gonococcal PID was found to be associated with a shorter symptom duration, fever and palpable adnexal mass more often than chlamydial PID which was more

frequently associated with abnormal uterine bleeding and an elevated ESR.[89]

A wet mount of vaginal secretions showing increased numbers of leukocytes is a very useful sign of acute PID as is the presence of mucopurulent cervicitis associated with chlamydial and gonococcal infection of cervix.[3,47,87,89] However in populations with a high prevalence of *C. trachomatis* and *N. gonorrhoeae*, cervicitis has a low positive predictive value for acute PID.[3] The absence of mucopurulent cervicitis and inflammatory cells in the wet mount of genital secretions has a good negative predictive value for ruling out PID. Although laparoscopy is currently the accepted 'gold standard' for diagnosis of acute PID, it is impractical to undertake this investigation in all patients.

Endometrial biopsy demonstrating endometrial inflammation has a good sensitivity and specificity rate for diagnosis of PID with a 90% correlation for histologic endometritis and laparoscopically confirmed salpingitis.[46,80,91] However, the clinical applicability of endometrial biopsy for diagnosis of PID is limited with its results not available for 2-3 days.

The role of sonography as a non-invasive diagnostic test for PID remains to be elucidated. Its clinical use is limited by its poor sensitivity (32%) although the specificity is excellent (97%). Thickened fluid filled tubes with or without free pelvic fluid are the suggestive features of acute PID on sonography.[92]

Laboratory tests such as antichymotrypsin, CA 125, tumour associated trypsin inhibitor and specific genital isoamylases are investigational and have not been shown to have a good positive predictive value.[3,80,89,93]

The clinician has to base the diagnosis of acute PID on clinical grounds in most situations. CDC has recommended a 'low threshold for diagnosis' of PID because of the potential damage to the reproductive health of women, if treatment is not instituted in time. The CDC recommends that in mild cases, treatment should be instituted on the basis of the minimum criteria with all three criteria being present i.e. lower abdominal tenderness, adnexal tenderness and cervical motion tenderness.[14] When more severe clinical findings are present, additional criteria which are more expensive and more invasive need to be looked at in order to avoid making an incorrect diagnosis and unnecessary morbidity. These additional criteria include – (a) oral temperature > (101°F) 38.3°C, (b) presence of white blood cells on saline microscopy in vaginal secretions, (c) elevated ESR (d) elevated C-reactive protein (e) laboratory documentation of cervical infection with *N. gonorrhoeae* or *C. trachomatis*, (f) abnormal cervical or vaginal discharge. CDC in 2002 guidelines, recommends following criteria are most specific for diagnosing PID. (g) histopathologic evidence of endometritis, (h) Transvaginal or magnetic resonance imaging techniques showing thickened, fluid filled tubes with or without free pelvic fluid or tuboovarian complex. (i) sonographic evidence of acute PID, (j) laparoscopic evidence of PID.[94]

Diagnosis of a tuboovarian abscess (TOA) may be difficult to make on clinical examination alone. Sonography and computed tomographic (CT) scanning and magnetic resonance (MR) imaging increases the diagnostic accuracy for a TOA and may be indicated if there is lack of response to antimicrobial therapy in the first two to three days.[95]

Sequelae of PID

Acute PID· is associated with significant sequelae that have an adverse effect on the general and reproductive health of young women.[3,12,14,18,78,96-101]

The short term consequences are perihepatitis (Fitz-Hugh and Curtis syndrome) which may occur in 7 to 16% of hospitalised cases of acute PID.[95] Mortality due to acute PID is not such a major problem in developed countries although it may be significant in countries where health care is not easily accessible. Rupture of a TOA with resultant generalized peritonitis is the most frequent cause of mortality (3 to 8%) associated with PID.[103]

The long term sequelae which develop in approximately 25% of women with acute PID are of more concern and these include infertility, ectopic pregnancy and chronic pelvic pain.[104-106] Unrecognized or 'silent' PID can also result in similar sequelae.[13]

Infertility

Tubal factor infertility (TFI) is the most common long term complication of acute PID.[8,96,99] In a large prospective study by Westrom et al[96] the reproductive events of patients with a laparoscopic diagnosis of PID were compared with controls. An infertility rate of 16% was found in those with PID whereas only 2.7% in control group failed to become pregnant. TFI was

confirmed in 10.8% in the PID group as compared to none in control group. The rate of infertility was found to be directly associated with number of episodes and severity of PID. Similar observations have been made by Lepine et al[107] more recently, however their data indicated disease severity at initial episode to be more important than the actual number of episodes. Poor outcome regarding fertility was observed in those cases where treatment of PID was delayed. Retrospective seroepidemiologic studies have demonstrated a strong and consistent association between previous chlamydial infection and TFI.[99] The relative risk of TFI is 3 to 8 in cases with past infection with *C. trachomatis*.[60,61,108,109] Most women with TFI and antichlamydial antibodies report no history of a diagnosis or treatment of PID, highlighting the concept of 'silent' PID resulting in tubal damage.[13] There is limited data relating to other organism such as *N. gonorrhoeae*, mycoplasmas and BV associated anaerobic-aerobic bacteria in their role in TFI.

Ectopic Pregnancy

Damage to the fallopian tube following PID is a well established cause of tubal pregnancy. An eight to ten-fold increase in the rate of ectopic pregnancy has been reported in those with PID.[96,98,100] A direct relationship between the number of episodes of PID and ectopic pregnancy has also been observed.[96] A significant association between ectopic pregnancy and previous chlamydial infection has also been demonstrated similar to TFI.[35,110-113] Role of nonchlamydial infections in ectopic pregnancy is not well studied although few studies have shown an association between *N. gonorrhoeae* and mycoplasmas and ectopic pregnancy[114,115].

Chronic Pelvic Pain

The cause of chronic pelvic pain is usually due to the presence of pelvic adhesions which result from the inflammatory response to acute PID. This entity is not as extensively studied. Chronic pelvic pain was found to be present in 18% of laparoscopically confirmed cases of PID versus 4% of controls by Westrom et al.[79] The severity and number of episodes of PID were found to be directly proportional to the rate of chronic pelvic pain. Chronic pelvic pain is also highly correlated with the extensive post PID adhesions.[116]

Treatment

Early diagnosis and treatment are crucial to the prevention of sequelae of PID. The effectiveness of therapy in prevention of these sequelae depends upon the interval between the onset of symptoms and the institution of treatment. It is important, therefore, not to rely on very strict criteria for the diagnosis of acute salpingitis and to institute early treatment based on a more flexible and realistic approach to diagnosis.

The aetiology of acute PID is polymicrobial and therefore for antibiotic therapy to be effective, a broader cover with antibiotics is required. Whether it is necessary to cover all the organisms implicated in the aetiology of PID is not proven. The clinician who diagnoses acute PID is often faced with the question of hospitalisation and oral versus parenteral therapy and the controversy in those aspects still exists. However CDC has recommended treatment schedules for acute PID and these are based on the premise that it is appropriate to cover all the major etiologic agents involved in acute PID including *N. gonorrhoeae*, *C. trachomatis*, anaerobes, gram negative enterococci, *G. vaginalis* and anaerobic streptococci.[94] No prospective data exists to address the issue of the clinical efficacy of oral (outpatient) versus parenteral (in patient) therapy of acute PID.

Indications for hospitalization of patients with acute PID as suggested in the guidelines by CDC[94] include the following:

1. Surgical emergencies eg. appendicitis clinically cannot be ruled out.
2. Patient is pregnant
3. Patient does not respond clinically or to oral antimicrobial therapy.
4. Patient unable to follow or tolerate outpatient oral regimen.
5. Patient with severe illness, nausea, vomiting or high fever.
6. Presence of TOA

In addition to the above, women using IUD should be treated on an in-patient basis because of a high co-existent rates of adnexal inflammation.

The major emphasis has been to use combinations of agents to provide empiric broad-spectrum coverage of the polymicrobial aetiology.

The CDC[94] recommends the following treatment schedules for oral treatment of acute PID:

Regimen A

Ofloxacin 400 mg po, bid for 14 days or Levofloxacin 500 mg orally od for 14 days with or without metronidazole 500 mg po bid for 14 days.

Regimen B (parenteral + oral)

Ceftriaxone 250 mg IM single dose or cefoxitin 2 g single dose IM plus probenecid 1g po in a single dose concurrently or third generation cephalosporins (eg. ceftizoxime or cefotaxime) plus doxycycline 100 mg po bid for 14 days with or without metronidazole 500 mg orally bid × 14 days.

Parenteral treatment.

Regimen A

Cefotetan 2 g IV every 12 hr or
Cefoxitin 2 g IV every 6 hr
    plus
Doxycycline 100 mg IV or po every 12 hr

Above regimen is given for atleast 24 hours after clinical improvement and then doxycycline continued 100 mg po bid for 14 days. Because of pain associated with infusion, doxycycline should be administered orally when possible, even when the patient is hospitalized. Oral and parenteral bioavailability for doxycycline is similar.

Regimen B

Clindamycin 900 mg IV every 8 hr
    plus

Gentamicin loading dose IV or IM (2 mg/kg) followed by maintenance dose (1.5 mg/kg) every 8 hrs

Above regimen is given for atleast 24 hours after clinical improvement and then doxycycline continued 100 mg po bid for 14 days or clindamycin 450 mg po qid for 14 days.

CDC has also suggested atleast three alternative parenteral regimens.[94] These are:

(i) Ofloxacin 400 mg IV every 12 hrs or Levofloxacin 500 mg IV od with or without metronidazole 500 mg IV every 8 hours or

(ii) Amplicillin—salbactum 3 g IV every 6 hrs plus doxycycline 100 mg IV or orally every 12 hrs

(iii) with or without metronidazole 500 mg IV every 8 hrs.

There are very few microbiologically controlled prospective studies comparing the various antibiotic regimens. Walker et al[117] performed a meta analysis of antimicrobial regimen efficacy for the treatment of acute PID with 21 studies meeting the criteria regarding appropriate system for making diagnosis of PID and assessment of clinical outcome. The pooled clinical cure rates ranged from 75% to 94% and pooled microbiological cure rates ranged from 71% to 100%. To ensure the best possible prognosis for fertility and to prevent other serious long-term sequelae, vigorous parenteral treatment with careful follow up of the patient is essential.

In those cases where TOA develops, but a rupture is not suspected, hospitalization and vigorous medical management with broad-spectrum antibiotics is instituted. A ruptured TOA is a surgical emergency, which may occur in 3 to 15% of all TOA.[118] Aggressive surgical intervention with hysterectomy and bilateral salpingo-oopherectomy results in more than 95% recovery rate. In unruptured TOA, if patients do not improve within 48 to 72 hours of antimicrobial therapy, surgical intervention needs to be undertaken and it may be possible to conserve reproductive function by aspiration and drainage of intra-abdominal abscesses.[119,120]

The role of steroids in preventing the subsequent adhesions, sterility and chronic pain is controversial. Although advocated by some in the past, no difference in the end results has been observed in a prospective study.[121]

Treatment of Sexual Partners

Appropriate management of acute PID includes examination and treatment of sexual partners of affected women, as the risk of additional episodes of PID will increase, if the male partner with asymptomatic *N. gonorrhoeae* and *C. trachomatis* infection are not treated. These partners should be treated with one of the regimens for uncomplicated gonorrhoeal or chlamydial infections, ceftriaxone 250 mg od followed by doxycycline 100 mg bid for 7 days or azithromycin 1 gm single dose.

PID and HIV Infection

The seroprevalence of HIV among women with PID is higher than that in women without PID.[122] It has been suggested that the clinical course of PID may be altered by symptomatic HIV infection and that these patients have blunted local mucosal immune responses leading to inadequate response to medical therapy.[123,124] HIV infected women with PID have been observed to have a more severe clinical illness with occurrence of TOA associated with microorganisms other than *N. gonorrhoeae* and *C. trachomatis*.[125,126] However the clinical response to CDC recommended antibiotics was the same in HIV infected and non-infected women.[126] Whether HIV infected women with acute PID require some aggressive interventions (eg, hospitilization or parenteral antimicrobial regimens) has not been determined.[94]

In conclusion, PID needs to be diagnosed early so that appropriate treatment can be instituted in order to prevent its medical and economic sequelae. A high index of clinical suspicion of acute PID has to be maintained. In cases of acute salpingitis, hospitalization and use of parenteral antibiotics, which have a broad-spectrum cover for the polymicrobial aetiology of the disease is of vital importance. Further, prevention of repeated infections is equally essential by treating the sexual partners of such women.

References

1. Centres for Disease Control and Prevention. 1993 Sexually transmitted diseases treatment guidelines. MMWR 1993; 42: 75.

2. Eschenbach DA. Epidemiology of pelvic inflammatory disease. In: Landers DV, Sweet RL, eds. Pelvic inflammatory disease. New York: Springer-Verlag 1997. p. 1-20.

3. Westrom L, Eschenbach DA. Pelvic inflammatory disease. In: Holmes KK, Sparling PF, Mardh PA et al, eds. Sexually transmitted diseases. 3rd Ed. New York: McGraw-Hill; 1999. p. 783-809.

4. Aggarwal AK, Kumar R. Study of reproductive tract infections and sexually transmitted diseases among ever married rural women aged 15-44 years. Integrated women Environment and Development project Report, Haryana 1997; 1-2.

5. Nandan D, Gupta YP, Krishnan V, Sharma A, Misra SK. Reproductive tract infection in women of reproductive age group in Sitapur/Shahjahanpur district of Uttar Pradesh. Indian J Public Health 2001; 45: 8-13.

6. Bhatti LI, Fikree FF. Health seeking behaviour of Karachi women with reproductive tract infections. Soc Sci Med 2002; 54: 105-117.

7. Eschenbach DA, Harnisch JP, Holmes KK. Pathogenesis

of acute pelvic inflammatory disease: role of contraception and other risk factors. Am J Obstet Gynecol 1977; 128: 838-850.

8. Westrom L. Incidence, prevalence and trends of acute pelvic inflammatory disease and its consequences in industrialized countries. Am J Obstet Gynecol 1980; 138: 880-892.

9. Jones OG, Saida AA, St. John RK. Frequency and distribution of salpingitis and pelvic inflammatory disease in short stay in hospitals in the United States. Am J Obstet Gynecol 1980; 138: 905-908.

10. Washington AE, Cates W, Zaidi AA. Hospitalizations for pelvic inflammatory disease. Epidemiology and trends in the United States, 1975 to 1981. JAMA 1984; 251: 2529-2533.

11. Rolfs RT, Galaid E, Zaidi AA. Epidemiology of pelvic inflammatory disease: trends in hospitalizations and office visits, 1979-1988. Paper presented at: Joint Meeting of the Centres for Disease Control and Prevention and the National Institutes of Health about Pelvic Inflammatory Disease Prevention, Management and Research in the 1990s; September 4-5, 1990; Bethesda, MD.

12. Rein DB, Kassler WJ, Irwin KL, Rabiee L. Direct medical cost of pelvic inflammatory disease and its sequelae: decreasing but still substantial. Obstet Gynecol 2000; 95: 397-402.

13. Wolner-Hanssen P, Kiviat NB, Holmes KK. Atypical pelvic inflammatory disease: subacute, chronic or subclinical upper genital tract infection in women. In: Holmes K, Mardh PA, Sparling PF, et al, eds. Sexually transmitted diseases. New York: McGraw-Hill; 1990. p. 615-620.

14. Centres for Disease Control and Prevention. Pelvic inflammatory disease: guidelines for prevention and management. MMWR 1991; 40: 1-25.

15. Washington AE, Aral SO, Wolner–Hanssen P, Grimes DA, Holmes KK. Assessing risk for pelvic inflammatory disease and its sequelae. JAMA 1991; 266: 2581-2586.

16. Padian N, Hitchcock PJ, Fullilove RE. Issues in defining behavioural risk factors and their distribution. Sex Transm Dis 1990; 7: 200-204.

17. Aral SO, Holmes KK. Descriptive epidemiology of sexual behaviour and sexually transmitted diseases. In: Holmes KK, Mardh PA, Sparling PF, et al eds. Sexually transmitted diseases. New York: McGraw-Hill; 1990. p. 19-36.

18. Westrom L, Mardh PA, Pelvic inflammatory disease: epidemiology, diagnosis, clinical manifestations and sequelae. In: Holmes KK, Mardh PA, Sparling PF eds. International perspectives on sexually transmitted diseases. Impact on venereology, fertility and maternal and infant health. Washington: Hemisphere Publishing; 1982. p. 251-268.

19. Jossens MOR, Schachter J, Sweet RL. Risk factors associated with pelvic inflammatory disease of differing microbial etiologies. Obstet Gynecol 1994; 83: 989-997.

20. Jossens MO, Eskenazi B, Schachter J. Risk factors for pelvic inflammatory disease: a case control study. Sex Transm Dis 1996; 23: 239-247.

21. Kani J, Adler MW. Epidemiology of pelvic inflammatory disease. In: Berger GS, Westrom LS, eds. Pelvic inflammatory disease. New York: Raven Press; 1992. p. 7-22.

22. Centres for Disease Control and Prevention. Condoms for prevention of sexually transmitted diseases. MMWR 1988; 37: 133-137.

23. Darrow WW. Condom use and use-effectiveness in high risk populations. Sex Transm Dis 1989; 16: 157-160.

24. Cramer DW, Goldman MB, Schiff I, et al. The relationship of tubal infertility to barrier method and oral contraceptive use. JAMA 1987; 257: 2446-2450.

25. Li DK, Daling JR, Stergachis AS, Stagno S, Cheeks J. Prior condom use and the risk of tubal pregnancy. Am J Public Health 1990; 80: 864-866.

26. Louv WC, Austin H, Alexander WJ, et al. A clinical trial of nonoxynol-9 for preventing gonococcal and chlamydial infections. J Infect Dis 1988; 158: 518-523.

27. World Health Organization. Mechanism of action, safety and efficacy of intrauterine devices. Geneva, Switzerland: World Health Organization; 1987. Technical report series 753.

28. Fairley TMM. Intrauterine devices and pelvic inflammatory disease: an international perspective. Lancet 1992; 339: 785.

29. Ness RB, Soper DE, Holley RL. Contraception and risk of PID in the PID evaluation and clinical health (PEACH) study. Am J Obstet Gynecol 2002 (in press).

30. Svensson L, Westrom L, Mardh P-A. Contraceptives and acute salpingitis. JAMA 1987; 251: 2553-2555.

31. Wolner-Hanssen P, Svensson L, Mardh PA, Westrom L. Laparoscopic findings and contraceptive use in women with signs and symptoms suggestive of acute salpingitis. Obstet Gynecol 1985; 66: 233-239.

32. Wolner-Hanssen P, Eschenbach DA, Paavonen J, et al. Association between vaginal douching and acute pelvic inflammatory disease. JAMA 1990; 263: 1936-1941.

33. Scholes D, Daling JR, Stergachis A, et al. Vaginal douching as a risk factor for acute pelvic inflammatory disease. Obstet Gynecol 1993; 81: 601-606.

34. Aral SO, Mosher WD, Cates W Jr. Self-reported pelvic inflammatory disease in the United States, 1988. JAMA 1991; 266: 2570-2573.

35. Chow JM, Yonekura L, Richwald GA, et al. The association between *Chlamydia trachomatis* and ectopic pregnancy: a matched-pair, case-control study. JAMA 1990; 263: 3164-3167.

36. Daling JR, Weiss NS, Schwart SM. Vaginal douching and the risk of tubal pregnancy. Epidemiology 1991; 2: 40-48.

37. Marchbanks PA, Lee NC, Peterson HB. Cigarette smoking as a risk factor for pelvic inflammatory disease. Am J Obstet Gynecol 1990; 162: 639-644.

38. Scholes D, Daling JR, Stergachis AS. Cigarette smoking and risk of pelvic inflammatory disease. Am J Epidemiol 1990; 132: 759.

39. Fullilove RE, Fullilove MT, Bowser BP, Gross SA. Risk of sexually transmitted diseases among black adolescent crack users in Oakland and San Francisco, CA. JAMA 1990; 263: 851-855.

40. Sweet RL, Blankfort-Doyle M, Robbie MO, Schacter J. The occurrence of chlamydial and gonococcal salpingitis during the menstrual cycle. JAMA 1986; 255: 2062-2064.

41. Mardh P-A, Lind I, Svensson L, Westrom L, Moller BR. Antibodies to *Chlamydia trachomatis*, *Mycoplasma hominis* and *Neisseria gonorrhoeae* in serum from patients with acute salpingitis. Br J Vener Dis 1981; 57: 125-129.

42. Sweet RL, Schachter J, Robbie MO. Failure of beta-lactam antibiotics to eradicate *Chlamydia trachomatis* in the endometrium despite apparent clinical cure of acute salpingitis. JAMA 1983; 250: 2641-2645.

43. Wasserheit JN, Bell TA, Kiviat NB, et al. Microbiological causes of proven pelvic inflammatory disease and efficacy of clindamycin and tobramycin. Ann Intern Med 1986; 104: 187-193.

44. Eschenbach DA, Buchanan T, Pollock HM, et al. Polymicrobial aetiology of acute pelvic inflammatory disease. N Engl J Med 1975; 293: 166-171.

45. Sweet RL, Draper DL, Schachter J, James J, Hadley WK, Brooks GF. Microbiology and pathogenesis of acute salpingitis as determined by laparoscopy: what is the appropriate site to sample? Am J Obstet Gynecol 1980; 138: 985-989.

46. Paavonen J, Teisala K, Heinonnen PK, et al. Microbiological and histopathological findings in acute pelvic inflammatory disease. Br J Obstet Gynaecol 1987; 94: 454-460.

47. Soper DE, Brockwell NJ, Dalton HP, Johnson D. Observations concerning the microbial aetiology of acute salpingitis. Am J Obstet Gynecol 1994; 170: 1008-1017.

48. Bukusi EA, Cohen CR, Stevens CE, et al. Effects of human immunodeficiency virus 1 infection in microbial origins of pelvic inflammatory disease and on efficacy of ambulatory oral therapy. Am J Obstet Gynecol 1999; 181: 1374-1381.

49. Rice PA, Schachter J. Pathogenesis of pelvic inflammatory disease. JAMA 1991; 266: 2587-2593.

50. Sweet RL. Role of bacterial vaginosis in pelvic inflammatory disease. Clin Infect Dis 1995; 20 (Suppl 2): S276-S285.

51. Hillier SL, Kiviat NB, Hawes SE, et al. Role of bacterial vaginosis-associated microorganisms in endometritis. Am J Obstet Gynecol 1996; 175: 435-441.

52. Eschenbach DA. Epidemiology and diagnosis of acute pelvic inflammatory disease. Obstet Gynecol 1980; 55 (Suppl): 142-153.

53. Cunningham FG, Hauth JC, Gilstrap LC, et al. The bacterial pathogenesis of acute pelvic inflammatory disease. Obstet Gynecol 1978; 52: 161-164.

54. Thompson SE, Hager WD, Wong KH, et al. The microbiology and therapy of acute pelvic inflammatory disease in hospitalized patients. Am J Obstet Gynecol 1980; 136: 179-186.

55. Westrom L, Eschenbach DA. Pelvic inflammatory disease. In: Holmes KK, Sparling PF, Mardh PA et al, eds. Sexually transmitted diseases. New York: Mc Graw- Hill; 1999. p. 783-809.

56. Rabe LK, Hillier SL, Wiesenfeld HC. Endometrial microbiology in women with pelvic inflammatory disease. In: Program and abstracts of the International Society of Sexually Transmitted Diseases Research; Denver, CO; July 11-14, 1999. Abstract 182.

57. Sweet RL, Gibbs RS. Infectious Diseases of the female genital tract, 4th ed. Philadelphia: Lippincott Williams and Wilkins; 2002. p. 368-412.

58. Svensson L, Westrom L, Ripa KT, Mardh PA. Differences in some clinical laboratory parameters in acute salpingitis related to culture and serologic findings. Am J Obstet Gynecol 1980; 138: 1017-1021.

59. Henry-Suchet J, Loffredo V, Sarfaty D. *Chlamydia trachomatis* and mycoplasma research by laparoscopy in cases of pelvic inflammatory disease and in cases of tubal obstruction. Am J Obstet Gynecol 1980; 138: 1022.

60. Jones RB, Ardery BR, Hui SL, Cleary RE. Correlation between serum antichlamydial antibodies and tubal factor as a cause of infertility. Fertil Steril 1982; 38: 553-558.

61. Moore DE, Spadoni LR, Foy HM, et al. Increased frequency of serum antibodies to *Chlamydia trachomatis* in infertility due to tubal disease. Lancet 1982; 2: 574-577.

62. Brunham RC, MacLean IW, Binns B, Peeling RW. *Chlamydia trachomatis*: its role in tubal infertility. J Infect Dis 1985; 152: 1275-577.

63. Hartford SL, Silva PD, diZerega GS, Yonekura ML. Serologic evidence of prior chlamydial infection in patients with tubal ectopic pregnancy and contralateral tubal disease. Fertil Steril 1987; 47: 118-121.

64. Wiesenfeld HC, Hillier SL, Krohn MA, et al. Lower genital tract infection and endometritis: insight into subclinical pelvic inflammatory disease. Obstet Gynaecol 2002; 100: 456-463.

65. Moller BR. The role of mycoplasmas in the upper genital tract of women. Sex Transm Dis 1983; 10 (Suppl): 281-284.

66. Mardh P-A, Lind I, Svensson L, Westrom L, Moller BR. Antibodies to *Chlamydia trachomatis, Mycoplasma hominis and Neisseria gonorrhoeae* in serum from patients with acute salpingitis. Br. J Vener Dis 1981; 57: 125-129.

67. Mardh PA, Westrom L. Tubal and cervical cultures in acute salpingitis with special reference to *Mycoplasma hominis* and T-strain mycoplasmas. Br J Vener Dis 1970; 46: 179-186.

68. Taylor-Robinson D, Carney FE. Growth and effect of mycoplasmas in fallopian tube organ cultures. Br J Vener Dis 1974; 50: 212-216.

69. Moller BR, Freundt EA, Black FT, Frederiksen P. Experimental infection of the genital tract of female Grivet monkeys for *Mycoplasma hominis*. Infect Immun 1978; 20: 248-257.

70. Palmer HM. Detection of *Mycoplasma genitalium* in the genitourinary tract of women by the polymerase chain reaction. Int J STD AIDS 1991; 2: 261-263.

71. Taylor-Robinson D. The history and rote of *Mycoplasma genitalium* in sexually transmitted diseases. Genitourin Med 1995; 71: 1-8.

72. Korn AP, Bolan G, Padian N, et al. Plasma cell endometritis in women with symptomatic bacterial vaginosis. Obstet Gyecol 1995; 85: 387-390.

73. Peipert JF, Montagno AB, Cooper AS, Sung CJ. Bacterial vaginosis as a risk factor for upper genital tract infection. Am J Obstet Gynecol 1997; 177: 1184-1187.

74. Korn AP, Hessol NA, Padian NS, et al. Risk factors for plasma cell endometritis among women with cervical *Neisseria gonorrhoeae*, cervical *Chlamydia trachomatis* or bacterial vaginosis. Am J Obstet Gynecol 1998; 178: 987-990.

75. Baveja G, Saini S, Sangwan K, Arora DR. A study of bacterial pathogens in acute pelvic inflammatory diseases. J Commun Dis. 2001; 33: 121-125.

76. Rice PA, Westrom LV. Pathogenesis and inflammatory response in pelvic inflammatory disease. New York: Raven Press, 1992: 35-47.

77. Paavonen J, Lehtinen M. Immunopathogenesis of chlamydial pelvic inflammatory disease: The role of heat shock proteins. In: infectious Diseases in Obstetrics and Gynaecology. New York: Wley-Liss 1994: 1-6.

78. Westrom LV, Berger GS. Consequences of pelvic inflammatory disease. In: Berger GS, Westrom LV eds. Pelvic inflammatory disease. New York: Raveri Press, 1992. 101-114.

79. Paavonen J, Westrom LV. Diagnosis of acute pelvic inflammatory disease. In: Berger GS, Westrom LV eds. Pelvic inflammatory disease. New York: Raven Press, 1992. p. 49-78.

80. Kahn JG, Walker CK, Washington AE, et al. Diagnosing pelvic inflammatory disease. A comprehensive analysis and considerations for developing a new model. JAMA 1991; 266: 2594-2604.

81. Sellors JW, Mahony JB, Chernesky MA, Rath DJ. Tubal factor infertility: an association with prior chlamydial infection and asymptomatic salpingitis. Fertil Steril 1988; 49: 451-457.

82. Paavonen J, Kiviat N, Brunham RC, et al. Prevalence and manifestations of endometritis among women with cervicitis. Am J Obstet Gynecol 1985; 152: 280-286.

83. Cleary RE, Jones RB. Recovery of *Chlamydia trachomatis* from the endometrium in infertile women with serum antichlamydial antibodies. Fertil Steril 1985; 44: 233-235.

84. Henry-Suchet J Catalan F, Loffredo V, et al. *Chlamydia trachomatis* associated with chronic inflammation in abdominal specimens from women selected for tuboplasty. Fertil Steril 1981; 35: 599-605.

85. Patton DL, Askienazy-Elbhar M, Henry-Suchet, et al. Detection of *Chlamydia trachomatis* in fallopian tube tissue in women with post infectious tubal infertility. Am J Obstet Gynecol 1994; 171: 95-101.

86. Wolner-Hanssen P. Silent pelvic inflammatory disease: is it overstarted? Obstet Gynecol 1995; 86: 321-325.

87. Jacobson L, Westrom L. Objectivized diagnosis of acute pelvic inflammatory disease. Am J Obstet Gynecol 1969; 105: 1088-1098.

88. Eschenbach DA, Wolner-Hanssen P, Hawes SE, Pavletic A, Paavonen J, Holmer KK. Acute pelvic inflammatory disease: association of clinical and laboratory findings with laparoscopic findings. Obstet Gynecol 1997; 89: 184-192.

89. Westrom L. Diagnosis, aetiology and prognosis of acute salpingitis (Thesis). Lund, Sweden: Student literature; 1997.

90. Hager WD, Eschenbach DA, Spence MR, Sweet RL. Criteria for diagnosis and grading of salpingitis. Obstet Gynecol 1983; 61: 113-114.

91. Paavonen J, Aine R, Teisala K, Heinonen PK, Punnonen R. Compairson of endometrial biopsy and peritoneal fluid cytology with laparoscopy in the diagnosis of acute pelvic inflammatory disease. Am J Obstet Gynecol 1985; 151: 645-650.

92. Boardman LA, Peipert JF, Brody JM, Cooper AS, Sung J. Endovaginal sonography for the diagnosis of upper genital tract infection. Obstet Gynecol 1997; 90: 54-57.

93. Pavonen J, Meittinen A, Heinonen PK, et al. Serum CA 125 levels in acute pelvic inflammatory disease. Br J Obstet Gynaecol 1989; 96: 574-579.

94. Centres for Disease Control and Prevention. Guidelines for treatment of sexually transmitted diseases. MMWR 2002; 55 (RR-6): 49-51.

95. Landers DV, Sweet RL. Tubo-ovarian abscess: contemporary approach to management. Rev Infect Dis 1983; 5: 876-884.

96. Westrom LV, Joesoef R, Reynolds G, Hagdu A, Thompson SE. Pelvic inflammatory disease and fertility. A cohort study of 1,8444 women with laparoscopically verified disease and 657 control women with normal laparoscopic results. Sex Transm Dis 1992; 19: 185-192.

97. Westrom LV. Sexually transmitted diseases and infertility. Sex Transm Dis 1994; 21 (Suppl): 532-537.

98. Safrin S, Schachter J, Dahrouge D, Sweet RL. Long term sequelae of acute pelvic inflammatory disease. Am J Obstet Gynecol 1992; 166: 1300-1305.

99. Chow JM, Schachter J. Long term sequelae of pelvic inflammatory disease: Infertility, ectopic pregnancy and chronic pelvic pain. In: Landers DC, Sweet RL eds. Pelvic inflammatory disease. New York, 1997: 152-169.

100. Buchan H, Vessex M, Goldacre M, Fairweather J. Morbidity following pelvic inflammatory disease. Br J Obstet Gynecol 1993; 100: 558-562.

101. Soper D, Ness RB. Pelvic inflammatory disease and involuntary infertility: prospective pilot observations. Infect Dis Obstet Gynecol 1995; 3: 145-148.

102. Fitz-Hugh T. Acute gonococcal peritonitis of the right upper quadrant in women. JAMA 1934; 102: 2984.

103. Pedowitz P, Bloomfield RD. Ruptured adnexal abscess with generalized peritonitis. Am J Obstet Gynecol 1964; 88: 721.

104. Westrom L, Wolner-Hanssen P. Pathogenesis of pelvic inflammatory disease. Genitourin Med 1993; 69: 9-17.

105. Mardh PA. Pelvic inflammatory disease and related

disorders; novel observations. Scan J Obstet Gynecol 1990; 69 (Suppl): 83-87.

106. McCormack WM. Pelvic inflammatory disease. N Engl J Med 1994; 330: 115-119.

107. Lepine LA, Hillis SD, Marchbanks PA, et al. Severity of pelvic inflammatory disease as a predictor of the probability of live birth. Am J Obstet Gynecol 1998; 178: 977-981.

108. Bjercke S, Purvis K. Chlamydial serology in the investigation of infertility. Hum Reprod 1992; 7: 621-624.

109. Reiners J, Collet M, Frost E. Chlamydial antibodies and tubal infertility. Int J Epidemiol 1989; 18: 261-263.

110. Walkers MD, Eddy CA, Gibbs RS. Antibodies to *Chlamydia trachomatis* and ectopic pregnancy. Am J Obstet Gynecol 1998; 259: 1823-1827.

111. Coste J, Job Spira N, Fernandez H, Papiernik E, Spira A. Risk factors for ectopic pregnancy: A case-control study in France, with special focus on infectious factors. Am J Epidemiol 1991; 133: 839-849.

112. Sheffield PA, Moore DE, Voight LF, et al. The association between *Chlamydia trachomatis* serology and pelvic damage in women with tubal ectopic gestations. Fertil Steril 1993; 60: 970-975.

113. Odland JO, Anestad G, Rasmussen S, Lundgren R, Dalaker K. Ectopic pregnancy and chlamydial serology. Int J Obstet Gynecol 1993; 43: 271-275.

114. Miettinen A, Heinonnen PK, Teisala K, Hakkarainen K, Punnonen R. Serologic evidence for the role of *Chlamydia trachomatis, Neisseria gonorrhoeae* and *Mycoplasma hominis* in the aetiology of tubal factor infertility and ectopic pregnancy. Sex Transm Dis 1990; 17: 10-14.

115. Robertson JN, Hogston P, Ward ME. Gonococcal and chlamydial antibodies in ectopic and intrauterine pregnancy. Br J Obstet Gynecol 1988; 95: 711-716.

116. Westrom L, Svensson L. Chronic pain after acute pelvic inflmmatory disease. In: Belfort P, Piotti JA, Eskes TKAB eds. Advances in gynaecology and obstetrics: Proceeding of the XII the World Congress of Gynaecology Obstetrics, Rio de Janeiro, October, 1988, vol 6: 265-272.

117. Walker CK, Kahn JG, Washington AE, Peterson HB, Sweet RL. Pelvic Inflammatory Disease: metaanalysis of antimicrobial regimen efficacy. J Infect Dis 1993; 168: 969-978.

114. Collins CG, Nix FC, Cerrha HT. Ruptured tubo-ovarian abscess. Am J Obstet Gynecol 1956; 72: 820.

115. McNeeley SG, Hendrix SL, Mazzoni MM, Konak DC, Ransom SB. Medically sound, cost effective treatment for pelvic inflammatory disease and tuboovarian abscess. Am J Obstet Gynecol 1998; 178: 1272-1278.

116. Gerzof SG, Robbins AH, Johnson WC, Birkett DH, Nabseth DC. Percutaneous catheter drainage of abdominal abscesses. N Engl J Med 1981; 305: 653-657.

117. Falk V. Treatment of acute nontuberculous salpingitis with antibiotics alone and in Combination with glucocorticoids. Acta Obstet Gynecol Scand 1965; 44: 3-18.

118. Sweet RL, Landers DV. Pelvic inflammatory disease in HIV-positive women. Lancet 1997; 349: 1265-1266.

119. Barbosa C, Macaat M, Brockman S, Sierra MF, Xia Z, Duerr A. Pelivic inflammatory disease and human immunodeficiency virus infection. Obstet Gynecol 1997; 89: 65-70.

120. Korn AP, Landers DV. Gynecologic disease in women infected with human immunodeficiency virus-1. Acquir Immuno Defic Syndr 1995; 9: 361-370.

121. Kamenga MC, De Cock KM, St. Louis ME, et al. The impact of human immunodeficiency virus infection on pelvic inflammatory disease: a case control study in Adidjan, Ivory Coast. Am J Obstet Gynecol 1995; 172: 919-925.

122. Cohen CR, Sinei S, Reilly M, et al. Effect of HIV-1 infection upon acute salpingitis: a laparoscopic study. J Infect Dis 1998; 178: 1352-1358.

123. Irwin KL, Moroman AC, O'Sullivan MJ, et al. Influence of human immunodeficiency virus infection on pelvic inflammatory disease. Obstet Gynecol 2000; 95: 525-534.

Chapter 30

Epididymitis and Prostatitis

Nitin S Walia

Epididymitis

Epididymitis is the clinical syndrome resulting from inflammation of the epididymis. Regardless of aetiology, the pain associated with both the acute and chronic condition can cause significant morbidity. As many as six million cases of epididymitis occur annually in the United States.[1] Researchers have reported that the incidence of epididymitis may range from one to four per 1000 men per year.[2]

Aetiopathogenesis

Until recently, this condition was considered idiopathic in at least 50 per cent of patients.[3] Indeed, even with the current state of research into the causes of epididymitis, specific infectious agents have been identified in only 80% of patients. Since the majority of epididymitis are attributed to an ascending infection from the urethra, prostate, and bladder (to the epididymis), the same considerations in the pathogenesis and clinical evaluation apply as to urethritis, cystitis, or prostatitis.

The sexually transmitted organisms N. gonorrhoeae and Chlamydia trachomatis have been clearly established to be the most common etiologic agents in sexually active heterosexual men under the age of 35 years (Table 1).[4] Although a history of sexual exposure can usually be elicited in men with Chlamydia trachomatis or N. gonorrhoeae, this exposure may be more than 30 days before the onset of symptoms. Watson found that one half of patients with epididymitis attributable to N. gonorrhoeae did not have urethral discharge.[5] In a small series of homosexual men under the age of 35 years with concomitant cystitis, the most common etiologic agent associated was E. coli.[6]

Coliform bacteria and pseudomonas (which are not

Table 1. Aetiology of Acute Epididymitis

1. Non-sexually transmitted pathogens:
   (a) Coliforms or *Pseudomonas aeruginosa*
   (b) *Mycobacterium tuberculosis*
   (c) *Miscellaneous*
   - *Schistosoma haematobium*
   - *Coccidioides immitis*
   - *Haemophilus inflenzae*
   - *Neisseria meningitidis*
   - *Brucella species*

2. Sexually Transmitted pathogens:
   (a) *Neisseria gonorrhoeae*
   (b) *Chlamydia trachomatis*
   (c) *Trichomonas vaginalis*

primarily sexually transmitted organisms) account for the aetiology of the majority of cases in men over 35 and in prepubertal boys. These patients often have either congenital or acquired structural urologic abnormalities. Reports implicating the following organisms in epididymitis have also been noted: *Trichomonas vaginalis, Schistosomia haematobium, Coccidioidis imitis, Haemophilus influenzae, Neisseria meningitidis,* and *Brucella* species.[7,8,9]

Before the availability of cultures for *Chlamydia trachomatis*, most epididymitis was thought to be caused by the reflux of sterile urine down the vas deferens while straining against a closed urethral sphincter. Voiding cystourethrography in the non-obstructed non-infected urinary tract has failed to show urethro-vasal reflux, even when straining caused intravesical pressure to exceed 70 cm H_2O pressure.[10] However, an inflamed or physically injured verumontanum may cause alterations in the vasal-urethral "valve", permitting bacterial entry into the vas.[11] Perhaps, straining may cause retrograde bacterial spread from an infected seminal vesicle into the vas and epididymis.

Diagnosis

Inflammation of the epididymis causes pain and swelling which is almost always unilateral and usually acute in onset. There may be a history of symptoms suggestive of urinary tract infection. Frequency, urgency and dysuria are common. On examination the scrotum on the affected side is erythematous, oedematous and tender.[12] The tail of the epididymis at the lower pole of the testis swells up first and later the swelling spreads to the head of the epididymis. The groove between the epididymis and testicle is maintained, unless concomitantly involved.

Gram stain, urine and urethral cultures will demonstrate the causative organism in the majority of cases of epididymitis. Serum micro immunofluorescence antibody titres to *Chlamydia trachomatis* will show a four-fold rise in titres when paired sera are tested, and they are more sensitive than culture. Cultures of epididymal aspirates should be used in only unusual circumstances like patients with indwelling Foley's catheter who have polymicrobial flora present in the urine, patients found at surgical exploration for torsion of testes to have epididymitis, and in patients who fail to respond or develop recurrent epididymitis with uncertain aetiologic agents.[13]

Conditions easily confused with epididymitis include torsion of the spermatic cord, testicular infarction, testicular tumour, torsion of the appendages, testicular abscess and traumatic rupture. None of these, except testicular abscess, will usually demonstrate pyuria or bacteriuria. Diagnosis can be confirmed by Doppler ultrasound,[14] or technetium 99 m radionuclide flow scan.[15] Colour coded Doppler ultrasonography has a sensitivity of 70% and specificity of 88%.[16] Since epididymitis is rare in prepubertal boys and torsion is relatively common, prompt surgical exploration is recommended to rule out torsion. Because torsion and epididymitis are common in men under the age of 35 years, Doppler or radionuclide scan should always be done to confirm the diagnosis of epididymitis.

In men or boys found to have coliform epididymitis, radiographic and cystoscopic evaluation should be performed to find a structural reason for the patient to have a urinary infection. Intravenous urography will disclose urologic abnormalities in 42 to 54 per cent of men with coliform epididymitis.[17] There may be prostatic calculi, benign prostatic hypertrophy, chronic bacterial prostatitis, neurogenic bladder or a history of recent urinary instrumentation. Intravenous urography in prepubertal children has shown colovesical fistula, reflux of urine into ejaculatory ducts, ectopic ejaculatory ducts, posterior urethral valves, bulbous urethral stricture, and neurogenic bladder.[18]

Complications of Acute Epididymitis

The most serious local complications are testicular infarction and abscess formation. Testicular infarction probably results from thrombosis of the spermatic vessels secondary to severe inflammation.[19] Infertility is a known complication of epididymitis as it may lead to bilateral occlusion of vas deferens. Decreased spermatogenesis, delayed sperm maturation and sperm antibodies may in addition cause infertility.[20]

Treatment

Therapy may be based on the clinical examination of urinary sediment and urethral swab. Treatment is directed to the specific etiologic organism suspected on initial evaluation and started immediately after collection of culture specimens. Therefore, when urethritis is associated with epididymitis, the treatment of choice is injection ceftriaxone 250 mg im followed by doxycycline 100 mg po bid or tetracycline 500 mg po qid for 10 days. When bacteriuria is present, treatment must be guided by sensitivity testing of the organisms. For epididymitis caused by enteric organisms, for patients allergic to cephalosporins and/or tetracyclines or for epididymitis in patients aged >35 years, either ofloxacin 300 mg orally bid or levofloxacin 500 mg orally once daily for 10 days is recommended.[21]

Supportive measures should include bed rest, scrotal elevation, and oral nonsteroidal anti-inflammatory drugs. In patients in whom the etiologic agent is a sexually transmitted pathogen, treatment is not complete without treatment of the sexual partner.

Chronic Epididymitis

Chronic epididymitis is defined as symptoms of discomfort and pain for a period of at least 3 months duration in the scrotum, testes and epididymis that is localized to 1 or each epididymis on clinical examination. It can interfere with the quality of life in upto one third of the cases.

Classification

Inflammatory Chronic Epididymitis

- Idiopathic
- Secondary
    Infective (Chlamydia)
    Post infective (after acute bacterial epididymitis)
    Tuberculosis
    Drug induced (amiodarone)

Obstructive Chronic Epididymitis

It is due to the congenital, acquired or iatrogenic obstruction of the epididymis or vas deferens.

Chronic Epididymalgia

It is characterized by pain or discomfort in the normal epididymis associated with no identifiable pathology.

In the management, it is mandatory to treat all the cases of chronic epididymitis with a course of antibiotics. Epididymectomy should be considered if there is no resolution after 4-6 weeks of conservative management. In cases of chronic tuberculous epididymitis, a course of anti-tuberculous therapy should be given but is less effective. If the lesions do not revolve by 2 months, epididymectomy is advised.

Prostatitis

Prostatitis is frequently regarded as an obscure ill-understood condition. This is due to a number of factors: the organ is deeply placed and poorly accessible to clinical examination, the aetiology is frequently unclear, the criteria for diagnosis are not accepted universally, investigation is difficult and therapy may be time-consuming and unsatisfactory.[23] This is unfortunate because inflammation of the prostate is common, making up a significant proportion of urologic practice.[24] Research in recent years has demonstrated that prostatitis is not one disease; rather it occurs in several distinct forms or syndromes. These prostatitis syndromes have distinctly different causes, manifestations and sequelae.[25] Moreover, proper clinical management and therapeutic outlook vary considerably among these different forms.

Anatomy

The prostate consists of acini draining into ducts, which in turn drain into the prostatic urethra and these are set in a stroma of collagen and muscle tissue. The gland can be divided into a small central zone around the prostatic urethra, and a larger peripheral zone forming 75% of the parenchyma of the gland. An important difference between the zones is that the ducts draining the central zone enter the prostatic urethra at an acute angle compared with the ducts draining the peripheral zone. Urine can thus, enter the peripheral zones more readily than the central zone ducts. Furthermore, contraction of the internal sphincter muscle will tend to compress the ducts of the central zone rather than those of the peripheral zone. During ejaculation, when the internal sphincter muscle is contracted, the intraurethral pressure rises dramatically and semen will enter the peripheral zone ducts more easily than the central zone ducts. (Fig. 1). Thus, the inflammatory process mainly affects the peripheral zone while the central zone around the urethra is relatively unaffected.[26,27]

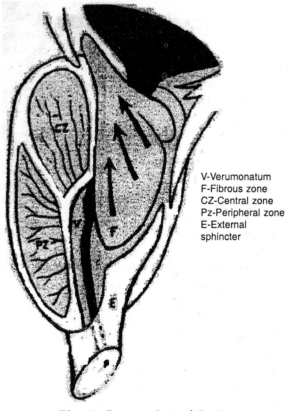

V-Verumonatum
F-Fibrous zone
CZ-Central zone
Pz-Peripheral zone
E-External sphincter

Fig. 1   Prostate Sagittal Section

Pathogenesis

The possible routes of infection in prostate include:

    (a) Ascending urethral infection
    (b) Reflux of infected urine into prostatic ducts that empty into the prostatic urethra
    (c) Invasion by rectal bacteria through direct extension or by lymphatic spread
    (d) Haematogenous spread

Kirby et al showed direct evidence of reflux into the prostate.[28] Carbon particles instilled into the bladder via a catheter were later found in the prostatic ducts of seven of the ten men in whom the experiment was carried out. This would also explain the observation that the organisms found in bacterial prostatitis do not differ significantly in type and prevalence from those causing other urinary tract infections.[29]

The constituents of the refluxing urine may contribute towards the formation of prostatic stones in some cases by precipitation of minerals upon existing corpora amylacea.

In addition, the refluxing urine by causing a chemical prostatitis may initiate and perpetuate the chronic inflammatory process in abacterial prostatitis and prostatodynia.[30,31] Rapid pressure within the prostatic urethra from failure of the external sphincter to relax completely during urination may be the cause of the reflux. Both indwelling urethral catheter and condom drainage system can lead to bacterial infection of the prostate because they are frequently associated with urethral colonization with pathogenic bacteria and ascending urinary tract infection. It is also commonly known that bacterial prostatitis can develop in men who have untreated infected urine immediately after transurethral prostatic resection.[32]

The prostate may be secondarily involved from another primary infection. Lymphatic drainage from nearby sources of infection such as the bladder, urethra or the rectum may influence inflammation of the prostate. There are few reports of the involvement of the prostate with proctocolitis especially in homosexual males.[33] Much less commonly, infection may be haematogenous, consequent upon septicemia or pyaemia; prostatitis is then a complication of another acute illness.[34]

Human immunodeficiency virus has given a new dimension to the frequency and spectrum of opportunistic infections. The prevalence of bacterial prostatitis among HIV-infected patients was reported to increase from 3% in asymptomatic carriers to 14% in patients with the acquired immunodeficiency syndrome.[35] Both B and T-cell dysfunction and local immunodeficiency of prostatic fluid can explain the abnormal susceptibility of patients to infections and favour prostatic abscess formation.[36]

Evaluation of Prostatitis

Detailed history is elicited paying particular attention to the symptoms. A history of previous urinary tract infections or genital symptoms is particularly helpful. Genital examination is performed to detect urethral discharge, to evaluate the scrotal contents and to elicit perineal tenderness. A rectal examination is performed in conjunction with the collection of specimens for laboratory evaluation. The specimen are collected sequentially in sterile containers to perform microbiologic studies.[29,37]

    (a) Collect the first 10-15 ml (VB1: voided bladder 1) of urine for culture and centrifuge 7 to 8 ml of urine to examine the sediment for pyuria.
    (b) Collect midstream urine (VB2) for culture and centrifuge 7 to 8 ml of urine to examine the specimen for pyuria.
    (c) Examine the prostate and then massage (except in acute prostatitis) the prostate in an attempt to express prostatic secretions for direct microscopy to evaluate for polymorphonuclear leukocytes, motile trichomonas and culture. More than 10 polymorphonuclear leukocytes per HPF is considered abnormal. Clumping of polymorphonuclear cells and a reduction in the number of lecithin bodies also indicate inflammation of the prostate. An additional finding is the presence of macrophages containing fat droplets, also called oval fat bodies.[38]
    (d) Collect the next 10-15 ml of urine for culture and centrifuge 10-15 ml of urine to examine for pyuria.

For the culture, the laboratory should be requested to inoculate media that will detect classical urinary tract pathogens and to use a 0.1 ml inoculum as well as the standard 0.001ml inoculum. The latter requirement facilitates the detection and quantification of specimens in low numbers. The specimens must be processed as soon as possible because prostatic fluid contains antibacterial substances that may inhibit growth.[39]

In conjunction with the urine specimens, some investigators prefer to have the patient provide an ejaculate rather than obtaining expressed prostatic secretions.[40] Bacterial concentrations 10 times higher in the post massage urine or prostatic secretions than in the midstream urine (bladder bacteriuria) provides proof that the prostate is infected.[24,41] If high numbers of organisms are present in the midstream urine (bladder bacteriuria) localization cannot be done.

If acute bacterial prostatitis is a possibility, blood culture specimen is obtained and the midstream urine sample alone is adequate. It is Gram stained as well as cultured. Urethroscopy or prostate biopsy is not by itself useful in the evaluation of prostatitis.[42,43]

Classification[44,45]

Based on localization studies Drach, Meares, Fair and Stamey proposed a classification separating prostatitis into four groups: Acute bacterial prostatitis (ABP), chronic bacterial prostatitis (CBP), chronic abacterial prostatitis (CAP) and prostatodynia (Pd) (Table 2).[44] The patients are categorized according to the cytological and microbiological findings in both the urine and expressed prostatic secretions.[24] According to this classification, only acute and chronic prostatitis are definitely caused by bacterial infection of the prostate as clearly demonstrated by positive urine and expressed prostatic secretion (EPS) cultures for pathogenic bacteria. The microscopic examination of the expressed prostatic secretions is however, similar in acute and chronic bacterial prostatitis as well as in non-bacterial prostatitis, showing evidence of inflammation by the presence of numerous white blood cells and lipid laden macrophages.[46]

Table 2. Classification of Prostatitis

Type	Aetiology	Evidence of Inflammation (EPS)	Culture positive (EPS)	Culture positive (bladder)	Common etiologic bacteria	Rectal Examination (prostate)
Acute Prostatitis	Bacterial	+	+	+★	Enterobacteriaceae	Abnormal
Chronic Prostatitis	Bacterial	+	+	+#	Enterobacteriaceae	Normal
Chronic Prostatitis	Bacterial	+	0	0	?	Normal
Prostatodynia		0	0	0	0	Normal

★ ABP is nearly always accompanied by a bladder infection.
characterized by recurrent bacteriuria, at varying intervals up to several months, after stopping antimicrobial therapy.

Both the microscopic examination of the expressed prostatic secretions as well as the bacterial localization cultures, are negative in prostatodynia.[47] Whereas acute and chronic bacterial prostatitis are well defined by objective evidence and specific treatment is available in the majority of patients, the last two entities are less well understood and no specific treatment is available.[48,49] The recent NIH classification of prostatitis syndrome is given in Table 3.[50]

Acute Bacterial Prostatitis

ABP is a well-established clinical entity and probably the easiest to diagnose, as well as to treat, among the different clinical entities in prostatitis. It is dramatic in its manifestations and presents the signs and symptoms of an acute septic process.[51] This entity is typified by

Table 3. NIH Classification of Prostatitis Syndromes

Category
I   Acute bacterial prostatitis
II Chronic bacterial prostatitis (CBP)
III Chronic pelvic pain syndrome (CPPS)
IIIA CPPS, inflammatory★ (formerly chronic non-bacterial prostatitis)
IIIB CPPS, non - inflammatory~ (formerly prostatodynia)
IV Asymptomatic inflammatory prostatitis★

★ Leucocytes in expressed prostatic secretions (EPS), postprostatic massage urine [voided bladder -3 (VB-3)], or semen.
~ Leucocytes not found in EPS, VB-3 or semen.
Adopted from GA Luzzi[50]

the sudden onset of high fever up to 40°C, chills, marked malaise and sometimes myalgia or arthralgia.[52]

Irritative micturition symptoms of frequency, urgency and dysuria soon develop and there may appear an associated urethral discharge. Difficulty in micturition or acute retention of urine may occur. There is usually a dull aching pain in the perineum, rectum or sacrococcygeal region.[53]

Rectal examination reveals a swollen, very tender and warm prostate; sometimes the prostate feels indurated with scattered soft areas. Prostatic massage will produce a thick purulent discharge full of white blood cells and oval fat bodies, which will grow large numbers of pathogens on culture. However, prostatic massage is both painful and dangerous to the patient as it may induce bacteremia in the acute stages of the disease. It is also unnecessary, as acute bacterial prostatitis is usually associated with a bladder infection by the same organism that is in the prostate, allowing for identification of the pathogen by culture of the voided urine, the urine obtained by suprapubic needle aspiration of the bladder, or the urethral discharge whenever present.[46]

The organisms causing acute bacterial prostatitis are usually those commonly found in urinary tract infections including the Gram-negative enteric bacteria or *Pseudomonas aeruginosa* as well as Gram-positive staphylococci and streptococci. Occasionally salmonella and anaerobic bacteria such as *Bacteroides fragilis* or *Clostridium perfringens* can also cause prostatitis.[54]

Therapy

At the beginning, the patient will require bed rest, adequate hydration, antipyretics, analgesics or spasmolytic drugs to alleviate the perineal or rectal pain and stool softeners. Urethral instrumentation should be avoided.[55] Parenteral broad-spectrum antibiotics should be instituted immediately after collection of urine and blood specimens for culture. A combination of aminoglycoside and ß- lactam antibiotic is the first choice. However, fluoroquinolones or third generation cephalosporins are alternative single drug therapies.[56,57] The intense diffuse inflammation enhances the passage of antimicrobial agents from plasma into the prostatic ducts and acini and the patient usually responds dramatically to therapy.

Acute bacterial prostatitis is a self- limiting disease and only rarely it will develop into a chronic prostatic infection. Some patients may continue to experience a certain degree of irritative micturition symptoms inspite of the bacteriological cure of the acute inflammatory process. Rectal examination may still reveal a hard prostate and several months may pass before the prostate returns to a normal consistency.

Prostatic abscess has become increasingly rare since the advent of effective antibacterial therapy. It should be suspected if a patient of acute bacterial prostatitis or urinary tract infection develops a spiking fever and fluctuation of the prostate inspite of adequate antibacterial therapy. These are caused mainly by *E. coli*. Sometimes metastatic abscess to the prostate may develop from a septic focus elsewhere and is caused mainly by Gram-positive organisms such as *Staphylococcus aureus*.[58] In rare instances, anaerobic bacteria or *Blastomyces dermatitidis* may cause an acute prostatic abscess.[59] Transrectal ultrasound and computerized tomography are helpful in early detection of prostatic abscess.[60,61] The main and definite treatment of an acute prostatic abscess is adequate surgical drainage by transurethral unroofing or perineal incision as soon as possible after adequate antimicrobial coverage.

Chronic Bacterial Prostatitis

The clinical picture of chronic bacterial prostatitis is quite variable and is typified by recurrent episodes of irritative voiding symptoms such as frequency, urgency and dysuria, associated occasionally with perineal discomfort, low back pain, myalgia or arthralgia and complicated sometimes by epididymitis.[62] Chills and fever are unusual, although post-ejaculatory pain and haemospermia occasionally occur. No findings on physical examination, rectal examination of the prostate, cystoscopy or urography are specifically diagnostic of chronic bacterial prostatitis. However, it is characterized by two basic features (a) recurrent urinary tract infections and (b) persistence of pathogenic bacteria in the prostatic fluid.[63] These are mainly Gram negative enterobacteria (*E. coli*, Proteus or Klebsiella) or *Pseudomonas aeruginosa* and are found only in small numbers in the prostate. Sterilization of urine generally affords relief of symptoms; however, when the patient stops taking the antibiotics the prostatic pathogen eventually reinfects the urine and symptoms return.[64]

Therapy

Chronic bacterial prostatitis poses a real therapeutic challenge to the treating physician. Neither short term nor long-term therapy with antibacterial drugs is able to cure the patients and this happens despite the pathogens being highly sensitive to the antibacterials and remains so at the end of the treatment. Stamey et al revealed that most of these drugs are unable to cross the electrically charged lipid membrane of the prostatic epithelium to reach therapeutic levels within the prostatic acini.[65]

Several antimicrobial agents are said to have some efficacy in the treatment of CBP. Trimethoprim-sulphamethoxazole (TMP-SMX) seemed promising but even long-term (4-16 weeks) therapy in full dosage effected a cure in only 33-55% of cases.[64,66] Other agents with reported efficacy include carbenicillin, erythromycin, minocycline, doxycycline and cephalexin. Newer quinolone derivatives like ciprofloxacin reach high concentrations in the prostatic secretions and have proved effective in prospective comparative studies. Recommended dosage is ciprofloxacin 500mg orally bid for 30 days, or norfloxacin 400mg orally bid for 30 days.[67,68]

Patients not cured by medical therapy can usually be managed satisfactorily by use of continuous suppressive therapy using low dose medication. Preferred regimens include TMP-SMX (one single-strength tablet daily), or nitrofurantoin 100 mg once or twice daily. Suppressive therapy generally controls symptoms and prevents bacteriuria. Even prolonged treatment however, fails to clear the pathogen from the prostate, and discontinuation of the medication eventually leads to recurrent symptoms and bacteriuria.[69]

Complete excision of the prostate, seminal vesicles and ampulla of vas deferens should uniformly cure all patients of refractory chronic bacterial prostatitis; however, the potential complications and consequences of this radical surgery seldom make this a reasonable choice unless associated pathologic conditions like prostatic calculi, benign prostatic hyperplasia, or adenocarcinoma of the prostate are also present.[70]

Non-Bacterial Prostatitis

Non-bacterial prostatitis (syn. abacterial prostatitis, prostatosis), the most common type of prostatitis syndrome, is an inflammatory condition of unknown cause. The findings of Schaeffer and co-workers suggest that the incidence of non-bacterial prostatitis exceed that of bacterial prostatitis by eight-fold.[71]

Patients with non-bacterial prostatitis have a large variety of symptoms referable to the genitalia (pain along the penis and in the testicles and scrotum, painful ejaculation), the musculoskeletal system (low back pain, perineal pain or discomfort, rectal pain, pain along the inner aspect of the thighs), the lower urinary tract (irritative: frequency, urgency, burning on micturition, suprapubic discomfort; or obstructive: hesitancy, decreased urinary stream) or have psychosexual symptoms (decreased libido, impotence). Physical examination is usually unremarkable, and the prostate is normal on rectal examination.[72]

Although many clinical features of chronic bacterial prostatitis and non-bacterial prostatitis are similar, one important difference bears emphasis; the patient with non-bacterial prostatitis has no history of documented urinary tract infection or positive cultures localizing a causative agent to the prostate. Like patients with chronic bacterial prostatitis, however, patients with non-bacterial prostatitis have excessive number of leukocytes and fat laden macrophages in their prostatic fluids.[73]

The aetiology of non-bacterial prostatitis is unclear. Extensive microbiologic studies by different investigators have excluded *Neisseria gonorrhoeae*, *Trichomonas vaginalis*, *Gardnerella vaginalis* and *Mycoplasma genitalium* as playing any role in the aetiology.[74] Other studies evaluated potential organisms like *Chlamydia trachomatis*, *Ureaplasma urealyticum* in addition to a host of fungi, viruses and anaerobic bacteria in men with persistent chronic non-bacterial prostatitis with no conclusive results.[75-77] Some workers have proposed prostaglandins, autoimmunity, neuromuscular dysfunction and psychological abnormalities as etiological factors.[78] It thus appears either that non- bacterial prostatitis is an infectious disease caused by yet unidentified pathogens or is a non-infectious inflammation of the prostate.

Therapy

In view of the fact that the cause of NBP is unknown, no specific therapy for this condition is available. The patient should be reassured, however, that in spite of unpleasant symptoms that would continue for an indefinite period, no serious condition is present and no complications are expected in the future, primarily no impairment of sexual ability and fertility.

A clinical trial of tetracycline or erythromycin 500mg qid orally for 14 days is indicated in symptomatic patients. Unless the clinical response is definitely favourable, additional treatment using antimicrobial agents is unwarranted.[79]

The main treatment plan should be to control symptoms. Normal sexual activity is encouraged and dietary restrictions imposed only if spicy foods or alcoholic beverages appear to cause or aggravate the symptoms. General relaxant measures such as hot Sitz baths and spasmolytics are indicated to relieve symptoms. Prostatic massage is probably therapeutic only in men who have congested prostates related to infrequent sexual activity. Pain and discomfort often respond to short courses of anti-inflammatory agents; irritative voiding dysfunction usually responds to the use of anticholinergics. The efficacy of oral zinc preparations and megavitamins remain unproved.[79]

Prostatodynia

In their classification of prostatitis, Drach and his associates applied the term 'Prostatodynia' to men in whom there were symptoms of urinary irritation, usually some frequency, mild dysuria, and perineal, penile, suprapubic, scrotal or urethral pain not necessarily related to voiding.[44] There may be variable signs of obstructive voiding dysfunction i.e. hesitancy, a weakened stream or an interrupted urinary flow. In addition to these irritative or obstructive symptoms, there is frequently impotence and painful ejaculation. Such cases require a full urological evaluation, both of the prostate and the outflow tract.

Typically, genitourinary examination reveals no specific abnormality. Bacterial culture is negative and microscopy of prostatic fluids is normal.[48]

These patients are difficult to treat and in most, there is a neurotic overlay of variable degree. This is easy to understand, as most would have undergone a multiplicity of antibiotic courses, invasive investigations and perhaps a transurethral resection during the course of their illness. Before concluding that the symptoms are entirely psychological, consideration should be given to the findings of Segure et al who observed that involuntary contractions of the pelvic floor might account for the pain and discomfort and the obstructive urinary symptoms.[78]

When there is functional disturbance in urinary flow, improvement may be obtained with alpha-adrenergic blocking agents in a dose sufficient to allow relaxation of the autonomic component of external sphincter without producing effects on the cardiovascular system.[80] Rectal diathermy and physiotherapy by neuro-muscular re-education of the muscles of the pelvic floor may be useful in some patients.[81]

Granulomatous Prostatitis

Granulomatous prostatitis is a characteristic reaction of the prostate to a variety of insults. On rectal examination, the prostate appears indurated and nodular. The histopathology shows a granulomatous reaction of lipid-laden histiocytes, plasma cells and scattered giant cells. A prominent eosinophilic infiltrate is apparent in some cases.[82]

A number of specific infections cause granulomatous reactions. Tuberculous prostatitis is usually secondary to tuberculosis elsewhere in the genital tract. Similarly, mycotic prostatitis is secondary to systemic involvement. Rare causes include actinomycosis, candidiasis and syphilis.[83] Recent reports suggest that HIV infection may be associated with an increased risk of granulomatous prostatitis and that the aetiology may include *Mycobacterium avium complex*. Rarely, granulomatous prostatitis has been associated with other rheumatoid disorders, particularly Wegener's granulomatosis.[84]

The differentiation from other causes of a hard, nodular prostate especially prostatic carcinoma is most important. Therapy is generally the specific treatment of the primary disease.

Conclusion

Several distinct types of prostatitis or prostatitis syndromes are now recognized. Accurate diagnosis is important to differentiate and identify the specific therapy for them. In contrast, urologic procedures and antimicrobials need to be judiciously used in the larger number of men suffering from chronic abacterial prostatitis. Reassurance and general supportive measures will often alleviate the condition remarkably in many patients.

References

1. Sufrin G. Acute epididymitis. Sex Transm Dis 1981; 8: 132: 29.
2. Drotman DP. Epidemiology and treatment of epididymitis. Rev Infect Dis 1982; 4: S 788-792.
3. Wolin LH. On the aetiology of epididymitis. J Urol 1971; 105: 531-533.
4. Berger RE, Alexander ER, Harnisch JP, et al: Aetiology, manifestations and therapy of acute epididymitis: prospective study of 50 cases. J Urol 1979; 121: 750-754.
5. Watson RA. Gonorrhoea and acute epididymitis. Milit Med 1979; 144:785-787.
6. Kessler DK, Berger RE, Holmes KK. Epididymitis in heterosexual and homosexual men. In: 5th meeting of

International Society of STD research; 1983 August; Seattle, Washington.

7. Fisher I, Morton RS. Epididymitis due to *Trichomonas vaginalis*.Br J Vener Dis 1969; 45: 252-253.

8. Gottesman JE. Coccidioidomycosis of prostate and epididymis with urethrocutaneous fistula. Urology 1974; 4:311.

9. Thomas D, Simpson K, Ostojich H. Bacteremic epididymo-orchitis due to *H. influenzae* type B. Br J Urol 1981; 126: 832.

10. Kohler PF. An inquiry into the aetiology of acute epididymitis. J Urol 1962; 87: 918.

11. Furness G, Kamat MH, Kaminski Z, Seebode JJ. The relationship of epididymitis to gonorrhoea. Invest Urol 1974; 11: 312-314.

12. Berger RE. Acute epididymitis. In: Holmes KK, Mardh PA, Sparling et al, Ed. Sexually Transmitted diseases. 3rd eds. New York Mc Graw Hill; 1999. p. 847-858.

13. Berger RE, Holmes KK, Mayo ME, et al. The clinical use of epididymal aspiration cultures in the management of selected patients with acute epididymitis. J Urol 1980; 124: 60-61.

14. Perri AJ, Slachta GA, Feldman AE, et al. The Doppler stethoscope and the diagnosis of the acute scrotum. J Urol 1976: 116: 598: 55.

15. Abu Sleiman R, Ho JE, Gregory JC. Scrotal scanning: Present value and limits of interpretation. Urology 1979; 13: 326-330.

16. Wilbert DM, Schaerfe CW, Stern WD, et al. Evaluation of the acute scrotum by colour-coded doppler ultrasonography. J Urol 1993; 149: 1475-1477.

17. Gislason T, Noronha RF, Gregory JG. Acute epididymitis in boys: a 5-year retrospective study. J Urol 1980; 124: 533-534.

18. Bullock KN, Hunt JM. The intravenous urogram in acute epididymo-orchitis. Br J Urol 1981; 53: 47-49.

19. Eisner DJ, Goldman SM, Petronis J, Millmond SH. Bilateral testicular infarction caused by epididymitis. Am J Roentgenol 1991; 157: 517-519.

20. Caldamone AA, Cockett AT. Review: There is a vast amount of evidence linking the presence of genitourinary, infertility and genitourinary infection. Urology 1978; 12: 304-312.

21. Centre for disease control and prevention. Sexually transmitted diseases. Treatment guidelines. MMWR. 2002: 51 (No: RR-6).

22. Nickel JC, Siemens DR, Nickel KR, Downey. The patients with chronic epididymitis: characterization of an enigmatic syndrome. J Urol 2002: 167; 1701-1704.

23. Thin RN. The diagnosis of prostatitis: A review. Genitourin Med 1991; 67: 279-283.

24. Krieger JN, McGonagle LA. Diagnostic considerations and interpretation of microbiological findings for evaluation of chronic prostatitis. J Clin Microbiol 1989; 27: 2240-2244.

25. Simmons PD, Thin RN. A method for recognizing non-bacterial prostatitis: Preliminary observations. Br J Venereal Dis 1983; 59: 306-310.

26. Blacklock NJ. The Prostate: Surgical Anatomy. In:

27. Chisholm G D, Fair W R, eds. Scientific Foundation of Urology. 3rd ed. London: Hienemann; 1990. p. 340-350.

27. Blacklock NJ. Anatomical factors in prostatitis. Br J Urol 1974; 46: 47-54.

28. Kirby RS, Lowe D, Bultitude MI, Shuttleworth KE. Intra-prostatic urinary reflux; an aetiological factor in abacterial prostatitis. Br J Urol 1982; 54: 729-731.

29. Stamey TA, Meares EM. Bacteriologic localization patterns in bacterial prostatitis and urethritis. Invest Urol 1968; 5: 492-518.

30. Ramirez CT, Reiz JA, Gomez AZ, et al: A crystallographic study of prostatic calculi. J Urol 1980; 124: 840-848.

31. Ekyn S, Bultitude MI, Mayo ME, et al. Prostatic calculi as a source of recurrent bacteriuria in the male. Br J Urol 1974; 46: 527-532.

32. Landes RR, French TN. Bacterial prostatitis: incidence in the obstructive prostate. J Urol 1973; 110: 427-428.

33. Berger RE, Alexander ER, Harnisch JP, et al. Aetiology, manifestations and therapy of acute epididymitis: prospective study of 50 cases. J Urol 1979; 121: 750-754.

34. Meares EM Jr. Prostatitis syndromes: new perspectives about old woes. J Urol 1980; 123: 141-147.

35. Lepont C, Rousseau F, Perronne C, et al. Bacterial prostatitis in patients infected with HIV. J Urol 1989; 141: 334-347.

36. Pahwa SG, Quilop MT, Lange M, Pahwa RN, Grieco MH. Defective B-lymphocyte function in homosexual men in relation to the acquired immuno deficiency syndrome. Ann Intern Med 1984; 101: 757-763.

37. Stames TA. Prostatitis. J R Soc Med 1981; 74: 22-40.

38. Oates JK. Prostatitis. Br J Hosp Med 1969; 2: 556-561.

39. Daniels GF, Grayhack JT. Physiology of prostatic secretions. In: Chisholm GD, Fair WR, eds. Scientific foundations of urology. 3rd ed. London: Heinemann; 1990. p. 351-358.

40. Mobley DF. Semen cultures in the diagnosis of bacterial prostatitis. J Urol 1975; 114: 83-85.

41. Krieger J N. Prostatitis syndromes: pathophysiology, differential diagnosis and treatment. Sex Trans Dis 1984; 11: 100.

42. Krieger J N, Hooton TM, Brus PJ. Evaluation of chronic urethritis: defining the role for endoscopic procedures. Arch Intern Med 1988; 148: 703-707.

43. Kohnen D W, Drach G W. Patterns of Inflammation in prostatic hyperplasia: A histologic and bacteriologic study. J Urol 1979; 121: 755.

44. Drach G W, Fair W R, Meares E M, Stamey T A. Classification of benign diseases associated with prostatic pain: prostatitis or prostatodynia? J Urol 1978; 120: 266.

45. Stamey TA. Pathogenesis and treatment of urinary tract infections. Baltimore: Williams and Wilkins. 1980.

46. Thin RN, Simmons PD. Chronic bacterial and non-bacterial prostatitis. Br J Urol 1983; 55: 513-518.

47. Anderson RU, Weller C. Prostatic secretion leukocyte studies in non-bacterial prostatitis (prostatosis). J Urol 1979; 121: 292-294.

48. Meares EM Jr. Prostatodynia: clinical findings and rationale for treatment. In: Weidner W, Brunner H, Krause W,

Rothauge CF eds. Therapy of prostatitis. San Francisco: W. Zuckschwerdt Verlag; 1986. p 207.

49. Meares EM Jr, Barbalias GA. Prostatitis: bacterial, non-bacterial and prostatodynia. Semin Urol 1983; 1: 146-154.

50. Luzzi GA. Chronic prostatitis and chronic pelvic pain in men: aetiology, diagnosis and management. JEADV 2002; 16: 253-256.

51. Meares EM Jr. Acute and chronic prostatitis: diagnosis and treatment. Infect Dis Clin North Am 1987; 1: 855-872.

52. Bowie WR. Men with urethritis and urologic complications of STD's. Med Clin North Am 1990; 74: 1551-1557.

53. Ireton RC, Berger RE. Prostatitis and Epididymitis. Urol Clin North Am 1984; 11: 83-94.

54. Drach GW. Trimethoprim-sulfamethoxazole therapy of chronic bacterial prostatitis. J Urol. 1974;111:637–639.

55. Krieger JN. Prostatitis, epididymitis and orchitis. Mandell GL, Bennett JE, Dolin R, eds. In: Mandell, Douglas and Bennet's Principles and practice of infectious diseases. 4th ed. New York: Churchill Livingstone; 1995. p. 1098.

56. Lipsky BA. Urinary tract infections in men. Epidemiology, pathophysiology, diagnosis and treatment. Ann Intern Med 1989; 110: 138-150.

57. Krieger JN. Prostatitis syndromes: pathophysiology, differential diagnosis and treatment. Sex Trans Dis 1984; 11: 100.

58. Weinberger M, Cytron S, Servadioc, et al. Prostatic abscess in the antibiotic era. Rev Infect Dis 1988; 10: 239-249.

59. Bergner DM, Kraus SD, Duck GB, Lewis R. Systemic blastomycosis presenting with acute prostatic abscess. Urol 1981; 126: 132-133.

60. Cyton S. Value of transrectal ultrasonography for diagnosis and treatment of prostatic abscess. Urol 1988; 32: 454.

61. Chia JK, Longfield RN, Cook DH, Flax BL. Computed axial tomography in the early diagnosis of prostatic abscess. Am J Med 1986; 81: 942-944.

62. Smart CJ, Jenkins JD, Lloyd RS. The painful prostate. Br J Urol 1976; 47: 861-869.

63. Pfau A. Prostatitis: A continuing enigma. Urol Clin North Am 1986; 695-715.

64. Pfau A, Sacks T. Chronic bacterial prostatitis: new therapeutic aspects. Br J Urol 1976; 48: 245-253.

65. Stamey TA, Meares EM Jr, Winningham DG. Chronic bacterial prostatitis and the diffusion of drugs into prostatic fluid. J Urol 1970; 103: 187-194.

66. Mc Gure ES, Lytton B. Bacterial prostatitis: treatment with trimethoprim-sulphamethoxazole. Urol 1976; 7: 499-500.

67. Baert L, Leonard A. Chronic bacterial prostatitis: 10 years of experience with local antibiotics. J Urol 1988; 140: 755-757.

68. Baert L. Re: a re-appraisal of treatment in chronic bacterial prostatitis. J Urol 1980; 123: 606-607.

69. Ristuccia AM, Cunha BA. Current concepts in antimicrobial therapy of prostatitis. Urol 1982; 20: 338.

70. Smart CJ, Jenkins JD. The role of transurethral prostatectomy in chronic prostatitis. Br J Urol 1973; 45: 654-662.

71. Schaeffer AJ, Wendel EF, Dunn JK Grayhack JT. Prevalence and significance of prostatic inflammation. J Urol 1981;125: 215-219.

72. Marmar JL, Katz S, Prais DE, et al. A protocol for evaluation of prostatitis. Urol 1980; 16: 261-265.

73. Miller HC. Stress prostatitis. Urology 1988; 32: 507-510.

74. Weidner W, Brunner H, Krause W. Quantitative culture of *Ureaplasma urealyticum* in-patients with chronic prostatitis or prostatosis. J Urol 1980; 124: 622-625.

75. Mardh PA, Colleen S. Search for uro-genital tract infections in patients with symptoms of prostatitis. Studies on aerobic and strictly anaerobic bacteria, mycoplasmas, fungi, trichomonads and viruses. Scand J Urol Nephrol 1975; 9: 8-16.

76. Bruce AW. The role of chlamydia in genitourinary disease. J Urol 1989; 126: 625-629.

77. Poletti F, Medici MC, Alinovi A, et al. Isolation of *Chlamydia trachomatis* from the prostatic cells in patients affected by nonacute bacterial prostatitis. J Urol 1985; 134: 691-693.

78. Segura JW, Opitz JL, Greene LF. Prostatosis, prostatitis or pelvic floor tension myalgia. J Urol 1979; 122: 168-171.

79. Meares EM Jr. Prostatitis. Med Clin North Am 1991: 405-424.

80. Barbalias GA, Meares EM Jr, Sant GR. Prostatodynia: Clinical and urodynamic characteristics. J Urol 1983; 130: 514-517.

81. Osborn DE, George NJ, Rao PN, et al. Prostatodynia-physiological characteristics and rational management with muscle relaxants. Br J Urol 1981; 53: 621-623.

82. Scmidt JD. Non-specific granulomatous prostatitis. Classification, reviews and report of cases. J Urol 1965; 607-615.

83. Towfighi J, Sadeghee S, Wheeler JE, et al. Granulomatous prostatitis with emphasis on the eosinophilic variety. Am J Clin Path 1972; 58: 630-641.

84. Murty GE, Powell PH. Wegener's granulomatosis presenting as prostatitis. Br J Urol 1991; 67: 107-108.

Chapter 31

Sexually Transmitted Diseases Associated Arthritis

Ashok Kumar

Introduction

STD associated arthritis is part of the broad category of 'Infection related arthritis'. The latter can be divided into 3 categories[1]:

1. Septic or invasive arthritis
2. Para-infectious arthritis
3. Post-infectious arthritis or 'Reactive' arthritis (Re A)

By definition, organisms can be demonstrated in the joint in the first category only. In the second category, organisms may be demonstrable in the blood or some extra-articular focus but not in the joint, *concurrently* with the arthritis. In reactive arthritis, on the other hand, the infective episode is supposed to have occurred in the *recent* past at a *remote* site. Organisms can no longer be isolated from the joint fluid or synovium. However, it is possible to demonstrate evidence of recent infection in most instances using serological tests.

The following arthritides may be associated with STD:

1. Reactive arthritis (Reiter's syndrome)
2. Gonococcal arthritis
3. Syphilitic arthritis
4. HIV-associated arthritis
5. HBV and HCV arthritis
6. LGV and arthritis

1. Sexually Acquired Reactive Arthritis (SARA)

Some recent evidence suggests that infectious particles or material derived from the pathogens may be present in the affected joint even in patients with reactive arthritis.[2] This has challenged the very concept of reactive arthritis. This is discussed further under aetiopathogenesis. In spite of the controversy raised by these new findings, the entity of reactive arthritis still exists. ReA can be considered both as an infection related arthritis and as a member of the seronegative spondyloarthropathies.

ReA is divided into 2 types based on the mode of acquiring the infection: sexually acquired or 'SARA' and enteric or 'enterically acquired reactive arthritis'. The latter is outside the scope of this chapter.

Nomenclature

Reactive arthritis is the new name for the old term Reiter's syndrome. The reasons in favour of this change in terminology are as follows[3]:

1. Hans Reiter was not the first to describe the syndrome,
2. The classical triad of arthritis, conjunctivitis and urethritis is not seen in the majority of patients.

Aetiopathogenesis

The Pathogens

The pathogens associated with SARA include Chlamydia and Ureaplasma. It appears that the bacteria or their products reach the synovium and then incite a specific immune response. There is definite evidence that live Chlamydia persists in the joint.[4-6] Chlamydia has also been demonstrated in the joint by PCR in 21% of patients with rheumatoid arthritis (RA) and 14% of patients with osteoarthritis (OA). The organisms are presumably transported to the joint by monocytes.

There is no study from India, focussing on the role of Chlamydia in SARA. However, two studies have looked at the bacterial triggers involved in the pathogenesis of sporadic reactive arthritis. Aggarwal et al[7] found antibodies to *Chlamydia trachomatis* in 2 out of 14 patients and none in the controls. Similarly, Joseph et al[8] did not find any sample positive for *Chlamydia trachomatis* antigen in the synovial fluid of 11 patients with reactive arthritis and 20 patients with undifferentiated arthritis. There is clearly a need to perform studies on microbiology of SARA.

Role of HLA B27

While the HLA B27 association in ankylosing spondylitis is very strong (~90%), it is much lower in the case of ReA. The frequency of B27 is only about 50% in Chlamydia induced ReA. There are 15 different subtypes or variants of HLA B27 that have been given the designations B*2701 to B*2715. The most widespread subtype in the world is B*2705. In northern India, the predominant subtypes are B*2705 (50%) and B*2704 (40%).[9]

Most of the current data suggest that HLA B27 functions as an antigen presenting molecule of a yet-unknown arthritogenic peptide. It is now known that a heterozygous state for the B27 gene is sufficient for the disease to develop. The susceptibility to disease is predominantly genetically determined (> 90%). However, HLA B27 gene contributes only about 36% to the genetic risk. Obviously other genes are involved. X chromosome does not appear to be involved in pathogenesis at all.

Cytokines in Reactive Arthritis

The Th1 cytokines such as IL-1, IFN-γ and TNF-α are crucial for the elimination of the bacteria implicated in the causation of ReA. A relatively low production of Th1 cytokines has been documented in ReA.[10] This might partly contribute to the bacterial persistence in the synovium. Quite paradoxically, however, anti-TNF-α therapy is beneficial in spondyloarthropathies. Study and interpretation of cytokine pattern in ReA is an area of active research, at present.

Role of Autoimmunity

Currently, there is no clear evidence of autoimmunity in ReA or other spondyloarthropathies, and there is no candidate autoantigen.

Epidemiology

No epidemiological data are available on SARA in India. In the southern part of Africa, reactive arthritis and undifferentiated spondyloarthropathies have become common only after the advent of AIDS epidemic.[11] It is not known what impact HIV has had on these disorders in India. A study has been reported from the armed forces wherein only 2 cases of SARA were identified out of 102 HIV patients.[12] In another study from Mumbai, 12/300 (4%) patients with HIV infection, had arthralgias/bone pain but no definite arthritis.[13] The same study also reported HIV positivity in 8/150 high risk individuals attending a rheumatology clinic. The diagnosis of the rheumatic disease in these 8 patients included: rheumatoid arthritis-1, ankylosing spondylitis-1, SARA-1, reactive arthritis in the remaining 5 patients.

Clinical Features

Classical picture consists of a sterile oligoarthritis involving large joints, 1-3 weeks following an infection in the urogenital tract (chlamydia, ureaplasma). As mentioned before, the typical triad of urethritis, conjunctivitis and arthritis (Reiter's syndrome) is rarely seen. Although urethral and gut infections are common in India and HLA B27 gene is prevalent in the population to the tune of 6%[14], there are limited published data on ReA. One possible reason may be under reporting of cases. The author, however, believes that clinically recognisable cases of classical ReA are uncommon. On the other hand, evidence of subclinical infections can be obtained with serology for the putative bacteria amongst patients labelled with undifferentiated spondyloarthropathy, as has been shown in a study from northern India.[7]

Prakash et al[15] described a series of 36 cases (29 men and 7 women, ratio 4:1) of Reiter's syndrome. The mean age of onset was 23.8 years. Clinical manifestations included non-specific urethritis (53%), dysentery and diarrhoea (33%), low back pain and stiffness (69%), heel pain (44%), conjunctivitis (39%), anterior uveitis (19%), mucosal ulcerations (17%), kidney disease

(14%), and keratoderma blenorrhagicum (8%). Peripheral arthritis was mono or oligoarthritis in 58% of patients, mainly affecting the large joints of lower extremities, and it was often asymmetric (mean degree of asymmetry = 0.37). Radiographic sacroiliitis was seen in 42%. HLA-B27 antigen was detected in 83% of 36 patients compared with 5.9% of 118 controls (relative risk 79).

The dermatologists in India often see cases of 'Reiter's syndrome' presenting with the hyperkeratotic skin lesions called keratoderma blenorrhagicum and an oligoarthritis. Sometimes, a previous history of sexual contact is also available. However, no sizeable series from India is published in the indexed literature. Only a few case reports have been published in Indian journals.[16] There is a need to systematically study ReA in India and report it. Clinical documentation of SARA in India is really scant.

Diagnosis

Currently, there are no established criteria for the diagnosis of SARA. There is no established method of testing for the identification of the causative bacteria. For chronic cases, IgA and IgG antibody is looked for. For Chlamydia, both serological tests and PCR are available. The latter is useful only on synovial fluid or tissue and is insensitive on blood.

Treatment

Role of Antibiotics

Since bacterial persistence is such a major issue in SARA, the role of antibiotics has been explored in its treatment. In case of *Chlamydia trachomatis* genital infection, antibiotic may prevent pelvic inflammatory disease, scarring, infertility, chronic pelvic pain and passage of the organism to the baby. There is no evidence that antibiotics even when administered in the long term modify the course of ReA. There is, rather, a theoretical concern that antibiotics may render the Chlamydia dormant, leading to a change in surface protein expression that enhance the arthritis. Thus, there is no established role of antibiotics in the treatment of SARA.

Symptomatic Therapy

NSAID should be used for symptomatic relief. Splinting of joints should be discouraged in patients with SARA as they have a tendency to develop contractures and ankylosis of splinted joints. Intra articular steroid injections and injections placed near sites of enthesitis are very helpful. Systemic steroids including dexamethasone pulse are also employed in severe or refractory cases. Hyperkeratotic skin lesions and balanitis respond to coal tar or topical steroid applications. Disease modifying anti-rheumatic drugs such as methotrexate and sulphasalazine have been used with good effect but no controlled trials are available to prove their efficacy in ReA. Physiotherapy plays a pivotal role in the management.

2. Gonococcal Arthritis[17]

Gonococcal arthritis occurs as part of the syndrome of disseminated gonococcal infection (DGI). It is the commonest form of acute bacterial arthritis in adults. About 1% of gonococcal infections are estimated to develop DGI.

Typical presentation comprises a 5-7 day history of fever with chills in a sexually active person who develops multiple skin lesions and fleeting polyarthralgias and tenosynovitis, finally resulting in a persistent, mono or oligoarthritis. The skin lesions include petechiae, papules, pustules, haemorrhagic bullae and necrotic lesions. Typically, the lesions begin as an erythematous macule which progresses to a papule and then a pustule with necrosis or ulceration. At any time, lesions may be present at different stages. They are distributed on the trunk and extremities, including palms and soles but spare the oral mucosa. Septic arthritis can occur in the small joints of hands, wrists, elbows, knees, ankles and rarely, the axial joints. Symptoms of genitourinary tract infection are generally absent in DGI. Women are often menstruating or pregnant.

Cultures of synovial fluid from joints with purulent gonococcal arthritis are usually positive. Similarly, fluid from skin lesions is also positive. Other suitable materials for culture include blood and swabs from urethra, cervix, rectum and pharynx. Culture can take about 24 hours but treatment must be started immediately on empirical basis. Initial treatment with ceftriaxone 1 gram daily is recommended. If the strain is sensitive to penicillin, one can shift to Inj. crystalline penicillin 10-20 million units daily for 7 days. Otherwise ceftriaxone can be continued for 7 days. Ampicillin 1g qid for 7 days is a good alternative. Synovial fluid may have to be frequently drained if it rapidly accumulates. Generally, gonococcal arthritis does not lead to permanent joint damage and complete recovery is the rule.

3. Syphilitic Arthritis

Treponema pallidum can cause joint disease. Arthritis is rare in primary and secondary syphilis. In tertiary syphilis, gummatous deposits can occur in the juxta-articular tissue, cartilage and bone. Large, painless effusions are characteristic of this condition. Charcot's joints are the result of neuropathic arthritis resulting from tabes dorsalis, primarily involving weight bearing joints (knee, hip and ankles). Since tertiary syphils is quite rare now, syphilitic arthritis has become a very rare entity.

Congenital syphilis is associated with two important syndromes: Parrot's pseudoparalysis, which is osteochondritis affecting the epiphysis and articular cartilage of the humerus or the tibia of neonates and infants within first 3 months of life. The other one is Clutton's joints which is a late sequelae of congenital syphilis presenting with chronic hydroarthrosis of one or both knees in children between the ages of 6 and 16 years.

4. HIV-Associated Arthritis[18]

A number of musculoskeletal syndromes have been described in patients with HIV infection. Whether HIV itself causes any arthritis is debatable. Psoriatic arthritis and reactive arthritis, particularly SARA, may occur more often in patients with HIV infection. SARA may occur in as many as 11% of patients with HIV. These patients may not have uveitis or sacroiliitis. Incomplete forms rather than the classical triad are more commonly seen. The prevalence of HLA B27 appears to be lower in HIV associated SARA than in ordinary SARA. The spectrum of HIV associated joint manifestations vary in different populations; implicating the role of co-factors. Thus, 40% of HIV patients with joint symptoms in Zimbabwe have classical SARA and another 40% have a pauci-articular presentation without the extra-articular manifestations of SARA. In the United States, psoriatic arthritis limited to oligoarticular pattern may occur in one-third of patients with HIV and psoriasis. However, the overall incidence of psoriasis does not appear to be increased.

Acute HIV 'seroconversion illness' may be associated with transient arthralgias. The concurrence of rheumatoid arthritis and HIV is thought to be rare. A picture of polyarthritis can occur with HIV but this is associated with periosteal new bone formation, which is not a feature of RA. A subacute oligoarthritis involving knees and ankles may cause severe arthralgias and disability but it is transient and peaks in intensity in 1-6 weeks and responds well to NSAID. The synovial fluid is non-inflammatory. About 10% of HIV patients suffer from 'painful articular syndrome' which lasts less than a day and involves shoulders, elbows and knees. The pain tends to be intense and incapacitating, requiring short term narcotic analgesics. The prevalence of fibromyalgia is reported to be as high as 29% in HIV patients.

5. HBV and HCV arthritis[17]

These 2 viruses may get transmitted sexually. HBV infection may cause immune complex mediated arthritis. This occurs early in the disease when significant viremia is present and anti-HBsAg antibodies are being produced. Usually, the clinical picture consists of an acute symmetrical polyarthritis but it can be migratory at onset. Hand and knee joints are most often involved. Urticaria may accompany. In general, arthritis is confined to the pre-icteric phase of hepatitis. Sometimes, it may persist even after icterus appears. Patients with chronic active hepatitis or those with chronic HBV viremia may have recurrent arthralgias or arthritis. Polyarteritis nodosa may be associated with chronic HBV viremia in 10-30% of cases. Hepatitis C virus is the commonest cause of essential mixed cryoglobulinemia, which classically presents with arthritis, palpable purpura and cryoglobulinemia.

6. Lymphogranuloma Venereum (LGV) and Arthritis

LGV is described in the 1940s with a syndrome resembling serum sickness including polyarthritis, rash, cryoglobulinemia and circulating rheumatoid factor. Such presentation is rare these days.

References

1. Kumar A, Chirkupalli R, Pande I, Malaviya AN. Infectious arthritis. A new perspective. JIRA 1994; 2: 32-34.
2. Beutle AM, Hudson AP, Whittum-Hudson JA, et al.

Chlamydia trachomatis can persist in joint tissue after antibiotic treatment in chronic Reiter's syndrome/reactive arthritis. J Clin Rheumatol 1997; 3: 125-130.

3. Siegal LH. Update on reactive arthritis. Bull Rheum Dis 2002; 50: 1-4.

4. Bas S, Griffais R, Kvien TK, Glennas A, Melby K, Vischer TL. Amplification of plasmid and chromosome Chlamydia DNA in synovial fluid of patients with reactive arthritis and undifferentiated seronegative oligoarthropathies. Arthritis Rheum 1995; 38: 1005-1013.

5. Branigan PJ, Gerard HC, Hudson AP, Schumacher HR Jr, Pando J. Comparison of synovial tissue and synovial fluid as the source of nucleic acids for detection of *Chlamydia trachomatis* by polymerase chain reaction. Arthritis Rheum 1996; 39: 1740-1746.

6. Wilkinson NZ, Kingsley GH, Sieper J, Braun J, Ward ME. Lack of correlation between detection of *Chlamydia trachomatis* DNA in synovial fluid from patients with a range of rheumatic diseases and the presence of antichlamydial immune response. Arthritis Rheum 1998; 41: 845-854.

7. Aggarwal A, Misra R, Chandrasekhar S, Prasad KN, Dayal R, Ayyagari A. Is undifferentiated seronegative spondyloarthropathy a forme fruste of reactive arthritis? Br J Rheumatol 1997; 36: 1001-1004.

8. Joseph J, Rodrigues C, Joshi VR. Bacterial DNA detection in spondyloarthropathies. In: CN Ramchand, Madhavan PN Nair, Bonny Pillo Eds. Recent advances in molecular biology, allergy and immunology. New Delhi: Allied Publishers Ltd, 2001; p. 26-37.

9. Kanga U, Mehra NK, Larrea CK, Lardy NM, Kumar A, Feltkamp TE. Seronegative spondyloarthropathies and HLA B27 subtypes: A study in Asian Indians. Clin Rheumatol 1996; 15 (Suppl 1): 13-18.

10. Yin Z, Braun J, Neure L, et al. Crucial role of interleukin-10/interleukin-12 balance in the regulation of the type 2 T helper cytokine response in reactive arthritis. Arthritis Rheum 1997; 40: 1788-1797.

11. Khan MA. Epidemiology of HLA-B27 and arthritis. Clin Rheumatol 1996; 15 (Suppl): 10-12.

12. Achuthan K, Uppal SS. Rheumatological manifestations in 102 cases of HIV infection. JIRA 1996; 4: 43-47.

13. Swati V, Samant RS, Nadkar MY, et al. HIV infection and rheumatological disorders. JIRA 1996; 4: 83-87.

14. Mehra NK, Taneja V, Kailash S, Raizada N, Vaidya MC. Distribution of HLA antigens in a sample of the North Indian Hindu population. Tissue Antigens 1986; 27: 64-74.

15. Prakash S, Mehra NK, Bhargava S, Malaviya AN. Reiter's disease in northern India. A clinical and immunogenetic study. Rheumatol Int 1983; 3: 101-104.

16. Singh M, Kaur S, Kumar B, Sharma VK, Kaur I. Reiter's disease-clinical profile of six cases. Indian J Dermatol Venereol Leprol. 1987; 53: 108-111.

17. Mahowald ML. Infectious disorders: A. Septic arthritis. In: Klippel JH, Weyand CM, Wortmann RL eds. Primer on the rheumatic diseases. 11th ed. Atlanta: Arthritis Foundation; p. 196-200.

18. Calabrese LH. Human immuno deficiency virus (HIV) infection and arthritis. Rheum Dis Clin North Am 1993; 19: 477-488.

PART V
Sexually Transmitted Diseases in Special Situations

Chapter 32

Sexually Transmitted Diseases in Children

S Murugan

Introduction

Sexually transmitted diseases (STD) in children (below 12 years of age) are a significant problem because of potential medical, legal, social and psychological consequences. STD in children especially the neonatal infections acquired from parental source are frequently missed due to low index of suspicion and lack of facilities for their detection.

In principle, STD in children are acquired through three different ways (1) transplacental transmission occurring in utero, intrapartum transmission (during labour and delivery) e.g. syphilis, HIV, CMV and human papilloma virus infection (HPV); (2) postnatal transmission (during breast-feeding, accidental and through sexual abuse) (3) in prepubertal children transmission is due to sexual abuse and (4) in sexually active adolescents, who are at risk of acquiring the STD as in adults. Rare cases of STD, due to accidental infection from mothers or nurses, through wet towels, bedding and sharing toilet seats have been reported.

Prevalence

Systemic perinatal bacterial infections that are acquired in utero or during delivery are seen in about 5 per 1000 live births.[1] Perinatal bacterial infections are two to three times more common than perinatal viral or protozoal infections. But it is very difficult to assess the exact prevalence of STD in children as they frequently go undiagnosed or unnotified.

Incidence of congenital syphilis was reported to be 1.4% in a study from a STD clinic in Delhi.[2] A study from Pondicherry, reported that congenital syphilis contributed for one third of childhood STD.[3] Prevalence of STD at various STD clinics in India is given in Table 1. With the advent of newer, effective antibiotics and proper antenatal care of the pregnant women, the incidence of bacterial STD in children have reduced. On the contrary, in the west the incidence of congenital syphilis has increased in last two decades.[4] The risk of perinatal transmission of HIV, and pediatric HIV infection are covered in detail in a separate chapter.

Table 1. Prevalence of STD in Children in India[3,4]

Disease	Garg et al. 1985 (n = 30) (n/%)	Pandhi et al. 1995 (n = 58) (n/%)	Mendiratta et al. 1996 (n = 49) (%)
Syphilis			
primary	—	3 (5.1)	—
secondary	9 (30.0)	11 (19.1)	77 (14.3)
congenital	10 (33.3)	2 (3.5)	28 (57.0)
Gonococcal infection	4 (12.6)	14 (24.1)	1 (2.05)
Non-gonococcal urethritis	—	1 (1.7)	—
Candidiasis	—	6 (10.3)	—
Chancroid	—	13 (22.4)	—
Genital warts	6 (18.7)	4 (6.9)	12 (24.5)
Herpes progenitalis	2 (6.2)	4 (6.9)	1 (2.05)

Risk Factors

Premature rupture of membranes, prolonged labour, instrumentation during labour, prematurity, and injury to the newborn during delivery appear to increase the transmission of STD from mother to infant.[5] Delivery by caesarean section has shown to reduce the risk of perinatal transmission in HIV, HPV and HSV infections.[5]

Child Sexual Abuse[6]

By definition, child sexual abuse is the use of a child as an object of gratification for adult sexual needs or desires. Sexual abuse ranges in severity from gentle fondling to forcible rape resulting in physical injury. The common sexual abuse encountered by girls are genital contact, masturbation, vaginal, oral or anal intercourse by a male perpetrator, while boys are subjected to felatio and anal intercourse. About half of child victims are involved in repeated incidents of sexual abuse. It is difficult to assess the prevalence in a society, as the offence is usually hidden due to fear of stigmatization.

Prevalence studies in the United States had estimated that 44,700 cases of sexual abuse occur in a 12 months period. The most sexual offenders against children are adult males. In a study, female offenders were 15% for female victims, 24% for male victims. Another study reported 2% intrafamilial and 6% extrafamilial sexual abuse cases. According to random community survey the male to female ratio of child abuse was 1:3. The rate of STD in sexually abused children has been reported to be approximately 5-20%. The peak age for sexual abuse for both girls and boys is between 7 and 13 years of age. The prevalence rates of various STD in prepubertal children evaluated for suspected sexual abuse in various studies were gonorrhoea (5-14.8%), syphilis (0.1-6%), chlamydia (1.2-6%), trichomonas (2-18%) and condylomata acuminata (2-5.6%).[6]

In orphanages, hostels and juvenile homes, older children and caretakers commonly indulge in sex abuse. Approximately 90 percent of perpetrators are males. In one study in an orphanage, 53 of 95 abused girls were infected with gonococcal infection.[7]

Clinical Features of Bacterial STD

Syphilis

Syphilis is transmitted transplacentally (congenital syphilis) and postnatally (acquired syphilis). Congenital syphilis is always caused by maternal syphilis whereas almost all acquired syphilis is due to sexual contact. Most of Indian studies have shown, that syphilis is the most common STD in children.[3,7,8]

Congenital Syphilis

The detailed features and laboratory diagnosis are described in a separate chapter.

Acquired Syphilis[9]

The transmission of acquired syphilis is almost always associated with sexual abuse, except when transmission is through breast-feeding and rarely due to extragenital primary chancre. Clinical features in children are almost similar as in adults. Initial presentation being primary chancre followed by secondary stage, latent stage and few of them develop tertiary syphilis. The incubation period is same as that of adults ranging from 19-90 days (average 3 weeks). In children, the chancres are said to be smaller and less likely to be recognized. So most children are found to have latent syphilis or secondary syphilis with mucocutaneous moist lesions either in vulva or in anus. Atypicality, multiplicity of ulcers have also been reported in literature. Secondary syphilis develops from 2 weeks to 6 months after primary chancre. All classical features like papular, papulosquamous with involvement of palms and soles, moist verrucous plaques in and around the genitalia and mucous patches have been described. Most common lesion in children is erythematous rash. The common differential for primary chancre would include a bacterial infection. Secondary syphilis is commonly confused with pityriasis rosea. Diagnosis is by demonstration of spirochete under dark ground microscopy, non-treponemal tests (VDRL, RPR) and treponemal tests (TPHA, MHA-TP, FT-ABS) as done in adults. No special tests or recommendation have been proposed for diagnosing acquired syphilis in children. Non-treponemal test if positive, should be confirmed by treponemal test like FTA-ABS, MHA-TP, IgG and IgM enzyme immunoassays and PCR.

Treatment of Acquired Syphilis[10]

CDC recommended regimens for children in primary, secondary and early latent syphilis

- Benzathine penicillin G 50,000 units/kg IM, upto the adult dose of 2.4 million units in a single dose.

In late latent syphilis or latent syphilis of unknown duration

- Benzathine penicillin G 50,000 units/kg, IM upto the adult dose of 2.4 million units administered as three doses at 1 week intervals.

Gonorrhoea

Gonococcal infections in children are acquired either perinatally or by intimate contact or through sexual abuse. Accidental infections are comparatively rare.

In neonates the transmission of gonococcal infection occurs due to direct contact with birth canal during delivery. It accounts for 42% of gonococcal conjunctivitis, 7% orogastric contamination, and disseminated infection are reported in <1% of neonates.[11] In 90-100% of cases of gonococcal infection below 12 years is due to sexual contact. The prevalence of *N. gonorrohoeae* in abused or sexually active and adolescent was reported to be 2.8 percent to 20 percent from various surveys.[12]

The clinical spectrum of gonococcal infection in children are conjunctivitis, asymptomatic pyuria, urethritis, vaginitis, proctitis, pharyngitis, rhinitis, scalp abscess, arthritis, sepsis of the newborn, and pelvic inflammatory disease (PID). In case of prepubertal girls, the most common form of gonorrhoea is vaginitis accounting for 75 percent of the infection. This is due to reduced estrogen load and alkaline vaginal pH of vaginal mucosa. It most commonly presents with profuse, purulent vaginal discharge, vulval erythema with dysuria and pruritus, rarely it can be asymptomatic. Very rarely ascending infection leading to salpingitis or peritonitis have been reported.

The frequency of infection in boys is less and usually presents with urethral discharge, asymptomatic pyuria, penile oedema (occasional), epididymitis, testicular swelling and conjunctivitis.

Pharyngeal and rectal infections are common in both the sexes. Pharyngitis occurs in 15-54% of gonococcal infection. The pharyngeal and rectal infections are mostly asymptomatic and anal infection is common in girls.

Gonococcal proctitis in female children results either from the spread of infection from the genital tract or by rectal intercourse. When there is profuse vaginal discharge it may dribble over the perineum and to the anal orifice and by sphincter action of anal canal, the organism reaches the rectum and produces gonococcal proctitis in female children. In male children it almost always occurs through anal coitus. The proctitis is usually asymptomatic. Some children may complain of discomfort, soreness or pain in the anus during defecation. The discharge is mucoid, purulent and bloodstained. Smears and cultures taken with platinum loop from rectum with the help of a proctoscope establish the diagnosis. Repeated examinations may be necessary for diagnosis.

Dissemination of gonorrhoea in infants and children is rare. It is often preceded by an asymptomatic genitourinary tract infection. Most commonly these children would present with polyarthralgia associated with systemic manifestations. The joints, which are commonly affected, are ankles, knees, wrists and hands. The other manifestations of disseminated disease are meningitis, sepsis of newborn and pseudoparesis of involved joints.[12]

Gonococcal arthritis in older children resembles that of adults and may be associated with cutaneous lesions. Involvement of the joint may include, suppurative arthritis, inflammation of periarticular surface and tenosynovitis of joints. Osteomyelitis has been occasionally reported.

Ophthalmia Neonatorum[9]

The Central Midwives Board in U.K. defines any inflammation that occurs in the eyes of an infant within 21 days of birth and that is accompanied by a discharge as ophthalmia neonatorum. The causes of purulent conjunctivitis of newborn children are gonococcal infection, chlamydial infection and other nonspecific organisms like streptococcus, staphylococcus, diphtheria, moraxenfield bacilli and irritation due to chemical instillation into the eyes. The risk for acquiring gonococcal ophthalmia neonatorum in a neonate born to a mother with untreated gonorrhoea is 10%. In a study from UAE, chlamydia and *N. gonorrhoea* accounted for less than 5% of cases of ophthalmia neonatorum.[13] In a sexually abused child, gonococcal ophthalmia may occur due to autoinoculation.

Gonococcal ophthalmia runs a more florid course in one or both eyes. The signs of infection usually appear on 3rd day of birth, whereas in chlamydia it may take 2 to 3 weeks to manifest (average 7 days). They manifest with profuse mucopurulent discharge, and on opening the lid forcibly, spurting of discharge is observed. The conjunctiva is congested and oedematous and if treatment is delayed, cornea may get perforated thus leading to blindness. The diagnosis is made by taking smears and cultures from the discharge and demonstrating gram negative intracellular diplococci. The infection in the mother's cervix can also be simultaneously established.

Prevention

All pregnant women at risk of acquiring infection should have endocervical culture examination for gonococci and other organisms during their antenatal care at least twice, once during their first trimester and second in last trimester and they should be treated if the culture is positive.

Recommended regimen for prevention at the time of delivery: (Crede's method)[14]

Step I: Wipe the discharge over the eyes immediately after birth with sterile cotton wipers from medial to lateral aspect as single stroke. If there is more discharge to be wiped fresh set of sterile wipers is recommended.[18]

Step II: Instillation of 1% silver nitrate (AgNO$_3$) solution in a single application. But this will be more effective only against gonococcal organisms.

As the other organisms causing ophthalmia neonatorum are more prevalent in present scenario, the American Academy of Paediatrics has recommended 1% tetracycline or 0.5% erythromycin ophthalmic preparations for prophylaxis.

Treatment[10]

CDC recommends 25-50 mg/kg IV or IM single dose not exceeding 125 mg ceftriaxone in uncomplicated gonococcal infections. For disseminated gonococcal infection and gonococcal scalp abscess, the recommended regimen is ceftriaxone 25-50 mg/kg/d IV/IM in a single dose for 7 days, 10-14 days if meningitis is documented or cefotaxime 25 mg/kg IV/IM every 12 hours for 7 days, with a duration of 10-14 days, if meningitis is documented.

Prophylactic treatment for infants, whose mother have gonococcal infection have been recommended with ceftriaxone 25-50 mg/kg/d IV or IM, not to exceed 125 mg in a single dose. If a child weights more than 45 kg, regular adult regimen can be advised. In cases, when the child is <45 kg, recommended regimen for uncomplicated gonococcal infection is ceftriaxone 125 mg in a single dose. Alternative regimen being spectinomycin 40 mg/kg (maximum dose of 2g) IM single dose. In bacteremia, arthritis, ceftriaxone 50 mg/kg (max 1g) IM/IV in a single dose daily for 7 days.

Bacterial Vaginosis

It is caused by *Gardnerella vaginalis*, mobiluncus, bacteroides, peptostreptococcus in prepubertal girls. The incidence of BV in prepubertal girls is low. Evidence of sexual abuse as a cause of BV in prepubertal girls is often inconclusive. Perinatal transmission of BV during vaginal delivery is unknown.

Most of the symptomatic children would present with gray white to yellow discharge with malodour. Determination of pH in prepubertal girls for diagnosing BV is not useful, because of alkaline pH of vaginal mucosa of prepubertal girls.

Vulvovaginitis due to Non-Venereal Causes

- Enterobius vemicularis infestation
- Candidial infection
- Dust and poor hygiene
- Foreign bodies (ex; pebbles, stones, peas, beans etc)

Other Bacterial STD

Diseases like chancroid, granuloma venereum, and mycoplasma infections have not been reported very often in children in recent years. The reasons are the decline in the general incidence of bacterial STD and poor availability of diagnostic facilities. Manifestation of chancroid reported in the children run a similar course to that in adults. Painful lesions like chancroid in female children can lead to acute retention of urine with distended bladder due to severe dysuria and present as an acute emergency in pediatric surgery department.

Trichomonal Infection[9]

Trichomonas vaginalis infection is observed in adolescent

girls or due to sexual abuse in prepubertal children. Though trichomonas can survive in fomites, transmission by fomites has not been reported in children. Studies have shown that the rate of perinatal transmission is nil to 0.6% when the infant is affected, they appear for a short duration and remits spontaneously. *Trichomonas vaginalis* infection in children more than 1 year of age is mostly due to sexual contact. Reported rates of *Trichomonas vaginalis* infection in possible sexually abused children was 0.4% because it is rarely seen before puberty. Hypertrophic epithelium, absence of glycogen and alkaline environment prevent the growth of trichomonas.

The sites of infection in infants are nose, throat and vagina. Clinical presentation may be asymptomatic, but transient vulvovaginitis is the commonest symptom in prepubertal children. These children present with greenish-white, frothy and offensive discharge from the vagina, but this appears to be a rare event. When the discharge is profuse, excoriations and vulval dermatitis may be noticed. Organisms can easily be demonstrated by mounting a saline preparation from the discharge when examined under the high power objective of a light microscope. Metronidazole (30 mg/kg/day in 3 doses × 7 days) or tinidazole (50-75 mg, single dose) preparation will cure the condition.

Chlamydial Infection

Pregnant women with cervical infection can transmit infection to neonates during vaginal delivery. About 50-75% infants born to infected mother develop conjunctival, nasopharyngeal infection, rectal and vaginal infection. Asymptomatic shedding by the affected child can occur for a long period (3 years). Any chlamydial infection after 3 years of age at vagina, rectum or pharyngeal sites, one should suspect a possibility of sexual abuse.[6]

Neonatal conjunctivitis is the major clinical presentation with chlamydial infection accounting for 30-50% of neonatal chlamydial infections and the symptoms develop within 3 weeks, presenting as mucopurulent discharge.[15] And in about 50% of the patients with conjunctivitis co-infection of nasopharynx is also seen.

The chlamydial infection was found to be far more prevalent than gonococcal infection in most studies in developed countries. In India, data on chlamydial infections in children is lacking because the isolation and the demonstration of the organism is difficult and serological tests are not available.

Premature rupture of membranes leads to earlier manifestation of the disease. The course will be usually less fulminant than that of gonococcal ophthalmia. Purulent discharge, chemosis, and pseudomembrane formation are seen. A follicular reaction like in adult trachoma is not seen in infants below 3 months of age, as they do not have the requisite lymphoid tissue. Corneal neovascularization and scarring can occur.[15]

Nasopharynx is the most frequent site of perinatally acquired chlamydial infection. Asymptomatic pneumonias occurs only in about 30% of infants with nasopharyngeal infection. The systemic infection usually develop between 4-12 weeks of age. Characteristic signs of chlamydial pneumonia in infants include (a) repetitive staccato cough with tachypnea and (b) hyperinflation and bilateral diffuse infiltrates on chest radiograph.[10] Fever, wheezing are distinctly absent. Laboratory abnormalities like eosinophilia (> 300 cells/cm) and raised immunoglobulin have been seen. In older children, vagina and rectum is commonly involved and rarely pharynx. Chlamydial otitis media occurs in infected infants by the spread from nasopharynx through eustachian tube to middle ear. It is described as serous otitis.

There are not many studies conducted in India on rectovaginal infections in older children due to sexual abuse, but incidence is likely to be more common than reported. The clinical features of chlamydial infection in children who are sexually abused are similar to that of infections in adults. Proctitis, pharyngeal infection in both sexes, vaginitis in female children, and urethritis in boys. The other manifestations are salpingitis and PID. The later two are more common among the adolescents. Disseminated disease is rare.

Manifestations of lymphogranuloma venereum in children resemble that in adults. Reiter's syndrome characterized by urethritis, arthritis and conjunctivitis occurs more in male children. Gastrointestinal infection is the most common predisposing factor. In children, conjunctivitis was most common initial complaint. Major symptoms occur after 2 weeks and persist at least for 2-3 months. The joint disease is asymmetric and usually involves larger, lower limb joints. Antimicrobial therapy has no proven benefit.[6]

Treatment[10]

Recommended regimens for neonatal conjunctivitis

and infantile pneumonia caused by *C. trachomatis* infection are treated with erythromycin base or ethyl succinate 50 mg/kg/d orally divided into four doses daily for 14 days.

In children who weigh less than 45 kgs are given erythromycin base/ethyl succinate at the same dose as mentioned above. Children who weigh ≥ 45 kgs, but who are less than 8 years of age, azithromycin 1g orally in a single dose is recommended, and in children who are > 8 years, azithromycin 1 g orally in a single dose or doxycycline 100 mg twice daily for 7 days is recommended.

Clinical Features of Viral STD

Paediatric HIV Infection is discussed in a separate chapter.

Herpesvirus Infections

Cytomegalovirus (CMV) and herpes simplex virus type 2 (HSV 2) can be transmitted transplacentally, during delivery, sexual contact, as ascending infection and non-sexual contact.

CMV infections are usually sub-clinical. Sources of virus include urine, oropharyngeal secretions, cervical and vaginal secretions, semen, milk, tears, blood and transplanted organs. Higher rates of sero-positivity have been observed in males and females with multiple sex partners and histories of STD. From these parents, children acquire the infection in utero or perinatally. Sexual transmission in children plays a minimal role as a mode of primary CMV infection.[16] In fact, no primary CMV infections in children due to sexual abuse have been reported from India.

Symptomatic infections show hepatomegaly, splenomegaly, microcephaly, jaundice and petechiae. Occasional clinical findings include hydrocephalus, haemolytic anaemia and pneumonitis. But 90 percent of infected infants remain asymptomatic.[16]

HSV 2 infections in children are common due to sexual abuse. The prevalence rate is 0.1-0.2% were seen in various studies on probable sexually abused children. It can occur due to autoinoculation from mouth to genitalia. In spite of HSV-2 infections being not uncommon among women, neonatal herpetic infections are rarely reported from developing countries, which may be due to non-recognition or lack of diagnostic facilities or passive transmission of HSV neutralizing maternal antibodies, which may protect the baby from manifesting the disease.

Clinical Features[9]

Neonatal HSV infections are almost invariably symptomatic and frequently lethal. Symptoms usually appear within the first week of life. Infection can involve multiple organs. If it is confined to the skin, eye and or mouth it is associated with a lower mortality. Clusters of vesicles on the presenting part of the body that was in direct contact with the virus during birth are the major features. With time, the rash may progress to involve other areas of the body as well. In 90% of children vesicles will occur over skin, eye or mouth. Vesicles usually erupt from an erythematous base and are 1-2 mm in diameter. They can progress to larger bullous lesions greater than 1 cm in diameter. Infections involving the eye may manifest as kerato-conjuctivitis or later chorioretinitis. Kerato-conjunctivitis is usually associated with microphthalmia, in the absence of therapy it can progress to chorioretinitis, cataract and retinal detachment.

Disseminated infection will have constitutional signs and symptoms including irritability, respiratory distress, jaundice, bleeding diathesis and shock along with exanthems. Liver and adrenals are the principal organs involved and elevation of SGOT, GGT, conjugated bilirubin, neutropenia, thrombocytopenia are common. The clinical manifestations of encephalitis include irritability, tremors, poor feeding, temperature instability, bulging fontanella and pyramidal tract signs. Culture of CSF yields HSV in 25 to 40% of all cases. CSF analysis will show pleocytosis and proteinosis (as high as 500 to 1000 mg/dl).

Prevention and Treatment

Infected mothers have viral shedding for a period of 3 weeks in case of primary infections and 2 to 5 days in a case of recurrent infections. So, if the women have the lesions in and around genitals after 32 weeks of gestation, the individual may be an ideal candidate for caesarian section to prevent neonatal infection.

In the treatment of neonatal HSV infection intravenous acyclovir when started earlier in the course of disease will prevent the mortality considerably in the dose of 20 mg/kg body weight intravenously every 8 hours for 21 days for CNS and disseminated disease or 14 days for disease limited to the skin and mucous membrane.[10]

Human Papilloma Virus Infection

The common human papilloma virus (HPV) type 6, 11, 16, 18 and 2 are responsible for causing most of the infection in children. The infection with HPV in below 3 years of age is considered to be due to vertical transmission.

The mode of infection is by hand to genital contact, non-sexual behaviours or inadequate hygiene. The average incubation period is about 3 months, but it could be upto 2 years.

HPV in children is reported by many Indian authors next only to syphilis.[3,7,8,17-22] Nonvenereal mode of transmission of condyloma acuminata especially in infants has been discussed by many authors.[19,20,23] Sexual abuse in pre-pubertal children and sexual contact in older children are probably common modes of transmission. Other methods of transmission suggested include direct contact with maternal warts during delivery. Tang et al reported a child with congenital condylomata acuminata whose mother had genital condylomata acuminata, wherein it was probably acquired through hematogenous spread.[23]

The viral warts in children are encountered in the mucocutaneous or in the intertrigenous area like anogenital area, perineum, labia, around the vaginal orifice, anus and in the rectum. It is rarely found intravaginally in young girls. Often the lesions are present around the mouth and between the toes. The warts in perianal area are about 57% in boys and 37% in girls. Labium is involved in 23% and penis in 17%. The viral warts are more frequently found in girls than boys. In case of juvenile papillomatosis the lesions are found in the oral cavity, vocal cord, epiglottis, trachea and lungs.[9]

These lesions can be treated either with chemical cauterization with 25% podophyllin solution in older children above 2 years or with cryosurgery in children below 2 years to avoid the possibility of neurotoxicity that may occur if it is absorbed through extensive area of application over the lesions. Laryngeal papillomata are acquired from mother's asymptomatic cervical infection during delivery. It comes to the notice of ENT surgeons when the patients are subjected for examination of the larynx for some other problem. Rarely it may lead to hoarseness of voice and obstruction to respiration.

Other STD like molluscum contagiosum, genital scabies may also occur in children due to sexual abuse, and the later may also spread through fomites and close contacts, especially in children in hostels and orphanages. The clinical features are not different from those in adult infection except that the complications due to genital scabies are more common in children than in adults.

Evaluation of Sexual Assault or Abuse of Children[10]

Identification of sexually transmitted agents in children beyond the neonatal period suggests sexual abuse. The investigation of sexual abuse among children should be conducted in compliance with recommendation by clinicians who have experience and training in all elements of the evaluation of child abuse, neglect and assault.

Postnatally acquired gonorrhoea, syphilis, chlamydia and non-transfusion, non-perinatally acquired HIV are usually diagnostic of sexual abuse. While confirmed trichomonas infection should be regarded with high suspicion of sexual abuse. Herpes genitalis, postnatally acquired ano-genital warts in a child, one should suspect sexual abuse whereas, presence of BV in a child is inconclusive evidence of sexual abuse.

Examination of children for sexual assault or abuse should be conducted so as to minimize pain and trauma to the child. Collection of vaginal samples in prepubertal children can be uncomfortable, so has to be done by an expert clinician.

The scheduling of examination should depend on the history of assault or abuse. If a recent exposure is documented, there could be insufficient concentration of organisms for a positive result. So in order to obtain sufficient evidence or follow up examination including the physical examination and collection of specimens has to be done after 2 weeks of recent exposure, and for antibodies to be detected in serum another follow up of 12 weeks is planned.

The following investigations are performed at initial and 2 weeks of follow up

- Visual inspection for bleeding, discharge, odour, irritation warts and ulcerative lesions.
- Swabs from the vesicular, ulcerative genital and perianal specimens should be sent for HSV culture.
- Specimen collection for culture for *N. gonorrhoeae* from the pharynx and anus in boys and girls, the vagina in girls and the urethra in boys. For

boys with urethral discharge a meatal sample is an adequate substitute for the isolation.

- Specimens for culture for *C. trachomatis* from specimens collected from the anus in both boys and girls and from the vagina in girls.
- Culture and wet mount of vaginal swab specimen for *T. vaginalis* infection and BV.
- Collection of serum for VDRL/RPR, FTA-ABS, HIV and HbsAg.

Examination at 12 Weeks after Assault

In circumstances in which transmission of syphilis, HIV or hepatitis B is a concern but baseline tests are negative, an examination at 12 weeks is appropriate as antibodies for the above disease may become positive. CDC does not recommend presumptive treatment in child acquiring a STD as a result of sexual abuse or assault because

(a) Prevalence of most STD is low following abuse/assault.

(b) Pre-pubertal girls appear to be at low risk for ascending infections than adolescent/adult women

(c) Regular follow up of children usually can be ensured

Parental concern regarding the possibility of STD in child may warrant presumptive treatment, only after adequate specimens are collected for diagnostic testing.

References

1. Seigel JD, MC Cracken GH: Sepsis neonatorum. N Eng J Med 1981; 304: 642.

2. Mendiratta V, Kumar V, Sharma RC, Koranne RC. Congenital syphilis. A clinical profile. Indian J Sex Transm Dis 1996; 17: 51-53.

3. Garg BR. Mohammed AS. Baruah MC. Sexually transmitted diseases in children. Indian J Sex Transm Dis 1986; 7: 11-13.

4. Pandhi RK, Khanna N, Sekhri R. Sexually transmitted diseases in children. Indian Pediatr 1995; 32: 27–30.

5. Sweet RL, Gibbs RS. Sexually transmitted diseases. In: Sweet RL, Gibbs RS, eds. Infectious disease of female genital tract. 4th Edn. Philadelphia: Lippincott Williams and Wilkins; 2002. p 118-175.

6. Chacko RM, Wood Jr CR. Gynecological infections in children and adolescents. In: Feigin RD, Cherry JD, eds. Text book of Paediatrics infection. 4th edn. Philadelphia: WB Saunders; 1998. p 509-547.

7. Murugan S, Raman LG, Solomon PJ, Kumarasamy. Morbidity pattern of STD in children of south Tamil Nadu Indian J sex Transm Dis 1987; 8: 47-50.

8. Kumar VM, Kumar AS, Kumar A, et al: Sexually Transmitted infections in child sexual abuse. Indian J Sex Transm Dis 2001; 22: 75-77.

9. Gutman LT. Sexually transmitted diseases. In: Feigin RD, Cherry JD, eds. Text book of paediatrics infection. 4th edn. Philadelphia: WB Saunders; 1998. p 548-561.

10. CDC. MMWR Sexually transmitted disease treatment guidelines 2002/51/RR-6.

11. Ahmed HJ, Ilard I, Antognoli A, et al. An epidemic of Neisseria gonorrhoeae from infants and children. Pediatr Infect Dis 1988; 7: 32.

12. Gutman LT. Gonococcal diseases in infants and children. In: Holmes KK, Mardh PA, Sparling PF, et al. eds. Sexually transmitted diseases. 3rd Edn. New York. Mc Graw Hill; 1999. p 1145-1153.

13. Nsanze H, Dawodu A, Usmani A, Sabarinathan K, Varady E. Ophthalmia neonatorum in United Arab Emirates. Ann Trop Paediatr 1996; 16: 27-32.

14. Nahmias AJ. Herpes Simplex. In: Remington JS and Klein JO eds. Infectious disease of foetus and newborn infants. Philadelphia: WB Saunders; 1983. p 636.

15. Hammerschlag MR. Chlamydial infections in infants and children. In: Holmes KK, Mardh PA, Sparling PF, et al, eds. Sexually transmitted diseases. 3rd Edn. New York: McGraw Hill; 1999. p 1155-1164.

16. Weller TH. Cytomegalovirus: a historical perspective. Herpes 2000; 7: 66-69.

17. Arora SK, Sardari Lal, Sharma RC, Bajaj P. Condyloma acuminata in a child. Indian J Sex Transm 1984; 5: 55-56.

18. Usman N, Gajendran K, Shakir FH. Anal Condylomata in an eleven month old infant. Indian J Sex Transm Dis 1985; 6: 61-62.

19. Koranne RV, Sundharam JA, Jagadish Rai, Gupta MM. Perianal condylomata acuminata in an eleven month old infant. Indian J Sex Transm Dis 1988; 8: 42-43.

20. Murugan S, Srinivasan G, Jafar Sadiq TSM, Kaleelulah MCA. Condyloma acuminata in children. Indian J Sex Transm Dis 1995; 16: 22-23.

21. Menditratta V, Kumar V, Sharma RC, Koranne RV. STD Profile in children. Indian J Sex Transm Dis 1996; 17: 1-3.

22. Weinstein LS, Golderring J, Carpenter S, Non-sexual transmission of sexually transmitted disease; an infrequent occurrence. Paediatrics 1985; 74: 67-76.

23. Tang CK, Shermeta DW, Wood C: Congenital Condylomata Acuminata. Am J Obstet Gynecol 1978; 131: 912-914.

Chapter 33

Sexually Transmitted Diseases in Women and Pregnancy

Usha Gupta

Introduction

Sexually transmitted diseases (STD) can affect women in the same way as they affect men. Women who are pregnant may become infected with the same STD as non-pregnant women. The consequences of STD are more serious, even life threatening for a woman and her baby if she becomes infected during pregnancy. Firstly, if the woman acquires the infection prior to pregnancy it can give rise to salpingitis and tubal blockage which can cause ectopic pregnancy or infertility. Secondly, immunological changes occurring during pregnancy can result in change in the severity of the disease e.g. viral warts may overgrow in size and shape. Thirdly, with untreated STD, the puerperal infections may be more severe.

As the number of STD continues to emerge especially in the HIV era, it is increasingly important that the women should be aware of the harmful effects of these diseases and how to protect themsclves. The outcome of pregnancy may also be affected as the newborn can get infected in utero via blood e.g. cytomegalovirus

infection and syphilis. Diseases like gonorrhoea and chlamydia infections can cause pelvic inflammatory disease (PID). Chlamydia infection may also cause pneumonia and ophthalmia neonatorum in neonate. Herpes virus can also infect the neonate during the passage through birth canal. STD may also cause premature rupture of membrane (PROM), still birth, low birth weight, neonatal sepsis, neurological damage (brain damage or motor disorders) and congenital abnormalities (including blindness, deafness and other organ damage). Acute hepatitis, meningitis, chronic liver disease and cirrhosis may also develop.

HIV infection is another cause of concern as it can be transmitted from mother to child. HIV infection may modify the course and treatment of other STD. Hence all pregnant women must undergo screening test for HIV.

The various STD syndromes and their complications in women are discussed in a separate chapter. The complications of STD pathogens in pregnant women and the prevalence of various STD in women in India are given in Table 1 and 2 respectively. It is apparent

Table 1. Complications of STD Pathogens in Pregnant Women

Pregnancy associated	
Chorioamnionitis	*N.gonorrhoeae, M. hominis,* Bacterial vaginosis-associated organisms
Spontaneous abortion/foetal wastage	Herpes Simplex Virus(HSV), *T.pallidum,* Bacterial vaginosis-associated organisms
Prematurity / PROM	Group B-streptococcus (GBS), *C. trachomatis, N.gonorrhoeae, T. pallidum,* Bacterial vaginosis-associated organisms
Postpartum endometritis	GBS, *N.gonorrhoea, M. hominis(?), C.trachomatis(?),* Bacterial vaginosis associated organisms
Congenital/perinatal infections	
TORCH syndrome	GBS, HSV, Cytomegalovirus (CMV), *T. pallidum,*
Sepsis/death	*C. trachomatis, N. gonorrhoeae*
Conjunctivitis	*C trachomatis,* GBS, *T pallidum, Ureaplasma urealyticum*
Neurological involvement	CMV, HSV, *T pallidum,* GBS.

Table 2.   Prevalence of STD in Women in India

Diseases	Kurnool 1992-1996 (%) (n = 990)	Pondicherry 1982-1990 (%) (n = 1884)	New Delhi 1983 (%)
Non gonococcal urethritis	19	—	—
Gonorrhoea	16.16	4.1	2.5
Syphilis	15	22.4	55
Herpes genitalis	14	12.3	17.3
Genital warts	3.2	10	10
Non venereal dermatoses	9.5	—	—
LGV	0.7	3.6	3.7
Molluscum contagiosum	1.7	60.3	1.65
HIV positive	0.4	—	—
Vulvovaginitis	21.18	12.3	11.5
Donovanosis	0.3	7.3	1.65
Chancroid	1.7	2.4	7.8
Psychosexual	2	—	—
Scabies	—	0.6	—

that syphilis, vulvovaginitis, herpes genitalis and gonorrhoea are common STD in women. The common clinical features of STD are similar in men and women and are described elsewhere and only the special features in women are emphasized in this chapter.

Syphilis

Syphilis is a STD caused by *T. pallidum*. Primary syphilis presents as a painless genital ulcer and in women the commonest site for a chancre is the cervix, (also during pregnancy) which may therefore pass unnoticed. The other sites are labia, fourchette, urethra and perineum. Extra genital sites for chancre include anus, mouth, oropharynx and nipple. Oedema induratum is a unilateral labial swelling with rubbery consistency and intact surface representing a deep-seated chancre. Kissing lesions may occur in areas of skin to skin contact as in vulva. The regional lymph nodes are often involved.[1,2] Secondary syphilis develops as the chancre disappears or upto 6 months later. It is manifested by asymptomatic to pruritic maculopapular rash predominantly affecting the palms & soles, mucous membrane lesions, condylomata lata. Secondary syphilis is a common mode of presentation in women. Syphilis may be detected in women with history of abortion or during antenatal check up. Neurosyphilis and cardiovascular syphilis are less common in women than men. However, benign tertiary syphilis was more frequently described in women than men.

Syphilis can affect the outcome of pregnancy depending upon the stage. Fimura et al,[3] in their observations regarding the outcome of pregnancy in relation to the stage of maternal syphilis, reported that among infants born to mothers with primary and secondary syphilis, half of them were premature, still born or died in the neonatal period and rest of them had congenital syphilis. With early latent syphilis, the transmission rate decreased to 40%, while 20% were premature, 4% died in the neonatal period and 10% were still born, 20% of them were normal and born at full term. In case of late latent syphilis 9% premature births, 11% of still births, and only 10% congenital syphilis were observed. With longer duration of untreated maternal syphilis the severity of effect in foetus will decrease. The mother who had congenital syphilis can hardly transmit the disease to the foetus.

The severity of disease in the foetus also varies, it is more severe in more recent infections and less so in long-standing disease (Kassowitz's law). However a patient who has had several miscarriages, still births and congenitally syphilitic children may give birth to healthy non infected child and again have a baby with congenital syphilis. Usually the last infant has fewer signs and symptoms of the disease.[3]

Routine antenatal screening with VDRL for all pregnant mothers should be done even when there is low prevalence as early diagnosis and treatment can prevent congenital syphilis. If the test is positive, then the possibility of biological false positive (BFP) reactions should be kept in mind. Usually BFP occurs at a titre of 1:8 or less. If the VDRL test is positive then it should be confirmed by specific test like TPHA or FTA-ABS test. If the confirmatory tests are negative an antibody screening like ANA and others should be done.[4]

The test for congenital syphilis in a newborn may be positive from the cord blood. This could be due to passive reaginemia. Even a positive FTA-ABS test may be found due to non-specific interference by the production of IgM and IgG antibody by the neonate. Therefore a positive serology at birth does not necessarily indicate the presence of infection. Hence routine screening of the newborn serum or umbilical cord blood is not recommended.

Treatment of Syphilis in Pregnancy

Appropriate penicillin regimen should be given during pregnancy depending upon the stage. Pregnant women who are allergic to penicillin should be desensitized and treated with penicillin. No alternatives to penicillin have been proved effective for the treatment of syphilis during pregnancy. The sexual partner should be examined and treated accordingly.[5] If the exact duration of the disease is not known, the patient's other children should also be investigated and treated.

While treating the pregnant woman with early syphilis the patient may experience Jarisch Herxheimer reaction. There is a risk of premature labour/foetal distress if the reaction takes place after 20 weeks of gestation. Hence an obstetrician should monitor the patient

Gonorrhoea

Gonorrhoea can manifest as cervicitis, urethritis, endometritis, salpingitis and perihepatitis in women. It can also cause conjunctivitis, tonsillitis and proctitis. Chronic asymptomatic infection is common in 50% of women. Almost all patients with gonococcal infection during pregnancy are asymptomatic. In the neonates, the passage through the birth canal of the infected mother can give rise to ophthalmia neonatorum, pharyngitis and proctitis. Meningitis as a complication of ophthalmia neonatorum has also been described.[2] The importance of gonorrhoea in women during pregnancy is that it may ruin the obstetric future by giving rise to complications like tubal blockage and ectopic pregnancy as a result of PID. Disseminated gonococcal infection and oropharyngeal infection (15-35%) are more common during pregnancy. Gonococcal infections may also lead to PROM, chorioamnionitis,

septic abortions, intrauterine growth retardation, prematurity and post partum sepsis.

Post abortal gonococcal endometritis and salpingitis are now well recognized complications of termination of pregnancy.[1] Patients undergoing therapeutic abortions who have untreated endocervicitis, have high risk of developing post abortal endometritis.[1] Various studies have shown that the perinatal outcome in mothers with untreated gonorrhoea would result in spontaneous abortion (11-35%), perinatal mortality (8-11%), prematurity (17-67%) and premature rupture of membranes (20-75%).[6] Because of these complications few experts suggest routine cultures at the initial prenatal visit and a repeat culture early in the third trimester.[7]

Risk of developing PID reduces during the first trimester of pregnancy because of cervical mucous plug which, forms a barrier and reduces the risk of anterograde transmission of infection. In the later part of pregnancy, chorion fuses with decidua blocking the uterine cavity, hence upward transmission of infection is prevented.

Treatment

Treatment of gonococcal infection is discussed in a separate chapter.

Uncomplicated gonococcal infection of urethra, cervix and rectum in pregnant women can be treated with one of the following regimens.[5]

Cefixime 400 mg orally in a single dose or

Ceftriaxone 125 mg IM in a single dose

PLUS azithromycin 1 g orally in a single dose or

Erythromycin stearate 500 mg orally qid for 7 days.

Pregnant women should not be given quinolones or tetracyclines. They should be treated with recommended or alternative cephalosporin. Women who cannot tolerate cephalosporin can be given spectinomycin 2 g IM single dose. Test for cure is no longer recommended, if they have received any of the CDC recommended regimens for gonorrhoea. Only those patients with persistent symptoms, a subsequent culture and antimicrobial susceptibility is tested after 1-2 months of treatment.[5]

Chlamydial Infection in Women

The clinical spectrum and epidemiology of *C. trachomatis* infection are many ways similar to that of gonococcal infection. But the differences are that *C. trachomatis* infection is less dramatic, more frequent, more asymptomatic or at times may exist with absence of signs of inflammation.[8] Thus, the presence of carrier state, long incubation period and frequent asymptomatic stages could place women at risk of ascending infection into the upper genital tract which would result in an adverse outcome of future reproductive health.

The clinical spectrum of chlamydial infection includes endocervicitis, bartholinitis, acute urethral syndrome, nonpuerperal endometritis and acute salpingitis. The most common type of presentation is endocervicitis, approximately two third of women with chlamydial infection are asymtomatic. In one third, it presents as mucopurulent cervicitis (MPC), acute urethral syndrome (by definition is characterized by acute dysuria, frequent urination in women with pyuria but whose voided urine is sterile or contains $<10^5$ microorganisms/ml). The sequelae of acute PID in these women would result in ectopic pregnancy, tubal factor infertility (TFI), and tubo ovarian abscess (TOA).[8]

Acute perihepatitis is a localized fibrinous inflammation affecting the anterior surface of the liver and the adjacent peritoneum. The sequelae of this are fibrous adhesions between the liver and diaphragm. If this condition is associated with acute salpingitis, it is called Fitz-Hugh curtis syndrome. The above syndrome is said to be most commonly caused by *C. trachomatis*.[9] The effect of the infection on pregnancy could be post partum endometritis, post abortal endometritis, spontaneous abortion and foetal deaths, prematurity, low birth weight and PROM.[10] It was noticed in a study that pregnant mother infected with chlamydia at or before 18 weeks gestation had higher incidence of prematurity, low birth weight infants, and perinatal deaths.[8]

Among babies born of infected mothers about, 60-70% of them have risk of acquiring infection during the passage through the birth canal, among which 20-50% will develop ophthalmia neonatorum in first 2 weeks and 10-20% would develop pneumonia within 3-4 months after birth.[11] The neonate may remain afebrile with paroxysmal cough and chest X-ray shows diffuse infiltration. In utero transmission is not known to occur. There is no evidence that additional therapy with a topical agent provides further benefit.

Treatment

CDC recommendations for chlamydia infection are covered elsewhere in the book. The recommendations during pregnancy are erythromycin 500 mg po qid for 7 days or amoxicillin 500 mg po tid for 7 days. Alternative regimens are erythromycin base 250 mg po qid for 14 days or erythromycin ethylsuccinate 800 mg po qid for 7 days or 400 mg of the same salt for 14 days or azithromycin 1g po in a single dose.[5]

CDC recommendations for prevention of chlamydial infection in women is universal screening of adolescents or young adults (<24 years) undergoing pelvic examination, annual testing for women with MPC, sexually active women <20 years old, 20-24 year old or more, inconsistent use of barrier contraceptive or new partner in past 3 months; screening of all pregnant women in first trimester, and in high risk women, rescreen in third trimester.[5]

Lymphogranuloma Venereum (LGV)

LGV is caused by *C.trachomatis*, serotypes L1, L2 and L3. The occurrences of acute LGV cases are more common in men than in women, in the ratio of 5:1 or more. On the other hand long term complications like ulceration, genital hypertrophy and rectal strictures are more common in women. Although transplacental congenital infection has not been reported, acquisition of infection during passage through an infected birth canal can occur.[12]

Treatment

Doxycycline 100 mg po bid for 21 days or erythromycin 500 mg po qid for 21 days. For treatment during pregnancy, erythromycin 500 mg qid is given for 21 days. Some authors even recommend azithromycin in multiple doses over a period of 2-3 weeks.[5]

Chancroid

Chancroid is caused by *H. ducreyi*. The most common site for 'soft chancre' is labia, clitoris and fourchette. The symptoms with which women present are dysuria, rectal bleeding, dyspareunia or vaginal discharge. The classic ulcer of a chancroid is superficial and shallow with ragged edge with an erythematous halo. Multiple ulcers are the rule in women in contrast to solitary ulcers in more than 50% of men.[1] Bubo formation classically described in men are rare in women.[13] CDC recommends that a probable diagnosis of chancroid can be made by following criteria.[5]

(a) If the individual has one/more painful genital ulcer.

(b) There is no evidence of syphilis on dark field examination or by serology at least 7 days after the onset of ulcers.

(c) Either the clinical presentation of the genital ulcers and inguinal lymphademopathy are typical for chancroid or tests for HSV are negative.

Treatment of chancroid remains the same as that of men, except in pregnant women where quinolonoes are contraindicated and, the safety of azithromycin has not been established. Ceftrioxone or erythromycin is the preferred regimen for pregnant and lactating women. No adverse affects of chancroid on pregnancy outcome or on foetus have been observed.[1,5]

Streptococcal—B Infection (GBS) (*Streptococcus agalactiae*)

GBS is known to colonize 5–25% females and rarely associated with vaginitis or cervicitis in non pregnant females. There are reports of GBS related infections in pregnancy e.g. chorioamnionitis, post partum wound infection and post partum endometritis. 1–2% of neonates born to GBS carrier mother develop the disease. The mortality rate is upto 50%. The risk is higher if the baby is premature or with low birth weight. The baby may develop pneumonia or septicemia within the first week. Late onset meningitis can also develop.

Treatment with erythromycin or ampicillin is effective. It is controversial whether treatment during pregnancy can eradicate the organism or prevent neonatal disease. Routine prophylactic treatment for exposed neonate is recommended.[1]

Donovanosis

A chronic progressively destructive infection of the genital area caused by *Calymmatobacterium granulomatis* ,a gram negative bacilli.In women,the usual sites of infection are labia and fourchette. The epithelium overlying the lesion subsequently enlarges to produce beefy, red velvety granulomatous ulcer. Untreated disease may involve groin and perianal area and bone

involvement has been described. In long standing cases, squamous cell carcinoma may develop.[14] O'Farrell has reported that during pregnancy donovanosis has a more aggressive course. The recommended regimen by CDC includes trimethoprim-sulfamethoxazole, or doxycycline for a minimum of three weeks. Alternative treatment regimens are ciprofloxacin, azithromycin and erythromycin. In pregnant and lactating women erythromycin is recommended with addition of parenteral gentamycin.[5]

Bacterial Vaginosis

Bacterial vaginosis may be associated with an increased incidence of adverse pregnancy outcomes (e.g. PROM, pre-term delivery and low birth weight). Rarely it can cause PID, puerperal pyrexia, septic abortion, neonatal bacteremia and cutaneous abscess. A symptomatic pregnant women should be treated, and those with a history of previous pre-term delivery should be screened to detect asymptomatic infections. Recommended treatment regimen is metronidazole 250 mg po tid for 7 days, alternative regimen include clindamycin 300 mg po bid for 7 days. Treatment with clindamycin vaginal cream is not recommended due to increase in preterm birth in women.[5] Women with high risk for preterm delivery should be considered for BV screening in early second trimester. If they have established or symptomatic BV then they should be treated with the above regimen, except with metronidazole gel.[15]

Genital Herpes

Genital Herpes is caused by HSV serotypes 2 and 1. Most cases of herpes genitalis is caused by HSV 2 and 15% of primary genital lesions are caused by HSV 1. Clinical manifestations of herpes infection can be broadly divided into three groups. (a) primary (b) recurrent and (c) non primary first episode. Primary herpes genitalis is characterized by marked local symptoms, with multiple vesicles rupture to form painful polycyclic erosions with associated systemic symptoms. There is usually a wide spread involvement of the vulva and vagina and also cervix. However it may pass completely unnoticed. Periurethral involvement in women may cause severe pain, dysuria dyspareunia and the involvement of the sacral nerves, which in turn leads to retention of urine in women. Primary pharyngeal and rectal infection are seen following oral or anal intercourse. Pregnancy does not influence the recurrence compared to the general population although it has been noticed that primary episode during pregnancy may be more severe than in non pregnant women.[2] Its importance in pregnancy is due to the devastating obstetric complications and neonatal infection.[16] The risk of transmission to the neonate is high (30-50%) if the women acquire genital herpes at the time of delivery and is low (<1%) among the women who acquire genital herpes during the first half of pregnancy. This may be due to type specific antibodies (maternal) that would protect the neonate.[17] Around 10% of the recurrent herpes infection is asymptomatic and it frequently affects perineum rather than cervix.[18]

The foetal infection occurs almost always due to viral shedding from the cervix or lower genital tract infection. The risk of perinatal infection due to asymptomatic shedding was found to be 4%.[18] The virus invades the uterus following the rupture of the membrane or when the foetus comes in contact with lesions during the time of delivery through the birth canal. Infection is rarely transmitted to the placenta, when the membrane is intact. The risk of neonate acquiring infection is more with primary maternal infection rather than with the recurrences. Nahmias reported a 50% risk of neonatal infection with primary disease but only 4-5% risk with recurrent infection. The risk of transplacental infection is high if the mother has primary infection.[19]

During pregnancy HSV may be acquired in utero, intrapartum or postpartum. About 5% of babies with neonatal herpes acquire the infection prior to labour. 85% of neonatal herpes occur due to direct contact with maternal genitalia or secretions during delivery, 5% cases occur due to intrauterine infection, 10% cases after birth due to direct contact with caretaker.[16]

Treatment

Acyclovir, valacyclovir and famciclovir are used for the treatment genital herpes in non-pregnant women. Acyclovir appears to be safe during pregnancy. CDC along with pharmaceutical company manufacturing acyclovir maintains the registry for exposure to this drug during pregnancy. More than 700 foetus were exposed to the acyclovir during the first trimester without any adverse effects. Episodic therapy with acyclovir may be useful in recurrent episodes and daily suppressive therapy with acyclovir may reduce the signs and symptoms but does not completely eliminate the viral shedding. According to the American College of Obstetrics and Gynaecology, caeserian delivery is indicated in women with active genital lesions or with typical prodrome. Caeserian delivery is performed only if the active lesions are present at the time of labour or within 4-6 hours of rupture of the membrane.[20]

Human Papilloma Virus

HPV types 6 and 11 usually cause anogenital wart. The most important sequelae are the development of cervical, vaginal and vulvar neoplasia.

The genital warts frequently increase in size and number during pregnancy sometime filling the entire vaginal canal or covering the perineum and thereby making vaginal delivery or episiotomy difficult. It is possibly the moistness due to constant leucorrhea throughout the pregnancy, offers favourable condition for the viral growth. Accelerated viral replication with advancing pregnancy has also been hypothesized. Most women with vulvar lesions also have cervical infection and vice versa due to the multifocal involvement and subclinical nature of the disease. Rarely it can cause life-threatening hemorrhage due to increased vascularity during pregnancy. The lesions usually improve after delivery possibly related to less amount of moisture, vascularity, and immunosuppression due to pregnancy.[1] The different treatment modalities during pregnancy include trichloro or dichloroacetic acid 80 to 90% once a week, cryotherapy, laser ablation, excision and electrocautery. Podophyllin, 5-FU, imiquimod and interferon are contraindicated during pregnancy.[20]

HPV can be transmitted perinataly. Aspiration of infected material at the time of vaginal delivery could cause laryngeal papillomatosis in infants. In a study of 301 pregnant women with HPV infection, 40% transmission of infection to the newborn was observed, and it was higher for those who delivered vaginally (51%) than with caesarian section (27%). Some authors prefer doing caesarian section if the wart is enormous in size and obstructs the vaginal canal.[21]

Cytomegalovirus Infection[22-25]

Cytomegalovirus (CMV) is double stranded DNA virus,

which has ability to remain latent within the host for years. CMV is transmitted through infected body fluids. Only the persons with immunosuppression are prone to get recurring illness. But for most people CMV is not a problem. However, CMV infection presents a specific challenge to the pregnant women because of the perinatal infection and mortality. So whenever a pregnant women experiences infectious mononucleosis like symptoms she should be evaluated for CMV infection. Cytomegalovirus infection is the most common perinatal infection and 40-50% infants born to mothers with primary CMV will have congenital infection. Of these 5 to 18% will be overtly symptomatic at birth and 80% of the survivors have severe neurological morbidity. Most of the congenitally infected infants are asymptomatic at birth and 10 to 15% of these children subsequently develop neurological sequelae.

The risk of foetal injury is higher with primary infection and is very low with recurrences or reactivated CMV infection. The virus can present itself in different strains. Boppana et al,[25] examined anti CMV antibodies from 46 pregnant women with preconceptual immunity to CMV. Of these 16 delivered CMV infected infants. They found that 62% of the mothers of infants with congenital CMV infection had acquired antibodies with new specificities as compared with 13% of the mothers whose infants were not infected. Earlier it has been thought that once an individual has been infected with CMV, that person is immune or protected against reinfection. But the current thinking is that even seropositive women can be re infected with different strains of CMV and can pass the newly acquired strain to the foetus and thereby causing serious injury. So whenever a pregnant mother acquires recurrent CMV infection the physician or the gynaecologist should be aware of the newly acquired primary infection with a different strain.

Diagnosis

Serological diagnosis of primary CMV in the mother is difficult because IgM antibodies persist for longer periods of time. For the best diagnostic result paired serum samples are taken for CMV antibodies. First sample is taken upon suspicion of CMV infection and another is taken within 2 weeks. If the tests show a fourfold rise in IgG and a significant level of IgM antibodies then it indicates an active infection.

Virus culture can be performed from the urine and throat.

Serologic testing: ELISA is the most commonly available test for measuring antibody to CMV which can be used to determine acute infection, prior infection or presence of passively acquired maternal antibody in infants. Other tests include various fluorescence assays, indirect haemagglutination and latex agglutinations. ELISA tests for CMV specific IgM is available. CMV specific IgM may be produced in low levels in reactivated CMV infection.

A more reliable diagnostic procedure to assess foetal infection is by polymerase chain reaction (PCR) and CMV culture performed in amniotic fluid at least 6 weeks following presumed maternal infection and past the 21st week of pregnancy.

Treatment

Currently no treatment exists for CMV infection. Ganciclovir is used for patients with immunosuppression. Vaccines are still in the research and developmental stage.

Recommendations for Pregnant Women (CDC)

1. Throughout the pregnancy, practice good personal hygiene, especially handwashing with soap and water, after contact with diapers or oral secretions (particularly with a child who is in day care).
2. Women who develop a mononucleosis-like illness during pregnancy should be evaluated for CMV infection and counseled about the possible risks to the unborn child.
3. Laboratory testing for antibody to CMV can be performed to determine if a women has already had CMV infection.
4. Recovery of CMV from the cervix or urine of women at or before the time of delivery does not warrant a caesarean section.
5. The demonstrated benefits of breast-feeding outweigh the minimal risk of acquiring CMV from the breast-breeding mother.
6. There is no need to either screen for CMV or exclude CMV-excreting children from schools or institutions because the virus is frequently found in many healthy children and adults.

Hepatitis B

Hepatitis B is caused by Hepatitis B virus, a DNA virus with three major antigens; surface antigen (Hbs Ag), core antigen (Hbc Ag), and 'e' antigen (Hbe Ag).

The natural course following an acute infection is that 85-90% experience complete resolution and develop protective antibodies, 10-15% would develop chronic infection, of which 15-30% would develop chronic active hepatitis / persistent hepatitis and about 20% of these patients would go on to develop hepatocellular carcinoma. Only less than 1% of patients with acute infection develop fulminant hepatitis leading to death.

The relevance of this infection during pregnancy is that infected mothers would perinatally transmit the infection to neonate, while the baby is traversing the birthcanal or when it comes in contact with genital secretions. Up to 90% of chronic carrier mothers can transmit the infections to the newborn at the time of delivery especially when the women are Hbs Ag and Hbe Ag positive.

Combination of active and passive immunization can prevent both vertical and horizontal transmission of hepatitis B infection. Neonatal immunoprophylaxis is 85-95% effective in preventing the neonatal hepatitis B infection. Thus CDC recommends an universal hepatitis B vaccination for all infants. The available vaccines are DNA recombinant vaccines, so do not carry risk of transmission of blood borne pathogen. All obstetricians must screen their patients for hepatitis B infection, because selective screening might miss out 30-50% of the infection.

Candidiasis

Higher glycogen content in the vaginal environment and enhanced adherence of Candida species to vaginal epithelial cells results in an increase risk of symptomatic vaginitis in pregnancy. The problem becomes more severe as pregnancy progresses. Local therapy with nystatin or imidazole vaginal pessaries can be used. Ketoconazole and itraconazole should not be used due to toxicity and risk of teratogenicity. Neonatal infections usually present with perioral or perianal rash or oral thrush. The details are given in chapter 27.

Trichomoniasis

Trichomoniasis infection in pregnancy is associated with puerperal maternal morbidity (postpartum fever) and a small but statistically significant increased risk of preterm delivery. There is increasing evidence of association between infection with *T. vaginalis* and PROM & low birth weight. Female neonates may acquire infection perinatally but this seems to be transient in most cases.[20] The details are given in chapter 28.

Scabies and Pediculosis

Scabies usually manifests with symptoms after 4-6 weeks of acquisition of infestation. The symptoms are predominantly pruritus, exacerbated during night time, with pleomorphic rash affecting characteristically the wrist, web space, flexures, groin and genitalia. There is no adverse outcome of pregnancy with scabies. CDC recommends 5% permethrin cream in pregnant and lactating women. Sulphur 6% can also be used in pregnancy. Sexual contacts and close household contacts should be treated as above.

Another infestation, which can be sexually transmitted, is pediculosis pubis, caused by phthirus pubis (crab louse). The incubation time of pediculosis is 30 days. Patients complain of irritation or pruritus. Treatment is with 1% permethrin rinse. It is to be applied for 10 minutes after first thoroughly washing the infested area and then gently rinsing that area off. It may be repeated after 7 days. Gamma-benzene hexachloride is not recommended and contraindicated in pregnant or lactating females and infants. This drug is lipid soluble and is neurotoxic. Vertigo, convulsion and mental confusion can occur as a result of systemic absorption. Other side effects include nausea, vomiting and blood dyscrasia.

HIV infection in pregnancy is discussed in chapter 7.

References

1. Sweet RL, Gibbs RS. Sexually transmitted diseases. In; Sweet RL, Gibbs RS eds. Infectious disease of female genital tract. 4th Edn. Philadelphia: Lippincott Williams and Wilkins; 2002. p. 118-175.
2. Infections in gynaecology In: Campbell S, Monga A

eds. Gynaecology by ten teachers. London: ELST; 2000: p. 183-204.

3. Radolf JD, Sanchez PJ, Schulz KF, Murphy FK. Congenital syphilis. In: Holmes KK, Sparling PF, Mardh PA, et al. eds. Sexually transmitted diseases. 3rd edn. New York: Mc-Graw Hill; 1999. p. 1165-1189.

4. Perinatal infections. In: Campbell S, Lees C, eds.Obstetric by ten teachers. London: ELST; 2000. p. 183-204.

5. Centre for disease control. Sexually transmitted diseases: Treatment guidelines. MMWR 2002: 51, 18-29

6. Edwards LE, Barrada MF, Hamman AA, et al. Gonorrhoea in pregnancy. Am J Obstet Gynecol 1978;132: 637-641.

7. Phillips RS, Hanff PA, Wertheimertt, Aronarson MD. Gonorrhoea in women sense for routine gynaecological care; criteria for testing. Am J Med 1985; 85: 177-182.

8. Sweet RL, Gibbs RS.Chlamydial infections. In; Sweet RL, Gibbs RS eds. Infectious diseases of female genital tract. 4th Edn. Philadelphia: Lippincott Williams and Wilkins; 2002: p. 57-100.

9. Wolner - Hanssen P,Westrom L, Mardh PA. Perihepatitis in chlamydial salphirgitis. Lancet 1980; 1: 901-904.

10. Gencay M, Koskiniemi M, Saikkn P, et al. *Chlamydia trachomatis* seropositivity during pregnancy is associated with perinatal complications. Clin Infect Dis 1995; 21: 424-426.

11. Alexander ER, Harrison R. Role of *Chlamydia trachomatis* in perinatal infection. Rev infect Dis 1983; 8: 713-719.

12. Perine PL, Stamm WR. Lymphogranloma venereum. In: Holmes KK, Sparling PF, Mardh PA, et al. eds. Sexually transmitted diseases. 3rd Edn. New York: Mc Graw Hill; 1999: p. 423-432.

13. Roral Ak, Albritton W. Chancroid and *Hemophilus ducreyi*. In: Holmes KK, Mardh PA, Sparling PF, et al. eds: Sexually transmitted diseases 3rd edn. NewYork: Mc Graw Hill; 1999: p. 515-523.

14. 'O' Farrell N. Donovanosis in pregnancy. Int J Sex Transm Dis AIDS 1991: 2: 447-448.

15. Sweet RL, Gibbs RS. Infections vulvovaginitis. In; Sweet RL, Gibbs RS, eds. Infectious diseases of female genital tract. 4th Edn. Philadelphia: Lippincott Williams and Wilkins; 2002. p. 337-354

16. Sweet RL, Gibbs RS. Herpes simplex virus. In; Sweet RL, Gibbs RS eds. Infectious disease of female genital tract. 4th Edn. Philadelphia: Lippincott Williams and Wilkins; 2002. p. 101-117.

17. Brown AZ, Voniver LA, Benedetti J, et al. Effects on infants of a first episode of genital herpes during pregnancy. N Engl J Med 1987; 317: 1246-1251.

18. Prober CG, Suependn WM, Xasukawa LL, et al. Low risk of herpes simplex virus infection in neonates exposed to the virus at the time of vaginal delivery to mothers with recurrent genital herpes simplex virus infections. N Engl J Med 1987; 316: 240-244.

19. Nahmias AJ, Josey WE, Naib ZM, et al. Perinatal risk associated with maternal genital herpes simplex virus infection. Am J Obstet Gynecol 1971; 110: 285.

20. Sexually transmitted diseases. In: Cunningham FG, Gant NF, Leveno KJ, Gilstrap LC, Hauth JC, Wenstorn KD, eds.Williams Obstetrics. New York: McGraw Hill; 2001. p. 1485-1516.

21. Maw DR. Treatment of anogenital warts. Dermatol Clin 1998; 16: 829-834.

22. Brown HL, Abernathy MP. Cytomegalovirus infection. Semin Perinatal 1998; 22: 260–6.

23. Ornoy A. The effects of cytomegalic virus (CMV) infection during pregnancy on the developing human foetus. Harefuah 2002; 141: 565–8, 577.

24. Gaytant MA, Steegers EA, Semmekrot BA, Merkus HM, Galama JM. Congenital cytomegalovirus infection: review of the epidemiology and outcome. Obstet Gynecol Surg 2002; 57: 245-256.

25. Boppana. Pregnant women can pass new CMV strains to foetus. N Engl J Med 2001; 344: 1366-1371.

Chapter 34

Sexual Assault and Sexually Transmitted Diseases

R K Sharma

Introduction

Sexual assault is an act of sexual intimacy done without the consent of the victim or where consent has been obtained by means of threat, fear or fraud. In our country sexual assault is a serious offence.

Sexual offence may be described as natural sexual offences like rape or unnatural sexual offences like sodomy, buccal coitus, tribadism, bestiality and certain sexual deviations.

Rape

Definition: Rape in India is defined (under Section 375 of Indian Penal Code) as unlawful sexual intercourse by a man,

- (i) With his own wife under the age of 15 years or
- (ii) With any other woman under the age of 16 years with or without her consent or
- (iii) With any other woman above the age of 16 years, against her will, without her consent or
- (iv) With her consent—when her consent has been obtained by putting her or any person in whom she is interested in fear of death or hurt or
- (v) With her consent—when the man knows that he is not her husband and the consent is given because she believes that he is another man to whom she is or believes herself to be lawfully married or
- (vi) With her consent—when at the time of giving such consent, by reason of unsoundness of mind or intoxication or the administration of any stupefying or unwholesome substance, she is

unable to understand the nature and consequence of that to which she has given consent.

Explanation

Penetration is sufficient to constitute the sexual intercourse necessary to the offence.

Punishment for Rape

Section 376 Indian Penal Code imposes a minimum term of seven years imprisonment and a maximum of life imprisonment for the offence of rape. However, a judge can award less sentence at his discretion.

Custodial Rape

It has been sometimes observed that women are sexually abused in jails, remand homes, hospital or where the woman is in custody and she is not in a position to render sufficient opposition to the act. In such cases, provisions of custodial rape are attracted under Section 376-C, 376-D Indian Penal Code.

Section 376-D IPC—Whoever, being on management of a hospital or being on the staff of a hospital takes advantage of his position and has sexual intercourse with any woman in that hospital, such sexual intercourse not amounting to the offence of rape, shall be punished with imprisonment of either description for a term which may extend to five years and shall also be liable to fine.

So, to constitute the offence of rape it is not necessary that there should be a complete penetration of penis. Partial penetration within labia majora, or even an attempt at penetration is quite sufficient for the purpose of law. So, it may be possible in a rape case that absence of injuries or seminal stains is there. Ideally, doctors should refrain from using the word 'rape' as it is a legal entity, not a medical condition. The doctors should only mention facts and condition of the victim and state that there is an evidence of sexual activity or not.

In cases where rape cannot be proved, it may be tried under less serious charge of indecent assault on a female committed with intent or knowledge to outrage her modesty. It is punishable under section 354 of Indian Penal Code by a term, which may extend upto two years, or fine, or with both. A woman may be accused of an indecent assault on a man but not rape.

Consent

According to law of India, a woman of sixteen years and above is capable of giving consent to the act of sexual intercourse. But the consent must be conscious, free, voluntary and given when she is mentally fit.

In certain sections of custodial rape [under clause (a) to (g) of subsection (2)] of section 376 of Indian Penal Code where sexual intercourse is proved and the question arises whether it was without the consent of the woman alleged to have been raped and she states in her evidence before court that she did not consent, the court shall presume that she did not consent (Section 114A, Indian Evidence Act). Thus the onus of proving consent shifts to accused from victim in such limited cases.

Prevalence of Rape

According to National Crime Records Bureau Report (1998), there were 15031 cases reported in India. Madhya Pradesh reported the highest incidence accounting for 22.3% of total cases. Among the cities, Delhi and Mumbai recorded more crimes numbering 365 and 118 respectively. In rates, Mizoram [9.3] led the table followed by Madhya Pradesh [4.3], Dadra and Nager haveli [3.9] & Delhi [3.4]

Victims of rape were maximum in age group of 16-30 years accounting for 8414 out of 15033 reported cases.

Age

No age is safe for rape. The children are easily abused as they can offer less resistance. Small infants even at the age of 4-6 months have also been abused. Even older women are not safe from rape. For committing rape, the law of India does not presume any limit under which a boy can be considered physically incapable of committing rape. In such cases, the development of child along with development of sexual organs has to be taken into consideration while deciding that he is capable of performing rape or not.

Socio-Economic Status

Incidence of rape is more reported from lower socio-economic status, as they tend to live in unsafe and crowded areas.

Examination of Victim

The examination of victim should be carefully done as per provisions of law as they are different from one state to another in India. As per the recent judgment of Punjab and Haryana High Court, it is mandatory to get the rape victim examined only by a female doctor. In Delhi, only a gynaecologist does the medical examination of rape victims. The examination of rape victim should be under supervision of a female medical practioner.

Consent

The consent to examine rape victim should be taken before commencement. It should be in writing. As per provisions of law, police or court has no power to compel a woman to submit private parts for examination to a medical practitioner, male or female.

Examination

After taking consent, the medical examination should be started in presence of a female attendant or witness while a male doctor examines the patient. No attempt should be made to undress the woman. She should be politely asked to remove clothes. The exact time of examination, name of the person who brought the victim, a short factual summary of incidence should be recorded in medico-legal report in the register, which has been approved by the state administration.

Two marks of identification of the victim should also be noted. A short description of place of occurrence of event, details of act, relative position of parties, whether ejaculation occurred or not, pain during act, loss of consciousness during act or efforts to resist should be recorded. The general behaviour and mental state of the victims should be noted. The detailed examination should begin in the following order.

1. Clothes: If clothes are same as those worn by her at the time of sexual assault, they should be carefully examined for the presence of blood or seminal stain or any other discharge. The clothes especially undergarments should be preserved for examination by Forensic Science Laboratory.

2. Injuries: The physical examination of body especially forearms, wrist, face, breasts, chest, inner aspects of thighs, and back should be done to look for scratches, abrasions or bruises caused as a result of struggle/ compression. Teeth marks if any may be observed on breasts, nipples, lips, or cheeks. Swabs from teeth bite should be taken for the presence of saliva.

3. Genitals: The examination should be preferably done in lithotomy position. The pubic hairs should be examined first, if they are found to be matted, they should be cut off with a pair of scissors to look for spermatozoa. They should be preserved in a dry bottle for examination at Forensic Science Laboratory. Dried seminal stains on external genitals/ thighs can be scrapped carefully or moistened with normal saline and slides may be made for microscopic examination. If bloodstains are present, they should also be preserved in a similar manner. Bruise or laceration if any on external genitalia may be carefully noted. The examination of hymen should be carefully done now. In a case of rape, hymen may have fresh radiate tears (more in posterior half), the edges of which may be red, swollen or painful if the examination of the victim is done within 24 hours. These tears heal within five to six days and looks like small tags of tissue after 10 days. Frequent sexual intercourse/ delivery completely destroys hymen. There may be cases where hymen may be found to be intact and not lacerated. In such cases, the distensibility of hymen can be recorded. The fourchette and posterior commissure are not usually injured in cases of sexual assault. The degree of injury is dependent on the force used.

In small children, the hymen usually escapes injury, as it is deep seated but becomes red and inflamed.

The vaginal secretions from the posterior fornix should be taken either by introducing a plain sterile cotton swab or by introducing 1 ml pipette and sucking the contents. The contents should be immediately transferred to a microscopic slide in a form of thin film and should be fixed. The slide can be viewed for spermatozoa. In married women, spermatozoa may be present because of previous sexual intercourse. The spermatozoa can be seen up to 17 days in vagina after last sexual intercourse. Even if spermatozoa is not present, the estimation of acid phosphatase level can be done in fluid obtained from posterior fornix to detect presence of seminal fluid.

Sexually Transmitted Disease

A woman can get venereal disease as a result of sexual assault if the person who committed sexual assault was suffering from such diseases. A discharge may be observed in cases of gonorrhoea. A thin film from the discharge may be made, fixed and stained with Gram's stain to see for gonococci under the microscope. The incubation period of gonorrhoea is about 2-8 days, so in a case of suspicion, another smear may be taken after few days to confirm. If syphilitic sores are seen or suspected, serum for dark ground examination for *Treponema pallidum* and blood for serological examination should be collected. The incubation period of syphilis vary from 9-90 days, so samples at a later date may be taken for confirmation. The sores on genitalia may be due to chancroid, which can also be confirmed by making smears to demonstrate Ducrey's bacillus, which is Gram-negative strepto–bacillus with rounded ends. The other common infection that is transmitted is chlamydial vaginitis and viral STD like herpes.

The most important sexually transmitted diseases is AIDS, which can be transmitted by sexual assault. The chances that a victim may get HIV infection in a single encounter are varied (3-5 percent). If it is suspected, relevant tests like ELISA or western blot may be done at repeated interval to confirm.

If sodomy has been attempted or performed, then anal swabs from around the anus and anal canal may be collected and looked for spermatozoa/seminal fluid.

Examination of the Accused

In India, the examination of the accused is done on a written request of the police. The person is brought under the custody of police to medical officer for examination. As per the law, whenever a person is arrested for committing sexual assault, a doctor should medically examine him as early as possible. In most of the states of India, the examination of the accused is conducted either by medical officers working in emergency services or dermatologist and venereologist is called upon for examination. In some centres where forensic experts are available, such cases are referred to them.

The examination of the accused should be recorded in medico-legal register duly authorized by state government. The police constable who has brought him should identify the accused. This should be recorded in the report. The consent of the accused is not necessary for examination as per the provisions of the law of India. In fact, a reasonable amount of force can also be applied to collect evidence from his person. The marks of identification should be noted and left thumb impression of the accused may be taken on medico-legal report itself. The medical officer should record preliminary data and then proceed for complete examination. Examination of clothes should be done to detect semen/bloodstain or tears. Undergarments should be especially looked for stains and should be preserved for examination by Forensic Science Laboratory. A complete physical examination involving all systems like cardiovascular, alimentary, respiratory and nervous system should follow. The complete body especially inner aspects of thighs should be examined for mud, blood or seminal stains. The genitalia should be examined. Pubic hair if matted should be cut and preserved. The penis should be examined for injury or some stain, circumcision, presence of smegma or discharge. The cremastric reflex may be elicited to rule out neuronal loss.

If, it is suspected that a person is suffering from STD, relevant evidence may be collected. After the examination is over, the doctor has to give opinion on two accounts.

1. Whether the person is capable of performing sexual intercourse or not?
2. Whether there is an evidence of recent sexual intercourse?

The capability to perform sexual intercourse depends on erection of the penis. It is naturally assumed that all normal males who have well developed sexual organs are capable of erection, thus can perform sexual intercourse. So, the opinion about capability to perform sexual intercourse is given in a double negative form like "There is nothing to suggest that this person is not capable of performing sexual intercourse".

If it is suspected that person may have some erectile dysfunction, he should be examined for chronic diseases like diabetes, hypertension, chronic alcoholism, neuropathies, or some psychic reasons. The opinion about recent sexual activity can be given if some stain/injury/redness is seen on penis/scrotum. Previously it was thought that absence of smegma could indicate recent sexual activity. Now it is not relied upon, as smegma collection depends on personal hygiene and circumcision.

Samples may be taken of vaginal epithelial cells, which adhere to penis during sexual intercourse, by taking a wet swab around penis and making microscopic slides. These vaginal cells are rich in glycogen and stain readily with iodine and can easily be inspected microscopically.

Previously, it was common to preserve semen in accused for which accused used to be asked to provide sample by masturbation. In non-cooperative accused, it was obtained by doing prostatic massage. Now this is not done. Sample of blood obtained from finger is preserved on a gauze piece and is dried and then sealed for examination by Forensic Science Laboratory.

Incest

Incest is defined as sexual intercourse between man and woman who are related with blood or by marriage i.e. within forbidden degrees of relationship like a daughter, grand-daughter, sister, step sister, niece, aunt or mother. In India, incest per se is not a crime unless it attracts provisions of rape. However, in many western countries, incest is recorded as a crime and is punishable.

Unnatural Sexual Offences

Section 377 of Indian Penal Code defines sexual offences relating to carnal intercourse against the order of nature with any man, woman or animal. Penetration is sufficient to prove the offence. The unnatural sexual offences are punishable with imprisonment of life or with a term of ten years and also with fine. These offences are classified as

1. Sodomy
2. Buccal coitus
3. Bestiality

Incidence

In India, unnatural sexual offences as mentioned above are quite less in percentage as compared to western countries.

The sodomy is frequent with small children working in tea stalls, workshop or offices. The sodomy has also been reported in prisoners or in armed forces especially those posted in the hilly areas.

Sodomy

It is also called buggery and is defined as anal intercourse between man and man or between man and woman. If the passive agent is a young child, it is called pedestry. The question of consent does not arise in sodomy, as it is punishable even if it is being done between two consenting adults. Marriage allows only normal intercourse not sodomy. If a couple is caught doing sodomy although they may be married to each other, it is punishable.

Buccal coitus

It is also called sin of Gommorrah when genitalia are stimulated by mouth or penis is introduced in mouth. Sudden deaths have been reported by impaction of penis into lower part of pharynx or aspiration of semen-ejaculate.

Bestiality

It is defined as when a lower animal is used for sexual gratification. The common animals, which are subjected to this cruelty, are dogs, sheeps, cats or sometime cows or buffalo. Usually penis is inserted into vagina or rectum of the animal. Cases have been reported when animals especially dogs have been stimulated to perform sexual intercourse by inserting their penises into vagina of woman.

Since these offences are punishable under law, they may be brought for medical examination to the doctor.

Examination of Victim or Passive Agent

Usually the police bring a victim or passive agent of sodomy for medical examination to the doctor. The consent of the victim or passive agent must be taken.

The examination should preferably be done in knee elbow position. Abrasion, contusion or laceration may be seen around anal sphincter and person may complain of severe pain. These injuries are more important if the victim is a small boy or girl as compared to the accused person and a great force has been used to penetrate. Blood or semen stains may be present around anus and they should be lifted as described earlier. Swabs from inside and around anus must be taken and examined microscopically.

In a person who is habituated to sodomy following features may be present

1. The shaving of anal hair may be seen.
2. A funnel shaped depression of buttocks toward anus may be seen.
3. There may be a complete relaxation of anal sphincter when lateral traction is applied on both buttocks.
4. The anus may be dilated and patulous with disappearance of radial folds. Prolapse of rectal mucosa may be seen.
5. Old lacerations may be seen around anus.
6. A complete absence of injuries may be there.
7. The presence of STD in form of discharge, chancre or wart may be seen.

Examination of Accused

The examination of accused is quite helpful if done within hours of act as the signs start decreasing with time. The examination of accused must be done on written request of police. Consent is not required. The marks of identifications must be noted. The complete physical examination, as in the case of accused of rape, must be done. There may be abrasion on the prepuce, glans penis or frenulum. Stains of faecal material may be seen on penis. The swabs must be taken from penis and around area to look for faecal material. The blood/semen stains may also be present and should be lifted as described earlier. There may be marks of struggle on the body. If the person is suspected/suffering from STD, the victim should also be examined for the same.

Bestiality is observed in villages in young shepherds who take animals for grazing and remain with them for almost whole day.

Lesbianism

This is female homosexuality which is practiced between

two females and mostly consists in friction of external genital organs by mutually body contact for sexual gratification. In some cases, the clitoris of the woman may be found to be enlarged. In some cases, artificial object may be used for stimulation.

Lesbianism is not punishable as it is not a crime under Section 377 of Indian Penal Code. It is usually found in females who are living together like in hostels or asylums.

Sexual Deviations

The common sexual deviations are described as follows:

1. **Sadism**: This is a sexual perversion where infliction of pain, torture and humiliation to partner, act as sexual stimulation. It may be seen in both sexes but is common in males. Male may inflict injuries by beating with hands or sticks or sometime sexual organs may be targeted, foreign bodies may be inserted in vagina and breast may be contused or sometimes, sadist may get so much excited, that he may murder her (lust murder) or he may eat her body (necrophagia) after raping her corpse (necrophilia).

2. **Masochism**: It is just opposite of sadism where gratification is obtained by getting beaten, tormented or humiliated by sexual partner. It is common in males but occurs in females also. The females may invite males to inflict pain on her or abuse her.

3. **Fetishism:** This perversion is seen in males only. In this male gets sexual gratification just by seeing some part of the woman or her article like undergarment, shoe, clothes etc.

4. **Transvestism:** It is the desire to wear the clothes of opposite sex. It is quite common in homosexuals. Some transvestites may seek medical treatment to change their gender.

5. **Exhibitionism:** it is a deviation in which exhibitionist get pleasure by showing his genitals to women, girls or small children. He may also make some lewd gesture. It is a punishable offence under Sec 294 of Indian Penal Code.

Sexual Harassment

Many cases are reported every day of sexual harassment of women at work places done by the superiors; such cases had created a strong public awareness to fight this evil.

Government of India has taken a serious view to fight this evil. A specific provision has been made in CCS (Conduct Rules), 1964, prohibiting sexual harassment of women by Government servants. This provision is Rule 3-C of CCS (Conduct Rules), 1964. Government against its employees can initiate severe penal action. In private institutions also, rules have been made to deal with this menace. The rules are based on guidelines and norms laid down by Supreme Court, which are as follows.

Guidelines and norms laid down by the Hon'ble Supreme Court in Vishaka and others v State of Rajasthan and others (JT 1997 (7) SC 384].

Having regard to the definition of 'human rights' in Section 2 (d) of the Protection of Human Rights Act, 1993, TAKING NOTE of the fact that the present civil and penal laws in India do not adequately provide for specific protection of women from sexual harassment in work places and that enactment of such legislation will take considerable time.

It is necessary and expedient for employers in work places as well as other responsible persons or institutions to observe certain guidelines to ensure the prevention of sexual harassment of women.

Definition

For this purpose, sexual harassment includes such unwelcome sexually determined behaviour (whether directly or by implication) as:

(a) Physical contact and advances;
(b) A demand or request for sexual favours;
(c) Sexually coloured remarks;
(d) Showing pornography;
(e) Any other unwelcome physical, verbal or non-verbal conduct of sexual nature.

Where any of these acts is committed in circumstances where under the victim of such conduct has a reasonable apprehension that in relation to the victim's employment or work whether she is drawing salary, or honorarium or voluntary, whether in Government, public or private enterprise, such conduct can be humiliating and may constitute a health and safety problem. It is discriminatory, for instance when the woman has reasonable grounds to believe that her objection would disadvantage her in connection with her employment or work including recruiting or promotion or when it creates a hostile work environment. Adverse consequences might be visited if the victim does not consent to the conduct in question or raises any objection thereto.

Criminal Proceedings

Where such conduct amounts to a specific offence under the Indian Penal Code or under any other law, the employer shall initiate appropriate action in accordance with law by making a complaint with the appropriate authority.

In particular, it should ensure that victims, or witnesses are not victimized or discriminated against while dealing with complaints of sexual harassment. The victims of sexual harassment should have the opinion to seek transfer of the perpetrator or their own transfer.

Medico-Legal Issues In AIDS and STD

AIDS and STD have raised a lot of medico-legal issues in India and abroad.
The issues can be divided into

- (a) Medical
- (b) Social
- (c) Ethical
- (d) Legal

Medical Issue

The issue, which often raises controversy, is rights of patients or victims of AIDS and STD. Every patient or victim has the right to receive treatment for the disease. AIDS testing is not compulsory in India. Nobody can be forced to go for such testing. However, government has the right to enforce it during screening tests for government jobs. It is common knowledge that hospital workers can get infected while treating AIDS patients and can bring lawsuits for compensation. The patients can be referred to designated hospitals in case of AIDS/STD where adequate facilities are provided to deal with such cases.

Social and Ethical Issues

In our society, carrying of AIDS/STD is a big stigma and doctors are duty bound to maintain secrecy to protect the identity of patients. They can disclose this information only after express consent of patients or relatives in case of deceased. However, in certain cases information can be divulged and this is called as Privilege Communication.

Privilege Communication

It is agreed that whatever information a doctor has acquired during treatment of that patient has to be kept confidential, but doctor has to perform his duty to society also. In such cases, disclosure of information is called privilege communication. In this regard, we have to understand what is absolute and privilege communication.

(a) Absolute Privilege

It applies to any statement made in court of law or parliament or state assembly. It also extends to statement made to lawyer during preparation for a court hearing as whatever has been said in these cases cannot be a ground for libel or slender.

(b) Qualified Privilege

Outside above any disclosure made by the doctor can be protected if following conditions are met:

1. The statement must not be malicious and must be in good faith to a person who has the right to receive it. Like if a person suffering from STD intends to use public swimming pool, the doctor can make disclosure about his disease to incharge of swimming pool but not to any other person.
2. Only relevant information needs to be conveyed to appropriate authority, not the whole medical history of the individual.

In 1998, the honourable Supreme Court of India passed an order in a case where a patient has sued the doctor as he has disclosed to his fiancée that he is suffering from AIDS and subsequently his marriage was cancelled on receipt of this information. The honourable Supreme Court observed 'So long as the person is not cured of the communicable venereal disease or impotency, the right to marry cannot be enforced through a court of law and shall be treated as suspended right and if a person suffering from the dreadful disease like AIDS, knowingly marries a woman and thereby transmits the infection to that woman, he would be guilty of offences under Section 269 IPC [negligent act likely to spread infection/disease dangerous to life] and Section 270 IPC [malignant act likely to spread infection/disease dangerous to life]. Moreover where there is a clash of the fundamental rights, as in this instant case, namely, the doctor's right to privacy as part of right of life and the bride's right to lead a healthy life, which is her fundamental right under Article 21, the right which would advance public morality or public interest, would alone be enforced through process of law.

(c) Legal Rights

Affliction of AIDS and STD raises a lot of legal rights of the victims. The victims may sue the assailant for damages and criminal intention. If a person in full knowledge of the fact that he is suffering from AIDS sexually assaults a woman/man with added intention to infect her/him so that she/he will die can also be booked under Section 307 [attempt to murder] or under Section 302 IPC [murder] if person dies because of that along with different sections likes 269 and 270 IPC.

The presence of STD/AIDS on the sexual partner in case of married couple can be taken by the other spouse as a ground of divorce as it can be granted easily if this plea is taken in court of law.

If a person gets AIDS during discharge of professional duties like as in hospital workers, he can sue hospital authorities if sufficient infrastructure facilities are not available. No worker can be discharged from services only on the fact that he is HIV positive, his other health parameters also have to be taken into consideration, if he is fit otherwise, he cannot be removed from service.

References

1. Crime in India 1998. National Crime Records Bureau, Govt.of India, New Delhi. p. 28-30.
2. Franklin CA. Modi's Medical Jurisprudence and Toxicology. 21st edition, Mumbai: N M Tripathi Ltd. 1988; p. 368–397.
3. Sharma R K. Legal aspects of patient care 1st edition, New Delhi: Modern Publishers; 2000. p. 11.

PART VI
Drug Resistance

Chapter 35

Drug Resistance in Sexually Transmitted Diseases

Meera Sharma, Sunil Sethi

Introduction

In all societies, sexually transmitted diseases (STD) are among the most common infections. In the developing countries, three bacterial STD gonorrhoea, chlamydial infections and syphilis rank amongst the top 10 to 20 diseases causing loss of healthy productive life due to major complications such as salpingitis, infertility, ectopic pregnancy and perinatal morbidity. Among the viral STD, infection with human immunodeficiency virus (HIV) has become the leading cause of death during the last two decades. Two other very important viral STD are hepatitis B virus (HBV) and human papilloma virus (HPV) infections. Although bacterial STD remain extremely common in all parts of the world, their incidence is decreasing in most of the developed countries, whereas on the other hand, the global spread of the HIV pandemic in a relentless manner further makes the situation even more grave. The problem has been further compounded by the emergence of drug resistance amongst various agents causing STD, particularly *Neisseria gonorrhoeae*, *Herpes simplex virus* and HIV. The emerging drug resistance warrants constant monitoring, need to look for the new drugs and change of operative plans to control the spread of STD.

Neisseria Gonorrhoeae

In most parts of the world gonococci are resistant to penicillins and tetracyclines, and resistance to multiple agents is also becoming very common. In some developed countries the penicillins are still used effectively, but major resistance problems exist in regions where gonorrhoea is most prevalent. Significant quinolone resistance has emerged in the WHO Regions of the Western Pacific and South-East Asia and has spread to countries on the Pacific rim. Although, there is no documented resistance to the third- generation cephalosporin antibiotics (cefixime–oral and ceftriaxone sodium–injectable), but the cost of these agents limits their use in many developing countries.[1]

Penicillin Resistance

Penicillin had been extensively used in the past for the treatment of gonorrhoea, but today in most parts of the world gonococci are resistant to penicillins and tetracyclines, and resistance to multiple agents is common[1]. Penicillin resistant strains of *N. gonorrhoeae* are more prevalent in developing countries where other effective antibiotics are either not available or are too expensive and contact tracing procedures are not developed. The problem has been further aggravated by appearance of penicillinase producing *N. gonorrhoeae* (PPNG).[2]

PPNG was first reported in 1976 simultaneously from UK and USA, which originated from Africa and South East Asia.[3,4] Most epidemiological investigations have indicated that Far East, Asia and West Africa had been the main foci of PPNG, from where the strains have been imported to other countries.[5] After its first documentation in 1976, has been extensively reported from Philippines, Singapore and West Africa.[5,6] Presently the PPNG are widely distributed throughout the globe; reports of PPNG from more than 40 countries are available in the literature. Resistance can be as high as 80% in some parts of the developing world. Although the true prevalence of penicillin resistance is unknown in the industrialized world. It is a problem in some parts of USA, whereas it is a major problem in the developing countries.[6]

Data from USA and Australia, where good surveillance programs exist have shown that the prevalence of PPNG infections was initially increasing slowly but has markedly increased in the recent years.[7] In the WHO Western Pacific Region, according to 1998 data from 16 countries, particularly high levels of resistance have been recorded in China (62%), Hong Kong (69%), Philippines (82%), Vietnam (77%), Singapore (59%), Republic of Korea (74%) and Mongolia (26%).[1]

In South East Asian Region countries also, PPNG are found in high prevalence. Studies from Thailand and Indonesia show high proportions of both PPNG and chromosomal mediated resistant *Neisseria gonorrhoeae* (CMRNG).[8,9] In India, the first case of PPNG was reported from Chennai in 1980[10] and later from Chandigarh in 1984.[11,12] In Delhi the resistance to penicillin rose from 12.8% in 1973 to 50.5%[13] in 1980 and in Bombay, penicillin resistance was seen in 56% cases in the same period.[14]

Studies from a number of African countries also indicated that a high proportion of isolates were penicillin resistant.[15]

After its first documentation in 1976, extensive research has been carried out on the mechanisms of development of drug resistance amongst *N. gonorrhoeae*. Antibiotic resistance in *N. gonorrhoeae* results from two different mechanisms: either due to mutation in the chromosomal genes or due to plasmid mediated β lactamase production.

In fully sensitive wild strains of *N. gonorrhoeae*, the minimal inhibiting concentration (MIC) for penicillin is <0.06 mg/l but mutation in a series of loci on the chromosome results in small additive increases in penicillin resistance MIC of 1 mg/l or greater. The currently recommended dose of penicillin becomes ineffective with MIC 1 mg/l. The main genetic loci that are involved in chromosomally mediated resistance are: *pen A, pen B and mtr*.[16] Mutation at pen A locus alone results in 8 fold increase in resistance,[17] *pen B* results in a 4 fold increase in resistance to penicillin and tetracycline. Mutation at mtr locus results in 2-4 fold increase in resistance to penicillin. The cumulative effect of these 3 mutations is a 128-fold increase in penicillin resistance.

There are 2 different types of resistance plasmids, viz. endogenous and exogenous plasmids. The endogenous plasmids are considered so because their GC ratio is indistinguishable from the chromosomal DNA of *N. gonorrhoeae*.

Endogenous Plasmids

1. 2.6 megadalton plasmid: No phenotypic character attributed, thus termed 'cryptic'
2. 7.8 megadalton plasmid: Described in 1983 and is again 'cryptic'.
3. 24.5 megadalton plasmid: It co-exists with the 2.6 megadalton plasmid. It is present only in 7–8% strains, although it may be present in as high as 40% strains from South East Asia. It has conjugative properties and is able to mobilize other plasmids like R plasmid.[6] Insertion of the resistance determinant *tetM* into this 24.5 megadalton plasmid results in a plasmid of 25.2 megadalton, thus giving rise to high-level tetracycline resistance.[18]

Exogenous Plasmids

Production of β lactamase (penicillinase) was first shown to be due to exogenous plasmids 3.2 megadalton in strains from Africa and UK and 4.4 megadalton from Asia and USA[3]. Initially, 24.5 megadalton plasmid was found only in 40% of the Asian strains. Because of the conjugative nature of the plasmid, within a very few years, 24.5 megadalton plasmid was found along with 3.2 megadalton plasmid. Another 2.9 megadalton plasmid has been found to code for β lactamase production. Therefore, irrespective of the size of the plasmid, β lactamase enzyme produced is identical and of TEM-1 type. DNA homology studies showed that these plasmids contain 40% of the transposable DNA sequence TnA, which contains the gene Tn2 coding for TEM β lactamase.[6]

Tetracycline Resistance

Although tetracyclines are not recommended for treatment of gonorrhoea, they are widely available and extensively used particularly in many developing countries.

In the WHO Western Pacific study, tetracycline resistant *Neisseria gonorrhoeae* (TRNG) were found to be widely present but unevenly distributed. In 1998, particularly high proportions of TRNG were seen in

Singapore (84%), the Solomon Islands (74%) and Vietnam (35.9%).[1]

TRNG are a significant problem in the WHO South East Asia Region (SEAR), particularly in Thailand and Indonesia.[9] In India, 28% of 50 consecutive isolates in New Delhi[19] and 10% of 94 isolates from Bangladesh were reported to be TRNG.[20]

Both chromosomal and plasmid-borne resistance against tetracyclines are found in gonococcal infection, the later being responsible for high level resistance.[16,18] Chromosomal resistance is linked to the *mtr* and *penB* gene alterations.[16] High-level tetracycline resistance in gonococci results from the acquisition of the *tetM* determinant and was first reported in 1986.[18] *tetM* in *N. gonorrhoeae* is located on a self-mobilizing plasmid and exists as 'Dutch' and 'American' types, which differ slightly.[21]

A steady rise in resistance to tetracycline occured from 5.6% in 1973 to 27.8% in 1982[22] and later 48.1% strains resistant to tetracycline were reported from North India.[23]

Spectinomycin Resistance

This injectable agent retains its activity against *N. gonorrhoeae* in most parts of the world. In the Western Pacific Region, 8% of strains from military personnel in the Philippines were spectinomycin-resistant.[24] In 1990, 8.9% strains from Thailand were spectinomycin-resistant, whereas no resistance was detected in 1994–1995.[24-25] In several African studies, all isolates have been reported to be susceptible to spectinomycin.[1] Therefore, although there have been several documented episodes of spectinomycin resistance in *N. gonorrhoeae* but it has not spread possibly because of the limited use of the antibiotic.

In *N. gonorrhoeae*, resistance to spectinomycin or to aminoglycosides usually occurs via a single-step chromosomal mutation, resulting in high-level resistance.[1]

Ciprofloxacin Resistance

As the gonococci were extremely susceptible to quinolones and these drugs were extensively recommended for the treatment of the drug resistant *N. gonorrhoeae*. Ciprofloxacin and ofloxacin are the primary treatment regime in a number of countries. However, gradually, quinolone-resistant gonococci

(QRNG) emerged and spread in areas with high burden of gonococcal disease. The development of resistance was mainly due to antibiotic overuse or misuse.[1] Resistance, which is exclusively chromosomally mediated, has developed incrementally. Recently a number of gonococcal strains have been identified with high level fluoroquinolone resistance. In the Western Pacific regions, the highest proportion of quinolone resistant strains were seen in the Philippines (63%), Hong Kong (48.8%), China (54.2%) and the Republic of Korea (11.2%).[1]

In South-East Asia, both low and high level QRNG have been detected including India, Sri Lanka, Myanmar and Nepal. This severely limits its therapeutic use.[1]

In Africa, quinolones are rarely used because they are generally not available, although there are very few available data of quinolone resistance.[1]

Quinolone resistant isolates have been reported from various parts of our country. In Delhi, 50% of the isolates showed resistance to ciprofloxacin in 1997.[26] Similarly, ciprofloxacin resistant strains have been reported from Mumbai.[27]

The targets of the quinolones are topoisomerases, including DNA gyrase. High-level resistance is mediated by alteration of the target sites, via mutation in the *gyrA* gene. Multiple mutations also occur in the *parC* gene, which codes for the production of topoisomerase IV, a secondary target for quinolones in gonococci. Quinolone resistance is almost exclusively mediated by chromosomal mutations, which affect either the target sites or access of the antibiotic to the cell.[1]

The first step towards diagnosis of drug resistant *N. gonorrhoeae* is clinical suspicion. Then further evaluation is necessary like laboratory tests, and if PPNG is isolated, proper treatment and follow up is necessary. There are various techniques for demonstration of β lactamase production, viz. acidometric test, rapid iodometric test or chromogenic cephalosporin method. With the emergence of PPNG, extensive research work was carried out on the drugs effective on them. Spectinomycin and aminoglycosides had been recommended for treatment of infection with the resistant strains. But with the development of resistance against these drugs as well, the drugs currently recommended are: ceftriaxone or cefixime. The ciprofloxacin is being used only in those areas where quinolone resistance has not yet been reported.[1]

Haemophilus Ducreyi

During 1930s, sulphonamides used to be very effective therapy for chancroid. In 1970, drug resistant strains of *H. ducreyi* started emerging leading to clinically significant treatment failures. For several years, *H. ducreyi* infections were treated with trimethoprim sulphamethoxazole combinations but resistance emerged against this regime also (initially in Thailand and subsequently in Kenya and Rwanda).[28] Erythromycin is still an effective treatment with no confirmed reports of emergence of resistance. Fluoroquinolones are now extensively being used for the treatment of chancroid.

Many isolates of *H. ducreyi* possess β lactamase, which is a TEM 1 β lactamase derived from Tn2 transposon. A 6000 kDa plasmid codes for this. Other plasmids 7300, 5700 and 3200 kDa have also been demonstrated. The larger plasmids are same with the 2 types of plasmids of *N. gonorrhoeae*. In Africa, all strains tested have been reported to produce penicillinase. Resistance to other antibiotics is also common. *TetM* resistance factor has been detected in *H. ducreyi*. It is located in a conjugative plasmid of 34000 kDa.[6]

Herpes Simplex Virus *(HSV)*

Drug resistance in viruses is defined as ED50 significantly higher than the normally achievable therapeutic concentration. Mostly, resistance is due to point mutations.

Strains resistant to any of the common drugs, nucleoside analogues or phosphonacetic acid have changes either in thymidine kinase (TK) or DNA polymerase genes.

Herpes virus TK is not essential for replication of the virus and therefore many different kinds of mutations are possible giving rise to lack of functional enzymes and hence to drug resistance. In contrast, DNA polymerase is always essential for replication of the virus and therefore only a few base substitutions leading to subtle changes in a functional protein are allowed, which does not compromise the normal functioning of the enzyme.[29]

It is not yet very clear, why the drug resistant strains are so rare among the clinical isolates. After more than 10 years of widespread use of acyclovir, the incidence of drug resistant strains has remained constant at <3%.[30]

Approximately 5% of immunocompromised subjects shed drug resistant virus. All the 3 different mechanisms play a role in development of drug resistance, viz. TK Tk^r and DNApol^r. Foscarnet resistance is selectively due to base substitution at DNA polymerase gene.

Therapy of acyclovir resistant HSV infection includes use of DNA polymerase inhibitors like foscarnet and nucleotide analogues like cidofovir. Bryant et al[31] reported resistance to both acyclovir and foscarnet in leukemic child.

Human Immunodeficiency Virus (HIV)[32–34]

There are mainly three groups of antiretroviral drugs used for the treatment of HIV infection. These are nucleoside analogue reverse transcriptase inhibitors, non-nucleoside analogue reverse transcriptase inhibitors and protease inhibitors. Among these nucleoside analogue reverse transcriptase inhibitors have been extensively studied and used for therapy in HIV infected patients.

Drug resistance was first demonstrated against zidovudine (AZT) and then subsequently it was shown against all other nucleoside inhibitors. Resistance to non-nucleoside reverse transcriptase inhibitors is even more common and the strains are cross-resistant. Resistance against various proteinase inhibitors has also been demonstrated.[29]

HIV-1 variants resistant to AZT have been described in many instances. The degree of resistance increases with the duration of treatment. It has been seen that, more than 16 weeks of AZT therapy leads to high-level resistance in 15% of patients. These HIV-1 variants, resistant to AZT are transmissible from person to person and thus the prevalence of resistance in HIV-1 in the population is increasing gradually. HIV-1 isolates resistant to didanosine (nucleoside analogue reverse transcriptase inhibitors) have also been described, especially with didanosine monotherapy. Resistance has been described with other nucleoside analogue reverse transcriptase inhibitors like zalcitabine, lamivudine and also occasionally with stavudine. Recently, HIV-1 variants resistant to multiple reverse transcriptase inhibitors have increasingly been described, particularly with prolonged therapy. HIV-1 isolates resistant to protease inhibitors like saquinavir and indinavir have also been reported. Resistance of HIV-1 to ritonavir has been well documented, both *in vitro* as well as *in vivo*.

Drug resistance in HIV is again due to point mutations giving rise to altered affinity of reverse transcriptase for its inhibitors. Point mutations and sometimes sequences of mutations lead to progressively increasing resistance. For example, resistance mutations during AZT therapy appear in an orderly fashion and mutations at two codons, at 41 and 215, are associated with highest levels of resistance and rapid progression of the disease. Resistance against didanosine involves mutation at codon 74. Mutation at codon 69 increases resistance against zalcitabine by almost five fold.[32] The replication of HIV, like any other retroviruses, is characterized by conversion of RNA into complementary single stranded DNA and then into double stranded DNA by the viral enzyme reverse transcriptase. All polymerases make base incorporation errors, but DNA dependant DNA polymerases 'proof read' and correct these errors. On the other hand, reverse transcriptase does not proof read and consequently, the fidelity of replication is low. The estimated error of reverse transcriptase is high, i.e. 10^{-4}/base, i.e. one base pair error per every 10,000 bases incorporated.

Combination chemotherapy (zidovudine plus didanosine; zidovudine plus lamivudine etc.) has been tried in several trials with success. Multi-drug therapy requires the virus to develop multiple separate mutations to develop resistance to all the anti-retroviral agents used and thereby, significantly increases the delay period in development of resistance. There is now little doubt about the necessity for use of combination of anti-retroviral drugs to achieve long-term suppression of HIV replication. Combination of different agents have shown to decrease HIV viral load by 2–3 logs and allow suppression of HIV RNA to below the threshold level for detection, for even more than 2 years.

Treponema Pallidum

Penicillin is the most effective drug in the treatment of syphilis and resistance is unknown. The co-infection of syphilis with HIV may cause problem in the management of syphilis. Crossen et al[34] report two patients with neurosyphilis who failed to respond to penicillin and were successfully treated with ceftriaxone. One of the patient had tested positive for CSF VDRL and was treated with weekly benzathine penicillin 2.4 MU for 4 weeks with good response. The CSF counts improved but CSF VDRL remained positive. The investigations for syphilis were normal but the patient developed psychiatric symptoms and was given injectable ceftriaxone 1000 mg/daily for 14 days with dramatic

improvement in symptoms. Second patient of untreated syphilis was given penicillin injection and his psychiatric symptoms improved but after few years he deteriorated without any sign of infection with syphilis. Because of the previous experience the patient was treated with ceftriaxone and had dramatic improvement in his condition. The above instances suggest failure of penicillin in neurosyphilis but it would require further studies to demonstrate whether it was due to resistance to penicillin or some other factors.

Human Papilloma Virus

The results of treatment of human papilloma virus with antiviral drugs are variable. Recently the resistance of HPV-6 to interferon-alpha have been suggested. Garcia Millian et al[35] proposed that HPV-6E$_7$ almost completely inhibits induction of interferon responsive element that promotes transient transinfection, there by resulting in ineffectiveness of the drug. They also demonstrated the absence of local immune response in the lesion of HPV by demonstrating absence of mRNA for interleukin-15 and IFN gamma. Further it was shown that HPV negative patients develop resistance to recombinant IFN- alpha-2b and increased level of antiIFN alpha 2b antibodies but responded to neutral IFN-alpha, suggesting the development of resistance to IFN is a complex phenomenon resulting from host and viral elements. Koonsaeng et al[36] reported similar drug resistance to IFN and isotretinoin while treating vulval intraepithelial neoplasia-III.

Chlamydia Trachomatis

Tetracycline is the first line drug till today in the most parts of the country for the treatment of chlamydial infection. The widespread and indiscriminate use of tetracycline has given rise to drug resistance. Lenart et al,[37] reported that chlamydial strains of human serovars L$_2$ (LGV-434) in a tissue culture treated with tetracycline developed complete absence of large aberrant reticulate bodies with increased concentration of tetracycline but on stoppage of tetracycline there was regrowth of chlamydia on the tissue culture, suggesting resistance to tetracycline. Somani et al[38] reported multi-drug resistance to doxycycline, azithromycin, and ofloxacin by identifying the identical genotypes of organism and suggested the cause could be widespread use of subtherapeutic doses of antibiotics. Stamm reported[39] antimicrobial resistance in patients who failed to respond to treatment or persistence of pneumonia by *Chlamydia trachomatis*.

Trichomonas Vaginalis

The widely used antibiotic for treatment of *T. vaginalis* is metronidazole. The resistance to metronidazole seems to be increasing with time. Schmid et al[40] did in vitro culture of vaginal discharge and correlated with the therapeutic outcome and found resistance of *T. vaginalis* metronidazoleo A Sobel et al[41] used tinidazole for treatment of 24 cases of metronidazole resistant *T. vaginalis*.

It is apparent from the above description that development of drug resistance is an ongoing process and constant monitoring is essential for treatment and control of all STD caused by bacterial, viral, chlamydial or trichomonal agents.

References

1. Antibiotic resistance in *Neisseria gonorrhoeae*. John T (ed). Antimicrobial resistance in Neisseria gonorrhoeae. WHO Collaborating Centre for STD and HIV, Sydney, Australia 2001.

2. Sethi S, Sharma M, Kumar B. Pencillinase producing Strains of *Neisseria gonorrhoeae*. Bull PGI; 1999; 33: 71-74.

3. Phillips I. Beta lactamase producing, penicillin resistant gonococcus. Lancet 1976; 2: 656-657.

4. Ashford WA, Golash RG, Hemming VG. Penicillinase-producing *Neisseria gonorrhoeae*. Lancet 1976; 2: 657-658.

5. Reyn A. Drug susceptibility pattern of *Neisseria gonorrhoeae*: A worldwide review. Asian J Infect Dis 1977; 1: 1-14.

6. Jephcott AE. Gonorrhoea, chancroid and granuloma venereum. In: Collier L, Balows A, Sussman M, eds. Topley and Wilson's Microbiology and Microbial Infections. 9th edn. London: Arnold; 1998. p. 623-640.

7. Lind I. Antimicrobial resistance in *Neisseria gonorrhoeae*. Clin Infect Dis 1997; 24: S93-S97

8. Lind I, Hutapea N. Antimicrobial resistance of *Neisseria gonorrhoeae* in Medan, North Sumatra, 1996. Abstract O145. *Proceedings International* Congress of Sexually Transmitted Diseases, Seville, 1997.

9. Knapp JS, Wongba C, Limpakarnjanarat K, et al. Antimicrobial susceptibilities of strains of *Neisseria gonorrhoeae* in Bangkok, Thailand: 1994-1995. Sex Transm Dis 1997; 24: 142-148

10. Vijayalakshmi K, Gopalan KN, Gopal Krishnan B, Mohan Ram CC. The first case of beta lactamase strain of *N. gonorrhoeae* from Madras. Indian J Sex Transm Dis 1982; 3: 13-14.

11. Sharma M, Kumar B, Agarwal KC, Sharma SK, Kaur S. Penicillinase producing strains of *Neisseria gonorrhoeae* from Chandigarh. Indian J Med Res 1984; 80: 512-515.

12. Sharma M. Agarwal KC, Kumar B, Sharma SK. Penicillin resistant gonococci. Indian J Dermatol Venereol Leprol 1985; 51: 22-25.

13. Masshoor K, Bhujwala RA, Pandhi RK, et al. Susceptibility of *Neisseria gonorrhoeae* to penicillin, ampicillin, tetracycline, erythromycin, cotrimoxazole and supristol-an in vitro study Indian J Pathol Microbiol 1980; 23: 171-175.

14. Moses JM, Desai MS, Bhosle CB, Tarasi MS. Present pattern of antibiotic sensitivity of gonococcal strains isolated in Bombay. Br J Vener Dis 1971; 47: 273-278.

15. Osoba AO, Path FRC. Overview of penicillinase producing *Neisseria gonorrhoeae* in Africa. African J of Sex Transm Dis 1986; 51-64.

16. Cannon JG, Sparling PF. The genetics of gonococcus. Ann Rev Microbiol. 1984; 38: 111-113.

17. Spratt BG. Hybrid penicillin binding proteins in penicillin resistant strains of *Neisseria gonorrhoea*. Nature 1988; 332: 173-176.

18. Morse SA, Johnson SR, Biddle JW, Roberts MC. High level Tetracycline resistance in *Neisseria gonorrhoeae* is result of acquisition of Streptococcal *tet M* determinant. Antimicrob Agents Chemother 1986; 30: 664-670.

19. Bhalla P, Sethi K, Reddy BS, Mathur MD et al. Antimicrobial susceptibility and plasmid profile of *Neisseria gonorrhoeae* in India [New Delhi] Sex Transm Inf 1998; 74: 210-212.

20. Bhuiyan BU, Rahman M, Miah NR. Antimicrobial susceptibilities and plasmid contents of *Neisseria gonorrhoeae* isolates from commercial sex workers in Dhaka, Bangladesh: emergence of high-level resistance to ciprofloxacin. J Clin Microbiol 1999; 37: 1130-1136.

21. Gascoyne-Binzi DM, Heritage J, Hawkey PM. Nucleotide sequences of the tet(M) genes from the American and Dutch type tetracycline resistance plasmids of *Neisseria gonorrhoeae*. J Antimicrob Chemother 1993; 32: 667-676.

22. Bhujwala RA, Pandhi RK, Bhargava NC, et al. *Neisseria gonorrhoeae* and its sensitivity to penicillin and tetracycline over a decade. Indian J Med Microbiol 1983; 1: 43.

23. Sharma M, Kumar B, Sharma SK, Kaur P, Agarwal KC. Antimicrobial susceptibility pattern of *N. gonorrhoeae* to penicillin, tetracycline and kanamycin. Indian J Med Microbiol 1986; 4: 111-114.

24. Clendennen TE, Echeverria P, Saengeur S, Kees ES, Beslego JW, Wignall FS. Antibiotic susceptibility survey of *Neisseria gonorrhoeae* in Thailand. Antimicrob Agents Chemother 1992; 36: 1682-1687.

25. Clendennen TE, Hames CS, Kees ES, et al. In vitro antibiotic susceptibilities of *Neisseria gonorrhoeae* isolates in the Philippines. Antimicrob Agents Chemother 1992; 36: 277-282.

26. Rattan A, Kumari S, Khanna N, Pandhi et al. Emergence

of fluoroquinolones resistant *Neisseria gonorrhoeae* in New Delhi, India Sex Transm Inf 1998; 74: 229.

27. Diveka A, Goga A. Ciprofloxacin resistance in *Neisseria gonorrhoeae* isolated in Mumbai (formerly Bombay). Indian Sex Transm Inf 1999; 75(2): 122.

28. Bogaerts J, Kestens L, Tello WM, et al. Failure of treatment for Chancroid in Rwanda is not related to HIV infection: in vitro resistance of *Haemophilus ducreyi* to trimethoprim sulphamethoxazole. Clin Infect Dis 1995; 20: 924-930.

29. Field HJ, Whitley RJ. Antiviral chemotherapy. In: Collier L, Balows A, Sussman M, eds. Topley and Wilson's Microbiology and Microbial Infections. 9th edn. London: Arnold; 1998. p. 989-1010.

30. Collins P, Ellis MN. Sensitivity monitoring of clinical isolates of herpes simplex virus to acyclovir. J Med Virol 1993; 1: 58-66.

31. Bryant P, Sasadeusz J, Carapetiz J, et al. Successful treatment of forcarnet-resistant herpes simplex stomatitis with intravenous cidofir in a child. Pediatr Infect Dis 2001; 20: 1083-1086.

32. Joseph JE Jr, Martin SH. Antiviral therapy of human immunodeficiency virus infection. In: Holmes KK, Mardh PA, Sparling PF, et al. eds. Sexually Transmitted Diseases, 3rd edn. New York: Mc Graw Hill; 1999. p. 1009-1030.

33. Ballard AL, Cane PA, Pillay D. HIV drug resistance: genotypic assays and their possible applications. Sex Transm Inf 1998; 74: 243-248.

34. Crossen WM, Nieku H, Nielson O, et al. Ceftriaxone treatment of penicillin resistant neurosyphilis in alcoholic patients. J Neurol Neurosurg Psychiatry 1995; 59: 194-195.

35. Garcia-Millian R, Santos A, Perea SE, et al. Molecular analysis of resistance of interferon in patients with laryngeal papillomatosis. Cytokines Cell Mol Ther 1999; 5: 79-85.

36. Koonsaeng S, Verschraegen C, Freedman R, et al. Successful treatment of recurrent vulvar intraepithelial neoplasia resistant to interferon and isotretinoin with cidofovir. J Med Virol 2001; 64: 195-198.

37. Lenart J, Andersen AA, Rockey DD. Growth and development of tetracycline – resistant *Chlamydia suis*. Antimicrob Agents Chemother 2001; 45: 2198-2203.

38. Somani J, Bhullar VB, Workowski KA, Farshy CE, Black CM. Multiple drug-resistant *Chlamydia trachomatis* associated with clinical treatment failure. J Infect Dis 2000; 181: 1421-1427.

39. Stamm WE. Potential for antimicrobial resistance in *Chlamydia pneumoniae*. J Infect Dis 2000; 181: S456-S459.

40. Schmid G, Narcisi E, Mosure D, et al. Prevalence of metronidazole-resistant *Trichomonas vaginalis* in gynaecology clinic. J Reprod Med 2001; 46: 545-549.

41. Sobel JD, Nyirjesy P, Brown W. Tinidazole therapy for metronidazole-resistant vaginal trichomoniasis. Clin Infect Dis 2001; 33: 1341-1346.

PART VII
Control of Sexually Transmitted Diseases

Chapter 36

Control of Sexually Transmitted Diseases

Neena Khanna

Introduction

Sexually transmitted diseases (STD) are considered a major global health problem, with more than 330 million cases being reported every year. Of these, over 80% of patients are believed to be from developing countries. In India, STD are one of the most prevalent communicable diseases,[1] though the data on the pattern of STD is likely to be fallacious due to a lack of comprehensive national registry, the inefficient reporting and data collection systems and the fact that the patients with STD seek help not from the public health facility but, from the private sector, reporting from where is understandably abysmal. The annual incidence rate of STD in India is estimated to be about 5%, with 3-4% of rural population being suspected to be infected with STD at any particular time. On an average, 40 million new cases of STD are estimated to occur every year.

STD pose an enormous public health problem in view of the large number of patients, the innumerable, mostly undocumented complications and the long term suffering. STD preferentially affect the economically productive sections of the society (20-40 years of age) causing loss of productive life measured as disability-adjusted-life-years (DALYS) lost.[2] The arrival of the human immune deficiency virus (HIV) pandemic has complicated the situation, especially in the background of amplified transmission of HIV infection in the presence of STD.

History of STD Control Programmes in India

Pre HIV Era

In 1949, independent India responded to the problem of venereal diseases (VD) by launching the National VD control programme with emphasis on the control of syphilis (Fig. 1). This eschewed focus on syphilis shifted in 1981-82 onto teaching, training and research in the various aspects of STD and the programme was renamed National STD control programme. To enhance the clinical and para-clinical aptitude of in-service doctors

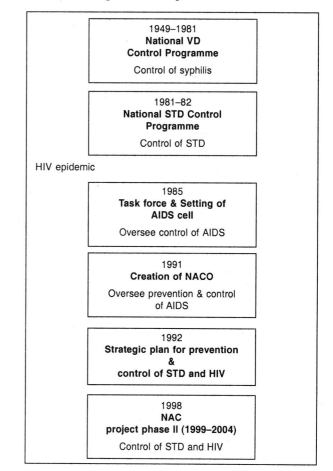

Fig. 1 History of VD/STD Control Programmes in India

and para-medical staff, two training centres were established one at Delhi and the other in Madras (now Chennai). The training facilities were augmented by establishing regional training centres in Calcutta (Kolkata), Nagpur and Hyderabad. Surveillance centres (27 in number) and research centres (40 in number) have also since been set up to enhance the skills of the concerned technical personnel.[4] STD clinics (504 in numbers) attached either to medical colleges and teaching hospitals or to the district hospitals are functioning in various parts of the country.

National AIDS Control Programme

The appearance of the HIV pandemic added a new dimension to the STD control programme. As the first reports of HIV infection began appearing, the initial response of the Government and community was almost hysterical, quite similar to what had happened in other parts of the world.[5] However, since the initial aberrant response, the Government of India in conjunction with ICMR is now genuinely committed to focus resources and priorities to contain the HIV epidemic in the country.[6] Thus, in 1985 the Government of India constituted a Task Force to look into the HIV epidemic and an AIDS cell was established in the Directorate of Health Services, New Delhi to co-ordinate activities pertaining to AIDS in the country. In 1991, National AIDS Control Organization (NACO) was officially created as the executive governmental organization to oversee the AIDS prevention and control efforts in India through the National AIDS Control Programme (NACP). To meet the onslaught of the HIV epidemic, in 1992 the Government of India drew up a "Strategic Plan for Prevention and Control of AIDS" for the period 1992-1997.[7] This strategic plan has received support from the World Bank (WB), the World Health Organization (WHO) and other international agencies. The aim of the plan was to establish a comprehensive, multi-sectoral programme for the prevention and control of AIDS in India, which would:

- Prevent HIV transmission.
- Decrease the morbidity and mortality associated with the infection.
- Minimise the socio-economic impact resulting from HIV infection.

Recognising the close relationship and the interaction between HIV and STD the implementation of the STD control programme was merged with NACP; certain components of the STD Control Programme like teaching, training and epidemiology, however, have remained independent.

Problems with the Strategic Plan for Prevention and Control of AIDS

Although the strategic plan was comprehensive, operationalizing was not easy because of several reasons:

- It failed to generate commitment and sense of urgency.
- Though the primary goal of the programme was to create awareness, the plan failed to do the same as cultural sensibilities hindered open discussion about sexuality.
- Denial of the problem of HIV continued, and this impeded the implementation of the programme. There were widely differing estimates about the magnitude of the problem and information collected from sero-surveillance, studies on the epidemiology of STD and behavioural patterns was not collated to construct a picture of the likely situation.
- Staffing was inadequate: key positions were not filled for long periods and there was a rapid turnover of officials, resulting in lack of continuity. Officials were over burdened with other responsibilities and failed to focus on the goals targeted by the NACP
- There were limitations of the methods used for IEC and there was lack of monitoring of the impact of these.
- Guidelines for Non Government Organization (NGO) failed to effectively mobilise NGO to participate in the National Programme because there was a lack of clarity of the roles and linkages between Centre, State and NGO.

National AIDS Control Project Phase II

However, in the last 3 years the situation has dramatically changed and the Government's response has moved into fast gear in an attempt to catch up with, and bring under control the fast growing epidemic. Phase II of the NAC Project (1999-2004) has been launched in 1999. It is a 100% centrally sponsored scheme implemented in 32 states/Union territories (UTs) and 3 principal corporations (Ahmedabad, Chennai and Mumbai) through AIDS control societies.

Strategies and Objectives of NAC Project Phase II

Aims, objectives, targets and components of NAC project phase II are described in detail in Chapter 3.

Achievements in Control of STD and HIV Infection

The National AIDS prevention and control strategy has been drafted to prevent the HIV infection from further spread and to reduce the socio-economic impact of HIV/AIDS. To achieve these goals the following targets have been attained:

- All district women's hospitals have been strengthened for management of reproductive tract infections (RTI) including STD. This is in addition to the already existing STD clinics functioning in medical colleges and district hospitals.
- Voluntary Counselling and Testing Centres (VCTC) have been established in medical colleges and major hospitals to facilitate testing for HIV with pre test and post test counselling. Districts are being covered in a phased manner to cover the whole country in 2-3 years.
- Financial support has been provided to all States for management of opportunistic infections for people living with HIV/AIDS.
- Annual round of Sentinel Surveillance for HIV infection is carried out during August-October at various sites (Antenatal Clinics, STD Clinics and Intravenous Drug Users) to understand the nature and progress of epidemic and to study the trend of the spread.
- Members of Parliament from Lok Sabha and Rajya Sabha and the Chief Ministers/Health Ministers of six high prevalence States have been sensitized to the enormous problem of HIV/ AIDS.
- An appeal has been made to the captains of

business houses in India to form a business coalition to deal with the problem of HIV/ AIDS effectively at workplaces in collaboration with the public and NGO.

- Targeted intervention projects for poor and marginalized high risk groups have been initiated in all States and Union Territories (UT). These projects are aimed at providing reproductive health care services, promoting the use of condom and counselling.
- Specific guidelines have been developed to encourage participation of NGO in the prevention and control of HIV/AIDS.
- For the expeditious flow of funds and implementation of the programmes, State AIDS Control Societies have been constituted in all States/UT with adequate technical and managerial staff.
- Community care centres have been established in States with high prevalence of HIV.
- For the protection of medical and para medical workers attending HIV/AIDS cases, from acquiring HIV infection in case they get accidental injury like needle prick/sharp injury, provision has been made to provide free post exposure prophylaxis (PEP) using antiretroviral drugs.
- Collaboration has been established with Ministries of Defence, Railways, Sports and Youth Affairs and organizations like Employees State Insurance and Steel Authority of India, etc. in prevention and control of HIV/AIDS.
- School AIDS Education Programmes have been initiated in all States/UT with the involvement of Ministry of Human Resource Development and some NGO.
- A National Family Health Awareness Campaign is conducted twice a year to sensitize the community, particularly in urban slums and rural areas about STD and HIV/AIDS.
- A comprehensive training programme for medical and para-medical workers has been initiated to train them in prevention and control of HIV/ AIDS.
- A feasibility study of prevention of Mother to Child Transmission (MCTC) of HIV by administering short course zidovudine has been implemented in 11 centres in states of Maharashtra, Tamil Nadu, Karnataka, Andhra Pradesh and Manipur

National AIDS Control Programme Hierarchy of Functioning (Fig. 2, 3)[6-8]

At the Head Quarters

At the national level, a National AIDS Committee, a National AIDS Control Board (NACB) and NACO were set up for policy formulation, technical advice and monitoring of the implementation of the NACP in India. NACO would operate through the AIDS Control Cells established in the States and Union Territories. An Empowered Committee and a Technical Advisory Committee were also constituted in every state for implementation of the programme.

The NACB at the Centre and the Empowered Committees at the State were set up to facilitate financial, technical and administrative work and to improve work relating to creation of posts, release of funds and appointment of staff. While the NACB at the centre has functioned effectively for the smoother implementation of the NACP, the Technical Advisory Committees and the Empowered Committees in the States have not been so effective in facilitating the programme at the state level.

Peripheral-Infrastructure

STD control activities can be delivered through a system which is either vertical or horizontal.[9] The vertical system has the advantage of delivering quality care but most often, these clinics are located in urban areas which are inaccessible to a majority of the population. The stigma of visiting a STD clinic further precludes their optimal utilization. A horizontal STD care facility which has been integrated into the primary health care facility has the tremendous advantage of being easily accessible to majority of the patients, of being non-stigmatizing, thereby increasing the acceptability of the service, more particularly to women. However, in the bargain the quality of service rendered is not quite the best, largely because the staff at such primary health care level is already over-burdened, is not optimally trained to handle STD patients and the attitude of the staff towards STD patients is often discriminatory; there is also the problem of inadequate drug supply and lack of laboratory back-up.

A combination of vertical and horizontal programme seems to be the ideal solution – the vertical component would be responsible for planning, co-ordination and development of new strategies and the horizontal limb would concentrate on implementation and integration at the first health care level.[8,9] The Ministry of Health and Family Welfare in India is now committed to integrate comprehensive STD control strategies in the existing health care system, both at the public and private health care facilities to provide non-stigmatized

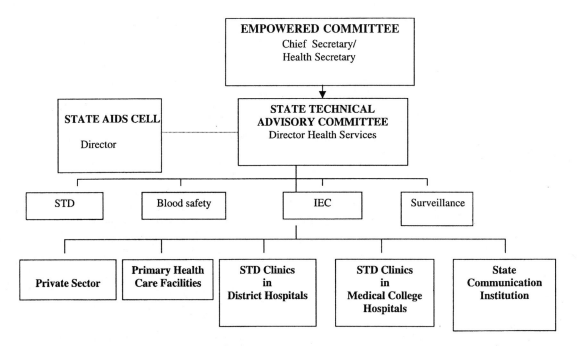

Fig. 2 Organization Structure of State AIDS Control Programme

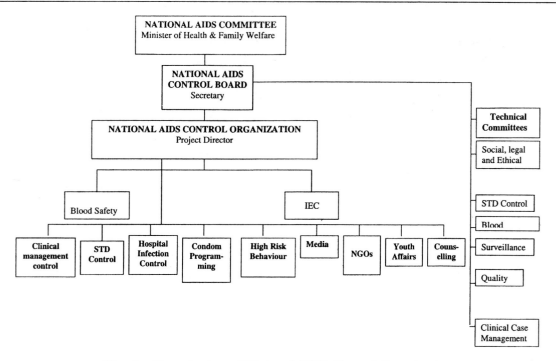

Fig. 3 Organization of National AIDS Control Organization

services with greater accessibility and acceptability to the patients.

Objectives of the STD Control Programme

The STD control component of the NACP has two major objectives:

- Reduce STD cases and thereby control HIV transmission by minimizing the risk factor
- Prevent the short term as well as long term morbidity and mortality due to STD.

The goal of STD control is to be established through developing and employing the following main strategies:

1. Effective and adequate programme management
2. Prevention of transmission of STD/HIV through IEC
3. Adequate and comprehensive case management
4. Increasing access to adequate health care for STD patients
5. Case finding and screening

The implementation of these strategies will be supported by :

i. Training of health care workers in comprehensive STD case management
ii. Development of appropriate laboratory services for diagnosis of STD
iii. Microbiological, socio-behavioural and operational research
iv. Surveillance to follow the epidemiological situation and to monitor and evaluate the implementation of STD control programmes and their effectiveness
v. Condom programming.

1. Effective and Adequate Programme Management

In the centre, for adequate and appropriate management of the programme, an STD consultant is employed by NACP to assist the Additional Project Director (Technical) in all its activities relating to the STD control programme. At the state level, the State AIDS programme officer is assisted by programme officers in the area of health education, STD surveillance and blood safety. The State AIDS cell is responsible for the day to day monitoring and supervision of the programme in each state. NACO supports the development, implementation and monitoring of state STD and AIDS control activities.

2. Prevention of Transmission of STD/HIV Infection Through IEC Activities

IEC activities have been developed for primary and secondary prevention of STD and HIV infection by improving the current awareness of STD and by promoting appropriate health seeking behaviour. The IEC materials provide:

- Basic information
- Modes of transmission of STD, including HIV
- Symptoms of STD
- Need for treatment compliance
- Partner notification
- Prevention of future infection
- Responsible sexual behaviour, safer sex and use of condom.

3. Adequate and Comprehensive STD Case Management

Since ulcerative STD and STD associated with genital discharges are associated with a significant increase in HIV transmission, vigorous control of STD would reduce rates of HIV transmission. NACO has decided to attack the problem of STD at 2 levels.

(a) Primary Health Care Level

To ensure the provision of good quality and effective STD management at the point of first contact health workers, (ANMS, MPW) and Aanganwadi workers are being trained to treat STD patients using a syndromic approach because this approach is effective, has a low cost and can be utilized at the periphery where laboratory facilities are scant; but this approach may result in over-treating patients with more than one antibiotic/chemotherapeutic agent.[10] A simplified module for syndromic management of STD has been prepared and several programmes have been conducted for orientation and training of private health care providers in STD case management by Indian Medical Association in collaboration with NACO.

(b) Specialist Facilities

The vertical arm of the programme exists in the form of 504 STD clinics in medical colleges and in district hospitals. These centres are being strengthened through the provision of laboratory equipment and training of manpower and subserve two main roles :

- Play a role in training of medical and paramedical personnel
- Act as referral centres for first level health care service providers in their catchment area.

4. Increasing Access to Adequate STD Care

The access of STD case management can be increased several folds if the facility is acceptable to the people. The following strategies have been adopted to achieve this:

- STD care services are being integrated into first level health care including MCH /FP and ANC and the number of specialized STD clinics is not being increased. Pilot projects have been conducted in two states (Orissa and Karnataka) to assess the feasibility of integrating STD control activities in the on-going family welfare services.
- A study on the health care seeking behaviour in relation to STD has been conducted to assist in formulation of guidelines for making existing facilities more acceptable and accessible to people with STD.
- Collaboration with other formal and informal health care providers including NGO is being encouraged.
- Providing STD care through mobile clinics is also being studied in order to improve STD case management.

5. Case Finding and Screening

In the absence of a simple diagnostic test for STD, the feasibility of case finding and screening is limited. Where required, a plan will be developed to implement universal screening for syphilis and subsequent treatment in all antenatal clinic attenders.

6. Training of Health Care Workers in Comprehensive STD Case Management

The following manuals have been prepared and circulated to train health care workers in comprehensive STD case management at different levels:

(a) Management of STD

A module, based on the syndromic approach to STD case management has been prepared for use by the first level health care worker. With the help of this module, the health worker should be able to manage 90-95% of all STD patients. The treatment regimes recommended in this publication are deemed to be effective in the Indian context. The syndromes for which recommendations are made include urethral discharge, vaginal discharge, genital ulcers, inguinal swelling, lower abdominal pain, scrotal swelling and ophthalmia neonatorum.

(b) STD Treatment Guidelines

This manual is meant for physicians at the secondary and tertiary care centres.

(c) Laboratory Diagnosis of STD

This manual is intended for use at referral centres.

7. Development of Laboratory Services for Diagnosis of STD

The quality control system for STD laboratories is being strengthened by upgrading the existing syphilis serology quality control system and establishing a quality assurance mechanism for the diagnosis of gonorrhoea. However, it is recognized that the management of STD patients will predominantly be on a clinical basis and lab support will be reserved for:

- Diagnosis of difficult cases.
- Management of treatment failures.
- Research and antibiotic susceptibility monitoring.

8. Research

The following epidemiological and operational research has been carried out:

- Research on prevalence of STD has been carried out in Tamil Nadu, Calcutta and Jaipur and is being conducted in Andhra Pradesh, Himachal Pradesh and Assam.
- A study on the prevalence of STD in pregnant and non-pregnant females attending Family Planning/Maternal and Child Health Clinic in East Delhi has also been undertaken.

- The feasibility of integrating STD services into MCH/FP and antenatal clinics both in the urban as well as in rural areas has been conducted in Orissa and Karnataka.
- The algorithms used in the syndromic approach have been validated
- Activities have been initiated on the development of an antibiotic susceptibility monitoring network for gonorrhoea.

9. Surveillance

This entails surveillance for STD and for HIV and AIDS.

(a) STD Surveillance

An STD surveillance protocol based on sentinel site reporting and epidemiological surveys in different states has been developed. Pilot work on this has been carried out in Tamil Nadu, West Bengal, Rajasthan, Karnataka and Maharashtra.

(b) HIV Surveillance

The objective of HIV surveillance has changed over the years depending on the changing needs and scenario in the country. The main objective of the current surveillance policy is to monitor trends in specific high-risk groups and also to monitor trends in groups considered to represent general populations such as antenatal clinic attenders. Different target groups identified for sentinel surveillance are STD clinic attenders, injecting drug users and pregnant women. The development of the sentinel surveillance system for tracking the progression of the HIV epidemic in India has given reliable information on dates and trends of infection. This has assisted the government to plan effective programmes and service delivery systems.

10. Condom Programming

Apart from abstinence and a mutually faithful monogamous relationship, consistent and proper use of an intact good quality latex rubber condom is a highly efficient mode of preventing transmission of STD and HIV. Recognizing this, the Government of India is strongly supporting the promotion of good quality, low cost condoms for the prevention of STD and HIV infection by:

- Providing technical assistance to manufacturers to produce condoms conforming with the international specifications laid down by the WHO.
- Modifying the Schedule R of Drugs and Cosmetics Act. This stipulates minimal quality standard for condoms manufactured in India.
- Phasing out the dry unlubricated condoms (e.g. Nirodh)
- Strengthening social marketing structures in the Department of Family Welfare as well as the management ability of PVO & NGO to promote and distribute condoms. Social marketing of condoms (where the user pays a subsidised price) is preferred to free distribution.
- Installing condom vending machines at strategic points.
- Interpolating the role of condoms in preventing HIV and STD infections in the IEC programmes of the Department of Family Welfare (which promotes the use of condoms for contraception).
- Supporting and strengthening the ICMR and population research centres for undertaking research on all aspects of condom use.

Intersectoral Collaboration

The challenges posed by HIV/AIDS have implications beyond the health sector. The responses to these challenges must therefore encompass the broadest base possible because the fight against HIV/AIDS/STD cannot succeed without intersectoral collaboration - this forms one of the key components of the second phase of NAC Project. Under this component, activities would be coordinated with other programmes within the Ministry of Health and Family Welfare and other Central Ministries and Departments, as well as those carried out by private corporations, individual groups, voluntary groups and in general society. Collaboration would focus on:

- Learning from the innovative HIV/AIDS programmes that exist in other sectors.
- Sharing in the work of generating awareness.
- Uniting in effort of advocacy and of delivering interventions.

NACO encourages the participation of NGO and Voluntary Organizations in spreading the much needed awareness, and in implementing various interventions in the care of support of the affected and marginalised populations. The State AIDS Control Societies are supporting the organizations with necessary infrastructure and capacity development.

Collaboration within the Government

Apart from Ministry of Health and Family Welfare, several other ministries have responded positively to the challenges posed by HIV/AIDS/STD.

Ministry of Youth Affairs

Ministry of Youth Affairs has several programmes to provide information about AIDS through the National Service Scheme to secondary schools and the university students.

Ministry of Human Resource Development

Ministry of Human Resource Development has initiated AIDS education for school students on a co-curricular basis.

Ministry of Information and Broadcasting

Ministry of Information and Broadcasting has given appropriate publicity to the cause of HIV through audio, audiovisual and multimedia mass communication. Several advertising agencies have also been roped in to create attractive information pamphlets.

Indian Council of Medical Research

Indian Council of Medical Research (ICMR) is actively focussed on control of STD/HIV. It has:

- Developed surveillance and research strategies.
- Developed programme for blood safety and laboratory development.
- Trained State AIDS programme officers and AIDS epidemiologists in the techniques of sentinel surveillance.
- Established the National AIDS Research Institute in Pune, to examine various biomedical and social aspects of HIV and AIDS in India.
- Encouraged pilot efforts to develop an anti HIV vaccine.

International Collaboration

A number of International development agencies are extending technical and financial support for implementation of projects for prevention and control of HIV/AIDS in India. Working together with NACO, the Joint United Nations Programme on HIV/AIDS (UNAIDS) and its 6 UN Co-sponsor agencies, the UNICEF, UNDP, UNFPA, UNESCO, WHO and World Bank are striving to combat the AIDS epidemic as a common effort (Table 1). The goal of the integrated UN work plan is to support a multisectoral response to HIV/AIDS epidemic in India (Table 2).

To facilitate the accessibility to technical resources, Technical Resource Groups (TRGs) have been constituted by NACO in major thematic areas :

- Epidemiology
- Targeted intervention
- Counselling
- Clinical management, TB and hospital infection control
- Blood safety

Table 1. Activities of Multilateral Agencies in Prevention and Control of HIV/AIDS in India

UNAIDS	• Coordinating, facilitating and monitoring inputs for activities of UN agencies. • Support of TRG. • Establish an information system linking the country to global efforts and trends on HIV/AIDS.
WHO	• Programme management • Surveillance • STD Control • Blood safety • Clinical management
UNFPA	• Integration of HIV/AIDS programme with that of the reproductive and child health programme
UNESCO	• Assisting school-based AIDS education • Assisting youth programmes • Prevention of mother to child transmission of HIV (MTCT) • Integration and support to state level IEC activities
World Bank	• Financial assistance in supporting the implementation of the program since 1992.

Table 2. Objects of UN Integrated Work Plan during NAC Project

Specific areas of Strengthening	Objectives
Advocacy	• Promote and maintain HIV/AIDS related issues as a priority on the national and state levels. • Sensitise decision-makers, programme planners and implementers on the issues related to the four cross-cutting themes and generate commitment in all areas of programming.
Surveillance	• Strengthening national and state level capacity in surveillance and monitoring of the epidemic. • Promote data collection on the factors related to risk vulnerability to the epidemic and the datas application for policy development, programming and evaluation for an expanded response to the epidemic.
Decentralization	• Strengthen the state level capacity in Programming and Management of HIV/AIDS prevention and care.
Difficult to reach and vulnerable populations	• Reduce the vulnerability of marginalized populations and to alleviate the impact of HIV/AIDS on them.
HIV/AIDS prevention for young people in particular for youth from low socio-economic strata, slums, and rural areas	• To reduce the vulnerability of youth to HIV/AIDS.
Impact Reduction	• Provide care, support and protection of human rights of people living with HIV/AIDS. • Mitigate the adverse health and socio-economic impact of HIV/AIDS epidemic.
Information Exchange Support	• Improve access to and more effective use of information available on HIV/AIDS nationally and globally.
Technical Resource Group	• Facilitate the accessibility of technical resources to the states.
Research	• Improve the quality of prevention and care interventions.

- STD and condom promotion
- Prevention at work place
- Injecting drug users
- Research and development
- Women and children

Bilateral Collaboration

In the past several years several Bilateral Agencies have shown their interest and have supported our effort for prevention and control of HIV/AIDS (Table 3)

Resource Allocation

Before 1992 most of the funds available were earmarked for screening for HIV, especially for blood safety. Since the inception of the NACP, the National Budget has supported the activities related to the prevention and control of AIDS. The signing of the credit agreement with World Bank in 1992, has substantially expanded the resources available for AIDS prevention and control at the National and State levels. The NACP now focuses on programme management, IEC and STD control.

Table 3.   Activities of Bilateral Agencies in Prevention and Control of HIV/AIDS in India

USAID	• Funding of AIDS Prevention and Control Project (APAC) in Chennai. The aim of this project is to introduce and re-inforce HIV prevention behaviour in high risk populations • Funding of AVERT Project in Maharashtra. This is being implemented with the objective to increase the use of effective and sustainable response to reduce transmission of STD/HIV/AIDS and related infectious diseases.
NORAD	• Support to several NGO in their fight against AIDS • Financial support to conduct National Physicians Training Programme.
ODA	• Intervention projects in several red light areas in Kolkata and other parts of West Bengal • Financial support to implement STD/HIV prevention and control programmes. • Develop IEC techniques. • Support to national IEC/STD project as the Truck Drivers Intervention Project.
DFID	• Financial support for sexual Health Project in West Bengal. • Fiancial support to "Healthy Highway project" with truckers • Formulation of partnership for Sexual health project for prevention and control of STD in Andhra Pradesh, Gujrat, Kerala and Orissa.

The NACP including the NAC Project Phase II and the related bilateral projects of USAID and DFID involve an outlay of Rs. 14.25 crores of which the World Bank aided NAC Project Phase–II accounts for Rs. 1155 crores. The component wise allocation of this amount is shown in Table 4.

UNAIDS Public Health Approach to STD Control

There is a strong link between STD and the sexual

Table 4.   Allocation of Funds for Different Activities of NAC Project – Phase II

Activity	Percentage allocation
Targeted intervention for high risk groups	23%
Preventive interventions for general community	34%
Institutional strengthening	25%
Low cost AIDS care	14%
Intersectoral collaboration	4%

transmission of HIV infection. The presence of an untreated STD can enhance both the acquisition and transmission of HIV by a factor of up to 10. Thus STD treatment is an important HIV prevention strategy in a general population.

The aim of STD prevention and care is to reduce the prevalence of STD through primary prevention and effective case management.

The magnitude of the problem of STD, and the strong association with HIV transmission, highlight the need to explore new and innovative approaches to prevent and control their spread. One such approach is the adoption of the "public health package". This package for STD control consists of the following components:

- Promoting safer sex behaviour
- Strengthening condom programming
- Promoting health-care-seeking behaviour
- Integrating STD control into primary health care and other health- care services
- Providing specific services for populations at increased risk

- Comprehensive case management
- Prevention and care of congenital syphilis and neonatal conjunctivitis
- Early detection of asymptomatic and symptomatic infections.

The traditional method of diagnosing STD is by laboratory tests. However, laboratory tests are often unavailable or too expensive. For this reason, syndromic diagnosis and management was developed. The syndromic approach consists of:

- Classification of the main causal pathogens by the syndromes they produce
- Use of flow charts to guide the management of a given syndrome
- Treatment of the syndrome, covering all the common pathogens with potential to cause grave manifestations and consequences
- Promoting treatment of sex partners.

References

1. India, 1994. A Reference Manual, New Delhi: Publications Divisions, Ministry of Information and Broadcasting, Government of India 1994.

2. Gerbase AC, Rowley JT, Mertens TE. Global epidemiology of sexually transmitted diseases. Lancet 1998; 351: 2-4.

3. Khanna N, Nadkarni V, Bhutani LK. India. In: Tan B, Chan R, Mugratitchian, eds. Sexually Transmitted Diseases in Asia and the Pacific. Melbourne: Venereology Publishing Inc, 1998: 114-137.

4. Park K. Health Programmes in India In: Park's Text Book of Socal and Preventive Medicine, 16th ed. Jabalpur: Banarasi Das Bhanot Publishers; 2000. p. 305-319.

5. Jayraman KS. Indian AIDS. Penalties and help for victims (news). Nature 1989; 341: 173.

6. Country Scenario 1997-98. National AIDS Control Organization, India, New Delhi: Ministry of Health and Family Welfare, Government of India.

7. Strategic plan for the control and prevention of AIDS in India, New Delhi, Ministry of Health and Family Welfare, 1991.

8. Combating HIV/AIDS in India 1999-2000, National AIDS Control Organization, New Delhi : Ministry of Health and Family Welfare. Government of India.

9. Piot P, Laga M. Current approaches to STD control in developing countries. Document written for study group on Integrated Behavioural Research for Prevention and Control of STDs, Bethesda 1990.

10. Pettitfor A, Walsh J, Wilkens V, et al. How effective is the syndromic management of STDs? Review of current studies. Sex Transm Disease 2000; 27: 371-385.

Chapter 37

Sexually Transmitted Diseases and Condoms

R D Mehta

Introduction

The golden rule 'Prevention is better than cure' stands true even today. With the advent of HIV one could even say that, 'Prevention is the only cure'. The barrier method of contraception 'Condom' has become an important tool of prevention against spread of sexually transmitted diseases (STD) and in turn HIV and AIDS. The cyber generation of this modern era finds no social, religious, ethical and moral barriers to uphold the Gandhian norms of forbearance, and abstinence. Sex is no more sanctity practice, the natural way of procreation. It has turned into a 'fad', a status symbol, or a symbol of being anti orthodox. Thus premarital and extramarital contacts whether heterosexual or homosexual are rising in number and so are the STD. The alarming increase in the prevalence rate of STD and HIV has prompted health managers and sociologists to focus on 'Condoms' and other barrier methods to checkmate the transmission of STD. The fact that STD facilitate HIV transmission has galvanised the development of newer biomedical preventive tools and improvising the existing methods. The developing world needs the barrier methods which are safe, cost effective and acceptable to promiscuous or sexually active persons with high risk behaviour.

Historical Overview

The Egyptians were the first to use colourful penile coverings as early as 1000 B.C. but these seem to have been more of decorative nature than as a barrier. Italian anatomist Gabrielle Fellopius described linen sheaths as preventive measures to protect against syphilis. In the 16th century, Dr. Condom, a physician in the Court of King Charles II of England first prepared the condom from the outer membrane of a sheep's intestine. The widespread use of condom started in 1844 when Goodyear and Hannock began to mass-produce vulcanized rubber condoms. Simultaneously cervical caps and diaphragm became available for use as pioneer female condoms in Germany between 1838-1860.

Barrier Methods

The physical and chemical barrier methods used as preventive measures include

- The male condom
- Sponge
- Cervical cap
- Microbicides
- The female condom,
- Diaphragm,
- Spermicides

These are effective against many of the STD pathogens including HIV 1 & 2.

Male Condom

The word 'Condom' has been derived either from 'Dr. Condom' the English Physician, or a 'Colonel Cundum' or the Latin word 'Condon' which means 'receptacle'. It is a protective device put by the male on an erect penis to cover the glans and shaft, the virtual entry or exit point for STD pathogens. It protects both the user and its partner if used prior to genital contact and remains intact during the sexual act. It must be used consistently if it is to be efficacious. There are different types of male condoms available commercially including those made from latex, natural membranes and polyurethane.

Latex Condom

This is the most widely used type of male condom. Latex condoms have been proven in different laboratory experiments and clinical studies to be effective barriers against various bacteria and viruses including HIV and Hepatitis B Virus (HBV).[2] Laboratory testing of latex condom simulating mechanical friction of coitus is performed to check its barrier effectiveness. In one study 30% of latex condoms tested allowed detectable leakage of particles sized similar to that of HIV,[3] however, the simulating conditions in the study were criticized later for being much harsher than actual sexual intercourse. More recent studies demonstrate the efficacy of latex condoms as mechanical barrier against transmission of HIV and other viral and bacterial microorganisms in protecting the users and their partners.[4,5,6]

It is most important to use the condom consistently and correctly for absolute protection. The latex device should cover the organ in such a way that genito-ulcerative diseases like syphilis, chancroid, granuloma inguinale, lymphogranuloma venereum (LGV), herpes progenitalis, condyloma accuminata etc, which require intimate mucocutaneous contact for transmission are prevented. Similarly the male urethral opening is also protected by the condom to check the diseases like gonococcal urethritis, NGU, trichomoniasis, HIV and HBV transmitted through seminal, urethral fluid or partner's infected vagino-cervical fluid. However, it must be remembered that areas such as the pubic region, upper inner thighs and oral cavity are left unprotected and are vulnerable to disease transmission.

Incorporation of spermicidals as lubricants in condoms may provide an added advantage, but this still remains to be proved. The efficacy of spermicidals like nonoxynol-9 is questionable as at the time of impregnation of lubricant the amount is too low to be effective and could further decrease shelf life.[7]

Allergic contact dermatitis to latex condom has been described.[8] Contact dermatitis to latex has been more frequently described in health care workers exposed to latex products in the form of gloves or in the latex industry. Prelubricated condoms with spermicidals further increase the allergenicity, and the prevalence rate of contact dermatitis ranges between 1% to 7%.[9]

Preventive Efficacy of Latex Condoms

Clinical studies provide evidence that consistent condom use protects the person from acquisition of HIV infection despite regular sexual exposure to their HIV positive partner. In a study on 123 couples discordant for HIV infection, the healthy partners remained seronegative over a two year span with the regular use of condoms. Among the inconsistent users 9.8% out of 122 turned seropositive.[10] Another study reported 1.8% seroconversion after consistent use of latex condom while 12% became HIV positive among those who used the condom irregularly.[11] It may be concluded that correct and consistent use of latex condoms provides virtually complete protection to both the partners. It has been shown that condom effectiveness for decreasing STD risk is affected by disease infectivity and number of exposures. Generalisation from low infectivity to highly infectious STD or short term to long term situations can overestimate the effectiveness.[12]

In underdeveloped countries the importance of consistent and correct use of condoms with risk reduction education strategies is being highlighted in order to decrease the prevalence and transmission of HIV. It is critical for health managers to realize and incorporate strategies to overcome barriers to condom use. A study of 49 women and 203 men from Mumbai highlighted the problem of privacy regarding condom purchase from stores and the social stigma associated with condom purchase and use.[13] Various studies emphasize the need to ease the social costs and constraints to safe sexual behaviour through acceptance and promotion of the regular use of condoms.

Mechanical failures of condoms may result in transmission of STD. In a study conducted in the United States to assess the incidence of mechanical failures of condoms using sexual diaries of 892 women it was estimated that 500 (2.3%) condoms broke during intercourse out of 21852 condoms used and another 290 (1.3%) slipped during usage. Breakage was more common with young, single or nulliparae while slippage was found more amongst married and multiparas.[14]

The condom needs to be popularized as a preventive tool against STD and HIV. The condom is still considered as the method of contraception even in the western world. In one study undertaken to assess the planned use of condom for prevention of STD among 2782 women, who were to undergo sterilization. Only 646 were using the condom prior to sterilization and half of them did not intend to use it after the surgical procedure, considering themselves safe against pregnancy. Thus 11% of study sample might have experienced high exposure risks to various STD organisms and HIV, if not counseled.[15] In another study of 966 sex workers in China the promotion of condom use and education regarding the mode of transmission of HIV resulted in an appreciable decrease in the incidence of STD. After counselling, the consistent use of condoms was found to increase from 30% to 81%, decreasing the incidence of STD (gonorrhoea, trichomoniasis and chlamydial infections from 17.5/100 persons per year to 3.0/100 persons per year.[16] Prevention of such conditions as herpes genitalis, which cannot be cured, is important, and its incidence can be decreased by improving condom use. Regular use of condoms is even more important for the male partners of pregnant women to prevent HSV-2 infection.[17]

Condom and Safe Sex

To the common man condoms only signify a means of contraception.[18] Its use as a barrier for prevention of STD and HIV in sexually active persons needs to be promoted and publicised.[19,20] The National AIDS Control Programme identifies the importance of condom promotion although socio-cultural factors may prevent its widespread acceptance.[21] The strengthening of IEC activities through Governmental agencies and Non Government Organizations (NGO) is to create public awareness about safe sex, which is the most important preventive action in curbing the rising incidence of STD and HIV.[22]

The predominant mode of transmisson of HIV in India is heterosexual.[23] It is estimated that ulcerative conditions of the genital tract increase the possibility of acquisition of HIV 10 fold, while STD presenting with a discharge increase transmission of HIV 5-fold.[24]

Although it may sound simple for community health workers to promote the already publicized method for birth spacing 'NIRODH' (the Sanskrit word for prevention), or condom for prevention of STD, unpublished observations of the author suggests that the acceptability of condom by sexually active persons with high risk behaviour is an uphill task.

The National AIDS Control Organization (NACO), New Delhi and different State AIDS Control Society (SACS) under various public health programmes have started free condom distribution at all the STD clinics and health centres promoting them as a preventive measure against spread of STD and HIV. Condom promotion is being done through wall messages at the roadsides and public places, posters, video-film shows, radio and television. However, in this campaign, reservations have been expressed that promotion of condoms to the young generation may promote 'Free Sex' rather than 'Safe sex'. 'NACO' through 'SACS' is ensuring easy access to good quality, affordable, acceptable condoms of international standards for safe sex. The government provides condoms at subsidized prices for distribution through the retail outlets. In year 2000-2001, 465.43 millions of condoms were distributed through social marketing strategy, while 627.42 million condoms were supplied through free distribution schemes.[25] Condoms are also available through commercial outlets at chemist shops, departmental stores etc. The concept of a 'Condom Club' in which a nurse interacted with teenagers and supplied condoms was also found acceptable to the younger generation.[26] This approach may be used by NGO in India.

Advantages of Latex Condoms

1. Cheap, safe, easy to use and readily available preventive measure.
2. Effective in preventing not only STD but also undesired pregnancy, hence makes the coitus hassle free.
3. May prolong erection and check the premature ejaculation making the act more enjoyable.
4. Decreases the messiness of intercourse.
5. Contained semen in the condom is an 'eye evidence' of protection.

Disadvantages of Latex Condoms

1. Many males complain, that it reduces the sensuality and sensitivity and thus the pleasure of intercourse.
2. It may break or slip during the act especially when used with oily lubricants as they cause the latex to deteriorate.
3. Every act requires a new condom.
4. Unpleasant latex odour.
5. It may cause premature ejaculation in some individuals owing to the time taken for wearing the condom over an erect organ thus decreasing the span for actual intercourse.

Social and Psychological Repercussions of the Condom

Condoms have embarrassing social connotations, as these are often perceived as being associated with, promiscuity and venereal disease. At a personal level condom are often perceived both by the male and female partners as a barrier to natural enjoyment. Even suggesting the use of condom to the male partner has been found insulting and offending. In sharp contrast among the sexually active generation in the West the use of the condom is now being seen as a measure of concern and care of the partner. Thus, the negative image of the latex condom is changing atleast in the west, although it may take somewhat longer in developing countries.

A newer consumer friendly version of the latex condom has become more popular now because it is loose at the tip and snug at the base.[27] It provides more friction and pleasure during coitus, being loose at the tip as compared to firm fitting traditional latex condom, making safe sex more enjoyable.

Failure of Condoms

1. Influence of alcohol may lead to its inadequate or improper use.
2. Improper storage of condom, heat, moisture and sunlight damage the condom, so storage must be in dry, dark and cool place.
3. Use of expired condoms.
4. Oil or petroleum based lubricants, which are sometimes used may cause it to slip during the act and also weaken the latex.
5. Breakage during coitus.

Natural Membrane Condom

Latex sensitivity led to the development of natural membrane condoms. These are also known as 'lambskin condoms'. These are porous and various in vitro studies showed easy passage of HIV, HSV, HBV etc.[28] Although seminal fluid dynamics during intercourse may not simulate the harsh mechanical methodology of testing the efficacy of membrane condoms in preventing transmission of STD.

The advantage of membrane over latex condoms is that it gives a more natural feel and sensuality. They are stronger, less elastic and hence are not likely to break during coitus. However, membranous condoms are considerably more expensive.

Polyurethane Condoms

These are also known as plastic condoms. Recent advances in technology have allowed the development of the thinner, yet stronger condom. Compared to the traditional latex condom, it allows better sensuality and sensitivity.[29] These are odourless and colourless and have a long shelf life. Oily lubricants do not damage the condom.

Disadvantages include the fact that these are more expensive as compared to latex condoms, require lubrication, and tend to be noisy during sexual intercourse.

Three newer thermoplastic varieties have been developed which are transparent, odourless & loose fitting. One is rolled on like the latex condom and the other one is slipped over the penis. The consumer friendly qualities find these newer types gaining popularity. The third variety is made of a synthetic thermoplastic elastomer material used for the manufacture of non-allergenic examination gloves.

The Female Condom

The female condom is a pre-lubricated, polyurethane sheath, which fits loosely into the vagina. It lines the vaginal walls from labia to cervix. The insertion methodology is same as of the traditional diaphragm. There are two flexible rings at both the ends, which help positioning the sheath. The first one at the closed end fits behind the pubic bone and second one, which is the open end, remain against the labia.

Preventive Efficacy of Female Condom

The female condom has been shown to be an effective mechanical barrier against HIV and other STD.[30] Consistent use is an important pre-requisite for sustained protection. In a study,[31] twenty consistent users had remained free from *Trichomonas vaginalis*, where as among inconsistent users the re-infection rate was 14.7% .

The use of the female condom needs to be popularized as a tool of women's empowerment. It helps them negotiate with their sexually active partners, preventing the transmission of HIV and STD with increase in sexual confidence and autonomy. Its development should receive high priority, more socio-political and scientific initiative as an important preventive technology against the dreaded epidemic.[32]

Advantages

1. It provides natural sexual pleasure to both the partners as compared to the male condom. The polyurethane material of the female condom also transmits the body heat unhindered.
2. The introitus is covered 'in toto', thus provides reliable protection.
3. Oil lubricants can be used concomitantly.

Disadvantages

1. Wearing of condom well in advance of intercourse may be undesirable.
2. Aesthetic appeal is lost after the insertion of condom.
3. Act of coitus is often noisy and embarrassing to the couple.
4. Slipping during the intercourse may occur.
5. It is expensive as compared to the male condom.

Female Condom Acceptance

The female condom shows good acceptability because they find a protective device over which they have the control. Many of the women in various studies feel that it is stronger than the male latex condom and found it more enjoyable.

Some women find discomfort and difficulty while putting it on. It also has a messy feel during the coital act and uneasy feel of outer and inner rings. Partner resistance to female condom may dampen the acceptability of the female condom. Recent studies, have shown that in urban Zimbabwe, washing and reuse was also acceptable.[33]

Other Barrier Devices

These include the sponge, the diaphragm and cervical caps. In addition spermicides and microbicides are the chemical barriers combating the microorganism transmission from one partner to the other.

Sponge

This is a flexible device with built in grooves for comfortable insertion and removal. These are impregnated with sodium cholate, non oxynol-9 and benzalkonium chloride. This combination has been found to be effective in inhibiting HIV reverse transcriptase[34] and inactivating microorganisms responsible for STD.[35]

Advantages

It is a cheaper and user friendly device and may be inserted prior to the act. The spermicidal impregnation makes it a multi use device which is disposable unlike cervical cap and diaphragm which are to be washed and stored after each use.

Disadvantages

It needs to be left in position for at least six hours after the intercourse. It is associated with higher vaginal infection rates, unpleasant odour and irritation.

However, the overall preference score is high because most of the women find it convenient to use and there is no associated discomfort.

Diaphragm

This barrier device, also known, as the 'Dutch Cap' is a shallow cup made of synthetic rubber or plastic with a flexible rim made of spring or metal. This reusable device covers the cervix and can be inserted six hours prior to the intercourse and hence can be used without partner's knowledge. The proper sized diaphragm (5-10 cm sizes are available) snugly fits between symphysis pubis and sacrum. Spring tension and vaginal muscle tone maintain the position of diaphragm.

It must always be used with a spermicide, which needs to be reapplied prior to each coitus. It provides protection only against those STD that primarily involve the cervix[36] such as *N. gonorrhoeae*, *Chlamydia trachomatis* and *Trichomonas vaginalis*. The protective efficacy is increased with the use of spermicides.

It is expensive and there is an associated risk of increased incidence of urinary tract infections because of the alterations caused in normal vaginal flora owing to the spermicides with which they are combined. The male partner may feel uncomfortable in its presence and the users may find the insertion and removal procedures tedious. Lax vaginal tone and improper fitting may cause its slipping during coital act. The latex device has an unpleasant odour and it cannot be used with oily lubricants. The acceptability of diaphragm is poor in the Indian women because of the skills required for insertion and removal and the lack of privacy for washing and storing in Indian context.[37]

Cervical Cap

These are smaller barrier devices as compared to the diaphragm. They are made of silicon and cover the cervix with a suction mechanism. It is to be combined with spermicide and can be left in place for 48 hours after the intercourse. It should be replaced every third year. Acceptability of cervical cap ranges from 75% to 89% but unwelcome odour, dislodgment during intercourse and partner discomfort were complained by users. There are no data supporting its efficacy in preventing STI and HIV.

Spermicides

These are chemical agents used for killing sperms and in addition they may inhibit STD pathogens. Various spermicides in use include nonoxynol-9, octoxynol, cholorhexidine, benzalkonium chloride and menfegol, gossypol, gramicidin and povidone iodine. These are available as foams, gels suppositories, foaming tablets and vaginal contraceptive films (VCF).

Preventive Efficacy of Nonoxynol-9 (N-9)

Laboratory animals as well as human studies have assessed the efficacy of N-9 in preventing STD microorganisms including HIV.[38] It is a non-ionic surfactant which destroys the lipid envelopes, and hence it is more effective against enveloped viruses like HBV. It has cidal effects against HIV, HBV, HSV, treponemes, gonococci, *H. ducreyi* and chlamydia.

The adverse effects of N-9 are associated with the frequency, concentration and amount used. In the terms of administration and contraception, negligible side effects are reported. However, the higher concentration amount necessary when used to prevent HIV/STD may prove more hazardous. It has been shown that frequent use of large amounts of N-9 may cause vagino-cervical ulceration. It is also found to be associated with a change in the vaginal flora that may facilitate the transmission of HIV and STD.

Advantages

It is easy to use, has a lubricant effect and can be used without the knowledge of the male partner. It is usually acceptable to both the partners. Spermicides are devoid of any long-term side effects.

Disadvantages

Planned activity is pre-requisite, as it requires at least 10 minutes for dissolution of spermicide. It may be messy especially if it leaks out of the vagina. A sensation of warmth, over lubrication and irritation may be felt by some users.

The acceptability of spermicide is increasing N-9 & menfegol foaming tablets are available with tolerable side effects such as burning, stinging and itching.

Microbicides

These chemicals are topically used to kill pathogens of STD or interfere with the mechanism of infection. Research activities are focused on products that may increase natural host defense mechanisms such as acid buffering agents, lactobacillus preparations, antimicrobial peptides (magainins, protegrins, defensins). Other compounds may interfere with viral entry to the target epithelial cells such as monoclonal antibodies,[39] sulfated polysaccharides and sulfonated polymers. A suppository made of extract from neem tree, soapnut (Reetha) and quinine hydrochloride is a promising device as a contraceptive and microbicide.

The sulfated polysaccharide, dextrin sulfate inhibits the adherence of HIV and chlamydia to epithelial cells. N- docosanol is a potent antiviral, which may inhibit the enveloped and non-enveloped virus even when applied topically. Squalamine is steriod-based compound, which has shown inhibitory effect against most of the STI pathogens including HIV. C31G is newer surfactant with a lower irritancy score as compared to N-9 and also appears to be more effective.

Conclusion

Barrier methods originally conceptualized, as contraceptive devices are becoming more popular as preventive measures against STD and HIV.[40] These have not yet gained momentum as the only 'preventive modality', in our country to combat the dreaded HIV and other STD. A lot needs to be done to promote safe sex, through consistent and proper use of condoms.

References

1. Conant MA, Hardy D, Sernatinger J, et al. Condoms prevent transmission of AIDS associated retrovirus. JAMA 1986; 255; 1706.

2. Judson FN, Ehret JM, Bodin GF, et al. In vitro evaluations of condom with and without Nonoxynol 9 as physical and chemical barriers against *Chlamydia trachomatis*, Herpes simplex virus type 2 and Human immunodeficiency virus. Sex Transm Dis 1989; 16:51-56.

3. Carey RF, Herman WA, Retta SM, et al. Effectiveness of latex condoms as a barrier to human immunodeficiency virus sized particles under conditions of simulated use. Sex Transm Dis 1992; 19: 230-234.

4. Carrey RF. Condom safety and HIV (Letter). Sex Transm Dis 1994 ; 26; 60.

5. Vail JG, Mercer DJ. Condom safety and HIV Comments from PATH (Letter). Sex Transm Dis 1994; 21; 61.

6. Stone KM, Timyan J, Thomas EL. Barrier Methods for the prevention of sexually transmitted diseases. In: Holmes KK, Mardh PA, Sparling PF et al, Eds. Sexually Transmitted Diseases.3rd Ed. New York: McGraw Hill; 1999. p. 1307-1322.

7. Smith N. Nonoxynol-9 in condoms. Int J STD AIDS 1990; 1; 449.

8. Rekart ML. The toxicity and local effects of the spermicide nonoxynol-9. J AIDS 1992; 5; 425.

9. Stratton P. Nonoxynol-9 lubricated condoms may increase release of natural rubber latex protein. XI International conference on AIDS.Vancouver: abstract Th C 433, 1996.

10. De Vincenzi I. A longitudinal study of human immunodeficiency virus transmission by heterosexual partners. N Eng J Med 1994; 331: 341-346.

11. Saracco A, Musicco M, Nicolosia A, et al. Man-to-woman sexual transmission of HIV: Longitudinal study of 343 steady partners of infected men. J AIDS 1993; 6; 497-502.

12. Man JR, Stine CC, Vessey J. The role of disease specific infectivity and number of disease exposures on long term effectiveness of the latex condom. Sex Transm Dis 2002; 29: 350-352.

13. Roth J, Krishnan SP, Bunch E. Barriers to condom use results from a study in Mumbai (India). AIDS education & prevention 2001; 13: 65-77.

14. Macaluso M, Kelaghan J, Artz L, et al. Mechanical failure of the latex condom in a cohort of women at high STD risk. Sex Transm Dis 1999; 26: 450-458.

15. Sangi-Haghpeykar H, Poindexter AN. Planned condom use among women undergoing tubal sterilization. Sex Transm Dis 1998; 25: 335-341.

16. Ma S, Dukers NH, van den Hoek A, et al. Decreasing STD incidence and increasing condom use among Chinese sex workers following a short term intervention: a prospective cohort study. Sex Trans Infect 2002; 78: 80-81.

17. Casper C, Wald A. Condom use and the prevention of genital herpes acquisition. Herpes 2002; 9: 10-14.

18. Misra RS. Sex, sexually transmitted diseases and AIDS, New Delhi: Vigyan Prasar; 1996: 124.

19. Cates W Jr, Steiner MJ. Dual protection against unintended pregnancy and sexually transmitted infections: what is the best contraceptive approach. Sex Transm Dis 2002; 29: 168-174.

20. Condom for prevention of HIV Transmission. In: NACO Training Module on HIV Infections and AIDS for Medical Officers. National AIDS Control Organization, Ministry of Health and Family Welfare, Government of India. 1999; 75-79.

21. Condom Promotion and Provision. In: AIDS- No time for complacency Regional Publication, SEARO No.26 World Health Organization, Geneva, AITBS Publishers and Distributors, New Delhi: 1999; 32.

22. Education on Risk Reduction and Condom Provision. In: Management of Sexually Transmitted Diseases at District and PHC levels. Regional publication, SEARO, No.25, World Health Organization Geneva, AITBS Publishers and Distributors, New Delhi. 1999; 5.

23. Health Programmes in India In: Park K, Editor. Park's Text Book of Preventive and Social Medicine.16th Ed. Jabalpur: Banarasi Das Bhanot; 2000. p. 310-311.

24. HIV Infection and Sexually Transmitted Diseases. In: NACO Training Module on HIV infection and AIDS for Medical Officers. National AIDS Control Organization. Ministry of Health and Family Welfare, Government of India 1999, 42.

25. Control of Sexually Transmitted Diseases (STD) Control and Condom Promotion. In: Combating HIV/AIDS In India. Ministry of Health And Family Welfare, National AIDS Control Organization, Government of India. 2000-2001, 23-24.

26. Thomson C, Smith H. 'Condom Club': an interface between teenage sex and genitourinary medicine. Int J STD AIDS 2001; 12: 475-478.

27. Roman M. What to wear to bed, Men's Health, July/August: 1994; 35.

28. Lytle CD, Carney PG, Vohra S, et al. Virus leakage through natural membrane condoms. Sex Transm Dis 1990 ; 17: 58-62.

29. Rosenberg MJ, Waugh MS, Solomon HM, et al. The male polyurethane condom: A review of current knowledge. Contraception 1996; 53; 141-146.

30. Drew WL, Blair M, Miner RC, et al. Evaluation of virus permeability of a new condom for women. Sex Trans Dis 1990; 17: 110-112.

31. Soper DE, Shupe D, Shangold GA, et al. Prevention of vaginal trichomonas by compliant use of the female condom. Sex Trans Dis 1993; 20; 137-139.

32. Gollub EL. The female condom: tool for women's empowerment. (Review) Am J Public Health 2000; 90: 1377-1381.

33. Pettifor AE, Beksinska ME, Rees HV, et al. The acceptability of reuse of the female condoms.among Urban South African Women. J Urban Health 2001; 78: 647-657.

34. Psychoyos A, Creatsas G, Hassan E, et al. Spermicidal and antiviral properties of cholic acid: Contraceptive efficacy of new vaginal sponge containing sodium cholate. Hum Repord 1993; 8: 866-869.

35. Cates W, Stone KM. Family Planning, STD & contraceptive choice: A literature update- PartI Fam Plann Perspect 1992; 24: 75-84.

36. Rosenberg MJ, Davidson AJ, Chen JH, Judson FN, Douglas JM. Barrier contraceptives and sexually transmitted disease in women: A comparison of female dependant methods and condoms. Am J Public Health 1992; 82: 669-674.

37. Park K. Demography and Family planning. In: Park K. editor. Park's Text Book of Preventive and Social Medicine. 16thEd. Jabalpur: Banarasi Das Bhanot; 2000. p. 332.

38. Feldbulum PJ, Weir SS. The protective effect of nonoxynol-9 against HIV infection. AmJ Public Health 1994; 84; 1032.

39. Cone RA. Whaley KJ. Monoclonal antibodies for reproductive health: Part-I Preventing sexual transmission of disease and pregnancy with topically applied antibodies. Am J Reprod Immunol 1994; 32: 144-151.

40. Weller S, Davis K.Condom effectiveness in reducing heterosexual HIV transmission. Cochrane Database Syst Rev 2002; (1): CD 003255.

PART VIII
Non-Venereal Skin Diseases of Genitalia

Chapter 38

Non-Venereal Diseases of Genitalia

Binod K Khaitan

Introduction

All lesions on genitalia are not sexually transmitted. A dermato-venereologist is usually familiar with diseases which are non-venereal and present on genitalia. There is no strict classification of such diseases. However, one can categorize these into three major groups.

1. Common dermatologic diseases with lesions on genitalia either exclusively or along with lesions elsewhere eg. vitiligo, psoriasis, lichen planus etc.
2. Diseases involving genitalia and considered to be physiological abnormalities eg. pearly penile papules, Fordyce spots etc.
3. Non-venereal diseases peculiar to genitalia. Some of the important conditions are as follows:

   (a) Peyronie's disease
   (b) Plasma cell balanitis
   (c) Lichen sclerosus et atrophicus
   (d) Lichen planus of the genitalia
   (e) Fixed drug eruption
   (f) Fournier's gangrene
   (g) Behcet's disease
   (h) Non-venereal sclerosing lymphangitis
   (i) Angiokeratoma of Fordyce
   (j) Phimosis and paraphimosis

Some of these diseases do occur elsewhere but have specific presentations on genitalia.

Common Dermatologic Diseases Affecting the Genitalia

These dermatologic diseases generally occur elsewhere and also involves the genitalia. When other sites are involved the diagnosis is straightforward. But, in rare situations, when the lesion is present exclusively on genitalia then the venereologist has to differentiate it from true sexually transmitted diseases (STD). The general principles of treatment in such situations are essentially same as for non-genital lesions.

Vitiligo, particularly acrofacial vitiligo patients may have depigmented macules on the glans, prepuce, penile shaft, scrotum, vulva and also in perianal area. These are asymptomatic and usually do not require any treatment.

Sometimes, the patients with psoriasis, post kala-azar dermal leishmaniasis, lepromatous leprosy, dermatophytic infection or other common dermatoses have lesions on genitalia, particularly in males. The lesions have same morphology as over the rest of the body and one should examine for the evidence of the respective disease process elsewhere on the body.

Among vesiculo-bullous diseases, pemphigus vulgaris involves oral mucosa in a large majority of the patients and genital mucosa, particularly glans penis and labia are also known to be affected. At the time of presentation, the commonest finding is superficial erosion or ulcer, however occasionally unruptured vesicles or bullae can be seen. The presence of oral ulcers of pemphigus and the flaccid bullae, crusts and ulcers on the other parts of the body make the clinical diagnosis easy. The presence of acantholytic cells on Tzanck smear and the classical histological and direct immunofluorescence findings make a definite diagnosis. The ulcerated vegetative plaques of pemphigus vegetans are rare as compared to ulcerative lesions of pemphigus vulgaris. These are seen characteristically on groins in both sexes and in labial sulci in females.

Bullous pemphigoid rarely may have genital lesions. Cicatricial pemphigoid, though a rare disease may have vesiculo-bullous lesions on genitalia healing with scarring. These vesiculo-bullous diseases sometimes need to be kept in mind to differentiate with ulcerative STD.

Developmental and Acquired Benign Lesions of Genitalia

Like any other part of the skin, some of the developmental defects or malformations may involve or encroach upon the genitalia viz. epidermal naevi, angiomas, lymphamgiomas, inclusion cysts, enlarged sebaceous glands and rarely benign appendageal tumours. The morphology of such lesions is similar as on other areas, except that due to maceration as in groins, coronal sulcus and subpreputial area. Some of these lesions may lead to venereophobia. Reassurance to the patient after clinical evaluation and when necessary histological confirmation is usually sufficient. The larger lesions need ablative therapy with electrodesiccation, surgical excision, laser ablation or other appropriate physical modalities of treatment.

Angiokeratoma of Fordyce

It is a distinct entity presenting as tiny erythematous, soft to firm, discrete papules of few mm size on the scrotal skin. Some lesions become brownish in colour with time. The lesions may bleed intermittently due to friction of undergarment or due to minor trauma. It requires ablative treatment with electrocautery or CO_2 laser.

Pearly Penile Papules

These are the manifestations of a harmless non-pathological process which may be the cause of worry to the affected persons mainly the young adults. These present as tiny 1-2 mm skin coloured or shiny papules arranged in a row or sometimes more than one row around the coronal sulcus and or as scattered lesions on the glans penis. These papules are barely elevated and considered to be physiological as these are prominent dermal papillae with slight hypertrophy. Rarely, pearly penile papules need to be differentiated with early lesions of condyloma acuminata, based on the dirty white colour and rough, verrucous or granular surface of the latter. Reassurance to the person about the physiological nature of the lesions is the only measure required.

Fordyce Spots

These are ectopic sebaceous glands present in the sub-preputial area of penis or on the vulva. These present as multiple, asymptomatic, discrete, randomly distributed tiny yellowish barely elevated papules. Similar lesions may be present over the lips. The harmless nature of these lesions needs to be explained to the person.

Lesions Due to Trauma

Self-inflicted traumatic lesions as a sexual behavioural aberration or trauma at the time of intercourse in situations such as a reluctant partner, inadequate spontaneous lubrication, inadequate penile erection etc. are not uncommon. The rupture of hymen leading to some amount of bleeding and sometimes discomfort in a young female either at the time of first intercourse or due to some other gratifying activities like masturbation is well known. Rape is another extreme situation, where the trauma can be minimal to extreme degree of laceration or mutilation of female genitalia depending upon the degree of coercion or violence used. In some communities or social groups, the mutilation of female genitalia as a ritualistic activity as a female counterpart of circumcision is also practised. This practice of genital mutilation is not prevalent in India.

In traumatic lesions, the diagnosis will depend on the reliable history and pattern of the lesions. The lesions may look bizarre in self-inflicted injuries or may present as bruises, lacerations, tear, tiny abrasions, asymmetrical or geometric erythematous sores. Associated oedema in both male and female genitalia, lesions developing within minutes or a few hours of intercourse, and a variety of permutations and combinations of several of the above mentioned findings suggest trauma. The treatment will depend upon the type of trauma and routine principles of prevention of secondary infection and rest to the part to promote healing will be applicable. In addition, it is important to look for the evidence of any 'real' STD at the time of examination and follow-up.

Non-Venereal Sclerosing Lymphangitis

It is an uncommon condition related to aggressive or rigorous intercourse leading to diffuse but subtle trauma to penis in young males. It is usually painless and presents as single or grouped cord-like soft to firm lesions arising from coronal sulcus and involving the dorsal parts of the penis. It is attributed to the thickened and sclerosed lymphatics, but there is some venous component as well. It regresses spontaneously within a few weeks.

Peyronie's Disease

Also known as penile fibromatosis or plastic induration of the penis, Peyronie's disease characteristically has one or more, indurated fibrous longitudinal cord-like subcutaneous plaques in the penile shaft.

Aetiology and Pathogenesis

The exact cause is unknown. In majority it occurs as an isolated abnormality. It may be associated with other fibromatous diseases, such as palmoplantar fibromatosis, knuckle pads and keloid. Atheromatous changes are known to be associated, as seen with the use of β-blockers.

The pathological changes are in the form of fibrous infiltration in the connective tissue of corpora cavernosa from the septum between the two corpora cavernosa comprising of fibroblastic tissue with dense collagen. Sometimes calcification and very rarely even ossification may occur. The changes may extend into the tunica albuginea.

Clinical Features

It presents usually in middle-aged men. Painful erection with varying degree of dorsal or lateral bending of the penis in erection is the main presenting feature. The firm to hard, cord-like longitudinal area or indurated localized area may sometimes be tender. The erectile deformity may lead to intercourse being painful, difficult or even impossible. The course is unpredictable and it may improve or remain unchanged after few months of progression.

High-resolution ultrasonography or MRI of erect penis may help in evaluating the severity.

Treatment

Spontaneous recovery is possible in 20-30% cases. The milder asymptomatic disease may not require any treatment. However, the persistent lesions with painful erection require treatment. Most of the cases report to the urologists and some of the treatment modalities are exclusively their domain. The following modalities have been tried with varying results:

(a) Intralesional corticosteroids

(b) Clostridial collagenase injections
(c) Intralesional injections of verapamil[1]
(d) Extracorporeal shock wave treatment with standard lithotriptor[2]
(e) Dexamethasone pulse therapy
(f) Nisbet's operation comprising of surgical removal of normal tunica albuginea opposite the point of maximum curvature
(g) Surgical correction of curvature with 16-dot plication technique[3]

Lichen Planus of the Genitalia

Lichen planus is a papulo-squamous disorder presenting characteristically when present on skin as violaceous flat-topped pruritic papules. There are several morphologic variants of lichen planus. In about 15% cases, lichen planus involves exclusively mucous membrane, either oral or genital or both. In addition, mucous membrane involvement is seen in upto 30-70% of cases along with cutaneous involvement.[4]

Clinical Features

On genitalia, if the lesion is present on penile skin, it presents as the lesions elsewhere i.e. violaceous flat-topped papules or plaques with different sizes with minimal scaling (**P XXIII, Fig. 91**). However the annular lesions are seen more frequently on genital skin. On the glans penis or preputial skin the lesions have whitish discoloration and the violaceous hue and hyperpigmentation is not uniform. Rarely, the lesions are also seen on scrotal skin. Ulceration of genital lichen planus is rare as compared to oral lichen planus. In female, the lesions are present on vulval skin and labia majora or sometimes on the inner aspect of labia minora. Mild lesions are small flat papules, usually multiple and grouped and the severe disease may be erosive with severe itching and pain. If the induration is present and the colour is ivory white, a biopsy is required to differentiate from lichen sclerosus et atrophicus. On healing, ulcerative lesions leave behind scarring. Occasionally, lesions of secondary syphilis may have a lichenoid presentation, but the lesions are present more on the folds with moist papules, its non-pruritic nature and other clinical evidence of secondary syphilis give the clue. However, in such cases, dark-ground microscopy and serological tests are essential.

In general, the genital lesions of lichen planus tend

to last longer than the skin lesions and recurrences are common.

Histology

A classical lesion of lichen planus shows hyperkeratosis and irregular acanthosis. There may be atrophy of the epidermis in late stages. There is damage to the basal keratinocytes with presence of cytoid bodies in the upper dermis and pigment incontinence along with predominant lymphohistiocytic infiltrate in a band-like pattern. The histology of genital lesion is similar to cutaneous lesions of lichen planus with certain differences due to the site. Apart from the non-keratinized or less keratinized epidermis with parakeratosis, the band-like infiltrate, which is otherwise lymphohistiocytic is rich in plasma cells. The cytoid bodies may be present but much less in number.

Treatment

Moderately potent topical corticosteroids are generally helpful in treating few lesions. If the lesions are persistent or recurrent, a course of oral corticosteroid may rarely be required. Symptomatic relief with antihistamines or analgesics is required in some patients.

Plasma Cell Balanitis

Also known as Zoon's balanitis or plasma cell mucositis, plasma cell balanitis is an idiopathic, benign disorder of the uncircumcised male genitalia.

Clinical Features

This condition presents with characteristic clinical features in middle aged or elderly uncircumcised men as a solitary, circumscribed, persistent plaque with a shiny smooth surface on glans penis (**P XXIII, Fig. 92**).[5] The plaque is moist with a glistening appearance and has minute red specks (cayenne pepper spots). The lesion is usually asymptomatic and single, though multiple lesions have been described. Some patients can have mild pruritus. Plasma cell balanitis most commonly involves glans penis. However, it may extend to involve inner surface of prepuce. Plasma cell balanitis has to be differentiated from Erythroplasia of Queyrat [squamous cell carcinoma (SCC) in-situ], which clinically has a velvety surface and shows features of SCC in-situ on histopathology.

Several variants of plasma cell balanitis have been described. In one, there is marked dermal oedema and predominantly lymphocytic infiltrate. Others are erosive and hypertrophic variants.

Histopathology

The epidermis is attenuated with absence of horny and granular layers. Suprabasal keratinocytes are diamond shaped which are also called "lozenge keratinocytes". Mild spongiosis with occasional dyskeratotic keratinocytes are observed. In the dermis there is dense mixed infiltrate with predominance of plasma cells, along with extravasated erythrocytes. Haemosiderin deposits and vascular proliferation are other histological features.

Treatment

Topical corticosteroids cause mild improvement, but the lesion usually recurs following discontinuation of treatment. Sometimes, it is frustrating. Superadded candidal infection may occur with prolonged use of topical corticosteroid and a combination with topical antifungal agents is sometimes helpful. Circumcision is curative.[6] Reports of treatment with CO_2 laser and copper vapour laser have appeared in literature.[7]

Fixed Drug Eruption (FDE)

It is a specific manifestation of drug reaction, where the lesions remain confined to certain areas and with each exposure of the particular drug, the lesions reappear on the same old sites of reaction, though in addition sometimes new areas may be involved with fresh episode. There are several drugs responsible for FDE. Analgesics, NSAIDS, antibiotics, sulphonamides, cotrimoxazole and tetracyclines are among the more frequent causes of FDE.[8]

Clinically in FDE, there is sharply demarcated, erythematous, oedematous plaques appearing within few hours of ingestion or injection of the offending drug. Sometimes, the lesions are so inflamed that bullous changes or ulceration can occur. Once the offending drug is withdrawn, the lesions heal in 5-10 days leaving behind dark-brown to black hyperpigmentation. Though FDE may present on any part of the body, the glans penis is a common site either exclusively or along with other sites on the body (**P XXIII, Fig. 93**).[8,9] The acute onset, the temporal relationship with drug intake, the well cirumscribed nature of the lesion and in subsequent episodes, acute changes occurring on a pre-existing hyperpigmented macule strongly suggests the diagnosis of FDE. On glans penis, the acute episode presents as a circular or oval superficial erythematous erosion or ulcer with minimal crust and underneath the crust the raw area is usually tender.

FDE on genitalia needs to be differentiated with other ulcerative STD as well as other causes of balanitis in male. Once the lesion heals, provocation with the suspected drug leading to re-appearance of the lesion gives the final proof. Usually application of potent topical corticosteroids for a few days is enough for healing. The residual hyperpigmentation is extremely difficult to treat and it may take several years for complete clearance.

Lichen Sclerosus et Atrophicus (LSA)

Lichen sclerosus et atrophicus (LSA) is a chronic inflammatory skin disease that causes substantial discomfort and morbidity, most commonly in adult women, but also in men and children. It is characterized by atrophic papules and plaques, occurring on any part of the skin and commonly on the anogenital skin of both sexes.

The first report of lichen sclerosus was by Hallopeau in 1887. The other synonyms are leucoplakia, lichen albus, hypoplastic dystrophy and kraurosis vulvae. The latter two exclusively used in LSA of female genitalia. The international society for the study of vulvovaginal disease favours the term lichen sclerosus. The dermatologists favour the term lichen sclerosus et atrophicus.

Epidemiology

The onset of LSA has been reported at all ages, although it is not common under 2 years of age. The mean age of onset in women is fifth or sixth decade. Studies have shown that LSA is more common in women than men at the ratio of 6:1 to even 10:1. Epidemiological surveys based on hospital referrals showed prevalence ranging from 1 in 300 to 1 in 1000 of all patients referred to dermatology. One study showed that there was a strong positive relation between the risk and age, highest risk being for 50-59 years and the incidence of LSA was 14 per 100,000/year.[10]

Aetiology

Familial LSA has been reported in identical as well as non-identical twins, sisters, mothers and daughters. In a study of histologically proven LSA of 84 patients showed positive correlation with class II antigens, HLA-DQ 7, and to a lesser extent to DQ8 and DQ9, but larger series have not found any correlation of class I antigens. The interleukin-1 receptor antagonist gene has been speculated to be a candidate gene for LSA. The association between autoimmunity and LSA has been described in several studies. In one study 40% of patients with LSA had thyroid and parietal cell autoantibodies. Other studies have shown association with alopecia areata, vitiligo, pernicious anaemia, diabetes mellitus and cicatricial pemphigoid. The association being more common in females compared to males. Several infective agents like pleomorphic acid fast bacilli, spirochaetes (borrelia) and human papilloma virus have been implicated, but none have been proved to be causal. Local factors such as trauma, constant friction and radiation treatment have been recognized as triggering factors.[10] It has also been observed that Koebner phenomenon can trigger LSA, like in post vulvectomy scars and circumcision scars.

Clinical Features in Females

LSA most commonly affects the anogenital region (85-98%), with extragenital lesions in 15-20% of patients. Most commonly affected non-genital areas are inner thighs, submammary area, neck, shoulders and wrists. Involvement of oral mucosa is rare. The most common symptom on genitalia is intractable pruritus. Other features are soreness of vulva and perianal area, dysuria, dyspareunia, and tenesmus. It may be totally asymptomatic, and diagnosed at routine examination. Painful traumatic fissures and tear may occur due to defecation and sexual intercourse. The skin changes are hypopigmented or depigmented small, polygonal papules or atrophic plaques with thin cellophane paper-like texture, wrinkled, fragile with telengiectasia, purpura, erosions, or tender fissures in the labial sulci and perianal area (**P XXIV, Fig. 94**). Some women may show areas of hyperkeratosis and sclerosis. The end stage is severe scarring and fusion of labia. Vagina is never involved in LSA.

Complications of LSA are complete fusion or resorption of labia minora, buried clitoris, narrow intriotus making intercourse impossible.

In prepubertal girls, pruritus and soreness are the

common symptoms, dysuria and painful anal fissures causing constipation is also observed. At menarche, the symptoms and signs spontaneously improve in some cases.

Clinical Features in Males

It is most common in middle aged men, but in a study of prepubertal boys who were circumcised for phimosis, 14% had LSA.

The glans penis and prepuce are the most commonly affected sites. The lesions are usually asymptomatic, but presenting symptoms if present are pruritus, dysuria, painful erection, and reduced sensation on the glans and reduction in urinary stream and calibre. In uncircumcised men, a sclerotic constricting band 1-2 cm distal to the prepuce develops resulting in phimosis. Examination would reveal initially only erythema, but with time, porcelain white macules, papules and sclerotic plaques are found. Older lesions become depressed. Rarely, purpura, ecchymosis and even hemorrhagic bullae within the lesion may develop. Involvement of the urethral meatus along with phimosis would result in difficulty in micturition. Most boys would present with meatal stenosis and phimosis, and involvement of the glans. Perianal involvement and extragenital lesions in males are rare. The end stage of LSA in men is balanitis xerotica obliterans (BXO) (**P XXIV, Fig. 95**). The onset and evolution of BXO is insidious, characterized by hypopigmented, thickened, contracted and fissured prepuce, fixed over the glans, and not retractable with moderate force.

Differential Diagnosis

In females, it has to be differentiated from nummular dermatitis, lichen simplex chronics, lichen planus, vitiligo, candidial vulvitis and cicatricial pemphigoid. In prepubertal girls, sexual abuse should be ruled out which may be co-existent and this could lead to LSA as a Koebner phenomenon in trauma scar.

In males, the differential diagnosis include vitiligo, post inflammatory hypopigmentation eg. repeated episodes of genital herpes or other ulcerative sexually transmitted diseases, and trauma.

Histopathology

The characteristic histopathological features are epidermal atrophy, basal cell degeneration, pale staining homogenous zone in the papillary and upper dermis due to oedema and or sclerosis and just below a band of inflammatory infiltrate comprising of CD4 and CD8 lymphocytes, in equal proportion, along with macrophages, mast cells and plasma cells (**P XXIV, Fig. 96**).

On hairy areas follicular plugging is also present. Squamous hyperplasia may be present due to chronic pruritus. Special stains show deposits of acid mucopolysaccharides in homogenous area and basement membrane. Electron microscopy shows structural changes in collagen. Immunohistochemistry reveals fewer elastin, fibrillin and increased expression of tenascin, an anti-adhesion molecule and reduced expression of fibronectin in the upper dermis.[11]

Management[10]

The following guidelines can be followed in the management of LSA.

- Confirm histology by a punch biopsy of affected area.
- Treat the patient, even if asymptomatic, with very potent topical corticosteroids twice daily for 3 months, then taper off gradually. Treatment may be repeated whenever necessary.
- Advice to avoid local irritants.
- Check for non-healing erosion or warty lesion that may indicate development of carcinoma.
- Patient is advised regarding need of surgery to relieve symptoms of scarring and to treat any possible malignant disorder.
- Long-term follow up.

Medical Treatment

Potent topical corticosteroids are the mainstay of therapy eg. 0.05% clobetasol propionate twice daily for 2-3 months and then gradually tapered as symptoms subside. Similar regimen can also be used in children. Androgens like 2% testosterone have been used in female patients. However a placebo-controlled trial showed no better results compared to emollients. In another study 2% progesterone, 2% testosterone and 0.05% clobetasol propionate were compared, and topical corticosteroid was found to be the treatment of choice. Topical retinoids are of no use and topical antibiotics or antifungals are indicated if there is associated secondary bacterial or fungal infection respectively. Oral antihistamines are given to control pruritus. Stool softening agents may be necessary in girls and occasionally in women with perianal LSA.

Surgical Treatment

Circumcision is the treatment of choice for phimosis in male patients and the procedure may be curative. Vulvectomy is no longer indicated if no malignancy is present. Surgical management in women may be necessary for dissection of a buried clitoris, division of fused labia, enlargement of narrowed intriotus. Other ablative techniques include cryotherapy and pulse dye laser.

In asymptmotic patients topical treatment may prevent progression of the disease and development of malignancy but side effects are also encountered. Each case has to be individualized and a long-term follow-up should be advised.

Prognosis

Studies of large group of women with LSA shows that 4.5% had risk of developing squamous cell carcinoma (SCC). Therefore, a long-term follow-up is necessary.[12] No median age for development of cancer has been established. Rarely, in men the LSA can transform into SCC.[13] Extragenital LSA does not carry any risk of malignant change.

Fournier's Gangrene (Idiopathic scrotal oedema, Synergistic gangrene)

It is an uncommon condition, which is due to vascular compromise following bacterial infection. It has been observed to follow minor trauma, some surgical procedures in perineal area, urethral dilatation, injections of hemorrhoids or opening of periurethral abscesses. The surgeons encounter this condition more frequently than the venereologists.

The organisms isolated from the gangrene are most commonly streptococcus, occasionally associated with staphylococcus, *E. coli* and *Clostridium welchii*. In about half the cases definite causative organism is not known. Clinically the patient presents with sudden pain in scrotum with swelling, and prostration, pallor and pyrexia. Initially only part of the scrotal skin is involved and rapidly within few hours or days it may involve the whole of scrotum, and the entire scrotal coverings would

slough off to expose the scrotal contents. The testis is healthy and unaffected by the process. Similar necrotizing process sometimes involves the lower abdominal wall. Histologically, a fulminating inflammation in the subcutaneous tissue, with necrosis associated with obliterating arteritis of the scrotal skin is seen.

Treatment

A swab from the necrosed area for culture and antibiotic sensitivity should be sent urgently. Usually the organisms are sensitive to gentamycin and cephalosporins and the parenteral antibiotics should be started immediately. The debridement in the form of wide excision of the sloughed/necrosed tissue is to be done. However, despite active treatment, the mortality is high.

Behcet's Disease

It is a chronic multisystemic disorder characterized by oral and genital aphthae, arthritis, variety of cutaneous lesions along with ocular, gastrointestinal and neurological manifestations. This condition was first described by Turkish dermatologist Hulusi Behcet in 1937.

Aetiology

Though, the exact cause is unknown, but there is strong genetic predisposition with association with HLA-B5 (Bw5I). In addition, there are various immunological abnormalities such as suppressor T-cell dysfunction, increased polymorphonuclear leucocyte motility and abnormal NK-cell activity. Circulating immune-complexes and vasculitis suggest some unknown antigenic trigger.

Clinical Features

The international study group criteria for the diagnosis for Behcet's disease are; the essential major criteria being presence of recurrent oral ulcers, minor, major or herpetiform aphthae observed by physician or patient, that has recurred at least 3 times in one year, plus two of the following criteria: recurrent genital ulceration, eye lesions as anterior uveitis, posterior uveitis or retinal vasculitis as observed by ophthalmologist, cutaneous lesions as erythema nodosum, pseudofolliculitis, papulopustular lesions or acneform nodules, and a positive pathergy test.[14]

Other cutaneous presentations are pyoderma-like lesions, necrotizing vasculitic ulcers and thrombophlebitis. The gastrointestinal and neurological manifestations are thrombosis of major vessels, gastroinstestinal perforations, meningomyelitis, brain stem syndrome and dementia.

Oral or genital aphthae are the required feature for the diagnosis of Behcet's disease, and they are often the presenting manifestations. The most common site for genital aphthae is on the scrotum in males and vulva in females (**P XXIV, XXV, Fig. 97, 98**). Other sites are shaft of the penis and perineum. The typical ulcer is painful, 1-3 cm in diameter, shallow or deep and have a yellow fibrous base. The other types of ulcers are major aphthae (large sized with necrotic changes) and herpetiform ulceration. The major aphthae heal with scarring. The minor aphthae and herpetiform aphthae subside within 1-3 weeks, whereas the larger ulcers subside over weeks to months.[14]

Differential Diagnosis

The ulcers have to be differentiated from common ulcerative STD like chancre, chancroid and herpes progenitalis. Some authors suggest that the initial presentation of Behcet's ulcer should be differentiated from ulcers of herpes with either culture or PCR. The other cutaneous manifestation associated with Behcet's disease also help in differentiating it from STD.

Histopathology

Vasculitis and thrombosis characterize the histologic features of Behcet's disease. Recent clinico-pathological analysis of cutaneous lesions from patients with Behcet's disease gathered from various centres around the world confirmed that the neutrophilic vasculitic reaction is the predominant histopathological finding.[14]

Treatment

If only mucocutaneous disease is present, then topical or intralesional corticosteroids are the treatment of choice. The other agents which are used according to the severity and availability are colchicine, dapsone, thalidomide, low dose methotrexate, prednisolone, interferon-alpha and combination of the above mentioned drugs. Severe disease or systemic involvement would warrant treatment with immunosuppressants like cyclophosphamide, chlorambucil and cyclosporine.

Prognosis of the disease varies as the disease is known for its chronicity. Mortality is low and occurs only in severe cases with pulmonary or central nervous system involvement. Morbidity is high as severe oral and genital ulceration may be debilitating due to its chronicity and recurrence and ocular involvement may lead to blindness.[14]

Phimosis and Paraphimosis

Phimosis is inability to retract the prepuce proximal to the coronal sulcus and paraphimosis is the inability to cover the glans again with prepuce after retracting it. Phimosis is caused by adhesion of prepuce over the glans due to a variety of reasons. In young boys, if the smegma is not cleaned periodically and the prepuce is not retracted to clean the glans, then the adhesion develop slowly over the years. This can be prevented by regular cleaning of the glans as part of bathing or if phimosis is still not too tight then gradual retraction over a few days. A jet of lukewarm water or saline through the nozzle of a syringe helps in gradual correction of phimosis. There are several non-venereal inflammatory or neoplastic condition which lead to phimosis such as LSA, recurrent balanitis or balanoposthitis eg. candidal balanitis in diabetes, squamous cell carcinoma or genital verrucous carcinoma, ulcerative STD such as primary chancre and also lead to phimosis which is temporaly related and is of acute onset. If phimosis is constricting as seen in some cases of LSA or causing discomfort or pain, then circumcision is the teatment of choice. Paraphimosis is seen with acute cases of ulcerative STD or balanoposthitis with some amount of oedema. Once the primary process is dealt with it can be corrected or in more severe cases, emergency circumcision may be required.

References

1. Levine LA, Goldman KE, Greenfield JM. Experience with intraplaque injection of verapamil for Peyronie's disease. J Urol 2002; 168: 621-625.
2. Lebret T, Loison G, Herve JM, et al. Extracorporeal shock wave therapy in the treatment of Peyronie's disease: experience with standard lithotriptor (siemens- multiline). Urology 2002; 59: 657-661.
3. Gholami SS, Lue TF. Correction of penile curvature using the 16-dot plication technique: A review of 132 patients. J Urol 2002, 167: 2066-2069.
4. Ive FA. The umbilical, perianal and genital regions. In, Champion RH, Burton JL, Burns DA, Breathnach SM.

eds. Rook/Wilkinson/Ebling Textbook of Dermatology. Sixth edition. Oxford: Blackwell Science;1998. p. 3163-3238.

5. Sonteyrand P, Wong E, MacDonald DM. Zoon's balanitis (balanitis circumscripta plasma cellularis). Br J Dermatol 1981; 105: 195-199.

6. Ferrandiz C, Ribera M. Zoon's balanitis treated by circumcision. J Dematol Surg Oncol 1984; 10: 622-625.

7. Baldwin HE, Geronemus RG. The treatment of Zoon's balanitis with the carbon dioxide laser. J Dematol Surg Oncol 1989; 15:491-494.

8. Sehgal VN, Gangwani OP. Genital fixed drug eruptions. Genitourin Med 1986; 62: 56-58.

9. Gaffoor PM, George WM. Fixed drug eruption occurring on the male genitalia. Cutis 1990; 45: 242-244.

10. Powell JJ, Wojnarowska F. Lichen sclerosus. Lancet 1999; 353: 1777-1783.

11. Fung MA, LeBiot PE. Light microscopic criteria for the diagnosis of early vulvar lichen sclerosus. A comparison with lichen planus. Am J Surg Pathol 1998; 22: 473-478.

12. Carlson JA, Ambros R, Malfetano J, et al. Vulvar lichen sclerosis and squamous cell carcinoma: A cohort case-control and investigational study with historical perspective and sclerosis in the development of neoplasia. Hum Pathol 1998; 29: 932-948.

13. Simonart T, Noel JC, De Dobbeleer, et al. Carcinoma of the glans penis arising after 20 years of lichen sclerosus. Dermatology 1998; 196: 337-338.

14. Ghate JV, Jori JL. Behcet's disease and complex aphthosis. J Am Acad Dermatol 1999; 40: 1-18.

Chapter 39

Premalignant and Malignant Lesions of Genitalia

M Ramam

Introduction

Even though sexually transmitted diseases (STD) are considered synonymous with infections, it is important for students of this discipline to be aware of genital neoplasms for two reasons. First, patients often report with genital malignancies to the STD practitioner and knowledge about these conditions will result in early diagnosis and appropriate management. Second, there is considerable evidence that sexual exposure is related to the development of genital neoplasms [1-3] and thus these conditions fall within the purview of STD.

Definition

There is no universally accepted definition of premalignant conditions and lately, some workers have contested the concept and stated that so-called precancers are in fact cancers that have an indolent course and a low potential for metastasis.[4,5] As a clinical concept, premalignancy is used to denote conditions that, if left untreated, progress to invasive malignancy with the potential for metastasis. Most genital conditions that are widely accepted as "premalignant" represent intraepidermal or intraepithelial neoplasias. In recent reports, they are referred to as intraepithelial neoplasias with a prefix indicating the site such as cervical, vulvar, vaginal, penile or anal. Older terms for these conditions include bowenoid papulosis, erythroplasia of Queyrat and Bowen's disease. Two other conditions have been included as premalignant conditions in this chapter: Buschke Lowenstein tumour, a disease whose position between infection and neoplasia is not settled and lichen

sclerosus et atrophicus, an inflammatory condition that may be associated with the development of neoplasia in some cases.

Squamous cell carcinomas are, by far, the commonest genital malignancy. Other malignant tumours that may develop on the genitals include basal cell carcinoma, malignant melanoma and sarcomas. A list of the premalignant and malignant conditions considered in this account is given in Table 1.

Table 1. Premalignant and Malignant Lesions of Genitalia

Premalignant
Erythroplasia of Queryrat
Bowenoid papulosis
Subclinical (colposcopically visualized) lesions
Extramammary Paget's disease
Buschke-Lowenstein tumour
Lichen sclerosus et atrophicans

Malignant
Squamous cell carcinoma
Basal cell carcinoma
Malignant melanoma
Connective tissue tumours ("sarcomas")

Aetiopathogenesis

The relation between genital malignancies and sexually transmitted agents is strongest for cervical cancer[1] but has also been implicated in cancer of the anus,[2] vulva,[3] and penis.[7] Nuns have a low mortality from cervical cancer,[1] there is a strong association between the total number of sex partners and cervical neoplasia[8] and also with the total number of sex partners of the husband.[9] Similar, but weaker, associations were noted for penile[7] and anal cancer.[2] These associations led to a search for the causative organism that is responsible and over the years many agents were considered including *Treponema pallidum*,[10] *Neisseria gonorrhoeae*,[11] *Trichomonas vaginalis*,[12] *Gardnerella vaginalis*,[13] and herpes simplex virus type 2 (HSV 2).[14] In the last 2 decades, evidence has accumulated linking the human papilloma virus (HPV) to genital neoplasia. HPV DNA has been demonstrated in most patients with invasive cervical cancer in many countries[15] including India.[16-18] The HPV types most frequently found in genital neoplasia are 16 and 18.[19]

It is recognized that only a small proportion of patients affected with the oncogenic HPV types go on to develop invasive neoplasias.[20] The reasons for this are not clear. An association with HIV co-infection has been reported in HPV induced genital cancers.[21] Different variants of HPV 16 have been described and it is unclear if some of these variants are more oncogenic than others.[22] The role of host factors has also been investigated and specific HLA class II alleles have been reported to be associated with both an increased risk and protection from HPV-associated cervical cancer.[23,24]

Premalignant Lesions

An account of the morphological variants of precancerous conditions follows. In the case of many conditions, older terminology has been retained because they are more familiar to venereologists and dermatologists.

Erythroplasia of Queyrat

Erythroplasia of Queyrat represents Bowen's disease on the genital mucosa. It is characterized by a well defined, erythematous, velvety plaque (**P XXV, Fig. 99**). On the penis, the lesion is usually situated on the glans. With time, the plaque may spread to involve the preputial skin. Similar lesions have been described on the vulva. The development of induration in the plaque signifies invasive carcinoma.

A biopsy reveals atypia of keratinocytes extending throughout a thickened epidermis. The keratinocytes are enlarged with large hyperchromatic nuclei and numerous mitotic figures. A number of dyskeratotic cells are seen. In about half the cases, the cells of the basal layer are not enlarged or atypical and form a palisade of small cells below the remainder of the atypical keratinocytes, the so-called eyeliner sign. The surface may be eroded or covered with a parakeratotic crust. A dense band of lymphocytes is frequently present in the papillary dermis.

There is temporary improvement with the application of topical corticosteroids. Other agents such as topical 5-fluorouracil, electrodessication, cryotherapy and radiotherapy have been reported to be useful. Excision of the lesion is the definitive treatment. Invasive carcinoma was concurrently found in 10% of cases in one series.[25] If invasion develops, the lesion should be treated like a squamous cell carcinoma.

Bowenoid Papulosis

Bowenoid papulosis is characterized by multiple, brown, small, 2-10 mm, slightly elevated papules. The colour may vary from skin coloured to brown, erythematous to violaceous (**P XXI, Fig. 82, 83**). The lesions are asymptomatic and have often been present for long periods of time before the patient comes to medical attention. The surface is slightly verrucous in some papules but may be smooth. Some papules coalesce to form small plaques and there may be mild scaling on the surface. In men, the papules are usually present on the penile shaft and glans and in women, on the perianal area and the vulva. Occasionally lesions may occur on the extragenital sites and even oral mucosa.[26-27]

Biopsy of a papule reveals unexpectedly atypical findings in these banal lesions. The epidermis is thickened and hyperkeratotic with focal parakeratosis. There are necrotic and dyskeratotic keratinocytes. There is crowding of the nuclei of keratinocytes which are large, hyperchromatic and pleomorphic. Mitoses are frequent and some are atypical. The histopathological features are identical to erythroplasia of Queyrat and Bowen's disease though some authors have stated that cytologic atypia is less severe in Bowenoid papulosis.[28]

Invasive carcinoma is distinctly rare[29] and spontaneous regression has been reported.[30]

The papules may be destroyed by any physical (electrocautery, cryotherapy, laser) or chemical (podophyllin, trichloroacetic acid) modality with equally good results. Recurrences may develop in some patients. The use of topical cidofovir[31] and imiquimod[32] have also been described recently but these compounds require further evaluation.

Colposcopically Visualized Lesions

Unaided visual examination of the genital tract has

been shown to have a low sensitivity for the detection of intraepithelial neoplasia especially in women. Colposcopic examination, with the application of acetic acid is useful in finding suspicious lesions, which may be further, investigated by exfoliative cytology or biopsy. If the dysplasia detected is low grade, no treatment is required and regular follow up is recommended. If high grade dysplasia including intraepithelial neoplasia is detected, excision by surgery or laser is the treatment of choice. Other modalities that have been described include application of 5-FU, electrodessication, cryotherapy and radiotherapy.

Extramammary Paget's Disease

This extremely rare condition presents as an itchy, red, scaly plaque in the anogenital region of patients who are usually older than 50. In most cases, the condition represents an intraepidermal adenocarcinoma with no other association; invasive carcinoma was reported in 12% and an associated vulval adenocarcinoma in 4%.[33] About 12% of patients have an associated underlying malignancy.[34]

Biopsy reveals large, pale atypical cells in the epidermis, arranged singly or in clusters. The nuclei of the cells are hyperchromatic and abnormal mitotic figures may be visible. The neoplastic cells may extend down the hair follicles and sweat glands.

The standard treatment is wide excision but recently, conservative vulva-sparing surgery has been recommended though recurrences are more frequent with the latter.[35] The prognosis is excellent in cases that are not associated with an underlying adnexal or visceral tumour.

Buschke-Lowenstein Tumour

Buschke-Lowenstein tumour otherwise known as giant condyloma accuminatum presents as an asymptomatic, papillomatous growth on the genitalia or the perianal area that grows to a large size (**P XXV, Fig. 100, 101**). Most of the lesions are 5 cm or more in diameter at the time of presentation. The surface and the consistency of the lesion is variegated: soft areas have a papillomatous surface while hard areas have a smoother surface. Typical cutaneous and mucosal warts may be present adjacent to the mass. Maceration and secondary infection are frequent in uncircumcised men. Local invasion of the tumour may lead to perforation of the prepuce and extension into the deeper structures of the glans leading

to induration. Giant condyloma acuminatum affecting urinary bladder in a patient with multiple sclerosis on immunosuppressives has been described.[36]

Biopsy shows massive epidermal hyperplasia without significant atypia. These patients often undergo multiple biopsies to rule out a malignancy. Human papilloma virus-induced changes of vacuolisation of the cells of the granular layer with clumping of coarse keratohyaline granules are usually absent in the main lesion but may be observed in the adjacent, smaller warts.

The exact position of the Buschke-Lowenstein tumour in the spectrum of benign and malignant lesions is not established. It grows larger than typical genital warts and tends to persist for longer. Rarely, invasive squamous cell carcinoma may supervene.[37]

In a study of 42 cases of Buschke-Lowenstein tumour affecting the anorectal and perianal region the tendency for local recurrence was seen in upto 66%. The recurrence was associated with longer duration of disease. Malignant transformation was reported in 56% and metastasis was rare.[38] Recently it has been proposed that if the tumours are confined to glans, a glansectomy to be carried out (in place of amputation) to preserve maximal penile length and functional integrity of corpora cavernosa. Patients were able to resume sexual activity one month post operatively and no recurrence was observed in 18 to 65 months follow up.[39] Other workers have administered interferon α post operatively or into the lesion to prevent the recurrence.[40] In our experience and that of others,[41] the lesion may respond partially to podophyllin. The frequency of applications may need to be increased above the once-weekly schedule for patients with ordinary genital warts and we have used alternate-day application in some patients. However, this course is not advisable for lesions in the perianal area or if the patient is unable to carry out instructions as misuse of the agent can lead to severe oedema and ulceration. There may be a reduction in the size of the tumour with this therapy. However, complete clearance with podophyllin alone is uncommon and the residual lesion may require excision or cryotherapy. In our opinion, amputation of the genitalia is unwarranted because of the benign course of the disease and the response to simpler modalities of treatment.

Lichen Sclerosus et Atrophicus

Lichen sclerosus et atrophicus is a disease of unknown aetiology with a predilection for genital skin. It occurs in both sexes but appears to be commoner in women. There are two age groups in which the disease is common: prepubertal children and older men and women.

The well-developed lesion is a shiny, hypopigmented atrophic plaque with underlying sclerosis. Telangiectasias and purpuras may be visible on the surface. The papules and plaques may enlarge and encircle the vulval orifice in women or the preputial opening in men. In men, this constriction leads to phimosis and predisposes to injury during coitus. There may be meatal stenosis with restriction of the urinary stream. In women, the mucosal surface may show fissuring. The perianal skin may also be affected. Some patients also have lesions at other, non-genital sites.

A skin biopsy reveals oedema and sclerosis of the papillary dermis. The overlying epidermis shows atrophy and follicular plugging. There is vacuolisation of the basal layer. A band-like infiltrate of lymphocytes is seen in the upper dermis just below the zone of oedema and sclerosis. In older lesions, oedema is less prominent, the basal layer is reconstituted, the infiltrate diminishes and sclerosis extends into the reticular dermis. At this stage, the changes may be indistinguishable from morphoea.

Early in disease, clobetasol propionate produces significant softening of the skin and may even reverse phimosis in men. Once symptoms and signs are relieved, therapy can be maintained with mild to moderate potency topical steroids. If the phimosis is unresponsive to treatment, circumcision may be considered so that the glans can be visualized and monitored.

The lesions must be monitored at regular intervals for the development of squamous cell carcinoma. The risk of developing cancer is widely recognized in women and a cohort study found that invasive carcinoma developed in 21% of women with symptomatic lichen sclerosus.[42] A recent study has suggested that men may also have an increased risk for developing squamous cell carcinoma.[43,44]

Malignant Lesions

Squamous Cell Carcinoma of Penis and Vulva

Squamous cell carcinoma is the commonest neoplasm of the genital tract in both men and women. The incidence of penile cancer varies consideraby from one population to another and is reported to be highest in

Uganda and lowest in Israel.[45] Epidemiological data for India is not available but the disease is not uncommon. The risk factors for developing penile cancer reported in different studies include phimosis, chronic balanoposthitis, lichen sclerosus et atrophicus, condyloma accuminata, multiple sexual partners and smoking. Neonatal circumcision is protective[7,46,50] but circumcision after the first year appears not to provide any significant reduction in risk. Treatments with PUVA and UVB have been associated with penile cancer in Western populations[51] but it is unlikely that these findings are relevant to Indian patients. HPV DNA has been detected in about 40% of cases.[6]

The condition presents as an asymptomatic, indurated papule or nodule that may be ulcerated. Early lesions may be mistaken for a sexually transmitted infection especially donovanosis and it is imperative to consider the diagnosis of penile cancer in patients with long standing ulcers or those recalcitrant to treatment. Neglected, the nodule progresses into an exophytic mass with necrosis and secondary infection (**P XXVI, Fig. 102, 103**).

Squamous cell carcinoma of the vulva presents with firm, indurated papules and nodules which may ulcerate. As in men, a high index of suspicion in ulcers that do not behave as expected will prevent misdiagnosis of vulval carcinoma.

Metastasis to the regional lymph nodes is common in both penile and vulval carcinoma and has been reported in about 60%[52] and 30%[53] of cases respectively.

The diagnosis is confirmed by biopsy which demonstrates atypical keratinocytes extending into the dermis (**P XXVI, Fig. 104**). The tumour shows varying degrees of differentiation; well differentiated tumours show mature keratinocytes with intercellular bridges and multiple horn pearls while undifferentiated tumours show cells with a high nuclear-cytoplasmic ratio, few intercellular bridges and little keratinization. There is often a dense infiltrate of lymphocytes in the dermis. The involvement of the regional lymph nodes can be assessed by fine needle aspiration cytology.

Treatment consists of excision of the tumour with a 2 cm margin. On the penis, this implies partial or complete amputation. If lymph nodes show metastatic disease, lymphadenectomy is indicated.

The prognosis depends on the tumour size and stage. Without metastasis, the 5-year survival rate in penile cancer is 60-90%, while it is 10-30% when nodal metastasis develops.[52] The 5-year survival rate for vulval carcinoma is about 70%.[54]

Other Malignancies

Malignancies of the genital tract other than squamous cell carcinoma are distinctly uncommon.

Basal Cell Carcinoma

Less than 200 cases of basal cell carcinomas have been reported on the genitals and perianal area and represent less than 1% of all basal cell carcinomas.[55,56] HPV does not appear to play a role in the development of these tumours.[55,57,58] The carcinoma occurs in older patients in the fifth to tenth decades. At presentation, the lesion is usually large in size and is ulcerated in about a third of patients. Biopsy reveals aggregates of basaloid cells with peripheral palisading and clefts between the aggregates and the stroma. Excision is the treatment of choice and the 5 year survival rate approaches 100%.[55]

Malignant Melanoma

Melanomas of the penis and vulva are rare and comprise about 1%[59] and 4-10%[60] of all malignancies at these sites respectively. The tumour usually presents as a pigmented macule or nodule; some lesions may be non-pigmented. Biopsy of the nodule reveals a poorly circumscribed lesion with atypical melanocytes within the epidermis and in irregular nests and aggregates in the dermis that vary in size and pigmentation. The melanocytes have large nuclei with prominent nucleoli and do not diminish in size with descent into the dermis. Wide local excision with a clear surgical margin is the treatment of choice. Lymphadenectomy is indicated if there is spread of disease to the lymph nodes. As with other cutaneous melanomas, prognosis depends on the stage of disease. The prognosis is good for stage I lesions with a 5-year survival rate of more than 90% and poor for patients with thick tumours and metastatic disease who have a 5-year survival rate of 30% or less.[61,62]

Sarcomas

Sarcomas of the genitals are extremely uncommon and are beyond the scope of this chapter. The interested reader is referred to a comprehensive account of these tumours.[63]

References

1. Fraumeni JF Jr, Lloyd JW, Smith EM, Wagoner JK. Cancer mortality among nuns: role of marital status in aetiology of neoplastic disease in women. J Natl Cancer Inst 1969; 42: 455-468.

2. Daling JR, Weiss NS, Hislop TG, et al. Sexual practices, sexually transmitted diseases, and the incidence of anal cancer. N Engl J Med 1987; 317: 973-977.

3. Newcomb PA, Weiss NS, Daling JR. Incidence of vulvar carcinoma in relation to menstrual, reproductive, and medical factors. J Natl Cancer Inst 1984; 73: 391-396.

4. Lober BA, Lober CW. Actinic keratosis is squamous cell carcinoma. South Med J 2000; 93: 650-655.

5. Ackerman AB, Vassallo. Conversion or transformation into cancer. In: Ackerman AB, Mones J. edrs Resolving quandaries in dermatology, pathology and dermatopathology. New York: Ardor Scribendi; 2001. p. 110-113.

6. Rubin MA, Kleter B, Zhou M, et al. Detection and typing of human papillomavirus DNA in penile carcinoma: evidence for multiple independent pathways of penile carcinogenesis. Am J Pathol 2001; 159: 1211-1218.

7. Maden C, Sherman KJ, Beckmann AM, et al. History of circumcision, medical conditions, and sexual activity and risk of penile cancer. J Natl Cancer Inst 1993, 85: 19-24.

8. Hulka BS. Risk factors for cervical cancer. J Chronic Dis 1982; 35: 3-11.

9. Buckley JD, Henderson BE, Morrow CP, et al. Case-control study of gestational choriocarcinoma. Cancer Res. 1988; 48: 1004-1010.

10. Rojel J. The interrelation between uterine cancer and syphilis: a pathodemographic study. Acta Pathol Microbiol Scand 1953; 97: 13.

11. Furgyik S, Astedt B. Gonorrhoeal infection followed by an increased frequency of cervical carcinoma. Acta Obstet Gynecol Scand 1980; 59: 521-524.

12. Zhang ZF, Graham S, Yu SZ, et al. *Trichomonas vaginalis* and cervical cancer. A prospective study in China. Ann Epidemiol. 1995; 5: 325-332.

13. Frega A, Stentella P, Spera G, et al. Cervical intraepithelial neoplasia and bacterial vaginosis: correlation or risk factor? Eur J Gynaecol Oncol 1997; 18: 76-77.

14. Olsen AO, Orstavik I, Dillner J, Vestergaard BF, Magnus P. Herpes simplex virus and human papillomavirus in a population-based case-control study of cervical intraepithelial neoplasia grade II-III. APMIS 1998; 106: 417-424.

15. Bosch FX, Manos MM, Munoz N, et al. Prevalence of human papillomavirus in cervical cancer: a worldwide perspective. International biological study on cervical cancer (IBSCC) study group. J Natl Cancer Inst 1995, 87: 796-802

16. Saranath D, Khan Z, Tandle AT, et al. HPV16/18 prevalence in cervical lesions/cancers and p53 genotypes

in cervical cancer patients from India. Gynecol Oncol 2002; 86: 157-162.

17. Gopalkrishna V, Aggarwal N, Malhotra VL, et al. *Chlamydia trachomatis* and human papillomavirus infection in Indian women with sexually transmitted diseases and cervical precancerous and cancerous lesions. Clin Microbiol Infect 2000; 6: 88-93.

18. Chatterjee R, Roy A, Basu S. Detection of type specific human papillomavirus (HPV) DNA in cervical cancers of Indian women. Indian J Pathol Microbiol 1995; 38: 33-42.

19. Wilczynski SP, Walker J, Liao SY, Bergen S, Berman M. Adenocarcinoma of the cervix associated with human papillomavirus. Cancer 1988; 62: 1331-1336.

20. Helmerhorst TJ, Meijer CJ. Cervical cancer should be considered as a rare complication of oncogenic HPV infection rather than a STD. Int J Gynecol Cancer 2002; 12: 235-236.

21. Frisch M, Biggar RJ, Goedert JJ. Human papillomavirus-associated cancers in patients with human immunodeficiency virus infection and acquired immunodeficiency syndrome. J Natl Cancer Inst 2000; 92: 1500-1510.

22. Da Costa MM, Hogeboom CJ, Holly EA, Palefsky JM. Increased risk of high-grade anal neoplasia associated with a human papillomavirus type 16 E6 sequence variant. J Infect Dis 2002; 185: 1229-1237.

23. Odunsi K, Ganesan T. Motif analysis of HLA class II molecules that determine the HPV associated risk of cervical carcinogenesis. Int J Mol Med 2001; 8: 405-412.

24. Odunsi K, Terry G, Ho L, et al. Susceptibility to human papillomavirus-associated cervical intra-epithelial neoplasia is determined by specific HLA DR-DQ alleles. Int J Cancer 1996; 67: 595-602.

25. Graham JH, Helwig EB. Erythroplasia of Queyrat. A clinicopathologic and histochemical study. Cancer 1973; 32: 1396-1414.

26. Popadopoulos AJ, Schwartz RA, Lefkowitz A, et al. Extragenital bowenoid papulosis associated with atypical human papilloma virus genotype. J Cutan Med Surg 2002; 6: 117-121.

27. Daley T, Birek C, Wysocki GP. Oral bowenoid lesions:differential diagnosis and pathogenetic insights. Oral Surg Oral Med Oral Pathol Oral Radiol Endod 2002; 90: 466-473.

28. Patterson JW, Kao GF, Graham JH, Helwig EB. Bowenoid papulosis. A clinicopathologic study with ultrastructural observations. Cancer 1986; 57: 823-836.

29. Yoneta A, Yamashita T, Jin HY, et al. Development of squamous cell carcinoma by two high-risk human papillomaviruses (HPVs), a novel HPV-67 and HPV-31 from bowenoid papulosis. Br J Dermatol 2000; 143: 604-608.

30. Eisen RF, Bhawan J, Cahn TH. Spontaneous regression of bowenoid papulosis of the penis. Cutis 1983; 32: 269-272.

31. Snoeck R, Van Laethem Y, De Clercq E, De Maubeuge J, Clumeck N. Treatment of a bowenoid papulosis of the penis with local applications of cidofovir in a patient with acquired immunodeficiency syndrome. Arch Intern Med 2001; 161: 2382-2384.

32. Petrow W, Gerdsen R, Uerlich M, Richter O, Bieber T. Successful topical immunotherapy of bowenoid papulosis with imiquimod. Br J Dermatol 2001; 145: 1022-1023.

33. Fanning J, Lambert HC, Hale TM, Morris PC, Schuerch C. Paget's disease of the vulva: prevalence of associated vulvar adenocarcinoma, invasive Paget's disease, and recurrence after surgical excision. Am J Obstet Gynecol 1999; 180: 24-27.

34. Chanda JJ. Extramammary Paget's disease: prognosis and relationship to internal malignancy. J Am Acad Dermatol 1985; 13: 1009-1014.

35. Louis-Sylvestre C, Haddad B, Paniel BJ. Paget's disease of the vulva: results of different conservative treatments. Eur J Obstet Gynecol Reprod Biol 2001; 99: 253-255.

36. Wioedemann A, Diekman WP, Holtmann G, Kracht H. Report of a case of giant condyloma(Buschke-Löwenstein tumour) localized in bladder. J Urol 1995; 153: 1222-1224.

37. Bjorck M, Athlin L, Lundskog B. Giant condyloma acuminatum (Buschke-Löwenstein tumour) of the anorectum with malignant transformation. Eur J Surg 1995; 161: 691-694.

38. Chu QD, Vezeridis MP, Libbey NP, Wanebo HJ. Giant condyloma acuminatum (Buschke-Löwenstein tumour) of anorectal and perianal region. Analysis of 42 cases. Dis Colon Rectum 1994; 37: 950-957.

39. Hatzichristu DG, Apostolidis A, Tzortzis V, et al. Glansectomy: an alternative surgical treatment of Buschke-Lowenstein tumour of the penis. Urology 2001; 57: 966-969.

40. Moreira PM, Perez LA, Colome EM. Giant inguinal condyloma (Buschke-Löwenstein tumour) with clinical aspect of squamous cell carcinoma. Rev Cubana Med Trop 2002; 52: 70-72.

41. Bedi TR, Pandhi RK. Buschke-Lowenstein's tumour presenting with urinary fistula. Br J Vener Dis 1977; 53: 200-202.

42. Carlson JA, Ambros R, Malfetano J, et al. Vulvar lichen sclerosus and squamous cell carcinoma: a cohort, case control, and investigational study with historical perspective; implications for chronic inflammation and sclerosis in the development of neoplasia. Hum Pathol 1998; 29: 932-948.

43. Powell J, Robson A, Cranston D, Wojnarowska F, Turner R. High incidence of lichen sclerosus in patients with squamous cell carcinoma of the penis. Br J Dermatol 2001; 145: 85-89.

44. Kanwar AJ, Thami GP, Kaur S, et al. Squamous cell carcinoma in long standing untreated lichen sclerosus et atrophicus of penis. Urol Int 2002; 68: 291-295.

45. Parkin DM, Whelan SL, Ferlay J, et al. editors. IARC Scientific Publications No. 143, Vol. VII, Cancer incidence in five continents. IARC Scientific Publications, Lyon, 1997.

46. Tsen HF, Morgenstern H, Mack T, Peters RK. Risk factors for penile cancer: results of a population-based case-control study in Los Angeles County (United States). Cancer Causes Control 2001; 12: 267-277.

47. Maiche AG. Epidemiological aspects of cancer of the penis in Finland. Eur J Cancer Prev 1992; 1: 153-158.

48. Daling JR, Sherman KJ, Hislop TG, et al. Cigarette smoking and the risk of anogenital cancer. Am J Epidemiol 1992; 135: 180-189.

49. Brinton LA, Li JY, Rong SD, et al. Risk factors for penile cancer: results from a case-control study in China. Int J Cancer 1991; 47: 504-509.

50. Hellberg D, Valentin J, Eklund T, Nilsson S. Penile cancer: is there an epidemiological role for smoking and sexual behaviour? Br Med J (Clin Res Ed). 1987; 295 (6609): 1306-1308.

51. Stern RS, Bagheri S, Nichols K. The persistent risk of genital tumours among men treated with psoralen plus ultraviolet A (PUVA) for psoriasis. J Am Acad Dermatol 2002; 47: 33-39.

52. Srinivas V, Morse MJ, Herr HW, Sogani PC, Whitmore WF Jr. Penile cancer: relation of extent of nodal metastasis to survival. J Urol 1987; 137: 880-882.

53. Binder SW, Huang I, Fu YS, Hacker NF, Berek JS. Risk factors for the development of lymph node metastasis in vulvar squamous cell carcinoma. Gynecol Oncol 1990; 37: 9-16.

54. Edwards CL, Tortolero-Luna G, Linares AC, et al. Vulvar intraepithelial neoplasia and vulvar cancer. Obstet Gynecol Clin North Am 1996; 23: 295-324.

55. Gibson GE, Ahmed I. Perianal and genital basal cell carcinoma: A clinicopathologic review of 51 cases. J Am Acad Dermatol 2001; 45: 68-71.

56. Betti R, Bruscagin C, Inselvini E, Crosti C. Basal cell carcinomas of covered and unusual sites of the body. Int J Dermatol 1997; 36: 503-505.

57. Nehal KS, Levine VJ, Ashinoff R. Basal cell carcinoma of the genitalia. Dermatol Surg. 1998; 24: 1361-1363.

58. Kort R, Fazaa B, Bouden S, et al. Perianal basal cell carcinoma. Int J Dermatol 1995; 34: 427-428.

59. Southwick A, Rigby O, Daily M, Noyes RD. Malignant melanoma of the penis and sentinel lymph node biopsy. J Urol 2001; 166: 1833.

60. Kendall Pierson K. Malignant melanoma and pigmented lesions of the vulva. In: Wilkinson EJ, edr. Pathology of the Vulva and Vagina. Edinburgh: Churchill Livingstone; 1987. p. 155-179.

61. Stillwell TJ, Zincke H, Gaffey TA, Woods JE. Malignant melanoma of the penis. J Urol. 1988; 140: 72-75.

62. Verschraegen CF, Benjapibal M, Supakarapongkul W, et al. Vulvar melanoma at the M. D. Anderson Cancer Centre: 25 years later. Int J Gynecol Cancer. 2001; 11: 359-64.

63. Weiss SW, Goldblum JR, Enzinger FM, eds. Enzinger and Weiss's Soft Tissue Tumours. 4th ed. St Louis: Mosby Inc; 2001.

PART IX
Psychological Aspects of Sexually Transmitted Diseases

Chapter 40

Sexual Behaviour and Sexually Transmitted Diseases

B M Tripathi, Sameer Malhotra

Introduction

Sexual behaviour includes all the activities related to expression and gratification of sexual needs. It is an important component of the expression of one's sexuality. The term 'sexuality' is often used to refer to its various aspects like sexual behaviour, sexual orientation, gender identification and role, social roles, relationships and eroticism. Sexuality is influenced by a number of social, cultural, psychological and biological factors and developmental experiences throughout the life cycle. Inherent complexities and issues of privacy make the study and understanding of the sensitive area of human sexual behaviours more difficult. Sexual behaviours have been studied in the context of sexual relationships and practices, reproductive health, sexually transmitted diseases (STD) and other reproductive tract infections, birth control and contraceptive decision making. Sexual behaviour and practices are linked to the acquisition and spread of STD including HIV/AIDS. In recent years a rising trend of STD and HIV infection has been observed in the country. The incidence rate of STD in India is estimated to be 5%, which means 40–50 million new infections every year.[1] Currently India is the country with largest HIV epidemic in the region[2-5]. STD and HIV infection are no longer restricted to the high risk groups but have spilled over to affect the general population as well.[6] In the current context, understanding of sexual behaviours in the general population as well as in high-risk groups, is important for prevention and treatment of STD and HIV/AIDS.

In this chapter, our discussion is restricted to the areas of: (i) sexual behaviour in Indian context-cultural and current perspective; (ii) sexual behaviour linked to sexual knowledge and attitude in general population and risk groups; (iii) factors associated with/ contributing to high-risk sexual behaviour and in turn to the risk of acquiring or spreading STD/HIV infection; and (iv) prevention of STD and HIV infection.

Sexuality and Sexual Behaviour in Indian Context

Ancient Hindu literature is rich in sexual symbolism and eroticism. Vatsyayana's *Kamasutra,* (a practical discourse on aspects of sexuality), erotic sculptures carved on the stone walls of the holy shrines of Khajuraho, Konark and many other Hindu temples of the medieval era, beautifully depict the various techniques of sexual acts, probably practiced during those times. Certain indications towards polygamous and polyandrous relationships from the famous Indian mythological scriptures, indicate a state of extraordinary openness in sexual matters in certain periods of Indian history, contrary to the periods of Muslim and British reigns and contemporary India. Prostitution as a profession has a long history in India and is mentioned in Kautilya's *Arthashastra (circa* 300 BC) and Vatsayana's *Kama Sutra*.[7-9] The *devadasi* (handmaiden of god) system of dedicating unmarried young girls to gods in Hindu temples, which often made them objects of sexual pleasure of temple priests and pilgrims, was an established custom in India by 300 AD. Prostitution was prevalent in large Indian cities during the eighteenth and the first half of the nineteenth centuries of British rule.[9]

The practice of homosexuality is also not new to India. Vatsayana's *Kama Sutra* refers to the practice of eunuchs and male servants giving oral sex to their male patrons and masters respectively.[7-9] Some erotic sculptures of medieval Hindu temples depict lesbian acts. The Muslim rulers in India are reported to have maintained harems of young boys. During the British rule sodomy (anal intercourse) was made illegal under section 377 of the Indian Penal Code enacted in 1861. Indian homosexual activists think that because of this legal provision, male homosexuals are often subjected to undue harassment and blackmail.

By and large Indian society is still rooted in traditions and people's attitude towards sex is influenced by values, which are peculiar to the traditional belief system. Marriage is a norm in India. Since the last few decades, the average age at marriage for both sexes has been rising by about a year per decade. As a result, a substantial proportion of boys and girls in contemporary India have to pass through a long period of heightened sexual desires.[9] The dominant value system strongly disapproves of premarital sexual relation amongst males and females, and fidelity within marriage is the ideal norm. Woman's virginity until marriage is still greatly valued. Even today in some sections of the population, particularly rural, boys and girls are betrothed at a young age and are allowed to have sex only after the bride attains menarche, when she is sent to stay with her husband (a practice called as 'gauna'). Although unmarried men have more opportunities for sexual adventures (often with married women/female sex workers) than unmarried women, there is no mainstream society in India that actually encourages men to have premarital sex.[10] As in the case of premarital sex, sanctions against extramarital affairs and sex are severer against women. The Hindu concept of 'pativrata'-the ideal for a woman to remain loyal to her husband under all circumstances has no counterpart for men.[9] Thus unmarried women for the fear of being called promiscuous find themselves unable to seek reproductive health services. However, women are now getting greater attention towards the emancipation of their sexuality. Sexual activity among unmarried adolescent women has been steadily increasing and so is the vulnerability towards STD including HIV. Many young girls are also at risk of sexual violence including rape. The issue of teenage pregnancy is of concern and is associated with significant morbidity and mortality in the mother and the child.

Gender relations in marriage are dynamic and continually negotiated. Women tend to use access to sex as a resource, a bargaining chip to reward/punish their husbands.[11] Sexual coercion occurs frequently in marriage.[12-13] However, women and men tend to differ in their perception of the nature of sexual coercion.[11]

The women consider sex to be coerced if the sexual relations with their husbands are against their wishes. The men in contrast feel that they have a right to demand sex in marriage and have right to access to their wives' body.

Engaging in sex frequently, having multiple sex partners, having many children and impregnating one's wife soon after marriage have been considered as significant indicators of masculinity/male characteristics.[10,14] Women are limited in their ability to control the interactions because of their low social status and economic dependence and also because of the power men have over women's sexuality.[15] Wife abuse appears to be common among men who have extramarital sex.[12] Women are often discriminated by their own kind.[16] In many cases the mother-in-law often takes the decision of marriage and first pregnancy.[17]

Diseases of the genitalia are regarded as *gupt rog* (secretive ailments); sex being considered a taboo and not a topic for open discussion in the society. Ignorance about sexual matters and illiteracy foster myths and prejudices towards sex. 'Virya' (semen) is considered to be the source of physical and spiritual strength. Loss of *virya* (through masturbation/nocturnal emissions or *swapnadosh*/wet dream) is considered harmful both physically and spiritually, and a cause of weakness.[7,9,18] This could be the reason for guilt feelings associated with pleasure during masturbation.[19] The traditional systems of medicine, both Ayurveda and Unani, lay emphasis on semen preservation, sexual restraint and diet. According to the metaphysical physiology, food is believed to be converted into blood and blood into semen. As a result there are many beliefs and practices prescribed to preserve and enhance the quality and quantity of semen. *Dhat syndrome*, a culture bound syndrome in India, is characterized by the guilt about loss of semen in young men, often leading to undue concern with its debilitating effect on physical and psychological health.[20-22]

Social and attitudinal changes and socio-economic developments during the post- independence period have lead to emergence of consumerist society and development of 'Western' oriented life styles. Western influence is evident in daily living, particularly in the urban areas amongst the youth. Pubs, late night parties and discotheques are often frequented by the young in major metropolitan cities, exposing this vulnerable population to risky behaviours. Recent years have seen developments in electronic media and sex entertainment is available through video, X-rated films and internet.

Indian society presents a contrasting picture of notions about sexuality, attitudes and sexual behaviour. The society can neither be regarded as rigid, nor permissive with regards to the area of sexuality, making generalizations difficult. The behaviour patterns vary across regions and states, gender, sub-populations, tribal and religious groups.

Sexual Knowledge, Attitude and Behaviour

Adult Population

There is a low level of knowledge about the body and reproductive health, including reproduction and contraception among men and women of all ages, marital status and geographical locations in the country. Young men and adult males, as compared to young women, usually know more about certain matters pertaining to sexuality like masturbation, orgasm, sexual intercourse, oral sex and contraception.

Traditionally sexual problems are known as *gupt rog* (secretive ailments), which refer to culturally defined illnesses of secret parts of the body and are therefore problems that are shameful and need to be kept a secret. Male sexual problems can be broadly categorized into contact problems (STD) which are referred to as *garmi* in local language and non-contact problems.[23-25] Men show great concern towards the non-contact problems viz., quality and quantity of semen, impotence/ erectile difficulties and premature ejaculation. Masturbation and nocturnal emissions (*swapnadosh*) are also frequently considered to be health problems. These sexual dysfunctions can have deep psychological impact, and can greatly influence the quality of married life, sexual behaviour and reproductive health. Males residing in slums, who have non-marital relations and those who spend more time with peers in male organizations and in smoking, drinking and gambling activities more often report non-contact problems. Having a non-contact problem is closely associated with having a contact problem.[25,26]

Women usually find their first sexual experience to be traumatic. Despite this first negative experience, majority of women develop a positive attitude towards sex as the marriage years progress. It has also been observed that women do communicate their sexual desire through direct physical contact or through various forms of verbal communication. It is quite contradictory to earlier notion that Indian women do no express their desire for sex.[27] Women are known to deny sex to their husbands if the husband is drinking (alcohol) heavily or not supporting the family. Physical violence is common amongst women who deny sex to their husbands. Abusive men are more likely to engage in extramarital sex and have STD symptoms, thereby placing their wives at risk for STD acquisition, sometimes via sexual abuse.[12]

Pre- and extra-marital relations are not socially approved but have been reported in many studies.[28,29] General population surveys have reported premarital sexual activity among 7-48% of male respondents and 3-10% of female respondents.[30-32] Men have a wide variety of premarital sex partners including sex workers, friends, relatives, and future spouses.[32] Premarital/ extramarital sexual encounters are significantly higher among unmarried, urban males. Almost half of those who have sex before or outside marriage report not using a condom during such encounters.[31]

Heterosexual relations with a person other than the legal spouse have also been reported amongst middle class professionals. In males, premarital sex is observed to increase the likelihood of extramarital sex.[33]

Fondling of breasts, kissing and vaginal penetrative sex are identified as the most common sexual acts in the minds of rural men and women. Sexuality and sexual behaviour in rural areas are expressed and practiced in a variety of contexts. Some factors and rituals that provide sexual contexts include (a) *Kumar Purnima* in Orissa which provides a unique opportunity to young and old women alike to share sexual knowledge and transmit certain sexual culture in an acceptable form; (b) *Gauna* (time gap between marriage and consummation of marriage) in North India is particularly a vulnerable period for young men; (c) the practice of *Kudike* (widow remarriage where widow is remarried but does not get the position of wife) adds another dimension to sexual context in rural Karnataka; (d) practice of commercial sex in a very non-commercial context in certain rural communities in Rajasthan and the practice of *Atta-satta* (practice of marrying on an exchange basis); and (e) pornographic literature and films which provide another explicit sexual context in the rural areas. Given a highly selective rural-urban migration and risky sexual behaviour of single migrant men, women in rural areas become vulnerable irrespective of their behaviour.[26]

A recent study on sexual behaviours and risk

perceptions among young men in the border towns of Nepal revealed the presence of risk behaviours in the migrant population (viz., Indian truck drivers and transportation workers) and the potential risk of HIV transmission across borders.[34]

The behavioural surveillance surveys (BSS) serve as early warning signals of the potential risk for HIV, can help explain trends in HIV prevalence in sub populations at high risk of infection, and reflect the impact of HIV prevention programme over time. Most recent rounds of BSS have been conducted by APAC (AIDS Prevention and Control) & FHI (Family Health International) and NACO (National AIDS Control Organization).[35-38] The APAC & FHI surveys in general population included auto-rickshaw drivers, diamond workers, industry workers, fishing industry workers, migrant workers, miners, plantation workers from many states of India. The reports suggest that many young men are involved in unprotected sex mostly with female commercial sex workers (CSW). The knowledge that consistent condom use prevents HIV/ AIDS does not necessarily translate into desired behaviour change. Though Behaviour Surveillance Surveys (BSS) have generally been conducted in the context of HIV infection, the findings are relevant for understanding sexual behaviours and prevention of STD and HIV/ AIDS.

The recent BSS findings reveal that more than three-fourth of the 84478 respondents across the country had at least heard of HIV/AIDS. More than 70% of the total respondents were also aware of the major routes of HIV/ AIDS transmission. However, the potential of mother to child transmission is still less known to respondents across the country. Less than one-third of the respondents had heard of STD and only one-fifth were aware of the linkage between STD and HIV throughout the country. There is low awareness about HIV/AIDS and its transmission amongst rural women in Bihar, Uttar Pradesh, Madhya Pradesh and West Bengal. Awareness about condom was less in rural areas and over one-third of rural females had neither seen nor heard about condom. The median age at first sex was 21 years for males and 18 years for females in the entire country. About 11.8% males and 2% females reported sex with non-regular partners in a 12-month recall period. Less than half of the males and about 60% females did not report using condom during the last sex encounter with their non-regular partners. Table-1 highlights the findings from nation wide baseline behavioural

Table 1.   Sexual Behaviour in the General Population

Information	N=	Urban		Rural	
		Male 20775	Female 21287	Male 20853	Female 21267
Age at first sex (in years)		21	18	20	18
Sex with non-regular partner (in last 12 months		12.6	2.3	11.4	1.8
Ever heard or seen a condom		94.7	86.2	84.5	69.5
Ever heard of STD other than HIV/AIDS		37.0	36.9	30.2	31.1
Genital discharge (in last 12 months)		1.0	4.3	1.7	5.5
Genital ulcers/sores (in last 12 months)		1.7	2.0	2.0	2.1
Awareness of link between STD & HIV		27.7	24.2	21.2	16.8
Ever heard of HIV		93.2	85.7	79.5	65.2
HIV can be transmitted through					
sexual contact		89.0	80.3	74.6	59.8
blood transmission		90.8	81.8	75.8	61.0
MTCT		81.7	77.8	68.2	58.7
Needle sharing		88.8	80.5	74.5	60.0
Breast feeding		62.4	63.2	55.3	49.7
HIV can be prevented through					
Consistent condom use		82.8	63.9	66.3	42.9
Faithfulness to the sexual partner		71.9	64.8	59.6	47.7

Total respondents = 84182 (Urban = 42062, Rural = 42120) (All India mean figures)
Source: National Baseline General Population Behavioural Surveillance Survey 2001 (*NACO 2002*)

surveillance survey amongst general population conducted in the year 2001.[38-39]

Adolescent Population

Much of the sexual behaviour is learned and early sexual experiences, particularly those in puberty and early adolescence, can have an effect on sexual behaviour during the later part of life. Sexual knowledge is often acquired through mass media and friends. Men report that they receive information about sexuality from their sisters-in-law (*bhabhis*), older brothers, 'instinct' and mass media. Other sources include peers, schoolbooks and teachers, community awareness programs. Parents are neither considered nor preferred as a source of such information by the adolescents. While girls feel masturbation causes weakness, disease, infertility and marital disharmony, boys feel that 'losing semen' leads to weakness.[10] Generally males have more knowledge about sex and masturbation is a source of sexual release in premarital years.[40] Substantial lacunae in knowledge of HIV/AIDS, STD and sexuality have been observed among college students,[41] particularly amongst girls from rural areas.[42] Although adolescents are somewhat aware of methods of contraception, they do not know how to use them effectively. Adolescent rural girls, because of their ignorance about sexuality, reproductive health and contraception, are vulnerable to suffer from various negative consequences. There is a relative lack of population education programs regarding sexuality and reproductive health in the country.[17] At times it has been found that the girls are unaware regarding the fact that sexual intercourse could result in pregnancy and STD; they are also at times unaware about the symptoms of STD.[38]

There is an increasing trend of risk behaviours among adolescents. More and more young people are becoming sexually active in their mid-teens.[43] Sexual activity begins as early as from 10 years of age among street boys to the mid- and late-teens among boys and girls in both rural as well as in urban areas. Surveys of adult students indicate that although premarital sexual experience among them is not as common as in Western countries, it is not as rare as perceived widely.[8] Peer group norms found to have significant association with intended sexual behaviour and actual sexual behaviour. Children of highly educated parents are less likely to engage in sexual activities in their adolescent years.[44] It is observed that boys tend to brag about their sexual experiences in-group, while they express fears and insecurities in private.[45,46] Adolescents especially in urban areas have favourable attitudes towards premarital and extramarital sex.[41,17] Recreational view of sexuality and sexual adventuring is noted in a considerable number of female college students in Delhi.[48] Interestingly, while students acknowledge deep personal interest in sexual gratification and liberal sexual standards before marriage, they consider monogamy as the cornerstone of the marital relationships.

In a study on sexual behaviours and their correlates among college students in Mumbai, it was found that some 47% male respondents and 13% female respondents had some sexual experience with the opposite gender; and 26% and 3%, respectively, had had intercourse. The strongest predictors of sexual behaviour were students' knowledge about sexuality-related issues, attitude towards sex, and levels of social interaction and exposure to erotic materials. For young women, the potential consequences of premarital sex, viz., pregnancy, desertion by one's future husband, domestic discord or loss of honor, often deter premarital sexual activity. Male students who initiate sexual activity appeared to do so at a young age.[49]

A high prevalence of risk behaviours, more or less similar to that of adolescents in other parts of the world, including drug intake, alcohol use, smoking, cannabis and premarital sex have been observed amongst rural and urban male adolescents in North India. Most of the risk behaviours are common in the urban adolescents.[50] Among predominantly unmarried school and college students (mostly in urban centres) premarital sex has been reported in 8-39% of male students and 1-20% of female students.[32] Heterosexual activity is more common in students who come from affluent homes.[51]

Sexual abuse has also been reported in adolescents. Rural boys are more likely to have experienced coercive sexual intercourse than urban boys and urban girls are more likely to have experienced any form of sexual abuse than rural girls.[52] Adolescent males, both in urban and rural areas, are particularly more prone to risky behaviours and vulnerable to STD and HIV infection.

There is very little information on the female sexual partners of unmarried male students. Neighbours, relatives, CSW, friends and fiancées have been mentioned as sexual partners. There is an indication that the premarital sexual partner of a male student is often a married (older) woman who may be a relative or neighbour.[9] This is somewhat expected because of the higher value placed on the premarital chastity of Indian women than that of men. A sizable proportion of unmarried male students visit CSW. Condoms are seldom used in premarital and extra marital sex, probably because of the mostly unplanned nature of such encounters and also because condoms are considered to interfere with sexual pleasure. Interestingly, adolescents residing in rural areas find it difficult to dispose of the condoms.[10]

Sexual Behaviour of High Risk Populations

Commercial Sex Workers (CSW)

Commercial sex contributes significantly to the spread of STD and HIV infection. HIV infection is high among sex workers and their clients.[53] Female sex workers can be broadly categorized into four groups: Brothel based, home based and part time, street based, and call girls.[54] Both, brothel and street based sex workers are referred to as 'direct sex workers'. Some women, who operate from home or work at stalls, nightclubs etc. sell sex to supplement their income. Such category of women are referred to as 'indirect sex workers' Brothel based sex workers tend to have a higher turnover of clients than street based sex workers, and they in turn have more clients than indirect sex workers.[37]

The findings of a few empirical studies in red-light areas of a few large cities in India corroborate the common knowledge that commercial sex workers, particularly those working in brothels, lead a poor standard of life in dilapidated and unhygienic environments.[55,56] The women are bonded to the brothel owners, who are unwilling to permit insistence on condoms. Brothel rules and client insistence on sex without condoms are upheld through the violence meted out by the pimps, police and local mafia. The competitive nature of the trade and resulting insecurity among the women is also found a constraint in adopting behavioural changes.[9,56] A large proportion of them suffers intermittently from various kinds of STD. The practice of oral sex has been reported among younger CSW, which is often unprotected. Pornographic film is a contributing factor for increase in such a sexual demand by the clients.[57]

CSW who are known as 'call-girls' are usually more educated and attractive than those living in brothels and are often engaged in some other occupation. They earn higher incomes and have some freedom in choosing

their clients, the latter mostly belonging to the middle and upper classes. Many of them have STD at one time or other and have undergone abortions. A high proportion of their clients prefers oral sex to vaginal intercourse.[9,58] Call girls belonging to the upper middle class are aware of AIDS and reject clients who refuse to use condoms.

Alcohol and drug use is common among CSW and has effect on sexual behaviour. A recent study of female sex workers found that HIV prevalence among injecting drug-using CSW was nine times higher than among non-injecting drug using CSW.[59]

Data from recent rounds of BSS show that a high percentage of direct sex workers reported condom use with their last client. However consistent condom use with all recent clients is comparatively low. Condom use with husbands or boy friends is rarely reported, perhaps in part to distinguish these personal partnerships from their professional relations. Lower condom use in noncommercial sex (when practiced by CSW or their client with other partners) is a potential for HIV spread from a higher into lower risk populations. Populations on a move, if engage in risk behaviours, can transport the STD and HIV infection from a high risk to a low risk population.

Clients of CSW

A few hundred thousand men have sexual relations with CSW every day in India but not much is known about their socio-economic characteristics, ways of life and sexual preferences. Clients frequently visiting CSW are low-level industrial workers living away from their families, transport workers, traders and customers in transitory markets, visitors to fairs, festivals and pilgrim centres, defense personnel living away from families, students, pimps and others who have some control over prostitutes, traders and service providers in red-light areas and professional blood donors. As in many other countries, Indian truck drivers and their helpers who spend the major part of the year on or near highways are generally known to visit many CSW during their stopovers.[9]

Men Having Sex With Men (MSM)

Prevalence of MSM has been reported to be 2-12 % in different population groups.[32] The findings of a study reveal that about 10% of the male respondents had their first sexual experience with another male. Many members of a culturally identifiable group known as 'hijra' in most parts of India are known to depend at least partly for their livelihood on working as male prostitutes. It has been observed that *hijras* engage themselves in sexual activity with men for money or for satisfying their own homosexual desires.[60]

Not much is known about the sexual techniques *hijras* practice or are asked to practice when they perform the role of a sex worker. They are often passive partners in anal intercourse without the use of condoms, making them vulnerable to HIV and other STD infections.[36,60]

Apart from *hijra* community, there are many full-time or part-time male sex workers. MSM in India have a great diversity and fluidity in social sexual and gender identities and behaviours as compared to the Western 'gay' experience. Vast majorities of MSM are married and are living with their wives reflecting the cultural situation in the South- Asian countries. Bisexuality tends to be practiced by men irrespective of their marital status.[61] MSM is often practiced without a 'homosexual identity' in covert manner and in discrete surroundings. Use of condom among them is relatively infrequent.[24,32] Discrimination and harassment, spread of sexual contacts, improper treatment seeking nature and risky sex practices (sex with multiple partners, group-sex and receptive anal sex) are some of the major risk factors for STD/HIV transmission in this group.[62] There is growing evidence that homosexuality may be more commonly practiced than is acknowledged. Situational homosexuality may occur in unequal (exploitative/potentially exploitative) relationships, defined by age (older men with adolescent boys, particularly hotel/restaurant workers), occupation (truck drivers with boy cleaners), or power (jail inmates).[19,36,60,63-65] They all form an important group at of risk of STD/HIV transmission.

Transport Workers and Migrant Population

Migrant workers and Indian truck drivers have high rate of contact with CSW; and STDs and HIV/AIDS [5,37,66]. Sexual partners among married truck drivers vary from 1-40. Married men have more sex encounters with commercial sex workers as compared to their wives. Predominant form of sexual activity with non-marital partners is vaginal intercourse followed by oral sex and anal intercourse. Interestingly, perceived risk for HIV is virtually non-existent in this high-risk group.

There is a denial of vulnerability to contract HIV and subsequent likelihood of spreading it on to their wives; although three-fourth believe that there is some chance that women they have sex with could have HIV/AIDS[66]. Condom use during commercial sex amongst this population has also been low (11-28%).[64,67]

Dhaba, a simple and inexpensive eating and drinking point, primarily meant for low income highway travelers serves as a halt place for the long distance truck drivers. Commercial sex activities flourish near halt places like Dhabas. CSW living nearby often visit these places in search of clients. Sometimes the truckers pick up the CSW waiting on the highways in search of clients and sexual acts in such cases take place within the trucks or in the roadside bushes. Truck drivers are known to visit villages adjacent to the national highway to obtain alcohol and women. Alcohol and substance use has effect on sexual behaviours and condom use. Some truck drivers also report their inability to visit a CSW unless inebriated with alcohol or opium. Truck drivers also have homosexual relationship with the 'helpers'.[63,64] Wives and steady sexual partners are at an increased risk of contracting HIV/STD.[68]

Other Risk Groups

High prevalence of STD and blood borne infections, sexual risk behaviours, alcohol/drug abuse and poor knowledge of HIV have been observed among the jail inmates.[65]

The social customs and sexual openness of certain Indian tribes, makes them freely indulge in premarital and extramarital sex. The outsiders sexually exploit the women from these tribes. As a result of this, prevalence of STD is high (8-30%) in some tribal groups.s[69]

Populations Attending STD Clinics

Most of patients attending STD clinics in different regions of the country are young males and have a history of contact with commercial sex partners. The first sexual encounter of male STD patients is often with a CSW. However, many male patients attribute their infection to sexual contact with acquaintances, friends, relatives or neighbors. The reason for male preponderance observed in such clinic based studies could be due to higher attendance to such clinics by males because of social reasons and also because of more painful symptoms of certain STD in males as compared to females. Thirty to forty percent of male STD patients visiting STD clinics are repeaters and the majority of them had their first sexual experience during their teenage[1]. It is estimates that only 5 to 10% of the people suffering from the disease attend public STD facilities.

Concomitant infection with STD, particularly those characterized by genital ulcers increases the chance of HIV infection. STD clinic attendees have high HIV prevalence (1- 64 % in major urban areas; 0-45% outside the major urban areas).[16,18,70,72] A person already having STD has a greater risk of acquiring HIV from an infected partner.

High-Risk Behaviour in Populations Affected with STD/HIV

A clinic-based study on a group of STD patients reveals that although knowledge about condom use is high in this group, the actual use of condom use has been low. Although STD patients are well informed about STD and know the methods to avoid infection, this knowledge has little impact on their behaviour.[73]

Although HIV-1 is still the predominant virus amongst the high risk HIV infected persons in Mumbai, dual HIV and 1.2 infections are increasing specially amongst the high risk group of promiscuous heterosexuals and FCSWs. Increases in HIV2 infections were observed later than dual HIV and 12 infections, indicating that it is the HIV-1 infected persons who through continued high risk behaviour got infected with HIV 2. The findings reflect that the high-risk behaviour continues in the promiscuous heterosexuals and CSW despite contracting the dreaded HIV infection and that it serves as a continuous source of spread of HIV. There is little information about the sexual behaviour of HIV infected persons. Considerable number of HIV positive men report bisexual preferences.[74]

Sexual Risk Behaviour Linked to Alcohol/ Substance Use

Alcohol and sexual behaviour has been studied from ethnographic, sociological and health perspective. Studies have demonstrated direct and indirect linkage between alcohol use and sexual behaviours but only few studies have specifically examined the nature of linkage and its effect on high risk behaviours and prevention of related health problems.[75] Intoxication has been connected with risky sexual behaviour and, failure to use condoms, with STD, and unplanned pregnancies.

It is observed that consumption of alcohol and visit to sex workers increases manifold during Indian festivals and celebrations. On the contrary during months of Shravana (observed by Hindus) and Ramzan (observed by Muslims), restraints on such vices help in decreasing/ preventing high-risk behaviours. The number of clients visiting the commercial sex workers decreases during the 'dry' (alcohol free) periods. An absence of or a reduction in alcohol use is associated with a decrease in high risk sexual behaviours and sexually transmitted diseases.[76-78] An observed association between drinking and high risk sexual activity could imply that these two behaviours are part of a larger risk taking tendency, or alcohol itself influences sexual risk taking or both. The larger control of HIV/STD during festivities could be achieved though an informed policy on dry alcohol days.[76]

Men who have been drinking alcohol report more contact and non-contact sexual problems as compared to those who do not use alcohol.[79] Association between alcohol and substance use and high risk sexual behaviours is more evident among high risk groups like CSW and truckers. The clients of CSW consume alcohol for sexual excitement. Alcohol use is strongly associated with high risk sexual behaviours for reasons like 'alcohol increases and sustains sexual drive', 'one can visit a CSW only when alcohol is consumed', 'it is difficult to engage in oral sex without alcohol consumption'; 'the CSW' demand alcohol for themselves'.

Condom use is low under the influence of alcohol.[63] In a study on assessment of the risk factors in STD, alcohol was one of the risk factors found to be significantly associated with the acquisition of STD.[80] Using in-depth interviews with men and women to learn about their sexual histories and recent sexual behaviours, a study described the use of alcohol particularly in group sex encounters in Haryana.[81] Alcohol use has been associated with extramarital sexual activities among women in Gujarat.[19]

There is increasing trend towards smoking, alcohol use, late night parties, sexual intercourse, adolescent pregnancies, STD and violence amongst the youth, particularly among those residing in urban metropolitan cities. Media also influences such high-risk behaviour.[50] Alcohol use and sexual experimentation during adolescence and youth are risk factors for acquiring sexually transmitted diseases.

Apart from alcohol, other substance use has also been linked to high-risk sexual behaviours. Substance users including injecting drug users commonly visit

CSW. In some areas, especially North-Eastern part of the country and metropolitan cities, IDU are reported to have high sero-positivity for HIV infection. These users are sexually active and can pass on the HIV infection in general population, fueling the HIV epidemic.[5]

Alcohol and substance use is common among youth and adolescents, high-risk groups like transport workers and migrant workers; commercial sex workers, jail inmates; and HIV infected persons. However, few studies have examined the triangular relationship between alcohol use; sexual behaviours; and sexually transmitted diseases including HIV infection in the high-risk and the general population.

Sexual Behaviour and Prevention of STD/AIDS

As STD and HIV prevalence rises in the population, the chance of someone encountering an infected partner close to the beginning of their sexual life also rises. It is therefore crucial to reach people with appropriate preventive interventions before their first sex encounter[82]. Adolescents have poor knowledge about issues related to sexuality. It is important that the adolescents receive age-appropriate and adequate information and education about issues related to sexuality from reliable and knowledgeable sources. Sex education should aim to increase the knowledge about sex and STD/HIV, to develop self-assertiveness and to develop positive attitudes towards sexuality. Education imparted in this way, will serve the two-fold purpose of satisfying their natural curiosity and protecting them from engaging in high-risk sexual behaviour. Though sex education is a part of university education, the curriculum rarely discusses issues related to reproductive health and sexuality. Many teachers in schools and colleges avoid teaching these topics as they find them too embarrassing.[83] Teaching adolescents about sex is not only an effective way to safeguard the future health of the nation, but also results in developing a stable value system and adoption of a responsible lifestyle. Young people can be agents of change and spearhead advocacy for sex education among peers, community members and parents.

Apart from students there is also a need to impart sex education to the general population and high-risk groups such as CSW, truck drivers, migrant workers, jail inmates and drug users. The sex education programs to these populations need to be tailored according to the specific needs of these groups.[84]

Research has shown that appropriately designed prevention programs, that provide a comprehensive range of coordinated services, can limit the further spread of HIV and other STD even when the latter are well established in a community. However in order to be effective, such prevention programs should be based on a thorough continuing assessment of local population needs and they should involve the local population in planning and implementing interventions and services. Such prevention programs have been shown to be cost effective.[84] Spread of HIV is influenced in short term by condom use and prevalence of STD, and these are the factors that can be manipulated to limit the spread of infection.[85]

Some well-designed and well-executed intervention programs by government and non-government agencies in a few red-light areas of the country have been carried out. One example is the STD/HIV Intervention Project, Sonagachi, Kolkata (Calcutta), initiated by NACO in the year 1992. The program focussed on promotion of condom use, AIDS awareness through peer educators and provision of STD treatment facility in the area. Such intervention programs have shown increase in condom use, improvement in knowledge about STD and reduction in the prevalence of STD among CSW.[23,37,86] One of the key factors in their success is peer-group education in raising AIDS awareness among prostitutes and motivating them to use condoms. However further improvements have been limited, both in terms of condom usage and STD prevalence. Even when health education programs succeed in motivating the CSW to use condoms, their customers, who usually have higher bargaining power, are often reluctant to use condoms. There is an indication that sex workers can control the behaviour of their clients to some extent by monetary bargaining.[57] However, the processes by which the CSW succeed/ fail in making the client use condoms in the above-mentioned programs are not very well understood.[9] The Sonagachi project findings, nevertheless, highlight the approach that can be utilized while addressing prevention programs in high-risk groups. The training and recruitment of a few selected CSW as peer educators in the program served as an important step towards the shift of the project's approach from a 'behavioural communication change model' to an 'empowerment model'. Working with and for their own group under supervision of experts proved to be an effective intervention strategy amongst these high-risk women. The HIV epidemic has been brought to a halt and maintained at low levels of transmission, even in situations of poverty in Kolkata because of the high level of organization among female sex workers which enables them to negotiate successfully for "protected sex only".[87]

In a recent review of published studies that evaluated different approaches to preventing STD/HIV transmission in heterosexual men (IDU, STD clinic patients, men in workplace and students), it was found that no single intervention could be identified as more effective than the other in reducing the incidence of STD/HIV in heterosexual men. In general, the studies had used either group-based or individual interventions. However, successful interventions included localized and national programs, video-based education programs, counselling and communication skill development, and long-term peer educators; a single approach is unlikely to be successful in any given setting.[88]

There is also a need to address masturbation and other semen loss concerns in sexual health campaigns in South Asia, keeping in mind the magnitude of these concerns, their potential to confound management of STDs and their significance as an idiom of psychosocial distress. Addressing such issues, lead to immediate identification among young men and provide an entry point for sexual health and safer sex education.[89]

Among Indian truck drivers, substantial deficits with respect to HIV prevention information, motivation and behavioural skills have been observed and have been found to be predictive of HIV risk and preventive behaviour.[66] There is a need to focus on higher levels of HIV prevention information, safer sex motivation (consisting of attitudes, social norms and perception of vulnerability to HIV) and safer behavioural skills, paralleling interventions with CSW.

It is seen that people tend to have safe sex with high risk partners and hish risk sex with safe partners, which predisposes the general population to the risk of infection.[90] Prevention programmes should also focus on the wives and steady sexual partners of the persons with high risk behaviours as the former are also at a high risk of acquiring STD and HIV/AIDS.[68]

Voluntary counselling and testing (VCT) is one of the essential components of various HIV prevention programs. VCT results in reduction of risk behaviours amongst the target groups but is not enough as a primary prevention strategy and other behavioural interventions are needed to bring an observable change.[91]

To convince people to adopt health behaviours, what is needed is the motivation to act and skills to translate knowledge into practice. Hence, apart from providing information it is also important to teach other skills. Sexual intercourse should be discussed displaying affection. Meta-analytic review reveals that service based prevention interventions have positive effects among population at risk through sexual transmission. The positive effects include both behavioural as well as biological prevention, such as reduction in STD.[92] Consistent and correct use of condoms coupled with risk reduction education strategies, have been vital for prevention of STDs and HIV transmission.[93,94] STD and HIV prevention strategies should target not only individuals, but also communities and social policies.

Acknowledgements: Our thanks are due to Drs.Peter Kok, Health Advisor, Cordaid; Shalini Bharat, Unit for Family Studies, Tata Institute of Social Sciences, Mumbai; Prabha Chandra, Dept. of Psychiatry, National Institute of Mental Health and Neuro-sciences, Bangalore; Ravi K. Verma, Horizons/Population Council, India, New Delhi. We sincerely thank Drs. Atul Ambekar and Avinash P, and Ms Suman Bhatia who have been helpful in collection of the review material and preparation of the document.

References

1. Ramasubban R. HIV/AIDS in India: Between Rhetoric and Reality. In: Pachauri, S Subramanian S. eds. Implementing a reproductive health agenda in India : the beginning. Population Council, South East Asia-Regional Office; 1999 p-347-376

2. MAP (Monitoring the AIDS Pandemic). The Status and Trends of HIV/AIDS/STI Epidemics in Asia and the Pacific. MAP. 2001

3. UNAIDS and WHO. India: Epidemiological Fact Sheet on HIV/AIDS and sexually transmitted infection. Geneva. 2001.

4. UNAIDS AIDS epidemic update-December 2001, UNAIDS/World Health Organization. 2001

5. Reid G, Costigan G, Revisiting the Hidden Epidemic-A situational assessment of Drug Use in Asia in the context of HIV/AIDS. The centre for Harm Reduction, The Burnet Institute, Australia 2002.

6. NACO National baseline general population behavioural surveillance survey -2001, New Delhi, NACO. Ministry of Health and Family Welfare, Government of India 2002.

7. Khazanchand (Kaviraj) ed. Indian Sexology: New Delhi: S.Chand & Co. ltd; 1972.

8. Nag M: Sexual behaviour in India with risk of HIV/AIDS transmission. Health Transit Rev 1995; 5: 293-305.

9. Nag M: Sexual Behaviour and AIDS in India, New Delhi, Vikas Publishing House 1996.

10. Chandiramani R, Kapadia S, Khanna R, Misra G. Critical review of studies on sexuality and sexual behaviour conducted in India from 1990 to 2000. Paper presented at the Reproductive health Research Review Dissemination Workshop, Dec. 2001, Mumbai.

11. George A. Differential perspectives of men and women in Mumbai, India on sexual relations and negotiations within marriage. Reprod Health Matters, 1998; 6, 87-96.

12. Martin SL, Kilgallen B, Tsui AO, Maitra K, Singh KK, K upper LL. Sexual behaviours and reproductive health outcomes-Associations with wife abuse in India. JAMA 1999; 282, 1967-1972.

13. Khanna R, Korrie K, Pongurlekar S et al.: Sexual coercion and reproductive health problems in slum women of Mumbai: Role of health care profile. Papers presented at Workshop on Reproductive Health in India: New Evidence and Issues, Pune, India 2000.

14. Mane P and Maitra SA. AIDS Prevention: the socio-cultural context in India. Bombay: Tata Institute of Social Sciences 1992.

15. Rao Gupta G. How men's power over women fuels the HIV epidemic. BMJ, 2002; 324, 183-184.

16. Thappa DM, Singh S and Singh A. HIV infection and sexually transmitted diseases in a referral STD centre in South India. Sex Transm Inf 1999; 75:191.

17. ICRW Adolescent sexuality and fertility in India-Preliminary Findings. Information Bulletin. International Centre for Research on Women, Washington, D.C., USA 1997.

18. Kar GC and Varma LP: Sexual problems of married male mental patients. Indian J Psychiat 1978; 20, 365-370.

19. Sharma, A, Sharma V: The Guilt and Pleasure of Masturbation: A study of college girls in Gujarat, India. Sex Marit Therap 1998; 13; 63-70.

20. Wig NN: Problems of mental health in India. J Clin Soc Psych 1960; 17; 48-53.

21. Malhotra HK, Wig NN Dhat syndrome: A culture bound neurosis of orient. Arch Sex Behav 1975; 4; 519-528.

22. Singh G: Dhat syndrome revisited. Indian J Psychiat 1985; 22, 419-122.

23. Pelto PJ. Sexuality and Sexual Behaviour: The Current Discourse. In: Saroj Pachauri, ed. Implementing a Reproductive Health Agenda in India: The Beginning, The Population Council, New Delhi, 1999; 539-585.

24. Pelto P J, Joshi A, Verma RK. Development of sexuality among men in India and its implications for reproductive health programmes: The Population Council, New Delhi 2000.

25. Verma R and Schensul SL. Male sexual problems in Bombay: Folk curiosities or Indicator of sexual risk? Paper presented at 4th APSSAM at Kandy, Sri Lanka 26-28 Oct. 2000. (cited with permission).

26. Verma R, Lhungdim H. Perception and practice of sexual acts: Findings based on key informant interviews and case studies in Rural India. Paper presented at national conference on sexual behaviour at TISS, Mumbai, 26-27 Dec. 2000.

27. Joshi A, Dhapola M, Kurien E, Pelto PJ. Rural Women's Experiences and Perceptions of Marital Sexual Relationships. Ford Foundation Working Papers Series 1998.

28. Basu D P. Appropriate Methodologies for Studying Sexual behaviour. The Indian J Soc Work, 1994; 573-588.

29. Savara M, Sridhar CR. Sexual behaviour amongst different occupational groups in Maharashtra India and the implications for AIDS education. Indian J Soc Work, 1994; 55: 617-632.

30. Carolina Population Centre Uttar Pradesh reproductive health survey 1995-1996. North Carolina, Carolina Population Centre 1997.

31. Kumar A, Mehra M, Badhan SK, Gulati N. Hetero sexual behaviour and condom usage in an urban population of Delhi, India. AIDS care 1997; 9: 311-318.

32. Hawkes S, Santhya KG. Diverse realities. STD and HIV in India. Sex Trans Infect 2002; 78(suppl):131-139.

33. Bhattacharjee J, Gupta RS, Kumar A, Jain DC. Pre and extramarital heterosexual behaviour of an urban community in Rajasthan, India J commun Dis 2000; 32: 33-39.

34. Tamang A, Nepal B, Puri M, Shrestha D. Sexual behaviour and risk perceptions among young men in bordered towns of Nepal. Asia Pacific Population Journal 2000; 16: 195-210.

35. APAC community prevalence of sexually transmitted diseases in Tamil Nadu 1998, Chennai, USAID, APAC, VHS 1998.

36. APAC HIV Risk Behaviour Surveillance Survey in Tamil Nadu- Report on Fifth Wave (2000), Chennai, USAID/AIDS Prevention and Control Project/Voluntary Health services 2001.

37. FHI What drives HIV in Asia? A summary of trends in sexual and drug-taking behaviours. FHI/DFID/USAID/Impact 2001.

38. NACO National HIV Sentinel behavioural surveillance survey -2001, New Delhi, NACO. Ministry of Health and Family Welfare, Government of India (www.naco.nic.in) 2002.

39. Pattanaik D, Lobo J, Kapoor SK, Menon PS. Knowledge and attitudes of rural adolescent girls regarding reproductive health issues. Natl Med J India, 2000; 13: 124-128.

40. Collumbien M, Bohidar N, Das R, Das B, Pelto, PJ. Male Sexual Health Concerns in Orissa: An Ethnic Perspective, AIMS Research Centre, Bhubaneshwar, Orissa. Continence, ed. WJ Robinson. New York: Critic and Guide Company 1998.

41. Sharma AK, Sehgal VN, Kant S, Choubey D, Bhardwaj A. Knowledge, attitude, belief and practice (KABP) on AIDS among senior secondary students. Indian Journal of Community Medicine, 1997; 22:168-171.

42. Lal SS, Vasan RS, Sarma PS, Thankappan KR. Knowledge

and attitudes of college students in Kerala towards HIV/ AIDS, sexually transmitted diseases and sexuality. Natl Med J India, 2000. 13, 231-236.

43. Kannan AT: Adolescent health: issues and concerns in India. Health for the Millions, 1995; 21: 29-30.

44. Selvan MS, Ross MW, Kapadia AS, Mathai R, Hira S. Study of perceived norms, beliefs and intended sexual behaviour among higher secondary school students in India. AIDS Care 2001; 13: 779-788.

45. Amin A, Fatula E , Khanna R: Attitudes and behaviours of men in relation to gender and sexuality: Evidence from qualitative studies conducted in the Santrampur taluka of Panchmahals district, Gujarat, Working Paper No. 4, SARTHI 1997.

46. Amin A. Fatula E, Grenon M. Men's Perceptions of the Illnesses of the Nether Area: Evidence from Qualitative Studies Conducted in the Santrampur Taluka of Panchmahals District, Gujarat,; Working Paper No. 3, SARTHI 1996.

47. Bhende AA. A study of sexuality of adolescent girls and boys in under privileged groups in Bombay. Indian J Soc Work, 1994; 55:557-571

48. Sachdev P. University Students in Delhi, India: Their Sexual Knowledge, Attitudes and Behaviour. The J Fam Welfare, 1997; 43,1-12.

49. Abraham L, Kumar KA. Sexual Experiences and their Correlates among College Students in Mumbai City, India. Internat Fam Plann Perspect, 1999; 25, 139-146.

50. Kishore J, Singh A, Grewal I, Singh SR, Roy K. Risk behaviour in an urban and a rural male adolescent population. Natl Med J India 1999; 12: 107-110.

51. Kaur U, Salim SP, Bambery P, et al. Sexual behaviour drug use and hepatitis B in Chandigarh student Natl Med J India 1996; 9: 156-159.

52. Patel V, Andrew G. Gender, sexual-abuse and risk behaviours in adolescents: A cross sectional survey in schools in Goa. Natl Med J India, 2001; 14: 263-7.

53. NACO. National HIV Sentinel behavioural surveillance survey -2000, New Delhi, NACO. Ministry of Health and Family Welfare, Government of India (www.naco.nic.in) 2001.

54. NACO. A summary of findings of the high risk behaviour study from 18 cities. New Delhi. Government of India, Ministry of Health and Family Welfare, NACO 1997.

55. Gilada IS (no date). Prostitution in India: causes, extent, prevention, rehabilitation. People Health Organization.

56. Gilada IS. AIDS and Sex Work: An Indian Perspective. In: M. Berer and S. Ray (eds.). Women and HIV/AIDS: An Indian Resource Book Information. Action and Resources on Women and HIV/AIDS. Reproductive Health and Sexual Relationship. London: Pandora Press 1993.

57. Bhattacharya S, Senapati SK. Sexual Practice of Sex Workers in a Red Light Area of Calcutta, The Indian Journal of Social Work LV 1994; 557-571.

58. Kapur P. The Life and World of Call Girls in India. New Delhi: Vikas Publishing House 1978.

59. Agarwal AK, Singh GB, Khundom KC, et al. The prevalence of HIV in female sex workers in Manipur. J Commun Dis. 1999; 31:23-28.

60. Nag M. Sexual Behaviour and AIDS in India: State-of -the-Art The Indian J Soc Work (Special Issues: Sexual Behaviour and AIDS in India) LV, 1994; 503-546.

61. Khan S. Cultural contexts of sexual behaviours and identities and their impact upon HIV prevention models: An overview of South Asian men who have sex with men. Indian J Soc Work, 1994; 55: 633-646.

62. Subramanian T, Suresh Kumar SK, Kachirayan M, Ramakrishnan R, Mohan DG. Risk of STD/AIDS in the sexual behaviour of eunuchs from Villupuram District. Indian J Sex Transm Dis; 1999; 20 (2): 47-53.

63. Rao A, Nag M, Mishra K, Dey A. Sexual behaviour pattern of truck drivers.and their helpers in relation to female sex workers. Indian J Soc Work 1994; 55,4:603-616.

64. Rao. KS, Pilli RD, Rao AS, Chalam PS. Sexual lifestyle of long distance lorry drivers in India Questionnaire survey. BMJ 1999; 318, 162-163.

65. Singh S, Prasad R, Mohanty A. High prevalence of sexually transmitted and blood borne infections amongst the inmates of a district jail in Northern India. Internat J STD & AIDS. 1999; 10: 475-478.

66. Bryan AD, Fisher JD, Joseph Benziger T. Determinants of HIV risk among Indian truck drivers. Social Sci & Med. 2001; 53, 1413-1426.

67. Singh IN, Malaviya AN. Long distance truck drivers in India: HIV infection and their possible role in disseminating HIV into rural areas. Internat J STD & AIDS 1994; 5, 137-138.

68. Bharat S, Aggleton P. Facing the challenge Household responses to HIV/AIDS in Mumbai, India. AIDS Care 1999; 11: 31-44.

69. Aswar NS, Wahab SN, Kale KM. Prevalence and some epidemiological factors of syphilis in Madia Tribe of Gadricholi District. Indian J of Sex Trans Dis 1998; 19:53-57

70. Jacob M, John TJ, George S et al. Increasing prevalence of human immuno-deficiency virus infection among patients attending a clinic for sexually transmitted diseases. Indian J Med Res. 1995; 101:6-9

71. Rodriguez JJ, Mehendale SM, Shafhard ME, et al. Risk factors for HIV infection in people attending clinics for sexually transmitted diseases in India. BMJ 1995; 311:283-286.

72. Kar HK, Jain RK, Sharma PK, et al. Increasing HIV prevalence in STD Clinic attendees in Delhi, India: 6 year (1995-2000) hospital based study results. Sex Transm Infect 2001; 77: 393.

73. Grover V, Kannan AT, Indrayam A, Sharma SC. Sexually transmitted diseases awareness and sexual behaviour-A study in clinical setting in an urban area of Delhi. Indian J Sex Trans Dis 1999; 20: 16-20.

74. Kamat HA, Banker DD, Koppikar GV. Increasing prevalence of HIV-2 and dual HIV 1-2 infections among patients attending various out door patient departments in Mumbai. Indian J Pub Health 1999; 43: 85-6.

75. Tripathi BM, Malhotra S. WHO Study on determinants of sexual risk behaviour among alcohol users in diverse cultural settings: a literature review of studies on alcohol use and sexual risk behaviours in India-Draft report 2002.

76. Ambwani PN and Gilada IS. Dry alcohol days during festivals to prevent HIV/AIDS. XII International Conference on AIDS, Geneva, 1998. AIDSLINE ICA 12/98410386. 1998.

77. Chandra PS, Bengal V, Ramkrishna J, Krishna VAS. Development and evaluation of a module for HIV/AIDS related risk reduction among patients with alcohol dependence (Project report). Bangalore, National Institute of Mental Health and Neurosciences 1999.

78. Alcohol policy and sexually transmitted disease rates-United States, 1981-1995. MMWR Weekly, 2000/49(16): 346-349.

79. Verma R, Sharma S, Singh R, Rangaiyan G, Pelto J. Beliefs concerning sexual health problems and treatment seeking among moan in an Indian slum community paper presented at the 3rd I ASSCS, 1-3 Oct. 2001, Melbourne, Australia (cited with permission) 2001.

80. Sharma AK, Chaubey D. Risk factors in sexually transmitted diseases. Indian J Sex Transm Dis 1996; 17: 8-10.

81. SWACH (Survival for Women and Children) Foundation: An in-depth study to understand men's reproductive health behaviour and feasibility of special intervention. Progress report. Ford Foundation, New Delhi, India 1998.

82. Pissani AIDS into 21st century: Some critical consideations. Reprod Health Matters, 2000; 8:63-76.

83. Jejeebhoy SJ. Adolescent sexual and reproductive behaviour. A review of the evidence from India. Social Scheme and Medicine. 1998; 46, 1275-1290..

84. NIDA: Principles of HIV prevention in drug using population- A research based guide, Washington DC, NIDA, US Department of Health and Human Services 2002.

85. Venkataramana CB, Sarada PV. Extent and speed of HIV infection in India through the commercial sex networks: a perspective. Trop Med Int Health, 2001; 6: 1040-1061

86. Nag M: Empowering female sex workers for AIDS prevention and far beyond: Sonagachi shows the way. Indian J Soc Work 2002. (in press)

87. Kok P: Dynamics of the HIV/AIDS Epidemic and its Implications for Prevention Programmes in Asia.(draft report) 2002.

88. Elwy AR, Hart GJ, Peticerw M. Effectiveness of intervention to prevent sexually transmitted infections and human immune deficiency virus in heterosexual men: A systematic review. Arch Int Med 2002; 162: 1818-30.

89. Lakhani A, Gandhi K, Collumbien M. Addressing semen loss concerns: Towards culturally appropriate HIV/AIDS intervention in Gujarat, India. Reprod Health Matters 2001; 9:49-59.

90. Peterman TA, Lin LS, Newman DR, et al. Does measured behaviour reflect STD risk? An analysis of data from a randomized controlled behavioural intervention study. Project RESPECT Study Group. Sex Transm Dis 2000; 27:446-451.

91. Tripathi, B.M. HIV Counselling and testing, National Inf Dis 1999; 1: 22-26.

92. Neumann MS, Johnson WD, Semaan S, et al. Review and meta-analysis of HIV prevention intervention research for heterosexual adult populations in the United States. J Acquir Immune Defic Syndr 2002; 1;30 Suppl 1:S106-17.

93. Roth J, Krishnan SP, Bunch E. Barriers to condom use: Results from a study in Mumbai (Bombay), India. AIDS Edu Prev 2001; 13:65-77.

94. Crosby R, DiClemente RJ, Holtgrave DR, Wingood GM. Design, measurement, and analytical considerations for testing hypotheses relative to condom effectiveness against non-viral STD. Sex Transm Infect 2002; 78:228-231.

Chapter 41

Psychosexual Disorders

Sameer Malhotra, Vinod K Sharma

Introduction

Sexuality is an important aspect of one's existence and health. Broadly speaking, it is influenced by physical as well as psycho-social factors. Biological factors, life-experiences, knowledge, attitude and behaviour, all contribute to the development of one's sexuality. Sexuality is considered to be abnormal if

a. The sexual behaviour is destructive
b. It cannot be directed towards the partner
c. Excludes stimulation of primary sex organs and
d. Is associated with inappropriate guilt and anxiety.[1]

Sexual disorders carry significant importance. They can have significant psychological, marital, social and legal implications for the individual. They are associated with significant distress and dysfunction in the individual as well as the partner.

The DSM (diagnostic and statistical manual of mental disorders) system (American Psychiatric Association, 1994) and the ICD classification of mental and behavioural disorders (World Health Organization, 1992) have described the psychosexual disorders.[2,3] Both these systems have discussed sexual disorders under different heads and subheads. A comprehensive list of sexual disorders as described in the two classification systems is shown in table 1.

Table 1. Classification of Psychosexual Disorders

DSM-IV classification	ICD-10 classification

Sexual and gender identity disorders
• Sexual dysfunctions
    Sexual desire disorders (hypoactive sexual desire disorder, sexual aversion)
    Sexual arousal disorders
    Orgasmic disorders
    (female and male orgasmic disorders, premature ejaculation)
    Sexual pain disorders
    (dyspareunia, vaginismus)
    Sexual dysfunction due to a general medical condition
    Substance induced sexual dysfunction
    Sexual dysfunction not otherwise specified
• Paraphilias
• Gender identity disorders
• Sexual disorder not otherwise specified (includes marked feelings of sexual inadequacy; persistent and marked distress about sexual orientation)
	Behavioural syndromes associated with physiological disturbance and physical factors include sexual dysfunctions
	• Sexual dysfunction, not caused by organic disorder or disease
	    Lack or loss of sexual desire
	    Sexual aversion and lack of sexual enjoyment
	    Failure of genital response
	    Orgasmic dysfunction
	    Premature ejaculation
	    Nonorganic vaginismus
	    Excessive sexual drive
	    Other sexual dysfunction, not due to organic disorder or disease
	    Unspecified sexual dysfunction
	Disorders of adult personality and behaviour
	• Gender identity disorders
	• Disorders of sexual preference (include paraphilias)
	• Psychological and behavioural disorders associated with sexual development and orientation (includes egodystonic homosexuality)
	    Other specified neurotic disorders
	• Dhat syndrome

The sexual response cycle consists of the phases of sexual desire, excitement, orgasm and resolution. Sexual dysfunction could result from the disturbances in one or more of these, or from pain associated with sexual intercourse (sexual pain disorders). Sexual dysfunctions are associated with marked distress and interpersonal difficulty (Table 2).[2]

The onset, context and etiological factors associated with sexual dysfunctions may vary. Accordingly, sexual dysfunction may be present since the onset of sexual functioning (primary) or may develop after a period of normal functioning (secondary); it may or may not be limited to certain types of stimulation, situations or partners; it may result from psychological factors, general

Table 2. Sexual-Response Cycle and Associated Disorders

Phase of Sexual cycle	Characteristics	Disorder
Desire	Fantasies about sexual activity & desire for sexual activity	Hypoactive sexual desire disorder; sexual aversion disorder
Excitement	Sexual pleasure and associated physiological changes. Penile tumescence and erection in males; pelvic vasocongestion, vaginal lubrication and expansion, swelling of external genitalia in females	Male erectile disorder (erectile impotence); female sexual arousal disorder
Orgasm	Peaking of sexual pleasure, release of sexual tension and rhythmic contraction of perineal muscles, anal sphincter and sex organs. In males: sense of ejaculatory inevitability followed by semen ejaculation; In females: contractions of the wall of the outer third of the vagina	Female orgasmic disorder; male orgasmic disorder (including anorgasmia); Premature ejaculation (PME)
Resolution	Sense of muscle relaxation & general well being. Males are physiologically refractory to further erection and orgasm for variable time periods.	Postcoital dysphoria Postcoital headache

Adapted from Sadock VA, 1995[1] & DSM-IV APA, 1994[2]

medical conditions, substance use or side effects of medication, specific physical deficits or a combination of these various factors.

Social, ethnic, religious and cultural factors influence sexual desire, attitudes, expectations and behaviour. Individual variations also account for the differences in sexual functioning.

The 'psychosexual' disorders are not better accounted for by major psychiatric ailments, general medical conditions and are not exclusively due to physiological effect of substance use. Mostly the definitions and descriptions as per globally recognized DSM-IV criteria have been followed in this chapter.[2] An attempt is made to be somewhat over-inclusive so as to provide a glimpse into the broad area of sexual disorders.

Though fewer in number, Indian studies are available on sexual dysfunctions in patients presenting to the psychiatric clinic of general hospital, psychosexual clinics and STD clinics.[4,5] A recent study conducted at the All India Institute of Medical Sciences (AIIMS), New Delhi, examined the clinical profile of psychosexual disorders in a thousand subjects attending a sex therapy clinic. The problems of premature ejaculation (77.6%), nocturnal emissions (71.3%), masturbatory guilt (33.4%), concern about the small penile size (30%), erectile dysfunction (23.6%) and venereophobia (13%) were prevalent in the study group.[5] The study highlights the relevance of the area of sexual disorders to dermato-venereologists and also the need for timely recognition, careful assessment as well as appropriate referral to the relevant specialists like psychiatrists, urologists and endocrinologists. Across various studies, erectile impotence and premature ejaculation are common amongst males: sexual desire and sexual pain disorders are common in females. The areas of female sexuality and associated disorders, sexual disorders other than sexual dysfunctions, the issues pertaining to management of sexual disorders have not been adequately addressed in the literature.

Sexual Dysfunctions

Disorders of Sexual Desire

Hypoactive Sexual Desire Disorder

It is seen in both sexes, more so in females. It is characterized by persistent or recurrent deficiency or absence of sexual fantasies, feelings and desire to indulge in sexual activity, inappropriate to the age and personal context. It manifests as decreased frequency and avoidance of sexual intercourse, or with complaints of a lack of desire. The disorder manifests around puberty and may remain lifelong. Sexual desire is influenced by biological drive and factors like self esteem, previous sex experience, availability of partner and appropriate circumstances, interpersonal factors and periods of abstinence. Biologically, hypoactive sexual desire may be associated with neurochemical (central dopaminergic blockade) or hormonal (decreased testosterone levels in males) disturbance. Psychodynamically, hypoactive desire may represent a defence against unconscious sexual fears.[1,2]

Sexual Aversion Disorder

It is characterized by a persistent or recurrent extreme aversion to and avoidance of all or almost all genital sexual contact with the sexual partner. At times it is difficult to distinguish between the hypoactive desire disorder and the sexual aversion disorder, and in some cases both can be co-existent. Previous traumatic sexual experiences viz., rape or child abuse, repeated painful experiences with coitus, interpersonal problems with the partner, early developmental conflicts in the unconscious, associating sexual intercourse with guilt, shame, pain and fear have been implicated as psychological etiological factors.[1,2] The disorder should be carefully assessed and the underlying cause should be appropriately treated. Mental and behavioural therapies are useful tools in management of such disorders.

Excessive Sexual Drive (Sex Addiction, Satyriasis)

Though it is not a universally accepted or recognized disorder, may be encountered in both the sexes, usually manifesting in late adolescence and young adulthood. It is referred to as "Don Juanism" in males and nymphomania in females.[1] The term sex addiction has often been used to describe persons who compulsively seek out sexual experiences and whose behaviour becomes impaired if unable to gratify their sexual impulses. Sex addicts are unable to control their sexual impulses and their entire life revolves around sex seeking behaviour and activities. A long-standing persistent or recurrent pattern of such behaviour and a history of several unsuccessful attempts to stop such behaviour are observed. The disorder manifests as out of control self-destructive or high risk sexual behaviour with persistence despite sexual adverse consequences (medical, legal and interpersonal domains); repeated attempts to stop or limit such behaviour; sexual fantasies and obsessions; need for increasing amounts of sexual activities; severe mood changes associated with sexual activity; substantial amount of time spent in such activities; and interference of sexual behaviour in socio-occupational life. It is commonly associated with impulse control and substance use problems. The behavioural manifestations often include paraphilias and compulsive masturbation. In order to diagnose it as an independent disorder, one should be able to rule out other possible etiologies like bipolar mood disorders and early stages of dementia. Psychotherapies and pharmacotherapies have been used to manage the disorder. Serotonin specific re-uptake inhibitors (SSRIs like fluoxetine) are known to reduce libido in some persons, a side effect that can be used therapeutically. Medroxyprogesterone acetate diminishes libido in men. Androgenic compounds contribute to sex drive in women, so antiandrogens (like cyproterone acetate) can be of benefit in reducing the sex drive in female patients.[1]

Sexual Arousal Disorders

These disorders are characterized by a persistent or recurrent, partial or complete failure to attain or maintain the sexual excitement response until the completion of the sexual act. The sexual excitement response refers to the lubrication and swelling response in females, and penile erection in males. The disorder is associated with marked distress and dysfunction.[2]

Female sexual arousal disorder can lead to painful coitus and associated problems like secondary dyspareunia, vaginismus and sexual desire problems. Vaginal dryness could result from psychological factors, infections, estrogen deficiency and use of anticholinergic medication.

Erectile dysfunction in males can be a cause of non-consummation of marriage, infertility and disruption of marital and sexual relationships. It may present as a primary or lifelong problem (if the male has never been able to attain or maintain an erection sufficient enough for successful sexual intromission or coital connection), or as a secondary or acquired one (following an initial period of normal functioning).

The problem may manifest or can be felt at different periods within the same phase of excitement viz. inability to attain the erection, ability to attain but inability to sustain the erection till penetration, ability to attain and sustain erection till penetration but inability to sustain it for a sufficient time following penetration. Impotence has been defined as an inability to attain and sustain an erection or for that matter satisfy the spouse at most attempts. It is often associated with premature ejaculation and may also be associated with sexual desire problems.

The coordination between the nervous system, vascular supply and the hormonal factors is required for smooth erectile function.[1,6] The disorder may result from a complex interplay of several physiological, biological, psychological, interpersonal and situational factors. Due to physiological reasons, it is difficult to attain erection soon after ejaculation. The quality and frequency of erections may also decline with advancing age.

The problem is likely to be psychogenic if erection occurs normally in certain situations like during masturbation, in sleep or with a different partner. Erectile dysfunction may manifest in a specific situational context or with a particular partner, thereby suggesting the role of external factors, both situational as well as interpersonal. Neurotransmitters like dopamine and ß adrenergic transmission have a facilitatory effect on erectile function while the – adrenergic transmission has an inhibitory effect.[1] Clinically the role of neurotransmitters is reflected by erectile dysfunction or impotence associated with antidopaminergic (antipsychotic) drugs and ß-blockers; and enhanced erection with dopaminergic agonists and priapism with trazodone (α1 blocker).

Neurohormonal disturbances, vascular etiologies and medical ailments can affect erectile function (Table 3).

Table 3. Disorders Associated with Male Erectile Dysfunction

Cardiovascular diseases
Atherosclerosis
Venous leakage syndrome
Coronary artery disease
Arterio-venous malformations
Aortic aneurysms
Cardiac failure

Endocrine disorders
Diabetes mellitus
Pituitary-adrenal-testes dysfunction
Acromegaly
Thyroid disturbance
Hyperprolactinaemia
Addison's disease
Cushing's syndrome
Adrenal neoplasia

Neurological disorders
Multiple sclerosis
Transverse myelitis
Parkinson's disease
Stroke
Temporal lobe epilepsy
Spinal cord injuries
Tumours of the CNS
Amyotrophic lateral sclerosis
Sensory neuropathies

Urological disorders
Peyronie's disease (fibrous bands in penile shaft)
Chronic renal failure
Hydrocoele

Varicocoele
Hepatic disorders (cirrhosis)
Pulmonary disorders (COPD, respiratory failure)
Infections (elephantiasis, leprosy, mumps)
Genetic disorders
(Klinefelter's syndrome, congenital penile vascular and structural abnormalties)
Nutritional disorders
Malnutrition
Vitamin and zinc deficiencies
Obesity
Psychiatric disorders
Depression
Anxiety
Substance use disorders (alcohol, opioids, cocaine, amphetamines, barbiturates, tobacco)
Pharmacological agents (drugs)
Antihypertensives
Psychotropics (antipsychotics and antidepressants)
Estrogens and anti-androgens
H-2 receptor antagonists,
Digoxin
Cytotoxic drugs
Poisonings (eg. lead, herbicides)
Surgical procedures (eg. certain abdomino-perineal surgeries)
Others (like radiation therapy, pelvic fracture, severe systemic debilitating disease)

Adapted from Saddock 1995 [1]

Atherosclerotic changes in the penile arteries and venous leaks (from corpora cavernosa) are the common vascular causes of male erectile dysfunction, particularly in middle-aged and elderly men. Medical illnesses associated with hypogonadism may predispose a person to erectile problems.

Diabetes mellitus, prolactinomas and thyroid dysfunction are commonly associated with erectile dysfunction. Vascular, hormonal and psychoneurogenic causes have been implicated as the major underlying factors.

Across different cultures, or manliness is equated to virility and sexual potency.[7,8] There is considerable stress, even if covert, on males to perform. A vicious cycle therefore sets in, with performance anxiety contributing to sexual dysfunction and the latter contributing or adding on to the former. Previous sexual experiences, if unpleasant or performed under stress, haste or with guilt or mixed feelings may also contribute. Unconscious fears, conflicts, sexual myths and beliefs also play an important role. Inadequate understanding and fear of stigmatization prevent early and appropriate help seeking from professionals and may add to the stress and anxiety and to the problem as a whole.

The disorder, like any other psychosexual disorder, requires adequate, careful and appropriate assessment. This requires for the clinician to be empathic, reassuring and competent. There is a need to ensure confidentiality and privacy, and to comfort the patient to establish mutual trust and rapport.

Assessment should include the patient's understanding about sexuality and the problem; assessment of patient's knowledge, beliefs and attitude, myths, pattern of sexual behaviour; defining the exact nature of the problem, pattern (since when, context), associated problems in other phases of the sexual response cycle; pressure of performance; liking of the sexual partner and the attitude towards her; the sexual understanding and attitude of the spouse or partner; previous sexual experiences (with spouse, partner, casual, commercial, masturbatory, paraphiliac) and the circumstances as well as the mindset under which performed viz. under the influence of substance or drugs, attempts to test potency, presence of guilt feelings with respect to masturbation or previous sex experiences; associated psychopathology or feelings of depression and anxiety; associated co-morbid physical ailments, substance abuse, medication history, history of spinal surgery or trauma.

Assessment of functioning should include a history of early morning erections, ability to attain some erection, history of masturbation or previous sexual functioning. A careful physical examination should include assessment of secondary sexual characteristics and genitalia (penile shaft, testicular size etc.). Cremasteric reflex and bulbocavernosal reflex should be checked to assess for neuropathies.

Investigations like penile blood pressure, nocturnal penile tumescence (NPT) studies using stamps or snap gauges at home or performed in sleep laboratories, papaverine induced penile erection (PIPE) test, computerized Doppler wave form analysis, colour coded duplex ultrasonography, cavernosography and endocrinological investigations like blood glucose, testosterone, luteinizing hormone, thyroid function and prolactin levels can be performed.[1,6]

Treatment: Psychological, medical and surgical interventions may be required depending on the underlying condition. In cases where a specific etiologic factor is identified, treatment involves management of the cause.

Medical: A variety of drugs have been used for correcting erectile impotence. Sildenafil citrate is a selective cyclic guanosine monophosphate (cGMP)-specific phosphodiesterase type 5 (PDE5) inhibitor. By inhibiting the enzyme, the drug allows increased levels of nitric oxide (NO) mediated cGMP in the corpus cavernosum, resulting in smooth muscle relaxation and blood inflow to the corpus cavernosum. The drug has no effect on absence of sexual stimulation and is contraindicated in persons taking nitrates viz. nitroglycerine.[9] It is available in the Indian market only on prescription of a psychiatrist, urologist, andrologist and dermatologists. The usual prescription dose is 50 mg PO, which is to be taken around an hour prior to the sexual act.

Other drugs used in the treatment of erectile dysfunction include trazodone (antidepressant with influence on α adrenergic and dopaminergic function), testosterone (oral as well as injectables), naltrexone (opiate antagonist), yohimbine (α2 adrenergic antagonist) and pentoxyphylline etc.[6]

Topical drugs like nitrates (vasodialating properties of nitroglycerine) and buccal preparation of phentolamine (α blocker) have also been used.

Amongst the injectable drugs, subcutaneous injections of apomorphine and intracavernous injections of papaverine (smooth muscle relaxant) and alprostadil (PGE1) are used.[10,11] Papaverine administration can lead to prolonged erection and priapism, which may merit necessary intervention; and repeated injections can also lead to fibrosis (corporosis).

Surgical: It includes prosthetic implants and penile revascularization surgery.[1,6]

Psychological: It includes sexual counselling, sex education and psychotherapies. The purpose is to allay myths and fears, educate regarding normal human sexual anatomy and physiology and to teach behavioural skills.

Conjoint marital unit therapy, as advocated by Master and Johnson, is based on the concept of marital unit or a dyad as the object of therapy. Both the partners need to actively participate in the therapy as both are considered to be involved in a sexually distressing relationship. The marital or interpersonal relationship as a whole is treated and specific emphasis is laid on sexual functioning. Individual sessions focus on understanding their current problem and their life style. Specific suggestions pertaining to sexual acts and lifestyle are followed by the couple. The problem can be effectively approached by team with male and female therapist.[7]

Behavioural exercises help in ameliorating fear of inadequate performance. Sexual dysfunction is assumed to be a learnt maladaptive behaviour and therefore through behavioural regimes efforts are made to unlearn the maladaptive patterns and to learn the adaptive ones. Relaxation exercises help in allaying anxiety. The couple is advised specific sexual play by the therapist. The therapy progresses in a graded fashion beginning with less demanding exercises (sensate focus exercises) that focus on sensory awareness to touch, site, sound and smell and ending up with satisfying sexual intercourse. Mastery of the initial less demanding assignments instills a sense of confidence and helps in dissociating anxiety from the sexual act.[7]

Depending on the dysfunction, specific exercises can be used for their management.

Other forms of psychotherapy like supportive psychotherapy and insight oriented psychotherapy can be incorporated in the treatment regime.[1]

Orgasmic Disorders

Orgasmic disorders include the male and the female orgasmic disorders and premature ejaculation in males.[2] Serotonin and $\alpha 1$ adrenergic transmission mediate orgasm and ejaculation. Drugs with $\alpha 1$ blocking properties may cause impaired ejaculation and serotonergic agents may inhibit orgasm.[1]

Female orgasmic disorder (inhibited female orgasm, anorgasmia) is defined as recurrent or persistent inhibition of the female orgasm. It manifests as the absence or delay in orgasm after a normal sexual excitement phase, as the clinician judges to be adequate in focus, intensity and duration. The diagnosis of the disorder should take into account factors like age, sexual experience and adequacy of sexual stimulation.

Male orgasmic disorder (inhibited male orgasm, retarded ejaculation) is characterized by persistent or recurrent delay or absence of orgasm following a normal sexual excitement phase during sexual activity. Before arriving at a diagnosis, the clinician needs to consider factors like the individual's age, focus, intensity and duration of the act.[2]

The condition is different from retrograde ejaculation, the latter being mostly organic. In retrograde ejaculation, the ejaculation occurs but the ejaculate passes backwards into the urinary bladder. Some men may have partial dysfunction or inhibition of orgasm and may experience a slow dribbling of ejaculate. They do not experience an orgasmic spurt and the pleasure associated with it.

Male orgasmic disorder is seen mostly following genitourinary surgeries (viz., prostatectomy), in elderly persons on drugs with anticholinergic side effects, use of antihypertensive drugs (methyl dopa, guanethidine monosulfate), phenothiazines, in disorders like parkinsonism and neurological disorders with lumbo-sacral spinal involvement. It is often associated with obsessive compulsive disorder or temperament. Transient retarded ejaculation is seen following heavy alcohol consumption or with hyperglycemia. Primary inhibited male orgasm may reflect unconscious conflicts or considering genitals and sex as dirty and sinful. Secondary inhibition may arise out of interpersonal difficulties with the partner and reflect a covert hostility towards the partner. Mutual agreement on issues pertaining to pregnancy, contraceptives, type and need for sex and satisfaction should be assessed.[1]

Pre-mature ejaculation (PME) is a condition in which a man recurrently achieves orgasm and ejaculation before he wishes to do so. It is difficult to define the time frame and no specific time duration in seconds or minutes has been defined to differentiate normal functioning from the dysfunction. The diagnosis is made when a male regularly (on a recurrent or persistent pattern) ejaculates on minimal sexual stimulation before or soon after entering the vagina.[2] Factors like age, novelty of the sexual partner, frequency and duration of coitus are factors that may affect the duration of the excitement phase and should be considered before making this diagnosis. In certain individuals, prolonged stimulation is required to attain an erection, and as a result the effective time interval between satisfactory erection and ejaculation may appear to be shortened; the primary diagnosis in such cases should be that of delayed erection.

The ICD-10 system of classification and Masters and Johnson have defined the disorder, taking into account both the partners rather than the individual alone.[3,7] Accordingly, the failure/inability to control ejaculation sufficiently for both the partners to enjoy sexual interaction is used to define the disorder. The diagnosis is made when the man cannot control ejaculation for sufficient period during intravaginal containment to satisfy the partner in about half of the episodes of coitus. This definition assumes that the female is capable of an orgasmic response. The problem can be related to the concern for partner satisfaction. The disorder is commonly associated with erectile dysfunction and sexual desire problems. In severe cases, ejaculation may occur prior to vaginal entry or in the absence of an erection.

Premature ejaculation is unlikely to be of organic origin, however it can be a result of a psychological reaction to organic impairments like erectile failure or pain.

Performance anxiety, performance in haste, unconscious fears about the vagina, fear of castration, previous sexual experiences (if performed in haste or under stress/fear of discovery leading to quick orgasm and ejaculation) and negative cultural conditioning are some of the factors that play an aetiological role in development of such a dysfunction. Partner role is very important and may exacerbate or help in the management of PME.

Sex counselling, behavioural exercises including relaxation techniques and adoption of specific postures during sexual play, help in management. The squeeze technique is typically used to raise the threshold of penile excitability. In this technique, the penis is stimulated until the initial sensation of impending orgasm and ejaculation are felt by the male. The male signals this to the female partner, who then stops the penile stimulation abruptly and forcibly squeezes the coronal ridge of the penis for a few seconds. The painful stimulus prevents orgasm and ejaculation in the male, and may lead to decline in erection. This technique is repeated several times during the sexual play.[7] In an alternative stop-start technique, stimulation is interrupted for some time and no squeeze is applied.

SSRIs and clomipramine (tricyclic antidepressant with serotonergic reuptake blockade) may be used to delay ejaculation.

Sexual Pain Disorders

Dyspareunia is characterized by recurrent or persistent pain during intercourse and can affect both males and females, mostly females. The pain is real and unbearable and can lead to subsequent avoidance of sexual act. In females it is often associated with vaginismus and both can result in one another.[1,2]

The causes are usually psychogenic or local infections or traumatic conditions. Female genital surgeries are often associated with temporary dyspareunia. Anxiety or fears about sex resulting in involuntary tension of vaginal muscles and previous traumatic sexual history of child abuse or rape could play an aetiological role in its development. It is important to rule out organic etiologies viz., pelvic inflammatory disease in females, infected hymenal remnants, episiotomy scars, Bartholin's gland infections, vaginitis, cervicitis, endometriosis, dermatological disorders viz. lichen sclerosis and other pelvic disorders. Irritation associated with improperly fitted or inadequately lubricated condoms and allergic reactions to the contents of contraceptive methods used may also contribute. Postmenopausal women may develop this problem because of atrophy of the vaginal mucosa and diminished lubrication.

The disorder though uncommon in males, is usually associated with Peyronie's disease, prostatitis, gonorrhoeal and herpetic infections. Post-ejaculatory pain may result from involuntary spasm of the perineal muscles due to psychological conflicts about the sex act or as a side effect of some medicines like antidepressants.

Vaginismus is the involuntary and persistent constriction of the outer third of the vagina that prevents penile insertion and intercourse.[1,2] It may reflect a general tendency or may be specific to coitus. In the former case, it may be demonstrated during gynaecological examination in which involuntary vaginal constriction prevents introduction of the speculum into the vagina. The disorder is usually seen in educated women of high socioeconomic status. The affected woman, may consciously wish to have coitus, but unconsciously prevents penile entry into her body. It may reflect strict religious upbringing equating sex to sin, previous life traumatic experiences, sexual conflicts, anticipation of pain and dyadic relationship problems with partner. Local causes presenting as vaginismus should be ruled out. Sex education, counselling and behaviour therapy are helpful in managing the disorder. Relaxation techniques help in allaying anxieties. The affected woman is advised to use her fingers or size graduated vaginal dialators to dialate the vaginal opening.

Sexual Dysfunction due to General Medical Diseases

In order to diagnose such a condition, there should be clear evidence (from history, physical examination and lab findings) that the distressing sexual dysfunction is due to direct physiological effects of a general medical condition.[2] Clues can be obtained from the temporal association between the onset, exacerbation or remission of the general medical condition and that of sexual dysfunction. The sexual dysfunction can affect various phases of the sexual-response cycle ranging from problems of desire to orgasm. The disturbance is not better accounted for by another mental disorder like major depression. A host of various medical conditions have been found to have direct physiological links with sexual dysfunctions and some of these have been described elsewhere in this chapter.

Substance Induced Sexual Dysfunction

Distressing sexual dysfunction is seen within a month of significant substance intoxication or withdrawal and is clearly linked to substance use problem.[2] Substances like alcohol, opioids, cocaine, amphetamines, hypnotic-sedatives are known to be associated with the dysfunction. The type of the dysfunction depends on the properties of the substance used and patterns of its use. In small amounts the substances can enhance sexual performance by disinhibiting, anxiolytic and euphorogenic properties. Continued chronic use can cause dysfunction in the various phases of the sexual-response cycle. For example alcohol can lead to sexual dysfunctions through a CNS depressant effect, direct gonadal effect or an indirect hormonal effect following compromised liver functioning. It is known to be associated with erectile disorders in men and tends to decrease testosterone levels in men. Opiod use can also lead to erectile dysfunction and decreased libido.

Paraphilias

Paraphilias are characterized by recurrent and intense sexual feelings, urges, fantasies and behaviours that involve unusual objects, activities or situations.[2] For example, they may involve non-human objects or children or non-consenting partners. They are usually associated with suffering or humiliation of self or the partner. The unusual fantasies are most of the times gratifying to the ego. They are associated with significant distress and dysfunction (Table. 4).

Unconscious sexual conflicts, child neglect or abuse, past traumatic sexual experiences, underlying personality and impulse contol problems (like borderline personality) and learning can contribute to development of paraphilias. In this regard, the role of pornographic literature and films can not be negated. There is also a need to carefully assess and rule out any other major psychiatric disorder.

Psychotherapeutic techniques have been frequently employed to manage such disorders. Behaviour therapy is used with a focus on unlearning of maladaptive patterns and learning of healthy and adaptive sexual patterns and practices. This is done by pairing of noxious (aversive) stimuli with the paraphillic urge, impulse and feelings. Desirable sexual feelings and behaviour are positively reinforced. Insight-oriented psychotherapy is used to deal with unconscious conflicts. Sex therapy can aid in managing associated sexual dysfunctions. Drugs like antipsychotics and antidepressants have also been used. Anti-androgens have been used in hypersexual paraphilias and SSRIs have been used for impulse control problems.[12]

Gender Identity Disorder

It is characterized by a strong and persistent cross-gender identification (not merely a desire for any perceived cultural advantages of being the other sex) and persistent discomfort with one's sex or sense of inappropriateness in the gender role of that sex.[2] In pure sense, it is not concurrent with physical intersex conditions like androgen insensitivity syndrome, congenital adrenal hyperplasia or ambiguous genitalia; nevertheless such conditions should be assessed before making a diagnosis. It is associated with significant

Table 4. Paraphilia and their Characteristic Features

Type of paraphilia	Characteristic features (manner in which sexual pleasure & excitement is obtained)
Exhibitionism	Exposure of one's genitals to an unsuspecting stranger
Fetishism	Sexual fantasies and behaviour involves the use of nonliving objects (fetish) like the female undergarments, belt and shoes. The sexual activity is directed to the nonliving object or the wearing of the inanimate object by the partner. The focus throughout the sexual cycle, from desire to orgasm, is on the inanimate object associated with the human body.
Sexual Sadism	Real acts involving psychological and physical suffering of the partner/victim; acts of humiliation of the partner or victim, restraint and blindfolding the victim, pinching, beating and inflicting injuries to the victim.
Sexual Masochism	Intense sexual urges, fantasies or behaviours involving the act (real, not simulated) of being humiliated, beaten, bound or other wise made to suffer.
Frotteurism	Touching and rubbing against a non-consenting person/stranger
Paedophilia	Sexual fantasies and behaviour involves sexual activity with pre-pubescent children. The person is at least 16 years of age and at least 5 years older than the child.
Transvestic Fetishism	Cross-dressing; while cross-dressed, the affected person usually indulges in sexual acts like masturbation, imagining himself to be the male subject as well as the female object of his fantasy. The condition is defined specifically for heterosexual males and therefore should not be confused with gender identity disorder.
Voyeurism	Act of observing an unsuspecting persons/strangers who are naked, removing their clothes or engaging in sexual acts. The observer gains sexual excitement from this observational (peeping) act, often fantasizes sexual experience with the observed person and hardly engages in a sex act with the latter. The observer is also referred to as 'peeping tom'
Others	Erotic excitement related to:
Coprophilia	Defaecating/faeces
Klismaphilia	Enemas
Urophilia	Urinating/urine
Telephone scatologia	Obscene phone calls
Zoophilia	Animals
Hypoxyphilia	Hypoxia (hanging, using plastic bag, suffocation)
Necrophilia	Dead or near dead
Partialism	Part of the body (foot)

distress and socio-occupational dysfunction. The cross-gender behaviour is generally apparent to the parents before 3 years of age. The childhood manifestations include repeated fantasies and stated desire or insistence that one is of the other sex, preference for cross-dressing with marked aversion towards normative sex clothing, intense desire to participate in the stereotypical games and pastimes of the other sex, preference for playmates of the opposite sex, assertion that one's genitalia are disgusting and that one would develop genitalia of the other sex. A boy with the disorder may insist to sit for urination and express the desire to get rid of his penis and testes and a young girl may stand to urinate and insist that she will grow a penis. In adolescents and adults, the manifestations include preoccupation to get rid of the primary and secondary sexual characteristics and requests for hormones and surgical interventions to physically alter the sexual characteristics to simulate the other sex. It is important to differentiate gender identity disorders (transsexualism) from transvestism,

homosexuality, psychotic and certain personality disorders.

Sexual Beliefs and Notions

Sexual myths and prejudices about sex abound. Indian society is deep rooted in traditions and sex is not openly discussed. Disorders of the genitalia are often referred to as *gupt rog* or secretive ailments. Amongst males, anxieties and concerns about semen loss, weakening of semen, loss of sexual vigour, *Kamzori* (weakness), nocturnal emissions (swapnadosh), masturbation, bent penis are common in the society.[4,13,14] Access to pornographic literature and films adds to the confusion. For details refer to chapter 40.

Masturbation is a common universal practice, more so in males than in females. Culturally and morally speaking, it is often considered a sin and a root cause of sexual, physical and mental ill health; and nevertheless is associated with significant guilt, worry and depression.[13,14] Despite strong cultural beliefs and irrespective of the frequency or the technique employed, masturbation has not been identified as a direct aetiological factor in sexual dysfunctions.[7] During the pubertal hormonal spurt and the associated physiological changes, masturbation is frequently accompanied by sexual fantasies and serves as a preparatory ground for adult interaction with the partner. Due to the rising age at marriage for both the genders, a significant proportion of young males and females have to pass through a long period of heightened sexual desires . Masturbation provides an acceptable release for heightened sexual impulses during this period. Even after permanent sexual relationship has been established, masturbation remains a healthy sexual activity during non-availability/illness of the partner. It is considered maladaptive, when it becomes compulsive, is performed in public and is preferred over partner interaction.[1]

Dhat Syndrome

Synonyms: Dhatu rog or shukrameha.

It is a commonly recognized problem in our culture and has been prevalent since ancient times. Dhat syndrome is characterized by vague somatic complaints (like fatigue and loss of appetite) and mental weakness ascribed to the loss of semen (whitish sticky fluid) in the urine as a result of excessive indulgence in masturbation or sexual activities or to nocturnal emissions.[13–20] The primary complaint of the affected person is the loss of semen. It is often associated with psychosexual dysfunctions like erectile impotence and premature ejaculation and with features of anxiety and or depression. The whitish discharge, though believed to be semen by the patient, is usually related to the presence of oxalates and phosphates in the urine. Ancient scriptures (like the Charak Samhita) and traditional systems of medicine (like the Ayurveda) have described this disorder and have laid emphasis on celibacy and avoidance of masturbation. According to a commonly held belief in the society, rich food gets converted into blood and blood gets converted into semen. Semen is regarded as an important dhatu (life elixir or vital force) and emphasis is laid on its preservation inorder to ensure mental as well as physical health. Such deep rooted beliefs give us clues to some understanding of the aetiology of the disorder.

The disorder has been subjected to clinical research and now also finds acceptance in the current ICD-10

classificatory system in the category of other neurotic disorders under the broad rubric of neurotic, stress related and somatoform disorders.[3] Strictly speaking it is not a sexual dysfunction, and is a sex related disorder – a sexual neuroses. Sex education, counselling and relaxation exercises are often used to address this problem. In sex education, emphasis is laid on the understanding of the normal human anatomy and physiological processes, particularly pertaining to the sex organs. Myths, prejudices, beliefs and attitudes towards sexuality are addressed. Co-morbid psychopathology should be explored, assessed and appropriately treated. The latter may require the use of anxiolytics and or antidepressants.

Homosexuality

It refers to sexual activity between persons of the same sex.[21] Sexual orientation is dynamic and therefore different categories ('homosexual', 'heterosexual') are not necessarily mutually exclusive and fixed. The issue to regard homosexuality as a mental illness is subject to significant controversies. Persistent and marked distress about sexual orientation (egodystonic homosexuality) is regarded as morbid.

Venereophobia

It is not a part of classification of psychosexual disorders but is a anxiety related disorder. Venereoneuroses may be divided into those neuroses that manifest with exposure to infection, including overreaction to infection, venereophobias and abnormal disease convictions, and factitious STD and AIDS. Some individuals may be unusually preoccupied with bodily processes, manifesting a genitally preoccupied hypochondriasis. There is irrational concern about appearance of genitals or sensation in genitals. Patient may self manipulate genitals to produce discharge and they may demand treatment. Demand of treatment in absence of demonstrable pathology is one indication of venereoneuroses and it is believed such patients are more seriously disturbed. Syphiliphobia was common in 20th century and in last 2 decades it was replaced by AIDS phobia. Many of these patient had single sexual act that makes them phobic of sex for life. Reassurance, counselling, sex education and treatment of underlying hypochondriasis are used for management.

Sex is a basic human, instinct end drive, and is inseparable from one's life. Sexual health is a very sensitive and important area, and is often ignored, dealt in a casual manner and full of controversies, myths and prejudices. Sexual disorders are a vast group of disorders. These disorders affect the individual's as well as the partner's life drastically and have significant medical, psychological, marital, social and legal implications.

There is a need to raise general awareness about sexual health in the society and to impart correct knowledge in an appropriate and healthy way. This shall help in prevention, early diagnosis and timely treatment of such problems. As clinicians, there is a need to approach the area sensitively, sensibly and with professional competence and ethics. There is a need for careful assessment and development, modification and utilization of effective interventions to deal with these disorders. Issues of privacy make the research into the area difficult. Systematic and careful research into such a sensitive area shall aid in enhancing the understanding and in management of such disorders.

References

1. Sadock VA. Normal human sexuality and sexual and gender identity disorders. In: Kaplan HI, Sadock BJ, eds. Comprehensive Text Book of Psychiatry. 6 th edn. Baltimore: Williams and Wilkins; 1995. p. 1295–1360.

2. American Psychiatric Association. Diagnostic and statistical manual of mental disorders. 4th edn., Washington DC: APA; 1994.

3. World Health Organization. The ICD-10 Classification of mental and behavioural disorders: Clinical description and diagnostic guidelines, WHO, Geneva.

4. Avasthi A, Nehra R. Sexual disorders: a review of Indian research. In: Murthy RS, eds. Mental health in India 1950–2000. Bangalore: PAMH; 2001.p. 42–53.

5. Verma KK, Khaitan BK, Singh OP. The frequency of sexual dysfunctions in patients attending a sex therapy clinic in North India. Arch Sex Behav 1998; 27: 309–313.

6. Vyas JN, Pandey SK Sexual disorders. In: Vyas JN, Ahiya N, eds. Textbook of Postgraduate psychiatry. 2nd edn. New Delhi: Jaypee Brothers; 1999. p. 333–344.

7. Masters WH, Johnson VE, eds. Human sexual inadequacy. London: J and A Churchill Ltd; 1970

8. Tripathi BM, Malhotra S. Study on determinants of sexual risk behaviours amongst alcohol users in diverse cultural settings, a report submitted to WHO, Geneva. 2002

9. McMahon CG. High dose sildenafil citrate as a salvage therapy for severe erectile dysfunction. Int J Impot Res 2002; 14: 533–538.

10. Mooradian AD, Morley JE, Kaiser FE, et al. The role of bi weekly intracavernous injection of papaverine in the treatment of erectile dysfunction. West J Med 1989; 151: 515-517.

11. Ishni N, Wanatabe H, Irisawa C, et al. Intra cavernous injection of prostaglandin E, for the treatment of erectile importence. J Urol 1989; 141: 323–325.

12. Meyer JK. Paraphilias. In: Kaplan HI , Sadok BJ, rds. Comprehensive text book of psychiatry. 6 th edn. Baltimore: Williams of Wilkins; 1995. p. 1334–1347.

13. Kaviraj Khazanchand, edr. Indian Sexology. New Delhi: S. Chand and Co; 1972.

14. Kulhara P, Avasthi A Sexual dysfunction in Indian subcontinent, Intervention. Review of Psychiatry 1995; 7: 231–239.

15. Wig NN. Problems of mental health in India. J Clin Social Psychiat 1960; 17: 48–53.

16. Malhotra HK, Wig NN. Dhat syndrome: A culture bound sex neurosis of orient. Arch Sex Behav 1975; 4: 519–528.

17. Behere PB, Natraj GS. Dhat syndrome: the phenomenology of a culture bound sex neurosis of the orient. Indian J of Psychiatry 1984;.26: 76–78.

18. Sing G. Dhat syndrome revisited. Indian J Psychiat 1985; 22: 119–122.

19. Chadda RK, Ahiya N. Dhat syndrome: a sex neurosis of the Indian subcontinent. Br J of Psychiat 1990; 156: 577–579.

20. Bhatia MS, Malik SC. Dhat syndrome – a useful diagnostic entity in Indian culture. Br J Psychiat 1991; 159: 691–695.

21. Gadpaille WJ. Homosexuality and homosexual activity. In: Kaplan HI, Sadock BJ, eds. Comprehensive Textbook of Psychiatry. 6th edn. Baltimore: Williams and Silkins; 1995. p. 1321–1333.

22. Ross MW. Psychological perspectives on sexuality and sexually transmitted disease. In Holmes KK, Sparling PF, Mardh PA, et al. eds. Sexually Transmitted Diseases. 3rd Edition. New York: Mc Graw Hill; 1999. p. 107–113.

PART X
General Guidelines in Clinical Approach to STD

Chapter 42

Clinical Approach to Genital Ulcer Disease

Vinod K Sharma, CS Sirka

Introduction

Genital ulcers are defined as breach in the continuity of genital mucosa and or skin. Genital ulcer disease (GUD) may be due to sexually transmitted diseases (STD) like syphilis, chancroid, donovanosis, lymphpogranuloma venereum (LGV), herpes genitalis, or non STD like traumatic ulcer, Behcet's disease, lichen planus, erythema multifome, lichen sclerosus et atrophicus, bullous diseases, Fournier's gangrene, squamous cell carcinoma etc.

GUD is the commonly encountered STD and it accounts for 1-70% of STD in different parts of the world with the lowest incidence in America.[1] The incidence of GUD differs from place to place because of the regional variation in the prevalence of etiological agents, sexual behaviour and sociocultural factors and possibly due to racial characteristics and genetic predisposition playing a role in acquiring the GUD. It has been observed that syphilis and chancroid are more prevalent in minority, blacks and hispanics, similarly the herpetic ulcers are more common in the whites. The civilization and economy has an influence in the different STD e.g. the developed countries have higher incidence of herpes genitalis than the developing country. Chancroid is common in the developing world, whereas the syphilis is common in both developing and industrialized countries. Donovanosis is encountered in some parts of Asia,[2] especially in the South India.

Genital ulcers are more frequently reported in men because they can be easily seen compared to women. Symptomatic genital ulcers like herpes genitalis have the same incidence in both the sexes. The non-tender GUD of cervix in female often remains unnoticed and are under reported. In some communities where the female prostitution is prevalent, there is increased incidence of GUD in male because of limited number of female act as the reservoir of the infection constantly infecting the male population.

The clinical diagnosis may be misleading because of the increasing HIV co-infection and mixed infection often alters the morphology of ulcer and the text book description of the various GUD may not be present.[3] The ulcers do not remain confined to the genitalia and may be seen in the extragenital sites, due to changing sexual behavioural pattern. It has also been observed that the clinical diagnosis is incorrect in about 40% of the GUD patients in comparison to laboratory tests.[1] The clinical sensitivity for the diagnosis of GUD like herpes genitalis is up to 67%,[4] chancroid 33-52.6%,[3,5] syphilis 55% and herpes genitalis is 22% respectively in a study at Johannesburg[6] and subsequently similar results were observed in the other cities of South Africa.[4] In practice the documentation of aetiological agent of the GUD remains difficult. The appropriate diagnostic tests are often not available, not properly utilized. Aetiological agent is not demonstrated due to the self-medication by the patient, or the ulcers are contaminated. However the bedside and laboratory tests are fairly sensitive and specific in early lesions. The dark ground illumination and Tzanck test are up to 80% positive in primary chancre and herpes genitalis respectively.[2,6] The culture for herpes is approximately 100% sensitive, at the vesicular stage and lower at the ulcerative stage.[7,8]

In the past few years the epidemic of the HIV has shown an impact on the course, treatment and transmission of GUD and there is possible impact of GUD on the spread and course of the HIV.

The common organisms causing genital ulcers are *Treponema pallidum* (syphilis), *Haemophilus ducreyi* (chancroid), *Herpes simplex virus (HSV)-2* and *HSV-1* (herpes genitalis), *Calymmatobacterium granulomatis* (donovanosis) and *Chlamydia trachomatis sero-type L1-L3* (LGV).

Diagnosis of Genital Ulcer

The approach to genital ulcer should include detailed history taking, thorough examination, bedside tests and laboratory investigations in all cases.

History

History taking is an important step in the GUD, which includes recording of age, sex, occupation and address to know the age group and sex most affected in the community and address for follow-up after treatment. The history of sexual contact (single or multiple), with exact date to estimate approximate incubation period. Whether the sexual act was under the influence of alcohol or drugs? Because the forceful sexual act under the influence of alcohol or drugs can give rise to immediate injury at frenulum. The history of sexual partner, whether male or female? Was it a vaginal, anal or oral intercourse? Promiscuity of the patient and the partner and drug abuse history is essential. History of present or past genital ulcer in the partner, if there was vesicle formation, duration of ulcer, if it has healed, how long did it take to heal, are required in all cases of GUD. In female patient, history of abortion or still birth and in children, history suggestive of sexual abuse need to be elicited. In all patients history of associated STD need to be enquired. As the GUD patients have the higher incidence of HIV infection, one should also ask about the associated symptoms of significant weight loss, frequent diarrhoea, persistent fever and chronic cough for more than one month to know about the immune status of the individual.

The healing time of the genital ulcer may suggest the diagnosis. For example the spontaneous healing time for the primary chancre is about 3-8 weeks, primary herpes genitalis is 14-21 days and recurrent herpes genitalis is about 10 days. LGV ulcers heal in 2-5 days and often it remains unnoticed by the patient, whereas the donovanosis and the chancroid rarely show tendency for spontaneous healing.[1] Incubation period and healing time are summarised in Table 1.

Examination

The examination of all the suspected GUD patients should be carried out wearing gloves. Complete evaluation should include examination of skin, oral cavity, lymphnode, liver and spleen, chest, cardiovascular system and neurological examination. In the examination of the lymphnodes, group involved, tenderness, consistency, overlying skin and attachment to the surrounding structure is important. Genital examination is followed by examination of the perianal area.

Inspection

Look for number, site, size, depth, presence of necrotic slough or granulation tissue on the floor of the ulcer margins and extension of erythema surrounding the ulcer. The primary chancre is usually solitary, where as the chancroid and herpetic ulcers are multiple. The classical ulcers of herpes and LGV are superficial, whereas the chancroid ulcers are relatively deep. Beefy granulation tissue on the surface of the ulcer is characteristic of donovanosis, whereas the chancroid ulcer is covered with necrotic slough and primary chancre is usually clean.

Palpation

In palpation the presence of tenderness, induration, bleeding on manipulation, attachment to the surrounding structure and per rectal examination findings are of help in diagnosis. Phimosis may cause difficulty in examining the lesion, the efforts should be made to

Table 1. Incubation Period and Healing Time in GUD

STD	Incubation Period	Spontaneous Healing time	Healing time on Treatment
Primary chancre	9-90 days (mean 21 days)	3-8 weeks, never exceeds 3 months	1-2 weeks
Chancroid	5-8 days (one to several weeks)	Self limiting but may persist for years	1-2 weeks
Herpes genitalis (primary)	5-7 days	14-21 days	16-12 days
LGV	10 days (5-30 days)	2-5 days (transient)	–
Donovanosis	9-50 days (probably)	No tendency for healing	3-4 weeks

retract the prepuce or palpate through the preputial skin. If it is not possible to examine due to phimosis, patient is advised frequent saline irrigation and examination of the lesion may be possible next day. If the prepuce is not retractable after the saline irrigation the dorsal slitting has been suggested but it is rarely needed. The tenderness is a feature of genital herpes and chancroid, whereas the primary chancre, donovanosis and LGV ulcers are relatively nontender. Primary chancre usually has button like induration but other GUD are non-indurated. Donovanosis bleeds on manipulation. The comparative features of different genital ulcers are summarised in Table-2. In mixed infection the picture is atypical and combination of diseases responsible for it eg. primary chancre and chancroid may result in indurated ulcer with an inflammatory bubo.

In female patient, examination of external genitalia is followed by speculum and per-vaginal examination. The appropriate samples for investigations are also collected during the examination. An effort is made to look for other STD that may be simultaneously present.

Investigations

Dark ground illumination, Tzanck smear, tissue smear and smear for Gram stain are mandatory for all genital ulcers. All the patients with GUD should be serologically tested for syphilis, HIV and preferably for hepatitis B and C. Other tests for chlamydial serology, culture for HSV, *H. ducreyi* and chlamydia are performed subject to availability.

The biopsy of ulcer is helpful in diagnosis of donovanosis and ruling out premalignant and malignant diseases of genitals.

Diagnosis of GUD

Primary Chancre

Definitive diagnosis of syphilis depends on the demonstration of *T. pallidum* by dark ground illumination (DGI) or fluorescence microscope examination. DGI is positive for *T. pallidum* in up to 80% of the primary

Table 2. Clinical Features of Common GUD

Characteristic	Syphilis	Herpes	Chancroid	LGV	Donovanosis
Primary lesions	Papule	Vesicle	Pustule	Papule, pustule, or vesicle	Papule
Number of lesions	Usually one, but in 1/3 cases it is >1	Multiple & may coalesce	Usually multiple & may coalesce	Usually one	Variable
Diameter	5-15 mm	1-2 mm	Variable	2-10 mm	Variable
Edges	Sharply demarcated, elevated, round, or oval	Erythematous, polycyclic	Undermined, ragged, irregular	Elevated, round, or oval	Elevated, irregular
Depth	Superficial or deep	Superficial	Excavated	Superficial or deep	Elevated
Base	Smooth, nonpurulent, covered with serous exudate	Erythematous	Purulent, bleeds easily	Variable	Red and velvety, bleeds readily
Induration	Button like	None	Soft	Occasionally firm	Firm
Pain	Uncommon, but tender on firm pressure	Frequently tender	Usually very tender	Variable	Uncommon
Lymphadenopathy	Firm, non-tender, bilateral & in 1/3 cases it may be tender	Firm, tender, often bilateral with initial episode	Tender, may suppurate, loculated, usually unilateral occasional cord like lymphangitis	Tender, may suppurate, loculated, usually unilateral	None, pseudobuboes (may be)
Recurrence	No	Yes, in 80%	No	No	No

chancre.[2] The DGI is conventionally recommended to be repeated for 3 consecutive days prior to giving negative result or starting treatment. In our experience the compliance for three day DGI test is poor so we prefer to repeat DGI twice in the first day itself and start the treatment. Nontreponemal test like VDRL, rapid plasma reagin (RPR) or toludine red unheated serum test (TRUST) are 75-85% sensitive in primary chancre.[1] And if the non-treponemal tests are positive, it should be confirmed by specific treponemal tests like FTA-Abs (Fluorescence treponemal antibody absorbent) or MHA-TP (Micro haemaggulutination assay for antibody to *T. pallidum*). These specific and non-treponemal test in combination gives 69-85% positivity in patients with primary chancre.[1] VDRL test is mandatory during follow up. The test is done on the first visit, if negative, repeated after 4-6 weeks of appearance of the ulcer. Recently the polymerase chain reaction (PCR) has been used in the detection of *T. pallidum* and the results were found to be similar to direct fluorescent antibody (DFA) test.[9] It is helpful to differentiate *T. pallidum* from the saprophytic spirochetes of oral cavity but it is not available in majority of laboratories.

Herpes Genitalis

The history of appearance of vesicles prior to the ulcer formation is definitive for the diagnosis of herpes. The Tzanck test is sensitive up to 80% and specificity is about 94%.[8] The immunofluorescence staining of slide is more sensitive than Tzanck test. For this type specific, fluorescein lebelled monoclonal antibody specific to HSV1 or HSV2 is added to the slide. The culture is the most sensitive and it is about 100% positive, the results are highly positive from vesicular lesion and least from the ulcerative lesion.[7,8] The viral culture is specific and shows cytopathic changes within 1-3 days.[1] Antigen detection test for HSV is positive even in healing ulcer and is an alternative test.[9] The PCR is more helpful as it can detect HSV DNA from the healing lesion.[10]

Antibodies to HSV 2 and 1 are not diagnostic as they may reflect previous infection and DNA hybridization and PCR are usually not available. In clinical practice the diagnosis is made on clinical grounds and Tzanck smear. Culture, serology, immuno-fluorescence, PCR are available only in research centres.

Chancroid

There is uncertainty in the accuracy of the different laboratory tests and the clinical diagnosis continues to be the mainstay of treatment. The gram stain sensitivity and specificity is variable from negligible to as high as 62% sensitive and 99% specific.[11] The other tests are fluorescein labelled monoclonal antibody for *H. ducreyi*, blot radioimmunoassay and DNA hybridization. Culture for *H. ducreyi* is positive in 0-80% of suspected cases of chancroid.[12] DNA probe and PCR are not available in most of the laboratories.

Lymphogranuloma Venereum

The diagnosis is based on the serology test and the positive serology >1: 64 with clinical feature supports the diagnosis but it is not specific of LGV. The infection by the other chlamydial species can also give the similar titre. The other sensitive test are direct fluorescence antibody staining, ELISA for chlamydial antigen[13] and IgG antibody to chlamydia (>1: 256). Culture for chlamydia, immunotyping, microimmunofluorescence serology, PCR, prove assay, chemiluminescence enhanced test, ligase chain reaction test (LCR), sero specific monoclonal antibody may be used.[13]

Donovanosis

Biopsy and tissue smear for the demonstration of donovan bodies are diagnostic. There is no serological test and the organism cannot be cultured in laboratory. In developing countries like India, specific tests are often not available for confirmation except in research or referral laboratories and most patients are treated on the basis of clinical diagnosis. The laboratory findings in GUD are summarised in Table 3.

It is clear from above description that specific test for etiological agent for GUD are frequently not available and there is coexistence of multiple organisms in a single ulcer. The use of multiplex PCR (M-PCR) amplification assay is used to detect simultaneous presence of multiple organism from a single specimen. Morse et al, observed the resolved sensitivity of M-PCR for *H. ducreyi* and *Herpes simplex* virus culture were 95% and 93% respectively, whereas the culture sensitivity of these organisms were 75% and 60%. The use of M-PCR reduces the indeterminate laboratory diagnosis from 35% to 6% and the detection of multiple agents from

Table 3. Lab Diagnosis of Genital Ulcers

Lab test	Syphilis	Chancroid	Herpes	LGV	Donovanosis
Microscopy	Darkfield Direct immunoflourence	Gram stain, Fluorescent labelled monoclonal antibody detection	Antigen detection by DFA. Immuno-peroxide staining & ELISA	Direct immuno-fluorescence staining, ELISA rapid assays like (1) Sure cell Chlamydia test (2) Clear view Chlamydia test (3) Test pack Chlamydia, Direct fluorescence for antibody to LGV, Immuno dot & micro immunofluorescence by ELISA	Giemsa stain tissue smears/ sections
Culture	Not available	Enriched Mueller-Hinton (MH) chocolate agar,Enriched gonococcal agar	Cell culture (vero cells/human diploid fibroblast(MCRC-5), Baby hamster kidney cells, rabbit kidney cells	Cell culture (HeLa-229, McCoy cells, Baby hamster kidney cell(BHK-21)	No
Collection/ Transport Media		Transport Media-Thioyoglycolate hemin medium containing L-glutamin & bovine albumin at 4°c	Swab-Wire Shaft with cotton tip *Transport media*-Viral transport media at 4°c, if time required for inoculation is >48 hours freeze at -70°c	Swab-Plastic shaft with Rayon swab & Cytobrush with plastic shaft	
Serology	Non-treponemal tests–VDRL/ RPR Treponemal test – ELISA,FTA-Abs, TPHA, MHA-TP, HATTS, Anti Treponemal IgM detection	ELISA, Immuno dot technique	Monoclonal antibodies to HSV 1 and 2, ELISA, DNA hybridization	CFT & immuno-flurescent antibody test	Experimental
Molecular techniques	PCR	PCR	PCR	PCR, LCR, Prove assay chemiluminescence-enhanced test in LGV. Immunotyping by PCR	Not available
Histop-athology	Perivascular infiltrate of lymphocyte, plasma cells accompanied by endarteritis obliterans	Surface zone- narrow consisting of neutrophils fibrin, erythrocytes, necrotic tissue. Middle zone – wide newly formed blood vessels with marked proliferation of their endothelial cells Deeper zone-dense inflammation of plasma cells and lymphoid cells	Degeneration of keratinocytes, resulting in acantholysis 2 types of degeneration • Ballooning • Reticular	Small area of necrosis with proliferating epitheloid & endothelial cell with stellate abscess	Acanthosis/ pseudocarcino—matous hyperplasia at edge of ulcer Dermis – dense inflammation of histiocytes plasma cells with absence of lymphocytes Small neutrophilic abscess Donovan bodies

Note: HIV ELISA should be done in every case of genital ulcer disease as genital ulcer can be a co-factor for HIV transmission.

the single ulcer increases from 4% to 18%.[14] In a study from Pune with multiplex PCR showed poor results in patients with suspected chancroid.[15]

Treatment

Often the immediate laboratory test are unrewarding and serology VDRL and HIV have been sent and the treatment administered is for the most likely clinical diagnosis and side lab investigations and the patient is reviewed after 7 days. If the symptomatic improvement is noticed by 3 days and treatment is continued. Donovanosis may take 5-7 days to respond. If the symptoms worsen the patient is re-evaluated. If the VDRL and HIV test are negative during the follow up, the test is repeated after 1 and 3 months. In case of HIV negative report the test has to be repeated after 6 months and 12 months of the last exposure. Patients with positive VDRL test having meningeal symptoms should be evaluated for CSF VDRL and in HIV positive patients with positive VDRL, the CSF VDRL is mandatory. The syndromic treatment is often used which includes treatment for syphilis and chancroid. In case of HIV positive patients there is no consensus regarding the change of treatment regimen for STD. However the treatment recommendations are similar to the CDC guideline in most of the GUD. It is also mandatory that the sexual partners of the STD patient should be examined, investigated and treated promptly.

Follow Up

Primary chancre: Post treatment VDRL is repeated at 3 month, 6 month and at one year.[16] In HIV positive patients with primary chancre the VDRL is repeated every month for the first 3 months and 3 monthly thereafter.[17]

Reference

1. Hoffman IF, Schmitz JL. Genital ulcer disease- Management in the HIV era. Post Grad Med 1995; 98: 67-82.
2. Schmid GP. Approach to the patient with genital ulcer disease. Med Clin North Am 1990; 74: 1559-1572.
3. Chapel TA, Brown WJ, Jeffres C, et al. How reliable is the morphological diagnosis of penile ulceration? Sex Transm Dis 1977; 4: 150-152.
4. O'Farrell N, Hoosen AA, Coetzee KD, et al. Genital ulcer disease: accuracy of clinical diagnosis and strategies to improve control in Durban, South Africa. Genitourin Med 1994; 70: 7-11.
5. Sturm AW, Stolting GJ, Cormane RH, et al. Clinical and microbiological evaluation of 46 episodes of genital ulceration. Genitourin Med 1987; 63: 98-101.
6. Dangor Y, Ballard RC, Exposto F, et al. Accuracy of clinical diagnosis of genital ulcer disease. Sex Transm Dis 1990; 17: 184-189.
7. Mosley RC, Corey L, Benjamin D, et al. Comparison of viral isolation, direct immunofluorescence and direct immunoperoxidase techniques for detection of genital herpes simplex virus infection. J Clin Microbiol 1981; 13: 913-918.
8. Solomon AR, Rasmussen JE, Varani J, et al. The Tzanck smear in the diagnosis of cutaneous herpes simplex. JAMA 1984; 251: 633-636.
9. Cone RW, Swenson PD, Hobson AC, et al. Herpes simplex virus detection from genitalia lesion: a comparative study using antigen detection (Herp Check) and culture. J Clin Microbiol 1993; 31: 1774-1776.
10. Dyck EV, Meheus AZ, Piot P. Genital Herpes :Laboratory diagnosis of Sexually Transmitted Diseases. WHO. Geneva 1999; p 50-56.
11. Taylor DN, Duangmani C, Suvongse C, et al. The role of *Haemophilus ducreyi* in penile ulcers in Bangkok, Thailand. Sex Transm Dis 1984; 11: 148-151.
12. Dyck EV, Meheus AZ, Piot P. Chancroid Laboratory diagnosis of Sexually Transmitted Diseases. WHO, Geneva 1999; p 57-66.
13. Dyck EV, Meheus AZ, Piot P. *Chlamydia trachomatis* infection : Laboratory diagnosis of Sexually Transmitted Diseases. WHO, Geneva 1999; p 22-35.
14. Morse SA, Trees DL, Htun Ye, et al. Comparison of clinical diagnosis and standard laboratory and molecular methods for the diagnosis of genital ulcer disease in Lesotho: Association with human immunodeficiency virus infection. J Infect Dis 1997; 175: 583-589.
15. Risbud A, Chan-Tack K, Gadkari D, et al. The aetiology of genital ulcer disease by multiplex polymerase chain reaction and relationship to HIV infection among patients attending STD clinics in Pune, India. Sex Trans Dis 1999; 26: 63-65.
16. Thappa DM. Current status of HIV modified Syphilis in Indian scenario. Indian J Sex Transm Dis 2002; 23: 1-13.
17. Siddappa K, Ravindra K. Syphilis and non venereal treponematosis. In: Valia RG, Valia AR, eds. IADVL Textbook and Atlas of Dermatology. Mumbai: Bhalani Publishing House; 2001. p. 1390-1422.

Chapter 43

Clinical Approach to Vaginal/Urethral Discharge

A J Kanwar

Vaginal Discharge

Vaginal discharge (VD) is one of the commonest presenting complaint in women attending the gynaecoloy & STD clinics, general practitioners and reproductive health clinics. For ages, the term VD has been used synonymously with leucorrhoea. It is defined as whitish discharge, which is not associated with menstruation. The symptoms and signs of vaginal discharge are observed in several physiological and pathological conditions, which may be both local and systemic. VD should be considered as abnormal (AVD) when anyone of the following feature is present.

1. Hypervaginal secretion not associated with menstruation
2. Offensive or malodorous discharge and
3. Yellowish discharge

Prevalence

It has been estimated that upto one third of females attending the gynaecology clinics have complaints of AVD. AVD can occur in women of all ages, however, it is quite common during pregnancy. In many clinics, more than 70% of pregnant women manifest AVD due to lower genital tract infections. The commonest causative organisms of AVD in females of reproductive age group are: Neisseria gonorrhoeae, Chlamydia trachomatis, Gardnerella vaginalis, Trichomonas vaginalis, and Candidiasis. Mixed infections are quite common.

Normal Vaginal Discharge

The normal vaginal discharge is whitish, non malodorous and floccular in consistency. Its amount varies considerably between individuals. It may result in only minimal staining of the undergarments to profuse discharge. The normal pH is acidic and ranges from 3.5 to 4.5 due to the activity of Doderlein's lactobacilli. These bacilli convert glycogen into lactic acid. The cellular contents of the discharge are composed of sloughed cells of cervical columnar and vaginal squamous epithelium. The bulk of discharge consists of serous vaginal transudate and cervical mucous.[1-3]

Aetiology of Vaginal Discharge

The symptoms and signs of AVD are attributable to vaginal infection. Increased profuse vaginal discharge is associated with trichomoniasis, bacterial vaginosis, vulvovaginal candidiasis (VVC) and in cases where there is coincidental sexual acquisition of cervical infection with N. gonorrhoeae and C. trachomatis.[4] It has been shown in several studies that there is no association of cervical infection with symptoms or signs of abnormally increased amount or abnormal odour of vaginal discharge.

The various causes of AVD can be broadly divided into physiological and pathological. The physiological causes are either age dependent (neonates, prepuberty, child bearing) or due to excessive secretion (pregnancy, sexual arousal). Table 1 lists the various pathological causes of AVD.

We shall first discuss the infective causes of abnormal vaginal discharge. Cervical infections associated with AVD are discussed elsewhere in this book.

Candidiasis

VVC is a frequent cause, affecting 15 to 30 percent of

Table 1.   Pathological Causes of AVD in Adolescents and Adult Women[5]

(a)   Infective
Vaginitis
- Bacterial vaginosis
- Vaginal candidiasis
- Vaginal trichomoniasis

Cervicitis:
- Mucopurulent cervicitis (MPC) due to *N. gonorrhoeae* and *C.trachomatis*

(b)   Non infective
Foreign bodies
- Intrauterine contraceptive device (IUCD)
- Tampons and other materials

Chemical irritants
- Antiseptics
- Deodorants
- Bath additives
- Detergent spermicide
- Douches
- Perfumed soaps

Gynaecological conditions
- Endocervical polyp
- Fistulae
- Radiation effects
- Post operative
- Tumours
- Medication and nutrition

women attending a gynaecology clinic for complaints of vaginal discharge. Majority of yeast strains (85-90%) isolated from the vagina are *Candida albicans*. The rest are non – albicans species, the chief among them being *Candida glabrata*. Recently there has been an increased incidence of vaginitis caused by non albicans species.[6,7]

C. albicans has an affinity to adhere to vaginal epithelial cells, although no epithelial cell receptor for candida have been identified. Only the germinative forms of *C. albicans* are able to produce VVC.

Pathogenic candida species secrete aspartyl proteinase.[8] This proteinase has been identified in vaginal secretion in women with symptomatic vaginitis only. Iron binding by candida organisms facilitates their virulence.[9] The ready availability of erythrocytes and haemoglobin in the vagina creates an ideal situation for yeast possessing erythrocyte-binding surface receptors.

Pathogenesis and Predisposing Factors

Candida organisms gain access to vaginal epithelium and secretions predominantly from adjacent perianal area. The mechanisms whereby asymptomatic colonization of the vagina changes to symptomatic VVC is not exactly clear.

Spontaneous phenotypic stretching occurs in colony morphology of most candida species when they are grown on amino acid rich agar in vitro at 24° C.[9] These variant phenotypes have a capacity to form mycelia spontaneously to express virulence factors, adherence and the capacity to invade and survive in diverse body sites as well as to cause disease. It is possible that such spontaneous phenotypic switching transforms asymptomatic colonization to symptomatic vaginitis. Various predisposing factors for VVC are listed in Table 2. Epidemiologic evidence for the role of sexual intercourse in transmission of VVC is lacking.

Table 2.   Predisposing Factors Associated with VVC[6]

- Pregnancy
- Uncontrolled diabetes mellitus
- Corticosteroid therapy
- Tight fitting synthetic underclothing
- Antimicrobial therapy
- Oestrogen therapy
- Contraceptives
  IUD
  Sponge
  Nonoxynol-9
  Diaphragm
  High dose estrogen oral contraceptive
- Increased frequency of coitus?
- Candy binge
- HIV infection
- Idiopathic

Sources of Infection

Persistent gastrointestinal tract carriage is a source of vaginal reinfection, as majority of candida strains isolated from the rectum and vagina are identical.[10] However, women prone to recurrent VVC are not known to suffer form perianal or rectal candidiasis. As already mentioned above the role of sexual spread of candidiasis is limited. It has been shown that vaginal relapse is responsible for recurrent VVC. Small numbers of candida organisms possibly survive temporarily within cervical or vaginal epithelial cells only to reemerge some weeks or months later. Fidel et al have shown that systemic cell mediated immunity (CMI) has only a minor role in providing a normal defense function at the level of vaginal mucosa. There is probably a local vaginal acquired defect in CMI predisposing to recurrent VCC.[9]

Probably the most important defense against both candidial colonization and symptomatic inflammation is the normal natural bacterial flora.

Candida organism in order to survive and persist must initially adhere to epithelial cells and then grow, proliferate and germinate, in order to colonize the vaginal mucosa successfully. Animal studies suggest that lactobacilli and candida frequently survive side by side.

Clinical Manifestations

Clinical spectrum of VVC varies from an acute florid exudative form with thick white vaginal discharge and large number of germinated yeast cells to other extremes of absent or minimal discharge, fewer organisms and pruritus. By and large, a quantitative relationship exists between signs and symptoms of VVC and the extent of yeast colonization.

The usual clinical presentation is acute pruritus and vaginal discharge. The discharge is classically described as typically cottage-cheese like in character. It may however at times be watery and homogenously thick. Odour is minimal and inoffensive. The patient complains of vaginal soreness, irritation, vulvar burning, dyspareunia and dysuria. Partners of patients with VVC may occasionally develop extensive balanoposthitis. More frequent however, is a transient rash, erythema and a burning sensation. All these symptoms are self limiting.

Diagnosis

A 10% KOH preparation would identify germinated yeast. Large number of WBC are usually absent in VCC and if present, indicate mixed infection. The vaginal pH is normal 4.0 to 4.5, if pH is more than 5, it indicates either bacterial vaginosis, trichomoniasis or a mixed infection. If the direct microscopy is positive, no culture is necessary. However, if it is negative and signs and symptoms suggest VVC, vaginal culture should be performed. Though vaginal culture is the most sensitive method for detection of candida, a positive culture does not necessarily indicate that the yeast is responsible for the vaginal symptoms.[9]

There is no reliable serologic test for diagnosis of VCC.

A latex agglutination slide technique which employs polyclonal antibodies reactive with multiple species of candida is commercially available. It has a reported sensitivity of 81% with a specificity of 98.5%.[9]

Treatment

The treatment modalities of VVC are given in appendix II.

Trichomoniasis

Trichomonas vaginalis is a flagellate pathogenic protozoan transmitted primarily by sexual contact. It causes vaginitis in women and urethritis in men. In addition to abnormal vaginal discharge, it is increasingly associated with preterm labour, premature rupture of membranes and post abortion or post caesarean infections. *T. vaginalis* is oval or fusiform in shape with a mean length of 15 μm. It has four anterior flagella which arise from an anterior kinetosomal complex. The cytoplasm is rich in glycogen granules, ribosomes, and large chromatin granules which are known as hydrogenosomes. The reproduction is by mitotic division and longitudinal fission. It occurs every 8 to 12 hours under optimal conditions (temperature between 35° C and 37° C and pH between 4.9 and 7.5).[11] *T. vaginalis* exists only in trophozoite form. It is capable of phagocytosis and is an aerotolerant anaerobe. At high oxygen tension, its growth is inhibited as it lacks catalase.[12] Numerous host macromolecules like alpha −1 antitrypsin, fibronectin lipoproteins and lipids coat the cell surface[13] of *T. vaginalis*. These molecules are important for the survival of the parasite in vivo and contribute to metabolism and pathogenicity of trichomoniasis.

Cellular, humoral and secretory immune responses are elicited after infection with *T. vaginalis*. These however, do not protect against repeated infection. The C3 component of the complement binds to receptors sites on the surface of *T. vaginalis* and leads to the death of the protozoan. The alternative complement pathway is involved.[14] It has been observed that symptoms of trichomoniasis are exacerbated shortly after menstruation, the time at which high levels of complement are found in vagina. *T. vaginalis* elicits predominantly a humoral response and the antibodies are directed against high molecular weight protein immunogen p 270[15] as well as also to cysteine proteinases.[11] For detailed information, refer to chapter 28.

Clinical Presentation

T. vaginalis primarily infects vaginal epithelium. Less commonly it is isolated from the cervix, urethra,

Bartholins and Skene's glands. Extravaginal sites are rarely infected. These include fallopian tubes, perinephric spaces and cerebrospinal fluid.

The clinical manifestations vary from asymptomatic carriage to severe vaginitis. Patients with vaginitis complain of vulvar itching and purulent yellow green colour discharge. The vulva may appear erythematous and oedematous with excoriations. As already mentioned discharge may be absent in a few percentage of cases. Cervix has small punctate haemorrhages with ulcerations. This is referred to as 'strawberry' cervix.

Diagnosis

Diagnosis based solely on clinical signs and symptoms are unreliable as the spectrum of infection is broad and other sexually transmitted pathogens may cause similar signs and symptoms.

Laboratory Diagnosis

Direct Microscopic Examination

A purulent yellow-green vaginal discharge is characteristic of trichomoniasis. As the discharge is absent in a varying percentage of cases, diagnosis of trichomoniasis depends on identification of *T. vaginalis* by wet mount, stains, culture, immunological and molecular methods.

Vaginal fluid or discharge is obtained during speculum examination using a cotton swab or wire loop. One drop of saline is placed on a microscopic slide and the vaginal sample mixed directly in the saline on the slide. Slightly warming the saline enhances the motility of *T. vaginalis*. The motility is best observed by using phase contrast microscopy. For this, either the condenser is brought down or diaphragm closed to increase the contrast. For the diagnosis, it requires identification of motile trichomonas with characteristic motility, size and morphology. In most cases, increased number of polymorphonuclear leucocytes are also present.

Identification of the protozoan on wet mount is better than various staining methods which include staining with Gram, Giemsa, neutral red, and other stains.[17,18] Wet mount preparations are also superior to Papanicolaou-stained smears which can detect *T vaginalis* in asymptomatic women during routine cytologic examination.[19] However, there is a high percentage of false positive and false negative results.[11]

If the wet mount examination is negative, culture is the 'gold-standard' for diagnosis of trichomoniasis. Of the various media available, the modified Diamond medium is the best as it allows more prolific growth.

Several serological techniques have also been described to diagnose trichomoniasis, but these are less sensitive than culture or even wet mount examination. Other tests are antigen detection immunoasssays using monoclonal antibodies and nuclear-acid based tests.

Treatment of Trichomoniasis

Metronidazole and related drugs are highly effective for treatment of trichomoniasis. The various treatment options are given in Appendix II.
Simultaneous treatment of sexual partners is recommended.

Other Therapies

Topical therapy: It should be reserved for clinical situations in which systemic metronidazole is contraindicated.

Topical preparation of metronidazole gel has low efficacy. Clotrimazole applied intravaginally for 6 days may have a role in the first trimester when metronidazole is not recommended. Though a vaccine for active immunization against trichomoniasis is commercially available, it has not been evaluated in well-controlled double blind prospective studies.

Bacterial Vaginosis

Bacterial vaginosis (BV) is an important cause of abnormal vaginal discharge and affects about 30-45% of women in the reproductive age group. It is a polymicrobial condition and the culture of vaginal fluid reveals mixed flora which includes genital mycoplasmas, *Gardnerella vaginalis*, anaerobic bacteria and Mobiluncus species.[20] There is a decrease in lactobacilli and increase in the total bacterial count from the normal of 10^5–10^6 cells/gm of secretion to 10^9–10^{11} organism/gm of secretion in patients of BV.

Clinical Features

Women with BV may be asymptomatic or may complain of increased vaginal discharge which is sticky and homogenous. It tends to adhere to the vaginal wall. The discharge has usually a fishy odour which is more noticeable after sexual intercourse. Pruritus is of only mild to moderate degree.

Diagnosis

In a patient suspected of BV, diagnosis can be made using Amsel's criteria[4] which are as follows

1. Nonviscous homogenous white uniformally adherent vaginal discharge.
2. High pH – Vaginal pH of more than 4.7 has high sensitivity and negative predictive value, but of low specificity.
3. Clue cells – vaginal squamous cells covered by bacterial rods. It leads to blurred border.
4. Whiff test: Adding 10% KOH to vaginal secretions produces an amine odour. It is due to production of cadaverine, putrescine and trimethylamine by enzymatic action of decarboxylases.
   If any 3 of the above criteria are present, a diagnosis of BV can be made.

The other details of BV and its management are discussed in a separate chapter.

Approach to a Patient with AVD

Symptoms and signs of AVD are mostly attributable to vaginal infection. Though in some studies an association between AVD and cervical infection has been found, by and large there is no association of cervical infection with symptoms or signs of AVD.

As in other patients with STD, the initial assessment in patients with AVD begins with history. In the history, the following points should be specifically enquired:

1. Is there an abnormal increase in the amount of vaginal discharge?
2. Is there an abnormal or unpleasant odour of vaginal discharge?
3. Is the colour of the discharge unusually yellow?
4. Abnormal ulcers or painful lesions over genitalia
5. Has the patient noticed any lumps or swellings?
6. Enquire specific details about the previous diagnosis, earlier treatments and their effects.
7. Ask about recent change of sexual partner or multiple sexual partners, history of STD in partner.

After history, one should proceed to examination. General and physical examination should precede the pelvic examination. Antiseptics should not be applied on external genitalia before pelvic examination to avoid vaginal contamination.

Speculum Examination

Warm water provides sufficient lubrication for speculum insertion. Following insertion, all aspects of vagina and cervix are assessed to see the presence or absence of mucopurulent cervicitis, ulceration, erythema and vesicular lesions of vulva or vagina. The amount, consistency and location of the discharge within the vagina should be noted. Also try to see for cervical motion tenderness.

Collection of Samples

The collection of vaginal discharge is done with a swab from the vaginal wall during speculum examination. Vaginal secretions can be taken without a speculum in prepubertal girls with swabs that have been moistened with saline. In cases of cervical discharge, wipe the ectocervix with large cotton swab and then collect the endocervical mucous on cotton tipped swab.

Appearance of Vaginal Discharge

The vaginal discharge is then examined with special attention to the amount, consistency, colour, odour and location of discharge within the vagina. The character of vaginal discharge can be classified as floccular, granular, homogenous (milky) and curdy. Normal vaginal discharge is floccular or granular.

Laboratory Evaluation

The colour of vaginal discharge should be noted in comparison with white colour of the swab.

The pH of the discharge is determined by directly rolling the swab containing the specimen on pH indicator paper. The pH indicator paper should show colour variation with pH above and below 4.5. An additional specimen removed with a swab is first mixed with a drop of saline and then with a drop of 10% KOH on a microscopic slide. An abnormal fishy or amine odour released on mixing of the specimen with KOH provides the usual basis for a clinical diagnosis of BV. Separate coverslips are placed on both saline and KŎH wet mounts for microscopic examination to detect the

(a) Presence and quantity of normal epithelial cells
(b) Clue cells
(c) Neutrophils
(d) Trichomonas – motile trophozoite forms
(e) Candidal hyphae and spores

In many of these patients, the symptoms and signs combined with risk assessment and with pH and amine tests and microscopic wet mount findings correspond to a consistent pattern and further studies are unnecessary. However, when the diagnosis can not be established, further microbiological studies are indicated. The nature and the choice of the study depend on the clinical findings. These may include

(a) Culture for *C. albicans*
(b) Culture for *T. vaginalis*
(c) Gram stain of vaginal fluid

It is important differentiate between normal flora and the flora characteristic of bacterial vaginosis. Here one should emphasize that in patients with prominent vaginal complaints but no abnormal findings,[21] all the 3 additional microbiological tests are indicated as at times the complaints may be functional. The endocervical mucous should be separately examined, apart from the vaginal discharge. The characteristics of endocervical secretion can be classified into mucoid, cloudy and mucopurulent. Yellowish colour on white-cotton tipped swab is considered as mucopus.

Endocervical Smear Stain

The swab is rolled onto an area of 1-2 square centimeter on a glass slide. The smeared secretion should be distributed in separated heterogenous islands.
The smear is heated dry and stained with

(a) Gram stain and
(b) Methylene blue

Emulsion oil is added and the microscopic slide is scanned to evaluate the presence of cervical mucous to look for contaminated squamous cells and microorganisms and to identify areas of mucous that contain inflammatory cells. Usually polymorphonuclear leucocytes are not uniformly distributed in the cervical mucous. Therefore, a representative area containing dense concentration of such leucocytes are selected. Presence

of 10 or more PMN leukocytes per field (1000 x) on a smear stained specimen of endocervical mucous at least in 5 separate areas is classified as mucopus. Demonstration of intracellular diplococci at least 3 pairs or more, is strongly suggestive of *N gonorrhoeae* infection. If there are only few leucocytes, it suggests physiological endocervical discharge.

The various causes of mucopurulent cervicits like *C. trachomatis* and *N. gonorrhoeae*, which can be associated with vaginal discharge, are referred to elsewhere in this book.

Urethral Discharge

Urethritis or inflammation of the urethra is characterized by the discharge of mucopurulent or purulent material associated with burning senstation during micturition. Asymptomatic infections are common. The only bacterial pathogens of proven clinical importance in men who have urethritis are *N. gonorrhoeae* and *C. trachomatis*. Accordingly urethritis is termed as gonococcal when *N. gonorrhoeae* is detected in urethral smears and non gonococcal urethritis (NGU) when this organism can not be visualized microscopically.

Aetiopathogenesis

Urethral discharge constitute 15 to 20% of patients attending STD clinics in India. Urethritis due to *N. gonorrhoeae* is the most common cause of urethral discharge in developing countries. It accounts for about 50% of the patients presenting with urethral discharge. NGU is diagnosed if gram negative intracellular organisms cannot be identified on Gram stains. *C. trachomatis* is the most frequent cause (5-15%) of NGU. Other pathogens are *Trichomonas vaginalis, Mycoplasma genitalium* and *Ureaplasma urealyticum*. Rarely urethral discharge can be caused by other organisms. The causes are listed in Table 3.

Approach to a Patient with Urethral Discharge

It is difficult to differentiate between gonococcal and NGU on clinical grounds. Both conditions present with urethral discharge, dysuria or urethral itching.[23] There are some differences. These are listed in table 4.

Table 3. Causes of Urethritis in Males[22]

(a) Infective
Gonococcal
- *Neisseria gonorrhoeae*
Non gonococcal
- *Chlamydia trachomatis*
- *Ureaplasma urealyticum*
- *Mycoplasma genitalium*
- *Trichomonas vaginalis*
- Yeasts
- Herpes simplex virus
- Adenoviruses
- Hemophilus spp
- Other bacteria

(b) Non infective
- Congenital anomalies of genitourinary tract
- Urethral stricture
- Phimosis
- Catheterization
- Chemical irritants
- Acute haemorrhagic cystitis
- Stevens Johnson syndrome
- Pemphigus

Table 4. Clinical Features of Gonococcal and Non Gonococcal Urethritis

Symptoms	Gonorrhoea	NGU
Discharge	Profuse, purulent and yellowish green	Scanty, mucoid or mucopurulent
Dysuria	Intense burning sensation	'Smarting' feeling in urethra on passing urine
Incubation period	2–5 days	2–3 weeks
Constitutional symptoms	Fever, malaise	Absent

(a) In many patients with NGU, the discharge many be absent while some may notice it only in the morning.
(b) It is not possible to differentiate between *C. trachomatis* positive and *C. trachomatis* negative NGU. In *C. trachomatis* negative urethritis, discharge may be more profuse and purulent.[22]
(c) *U. urealyticum* infection may be associated in some cases with only dysuria and no discharge.[22]
(d) Some patients may present with other manifestations of NGU. These include

(i) Chlamydial conjunctivitis

(ii) Epididymitis
(iii) Prostatitits
(iv) Reiter's syndrome

Laboratory Approach to a Patient with Urethral Discharge

Collection of Sample

Urethral material is obtained with meatal or intra urethral swabs; the choice depends on the organisms and the amount of urethral discharge. In males, detection of urethral discharge can be enhanced by milking the penis from the base to the glans. Meatal discharge is an appropriate specimen for detection of *N. gonorrhoeae*. If there is no meatal exudate, an intraurethral swab should be used. It is important that patient should not have passed urine for at least 2 hours. The swab is introduced slowly for about 2–3 cms, rotated and then withdrawn gradually.[24]

In patients when there is no discharge, early morning urine sample or urine voided at least after 4 hours of retention should be collected and centrifuged for at least 10 minutes. The superficial part is decanted and the sediment is used as the specimen.

Gram Stain

The swab is rolled onto the slide which is then air fixed or passed through a flame. It is then stained with Grams' stain. The slide is examined under 100 × magnification. Area that shows maximum number of polymorphonuclear leucocytes (PMNL) is then examined under oil immersion (1000 ×). Presence or absence of diplococci and the number of PMNL in each field is noted.

1. Interpretation of slide: Detection of gram negative diplococci inside PMNL is diagnostic of gonococcal urethritis. In presence of only extracellular gram-negative diplococci, the diagnosis of gonorrhoea should be confirmed by culture.
2. Presence of greater than or equal to 5 WBC per oil immersion field in the absence of gram negative diplococci is diagnostic of NGU.[25]
3. When the results of smear are equivocal with finding of only extracellular or atypical diplococci, it is imperative to do cultures.[22,25]
4. Cultures of *C. trachomatis* and *U. urealyticum* are

not universally available. Cultivation of *C. trachomatis* in tissue culture requires the support of a well equipped laboratory.

5. Positive leucocyte esterase test[26] on first void urine or microscopic examination of first void urine demonstrating greater than or equal to 10 WBC per HPF is diagnostic of NGU. Various culture media used and other diagnostic tests employed for gonorrhoea and NGU are discussed elsewhere in this book.

Treatment Guidelines

Refer to chapter 44 and Appendix II.

References

1. Salerno LJ. Leukorrhoea. In: Sciarra JJ, Mc Elin TW, eds. Gynaecology and Obstetrics. Hagerstown: Harper and ROW Publishers; 1981. p. 1-5.

2. Siemmens JP, Wegner G. Estrogen deprivation and vaginal function in post menopausal women. JAMA 1982; 2481: 445-448.

3. Eschenbach DA. Infectious vaginitis. In: Sciarra JJ (CD-ROM 2000 edition). Gynaecology and Obstetrics. Lipincott Williams and Wilkins. Vol 1. Chapter 40.

4. Holmes KK, Stamm WE, et al. Lower genital tract infection syndrome in women. In: Holmes KK, Sparling PF, Mardh PA, et al. 3rd ed. Sexually Transmitted Diseases. McGraw Hill, New York: 1999; p 761-781.

5. Blackwell A. Management of vaginal discharge. Med Digest Asia 1983; 1: 12-20.

6. Sobel JD. Epidemiology and pathogenesis of recurrent vulvo-vaginal candidiasis. Am J Obstet Gynaecol 1985; 152: 926-929.

7. Morton RS, Rashid S. Candidal vaginitis: Natural history, predisposing factors and prevention. Proc R Soc Physc 1970; 70 (suppl 4): 3.

8. De Bernardis F. Evidence for a role for secreted aspartate proteinase of *Candida albicans*, in vulvo-vaginal candidiasis. J Infect Dis 1990; 161: 1276-1278.

9. Sobel JD. Vulvovaginal candidiasis. In: Holmes KK, Sparling PF, Mardh PA, et al, eds. 3rd ed. Sexually Transmitted Diseases. New York: McGraw Hill; 1999. p. 629-639.

10. Meinhof WL. Demonstration of typical features of individual *C. albicans* strains as a means of studying sources of infection. Chemotherapy 1982; 28 (1): 51-55.

11. Krieger JN, Aldrete JF. *Trichomonas vaginalis* and Trichomoniasis. In: Holmes KK, Sparling PF, Mardh PA, et al. eds. 3rd ed. Sexually Transmitted Diseases. New York: McGraw Hill, 1999. p.587-604.

12. Honigberg BM. Trichomonads, Parasitic in humans. London, Springer Verlag 1989: p. 24.

13. Peterson KM, Aldrete JF. Host plasma proteins on the surface of pathogenic. *Trichomonas vaginalis*. Infect Immun 1982; 37: 755-762.

14. Gillin F, Sher H. Activation of alternate complement pathway by *Trichomonas vaginalis*. Infect Immun 1981; 34: 268-272.

15. Aldrete JF. Alternating phenotypic expression of two classes of *Trichomas vaginalis* surfaces markers. Rev Infect Dis 1988; 10 S: 408.

16. Wasserheit JN. Epidemiological synergy: Inter relationship between human immunodeficiency virus infection and other sexually transmitted diseases. Sex Trans Dis 1992; 19: 61-65.

17. Quinn TC, Krieger JN. Trichomoniasis. In: KS Warren, AAF Mahmoud eds Tropical and Geographic medicine. 2nd ed. New York: McGraw Hill: 1990; p. 358.

18. Nielsen R. *Trichomonas vaginalis:* II Lab investigations in trichomoniasis. Br J Vener Dis 1973; 49: 531-534.

19. Weinberger MW, Harger JH. Accuracy of Papanicolaou smear in the diagnosis of asymptomatic infection with *Trichomonas vaginalis*. Obstet Gyanecol 1993; 82: 425-428.

20. Hill GB. The microbiology of bacterial vaginosis. Am J Obstet Gyanecol 1993; 169: 450-454.

21. Hillier S, Holmes KK. Bacterial vaginosis In: Holmes KK, Sparling PF, Mardh PA, et al eds. 3rd ed. Sexually Transmitted diseases. New York: McGraw Hill; 1999: p. 563-586.

22. Martin DH, Bowie WR. Urethritis in males. In: Holmes KK, Sparling PF, Mardh PA, et al. 3rd ed. Sexually transmitted diseases. McGraw Hill, New York 1999: p 833-845.

23. Munday PE, Attman DG, Taylor RD. Urinary abnormalities in non-gonococcal urethritis. Br J Vener Dis 1981; 57: 387-90.

24. Dyck K EV, Meheus AZ, Piot P. In: Laboratory diagnosis of sexually transmitted diseases. Genera WHO: 1999. p. 1-2

25. Jacobs NF, Kraus SJ. Gonococcal and non gonococcal urethritis in men. Clinical and laboratory differentiation. Ann Intern Med 1975; 82: 7-14.

26. Patrick DM, Rekart ML, Knowles L. Unsatisfactory performance of leukocyte esterase test of first voided urine for rapid diagosis of urethritis. Genitourin Med 1994; 70: 187-190.

Chapter 44

Critical Evaluation of Syndromic Management of Sexually Transmitted Diseases

B Loganathan

Introduction

Sexually transmitted diseases (STD) is not only a medical problem but also causes significant social stigma. Most of the STD are curable after adequate treatment. Treatment forms an important component of control and prevention of any communicable disease. Early diagnosis and appropriate treatment of other STD will definitely curb the transmission of HIV/AIDS. These concepts have been proved true by a recent report from Tanzania, which says, "Inspite of sexual behaviour practices such as low usage of condoms or number of sexual partners remaining unchanged, the incidence of HIV infection in the community is reduced by effective STD intervention program which focuses on early diagnosis and treatment of STD".

To achieve this, the new concept of **Syndromic Approach to STD Management** came into effect. The syndromic approach is an approach where the health care providers (HCP) diagnose and treat patients on the basis of groups of symptoms or signs (syndromes) rather than for a specific STD. Many STD can cause a particular syndrome and therefore HCP may need to treat for several STD at the same time. Thus, a genital ulcer, which is a symptom of both chancroid and syphilis, is treated for both syphilis and chancroid in an area where both are prevalent. Similarly, vaginal discharge which is a symptom of bacterial vaginosis, candidiasis, chlamydia, gonorrhoea and trichomoniasis, all these conditions need to be treated.

Syndromic Management: Promoting Effective STD/HIV Control[1,2]

Sexually transmitted diseases are unique among infectious diseases due to the stigma attached to the word "sex" in this country. Disease perception among the population is very low, as the people lack the necessary education on the problems of STD and also it affects more often certain marginalised group such as commercial sex workers (CSW) intravenous drug addicts and certain inaccessible populations. Many STD cases remain undetected because they are asymptomatic. Assessment of exact disease load in India is made difficult as most of these STD patients seek treatment either from private clinics or from traditional healers.

"WHO recognizes that the control of sexually transmitted diseases is an intervention which improves the health status of the population and prevents HIV transmission" (WHO/GPA/STD/1993). Primary prevention includes such activities as promotion of safer sexual behaviour and provision of condoms. Secondary prevention consists of promotion of health seeking behaviour and the provision of accessible, effective and acceptable treatment services.

The STD case management should provide treatment which must result in a cure. It must also underline the importance of bringing the partners for treatment and prevent the risk taking behaviour.

There are three approaches to diagnose and treat STD: (a) Aetiological Diagnosis (b) Clinical Diagnosis and (c) Syndromic approach.

Problems with Aetiological Diagnosis

Aetiological diagnosis is based on identifying the aetiological agent by laboratory test.

- Skilled personnel and sophisticated equipments are needed to identify the causative agents of STD

- Lab tests for diagnosis are expensive and time-consuming
- Treatment does not begin until the results are obtained
- Testing facilities are not available at the primary health care level where many people with STD seek care

Problems with Clinical Diagnosis

Clinical diagnosis is based on identifying STD based on the clinician's experience. It is well known that even experienced STD clinicians may miss concurrent infections. Studies have shown that clinicians correctly identified only one-third of the cases of chancroid and syphillis, half of the cases in women, and less than 10% of mixed infections.

- Clinical diagnosis is only accurate for 50% of STD cases.
- Mixed infections are not usually considered.
- Mistreated and untreated infections can lead to complications and continued transmission.

STD Associated Syndromes[1,2]

The syndromic approach is based on treating patients of STD on the basis of group of symptoms or syndromes as given below:

STD Syndrome	Possible Causes
• Urethral discharge (Fig. 1, 2)	*Neisseria gonorrhoeae (N. gonorrhoeae) Chlamydial trachomatis (C. trachomatis)* D to K
• Genital ulcer disease (Fig. 3)	*Treponema pallidum, Haemophilus ducreyi, C. trachomatis* (L_1, L_2, L_3) *Calymmatobacterium granulomatis,* Herpes simplex virus
• Vaginal discharge (Fig. 4, 5, 6)	*Trichomonas vaginalis, Candida albicans, Gardnerella vaginalis N. gonorrhoeae, C. trachomatis,* Anaerobes.
• Lower abdominal pain (Fig. 7)	*N. gonorrhoeae, C. trachomatis,* Anaerobes.
• Inguinal Bubo (Fig. 8)	*H. ducreyi, C. trachomatis* (L_1, L_2, L_3)
• Scrotal swelling (Fig. 9)	*N. gonorrhoeae, C. trachomatis,* viruses and surgical conditions
• Ophthalmia neonatorum (Fig. 10)	*N. gonorrhoeae, C. trachomatis*

Criticisms of the Syndromic Approach

- The syndromic approach is not a scientific procedure.
- Syndromic diagnosis is too simple for a physician to use, and approach does not use a provider's clinical skills and experience.
- Some physicians still feel better treating according to clinical diagnosis in the absence of lab facilities and then, if symptoms do not improve, treating for another cause.
- The syndromic approach wastes a lot of drugs.
- It promotes the development of antibiotic resistance.
- Simple laboratory tests should be included.

STD Case Management[1,2]

When a patient with STD complaint comes to the clinic, he or she must be treated effectively. So the health care provider must be knowledgeable about STD. Lack of perception or recognition of symptoms leads to deferment of treatment. To ensure this simplest and least expensive method, syndromic approach may be best suited at this level. To make STD care available at primary health centre, it may be necessary to integerate STD care at the primary care level.

Diagnosing Syndromes[1,2]

The clinician's diagnosis is based on the combination of clinical findings and patient symptoms. When a patient complains of urethral discharge, treatment is given for gonorrhoea and chlamydia infections. Since treatments are offered for all likely causes, the likelihood of a cure for STD causing discharge is greatly enhanced.

Simple flow charts by WHO provide the information to institute treatment based on the symptoms. These flow charts are prepared based on the STD prevalence and drug availability in that area. They are displayed as posters or as pamphlets for the easy reference of the provider (Fig. 1–10).

The flow chart for genital ulcers helps to explain how the algorithms work. When a patient complains of a "Genital sore", the provider consults the flow chart for genital ulcers—a syndrome usually caused by syphilis, chancroid or herpes. Since an examination alone is not a reliable way to differentiate the causes of

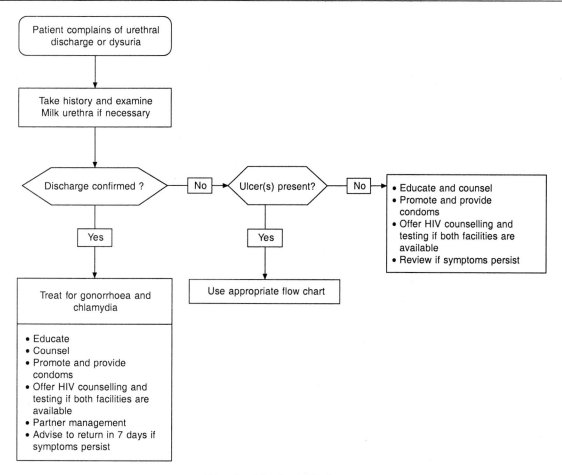

Fig. 1 Urethral Discharge

such "sores" the algorithm on the flowchart helps the providers to decide whether to treat presumptively for syphilis and chancroid (Fig. 3).

The first step is to examine the external genitals in men and the outer and inner surfaces of the labia in women. If the "sore" is in fact an ulcer, the provider is advised to treat for both syphilis and chancroid. The chart also reminds providers to educate patients about the treatment and how to prevent further transmission, including condom use and referring partners for treatment, and to explain how patients will know whether a follow-up visit is necessary. If the provider instead observes small, fluid filled (vesicular) lesions, the next step is to treat to relieve the symptoms of herpes, provide education and counselling about the disease and its prevention, and encourage the patients to use condoms.

Syndromic management flow charts are designed to follow a diagnostic logic close to the provider's own thought processes. "This is, in fact, the approach that many doctors follow naturally and subconsciously," says

Dr. Johannes van Dam of the Joint United Nations Programme on AIDS (UNAIDS), "It simply provides a rational basis for a diagnosis or for a therapeutic decision by offering correct information based on the latest possible data".

In syndromic case management, the provider is less dependent on laboratory tests. The tests are expensive and are unavailable in many settings. It may take weeks to get the result from the lab, which may delay the starting of appropriate treatment. The test may not be reliable. The patient might be living far away from the clinical facility and find it difficult to repeatedly come for the lab result and treatment. Adopting the syndromic approach allocates more funds for drugs for STD treatment.

The simplified procedure of the syndromic approach gives a readymade tool to health workers, and it enlarges the number of providers for STD care. The services will be available on a wider scale, and reduce the prevalence of STD in a shorter time period.

"Patients like the idea of being treated at first visit,

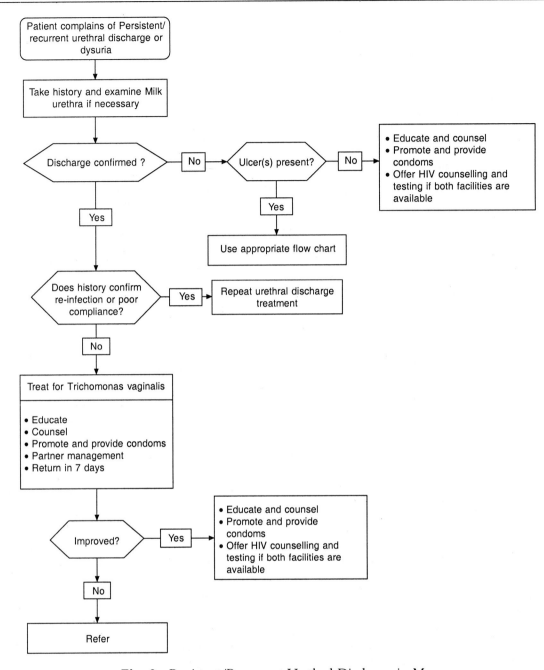

Fig. 2   Persistent/Recurrent Urethral Discharge in Men

and because syndromic management is more efficient, the waiting time for clinic visits is much shorter", says Dr. Alfred Brathwaite of the Jamaican Ministry of Health, which has implemented syndromic management in many of the country's STD clinics.

The cure rates are more, and infection spread curtailed by reducing the length of illness. This approach also includes prevention education, which includes counselling for behaviour change, condom use, and

improvement in health-seeking behaviour.

Treatment of Individual STD Syndrome
Refer to Appendix III

Validity of the Syndromic Approach[1,2]

The validity of the syndromic approach depends on:

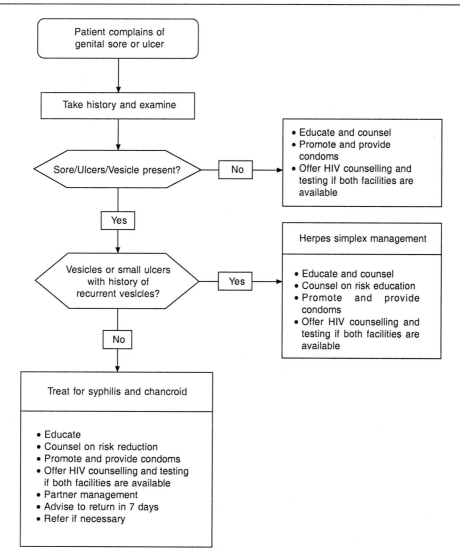

Fig. 3   Genital Ulcers

- Efficacy of the drugs chosen against STD pathogens
- The pathogens causing the diseases included in the syndrome
- Diagnostic validity
- Assessing the cure rate and compliance of treatment
- Immunological status

Challenges

- Syndromic algorithms must incorporate local data on STD prevalence
- Affordable drugs must be prescribed on the flow chart.

- May need modification based on new treatment strategies
- Development of algorithms for different situations and locations.
- Challenges from Medical Schools, which perceive it as inferior quality.
- Resistance from physicians as ordering laboratory tests is considered a matter of prestige.
- Asymptomatic patients—Health workers must be trained to identify such cases.

Critical Evaluation of Syndromic Approach

Since the introduction of the syndromic approach in

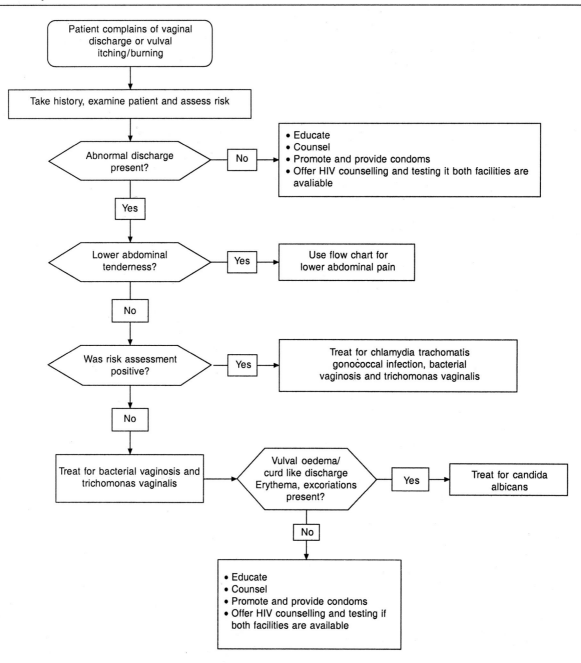

Fig. 4 Vaginal Discharge

1991 by the WHO, most the centres across the world have been using this approach. However, there has been some controversy regarding the use of this approach. The operational performances of syndromic approach, its usefulness in the diagnosis treatment and prevention of various STD and the sensitivity of syndromic approach have been studied in various centres.

Campbell and Plumb[3] from Canada have undertaken a Medline-based study to understand the use of the syndromic approach in managing STD in low-income countries, and to determine if evidence supports its continued use. In resource poor countries the use of syndromic approach is appropriate for high-risk groups and for symptomatic individuals. However, it is still a poor screening approach when applied to asymptomatic cases, particularly in women. Risk scoring and simple laboratory tests help to increase the algorithmic sensitivity of the syndromic approach. The authors conclude that

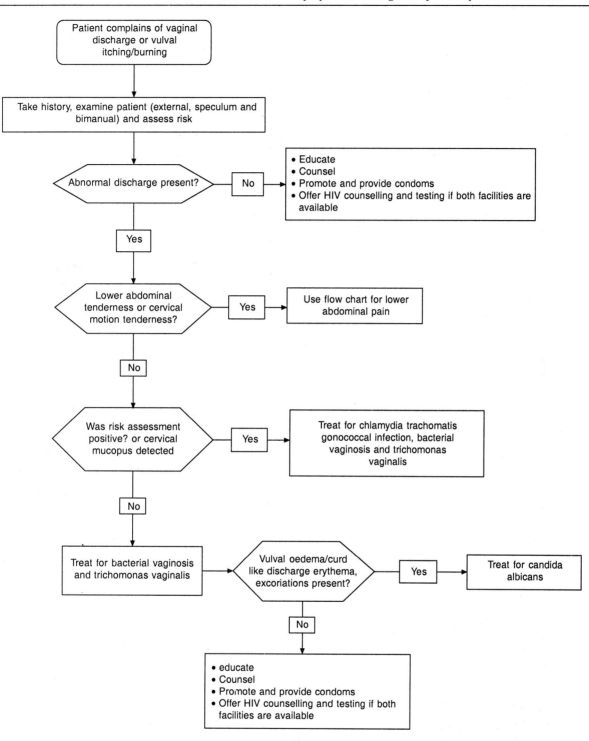

Fig. 5 Vaginal Discharge (Speculum and Bimanual)

until inexpensive, simple and accurate STD diagnostic tests are developed and made available for use in low income countries, a modified syndromic approach is the most feasible method of STD management in low income countries.

In a report from South Africa,[4] the sensitivity of a syndromic management approach in detecting STD in patients at a public health clinic was evaluated. All new patients attending the STD clinic were sampled systematically by gender over a 6 weeks period. All the

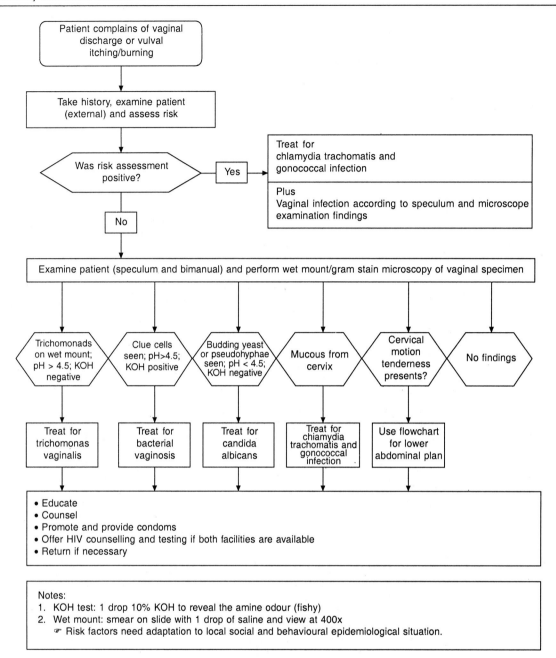

Fig. 6 Vaginal Discharge (Speculum and Microscope)

patients were examined thoroughly and specimens were collected for laboratory tests. In a retrospective simulation clinicians syndromic diagnosis were validated against the laboratory findings or for genital ulcer syndrome against the findings of the research physicians. There were 170 men and 161 women. Syndromic diagnostic procedures achieved reasonable levels of sensitivity in detecting *N.gonorrhoea and C.trachomatis* in men and women and in detecting *Trichomonas vaginalis* and bacterial

vaginosis in women. However the sensitivity of detecting genital ulcers in women was only 36.4% and *Candida albicans* 0-12.3%. With syndromic approach 8.2% of men and 32.9% of women would leave the clinic with at least one infection inadequately treated. The authors have concluded that a proportion of STD and genital tract infections are not being detected and treated owing to the high prevalence of multiple syndromes and mixed infections, both symptomatic and asymptomatic.

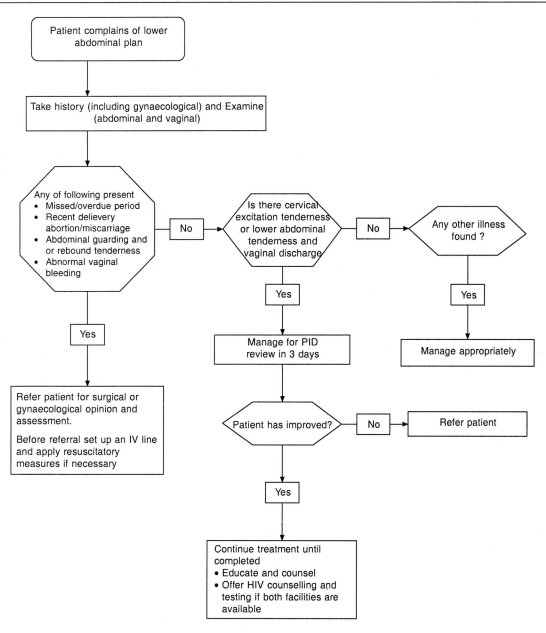

Fig. 7   Lower Abdominal Pain

In a study by Hanson et al[5] from Zambia the algorithms for the treatment of STD syndromes were evaluated. A total of 436 patients were followed up. The cure rate for the discharge syndrome was 97–98% for both the sexes and for genital ulcer diseases, 83% for female and 69% for male patients. The large proportions of treatment failures especially in males were possibly related to decreased susceptibility of *Haemophilus ducreyi* to co-trimoxazole.

In a report of operational performance of a STD control programme in Tanzania by Grosskurth et al[6],

during a 2 year period, 12,895 STD syndromes were treated at 25 intervention health units. The most common syndromes were urethral discharge (67%), and genital ulcers (26%) in men and vaginal discharge (50%) in women. Based on various approaches, utilisation of the improved health units by symptomatic STD patients in these communities was estimated at between 50% and 75%. During the first 6 months of intervention attendance at intervention units increased by 53%. Thereafter, the average attendance rate was about 25% higher than in comparison communities.

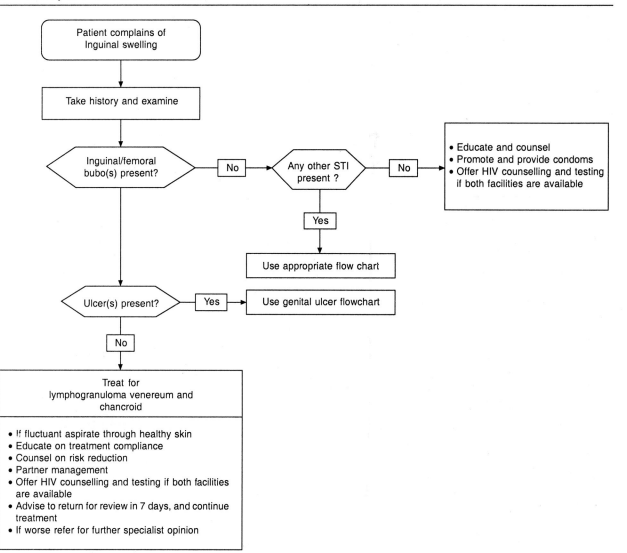

Fig. 8   Inguinal Bubo

Home visits to 367 non-returners revealed that 89% had been free of symptoms after treatment, but 28% became symptomatic again within 3 months of treatment. 100% of these patients reported that they had received treatment, but only 74% had been examined, only 57% had been given health education, and only 30% were offered condoms. Patients did not fully recall which treatment they had been given, but possibly only 63% had been treated exactly according to guidelines. The authors have concluded that the syndromic approach to STD control should be supported by at least one reference clinic and laboratory per country to ensure monitoring of prevalent aetiologies, of the development of bacterial resistance, and of the effectiveness of the syndromic algorithms in use.[6]

Daly et al[7] in their report from Malawi compared the actual cost of observed antibiotics treatment for 144 patients receiving same day treatment for two STD syndromes with that of the syndromic approach for the management of STD. The costs of drug treatment in both the categories were similar. The authors have concluded that syndromic management of STD would result in more effective treatment of STD at no additional cost.

In a study of observations of STD consultation in India by Mertens et al,[8] structured observations of consultation for STD in health care facilities were

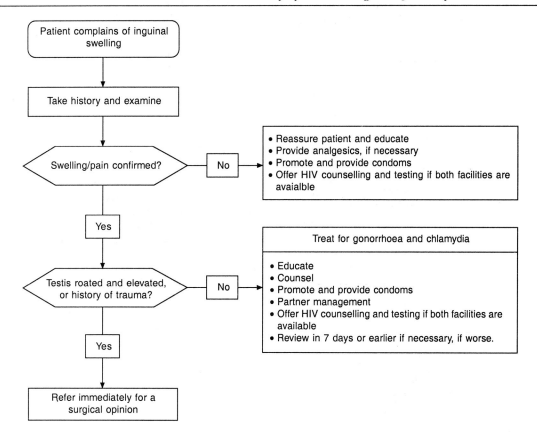

Fig. 9 Scrotal Swelling

undertaken. With STD treatment adequacy scored against the Indian national guidelines, history taking, examination and treatment were satisfactory in 76 out of 108 (70%) of observed consultation. However, the scoring with respect to syndromic approach towards selected STD (male urethritis and non herpetic genital ulcer in both the sexes), only 8 out of 81 (10%) patients had satisfactory management. This suggests that further improvement is required in the form of simplifying the existing treatment guidelines and periodic assessment and feedback on the quality of STD care.

Conclusion

Sexually transmitted diseases impose an enormous burden of morbidity and mortality in many developing countries. These once neglected diseases have come to the centre stage with the spread of HIV infection. However, simple STD control measures have not received adequate attention, even from many of those within the health care delivery system. It is easy to draft an STD

programme, on the primary approach. Improved clinical services for STD can significantly reduce HIV infection and this can be achieved by cost-effective, sustainable, and simple technology.

References

1. WHO. Guidelines for the management of sexually transmitted infection 2001. WHO/RHR/01.10.
2. NACO. STD Treatment Recommendation. 2002.
3. Campbell RL, Plumb J. The syndromic approach to treatment of sexually transmitted diseases in low-income countries. issues, challenges, and future direcions. J Obstet Gynaecol Can 2002; 24: 417-424.
4. Mathews C, van Rensburg A, Coetzee N. The sensitivity of a syndromic management approach in detecting sexually transmitted diseases in patients at a public health clinic in Cape Town. S Afr Med J 1998; 88: 1337-1340.
5. Hanson S, Sunkutu RM, Kamanga J, Hojer B, Sandstrom E. STD care in Zambia: an evaluation of the guidelines for case management through a syndromic approach. Int J STD AIDS 1996; 7: 324-332.

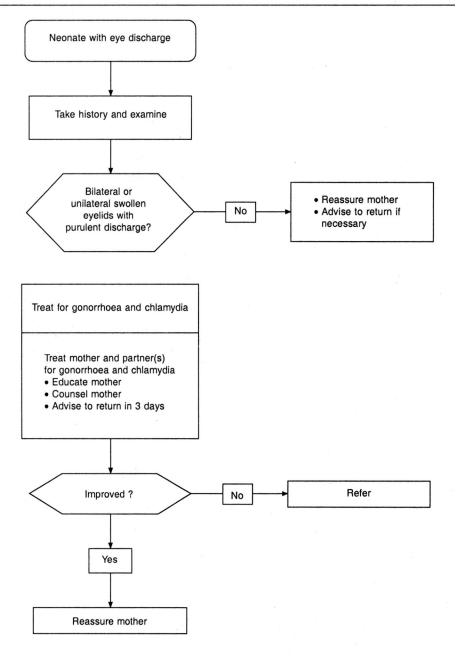

Fig. 10 Neonatal Conjunctivitis

6. Gorsskurth H, Mwijarubi E, Todd J, et al. Operational performance of an STD control programme in Mwanza Region, Tanzania. Sex Transm Infect 2000; 76: 426–436.

7. Daly CC, Franco L, Chilongozi DA, Dallabetta G. A cost comparison of approaches to sexually transmitted disease treatment in Malawi. Health Policy Plan 1998; 13: 87–93.

8. Mertens TE, Smith GD, Kantharaj K, Mugrditchian D, Radhakrishnan KM. Observation of sexually transmitted disease consultations in India. Public Health 1998; 112: 123–128.

PART XI

Colour Atlas of Sexually Transmitted Diseases and HIV/AIDS

P I
HIV/AIDS

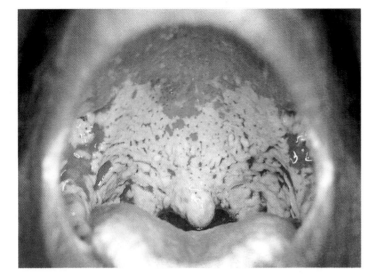

Fig. 1. Oral candidiasis in HIV positive patient

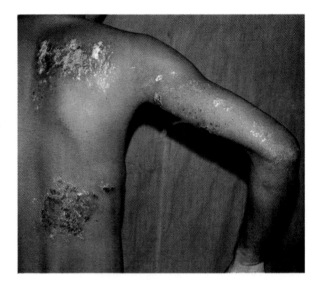

Fig. 2. Multidermatomal herpes zoster in HIV positive patient

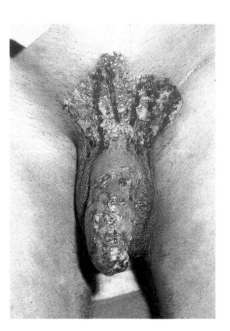

Fig. 3. Genital herpes in HIV positive patient

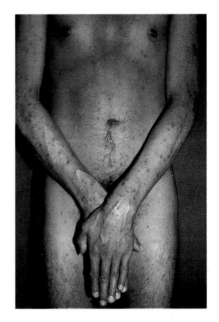

Fig. 4. Pruritic papular eruptions in HIV positive patient

P II
HIV/AIDS

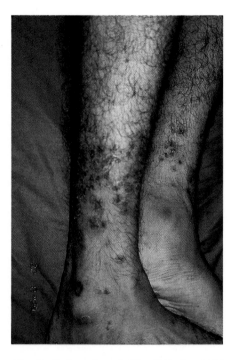

Fig. 5. Extensive folliculitis in HIV positive patient

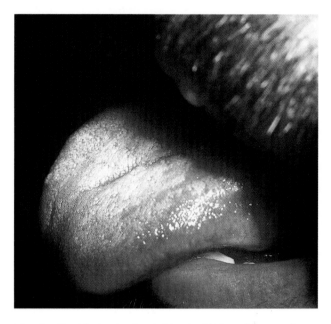

Fig. 6. Oral hairy leukoplakia in HIV positive patient

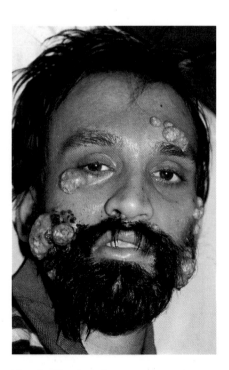

Fig. 7. Giant molluscum contagiosum in HIV positive patient

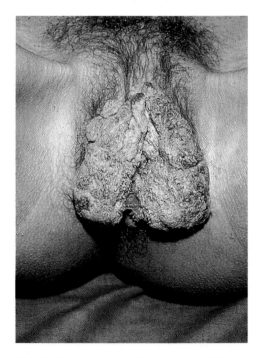

Fig. 8. Exuberant genital warts in HIV positive patient

P III
HIV/AIDS

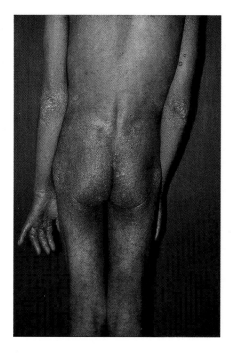

Fig. 9. Norwegian scabies in HIV
positive patient

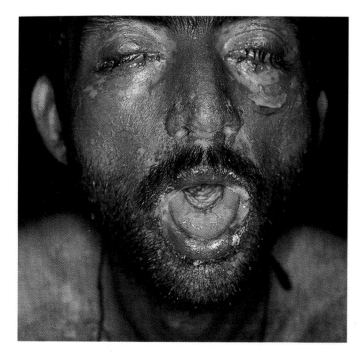

Fig. 10. Stevens Johnson syndrome in HIV positive patient

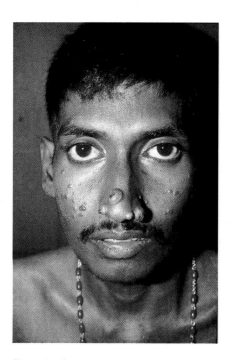

Fig. 11. Cutaneous cryptoccosis in
HIV positive patient

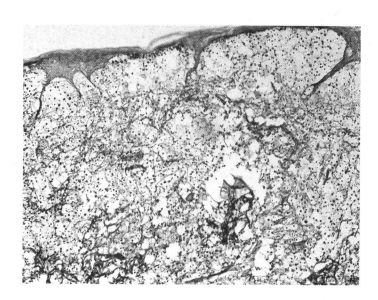

Fig. 12. Cryptococcosis (H & E) photomicrograph showing
granulomatous infiltrate with numerous spores

P IV
HIV/AIDS

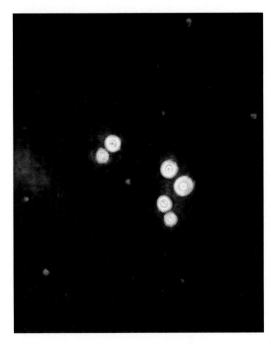

Fig. 13. Cryptococcosis (India ink preparation)

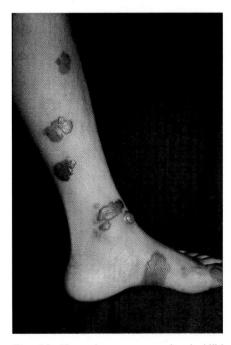

Fig. 14. Kaposi sarcoma on leg in HIV positive female patient

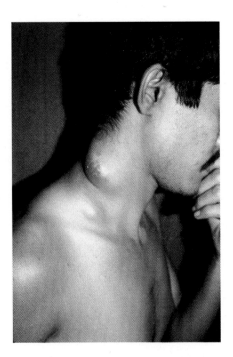

Fig. 15. Tuberculosis of lymph nodes in HIV positive patient

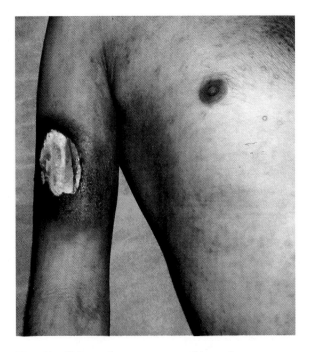

Fig. 16. Tuberculous gumma with molluscum contagiosum in HIV positive patient

P V
HIV/AIDS

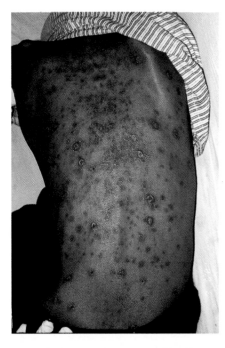

Fig. 17. Secondary syphilis (Lues Maligna) in HIV positive patient

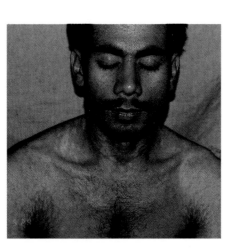

Fig. 18. Xerosis, icthyosis in HIV positive patient

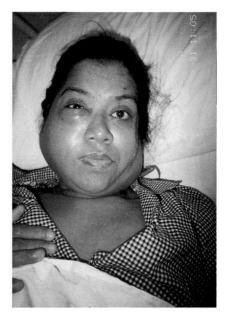

Fig. 19. Parotitis in HIV positive patient

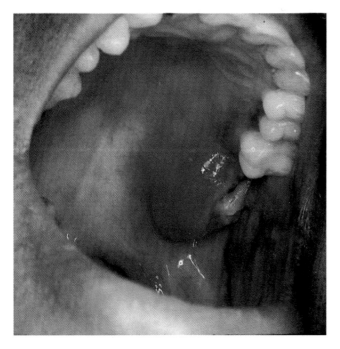

Fig. 20. B cell lymphoma in oral cavity of HIV positive patient

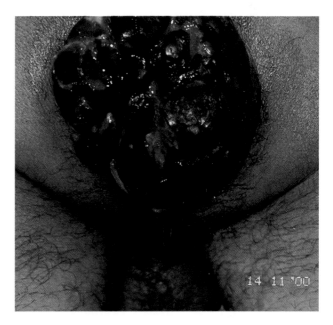

Fig. 21. Lymphoma in HIV positive patient

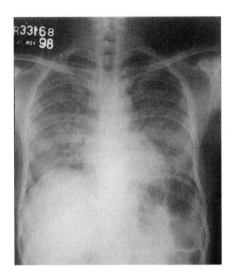

Fig. 22. X-ray chest (Soap bubble
appearance) *Pneumocystis
carinii* pneumonia

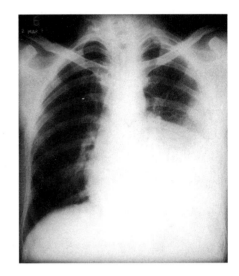

Fig. 23. X-ray chest, Pleural effusion
(Tuberculosis)

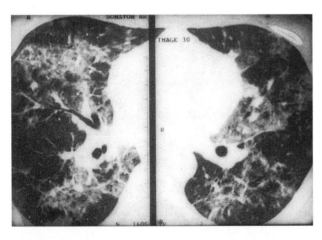

Fig. 24. CECT chest *Pneumocystis carinii* pneumonia

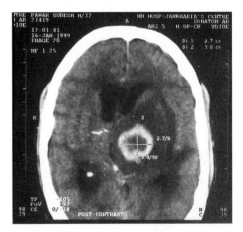

Fig. 25. CECT head, ring enhancing
lesion (Toxoplasmosis)

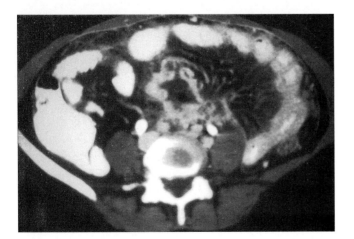

Fig. 26. CECT abdomen (Abdominal Tuberculosis)

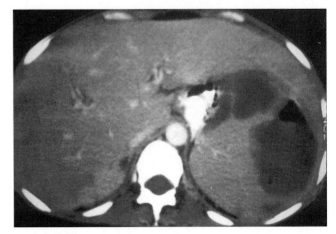

Fig. 27. CECT abdomen (Splenic abscess)

P VII

HIV/AIDS

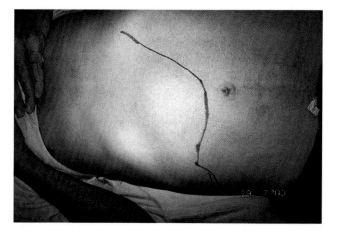

Fig. 28. Hepatomegaly (Tuberculosis of liver) in HIV positive patient

Syphilis

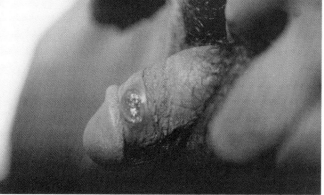

Fig. 29. Single, well defined, clean ulcer—Primary chancre

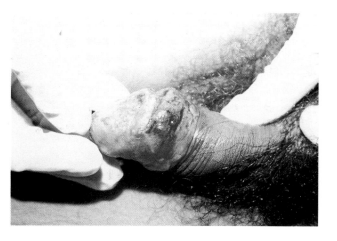

Fig. 30. Atypical primary chancre in HIV positive patient

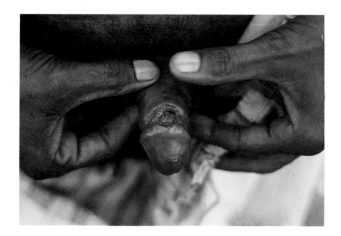

Fig. 31. Hunterian chancre

P VIII
Syphilis

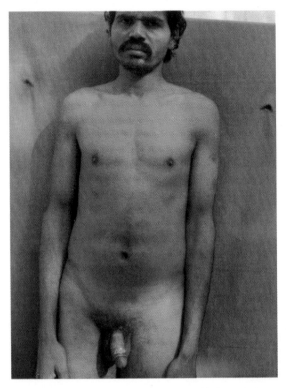

Fig. 32. Primary chancre, genital and lip lesions

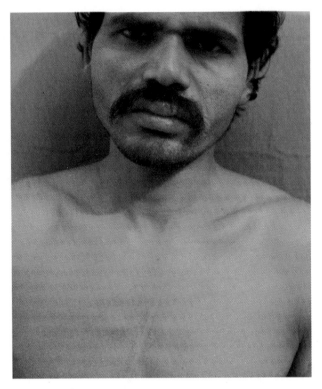

Fig. 33. Primary chancre, lip lesion

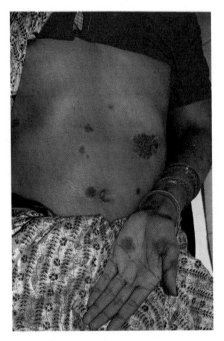

Fig. 34. Secondary syphilis - Lichenoid variety

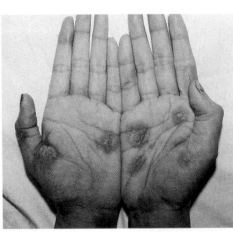

Fig. 35. Secondary syphilis, lesions on the palms

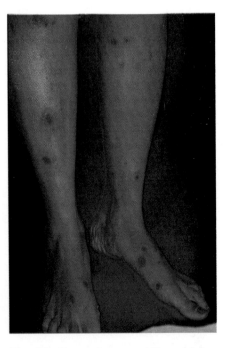

Fig. 36. Secondary syphilis - Lichenoid variety

P IX
Syphilis

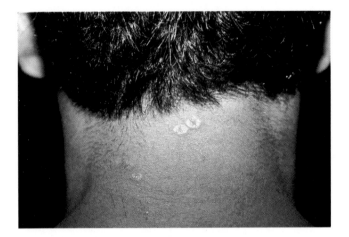

Fig. 37. Secondary syphilis - Annular variety

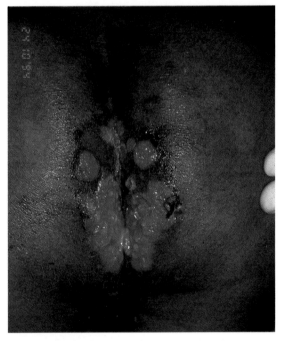

Fig. 38. Secondary syphilis - Perianal condylomata lata

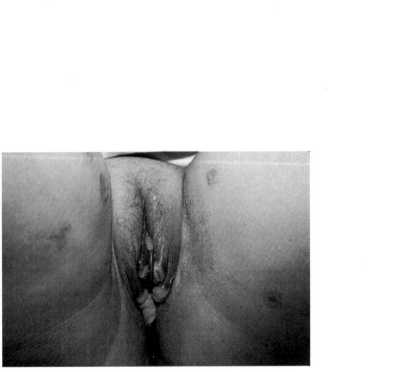

Fig. 39. Secondary syphilis - Vulval condylomata lata

P X
Syphilis

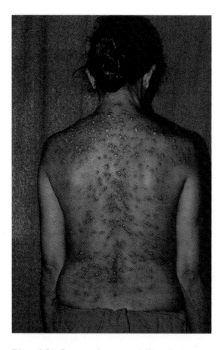

Fig. 40. Secondary syphilis - Pustular variety

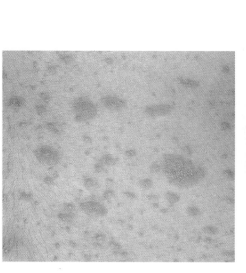

Fig. 41. Secondary syphilis - Papulo pustular variety

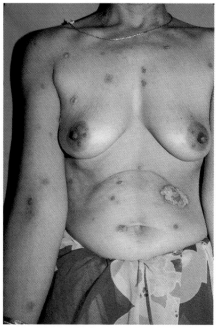

Fig. 42. Secondary syphilis - Pustular variety

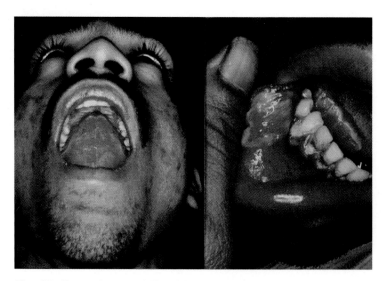

Fig. 43. Secondary syphilis - Mucous patches

P XI
Syphilis

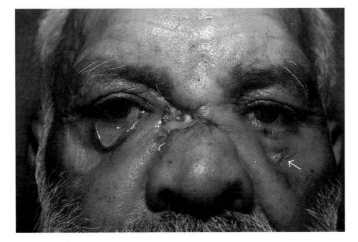

Fig. 44. Tertiary syphilis - Gummatous ulcer on the nose and scar as indicated by arrow

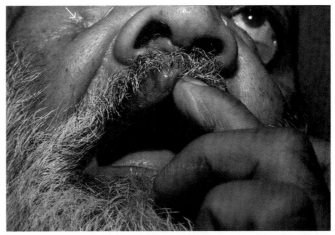

Fig. 45. Tertiary syphilis - Gummatous ulcer on the upper lip and scar as indicated by arrow

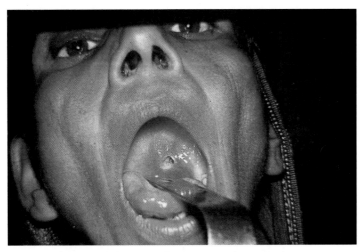

Fig. 46. Tertiary Syphilis - Gumma on the palate

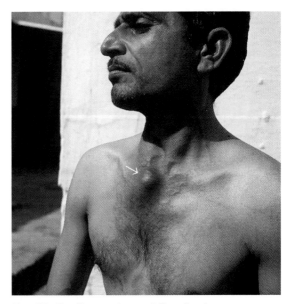

Fig. 47. Cardiovascular syphilis - Aortic aneurysum

P XII
Syphilis

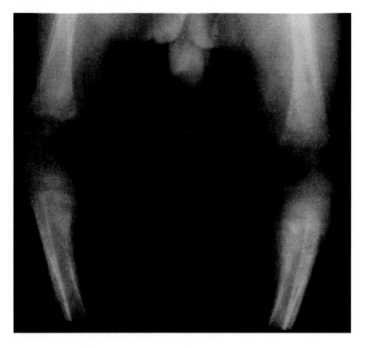

Fig. 48. Congenital syphilis - X-ray of lower limbs showing 'Wimberger sign'

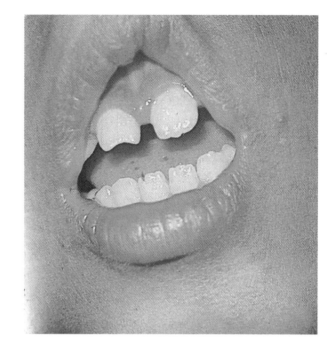

Fig. 49. Congenital syphilis - Hutchinson's teeth

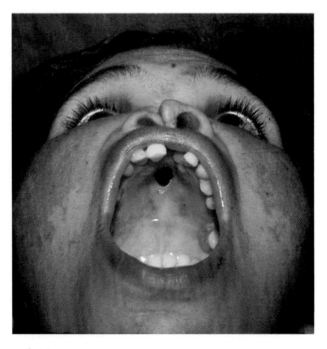

Fig. 50. Congenital syphilis - Palatal perforation

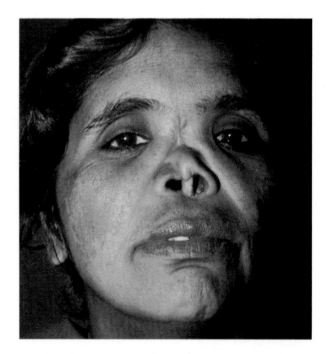

Fig. 51. Congenital syphilis - Saddle nose deformity

P XIII
Chancroid

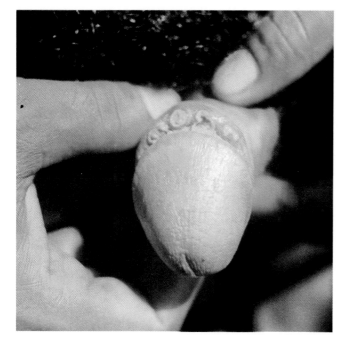

Fig. 52. Chancroid - Multiple, ragged edge ulcers on the coronal sulcus

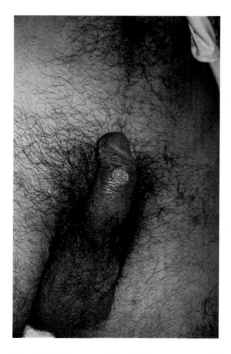

Fig. 53. Chancroid - Solitary, ragged edge ulcer on the shaft of penis

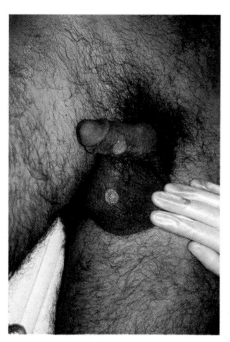

Fig. 54. Chancroid - 'Kissing ulcers'

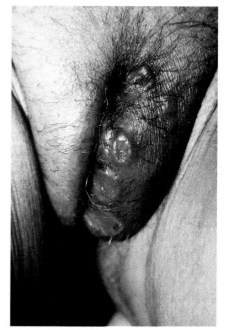

Fig. 55. Chancroid - Multiple, ragged edge ulcers on the labia majora

P XIV
Chancroid

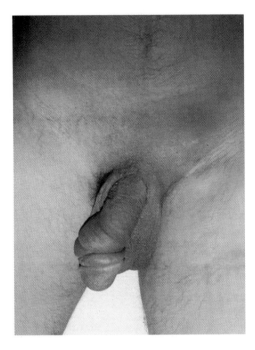

Fig. 56. Chancroid with penile edema and unilateral bubo showing groove sign

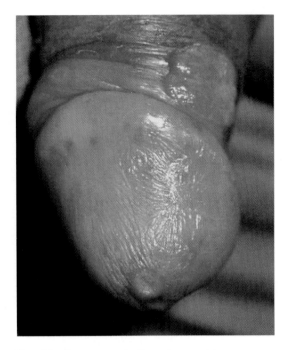

Fig. 57. Donovanosis like chancroid

Donovanosis

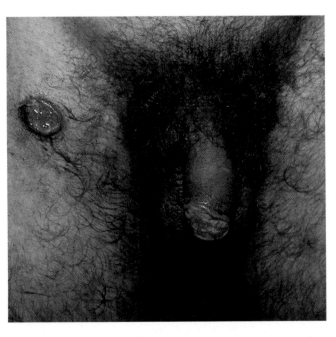

Fig. 58. Donovanosis - Ulcerogranulomatous variety, lesion on the glans penis and inguinal region

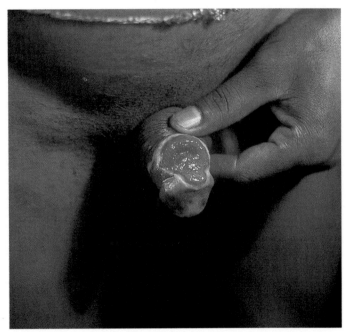

Fig. 59. Donovanosis - Ulcerogranulomatous variety

P XV

Donovanosis

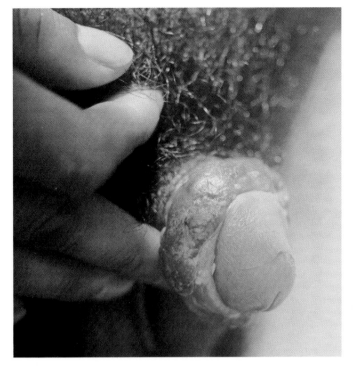

Fig. 60. Donovanosis - Hypertrophic variety

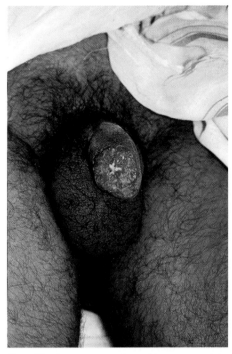

Fig. 61. Donovanosis - Hypertrophic variety

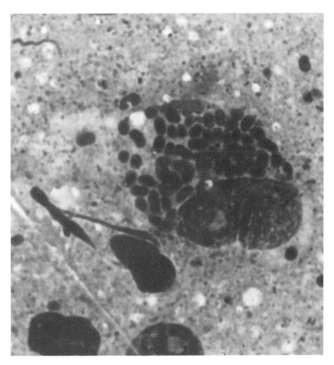

Fig. 62. 'Donovan bodies' (H & E) 100X

P XVI
Gonorrhoea

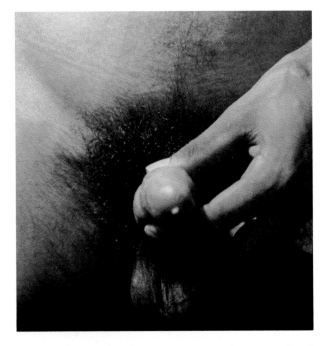

Fig. 63. Gonorrhoea - Muco-purulent urethral discharge

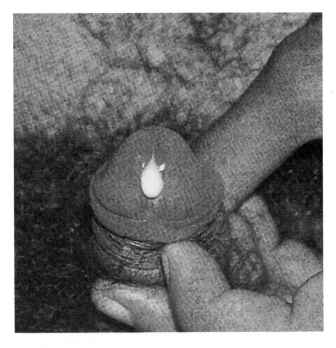

Fig. 64. Gonorrhoea - Copious purulent discharge from urethra

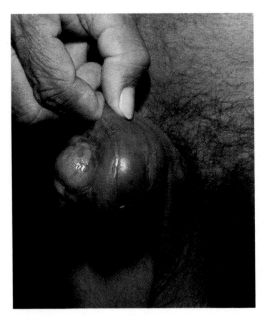

Fig. 65. Gonorrhoea - Periurethral abscess

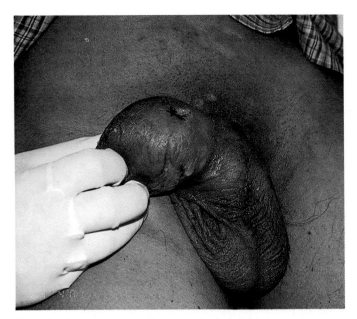

Fig. 66. Gonorrhoea - 'Water can' perineum

P XVII
Gonorrhoea

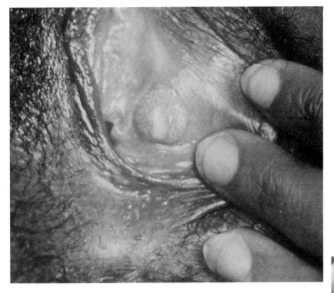

Fig. 67. Gonorrhoea - Pus at the opening of Bartholin's duct

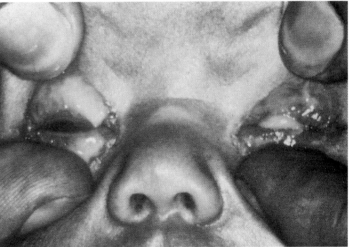

Fig. 68. Ophthalmia neonatorum

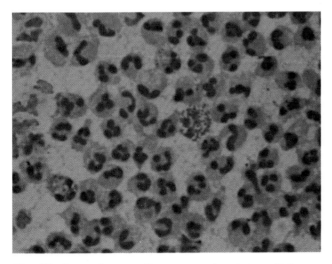

Fig. 69. Gonorrhoea - Gram negative intracellular diplococci (Gram stain, X100)

P XVIII
Lymphogranuloma Venereum

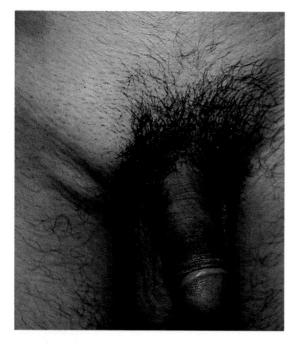

Fig. 70. Lymphogranuloma venereum - Unilateral bubo

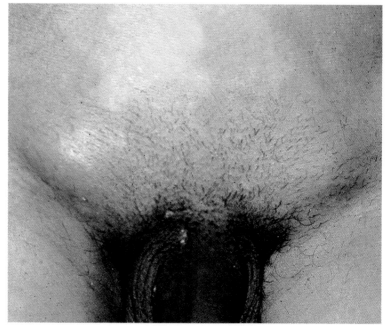

Fig. 71. Lymphogranuloma venereum - Bilateral bubo

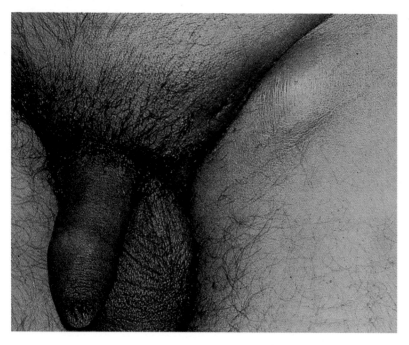

Fig. 72. Lymphogranuloma venereum - 'Groove sign'

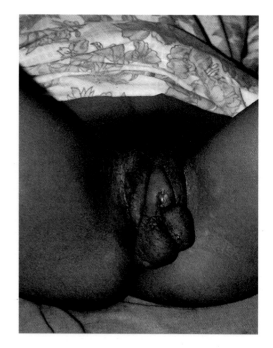

Fig. 73. Lymphogranuloma venereum - Esthiomene

P XIX
Bacterial Vaginosis - Genital herpes

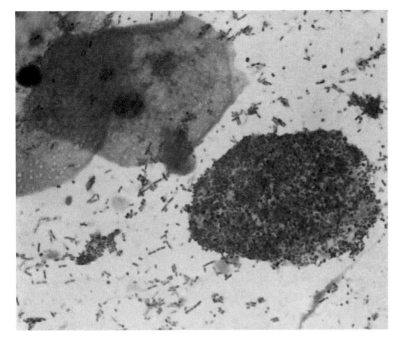

Fig. 74. Bacterial vaginosis - 'Clue cell', Gram stain(100x)

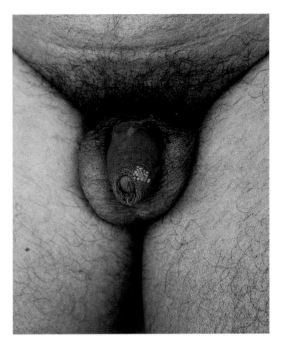

Fig. 75. Genital herpes - Vesicular stage

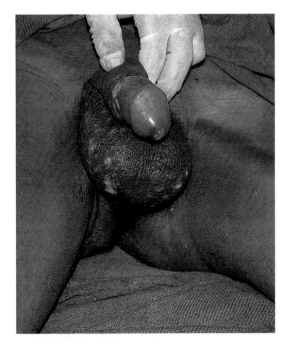

Fig. 76. Genital herpes - Multiple polycyclic, superficial ulcers

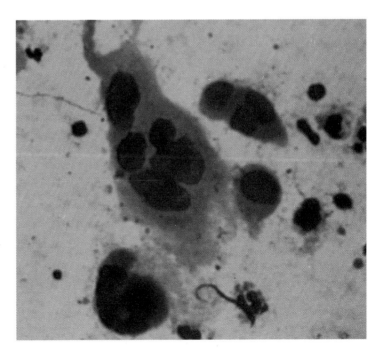

Fig. 77. Genital herpes - Multinucleated giant cells Giemsa stain(100X)

P XX
Anogenital Warts

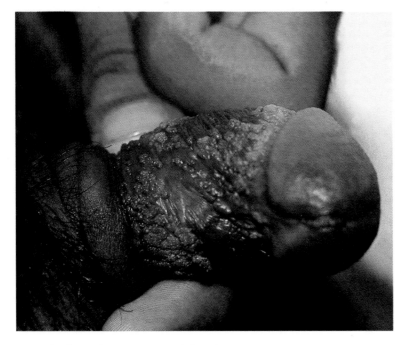

Fig. 78. Genital warts, preputial region

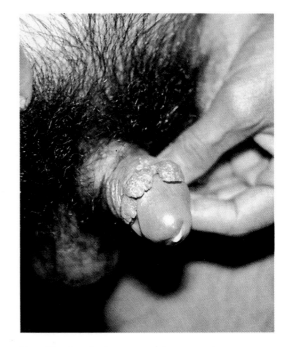

Fig. 79. Genital warts with gonorrhoea

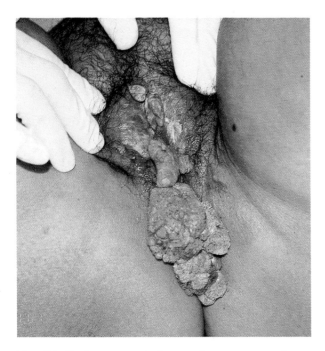

Fig. 80. Exuberant genital warts in pregnant woman

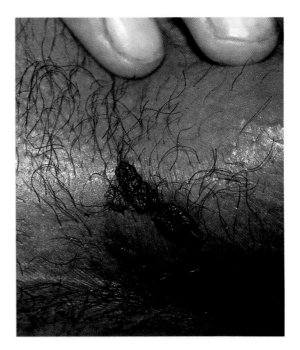

Fig. 81. Genital warts in the groin region

P XXI

Anogenital Warts

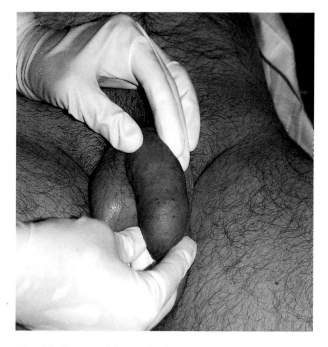

Fig. 82. Bowenoid papulosis

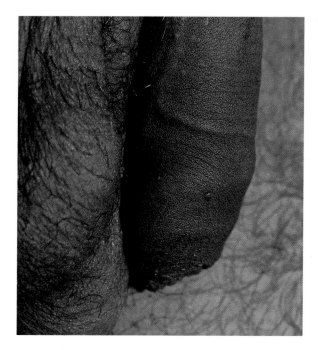

Fig. 83. Bowenoid papulosis

Balanoposthitis

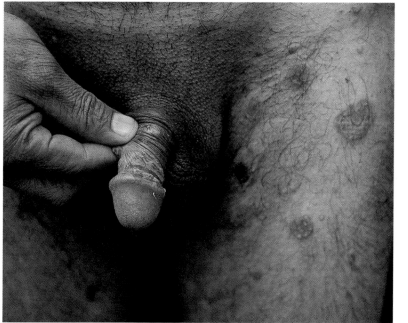

Fig. 84. Pemphigus vulgaris with genital involvement

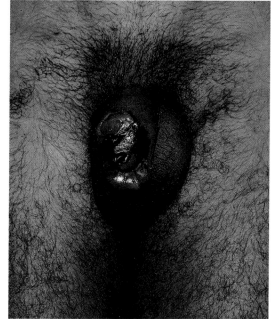

Fig. 85. Phagedena

Miscellaneous Sexually Transmitted Diseases

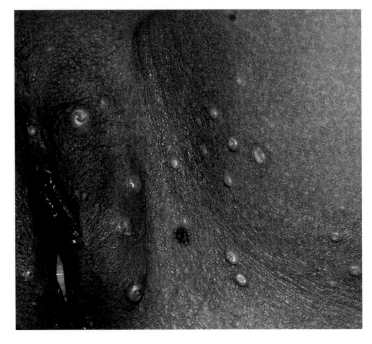

Fig. 86. Molluscum contagiosum - Umbilicated papules

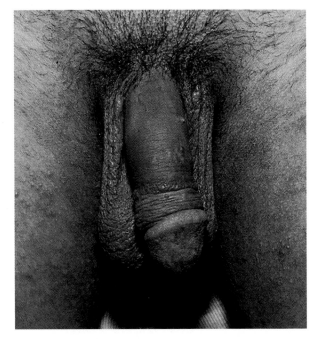

Fig. 87. Scabies - Burrows and papules

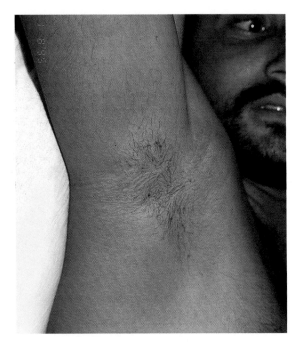

Fig. 88. Pediculosis pubis, axilla

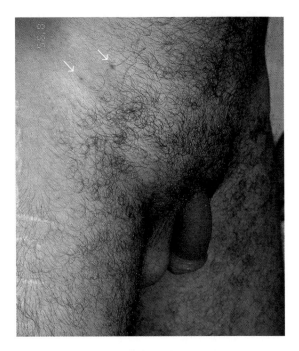

Fig. 89. Pediculosis pubis - Maculae caeruleae

Miscellaneous STD - Non - Venereal Diseases

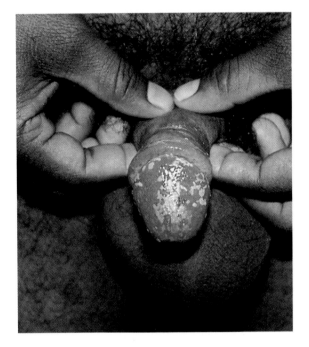

Fig. 90. Candidial balanoposthitis

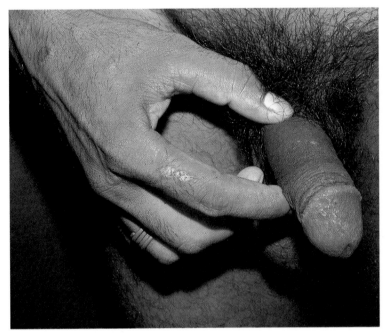

Fig. 91. Lichen planus of penis

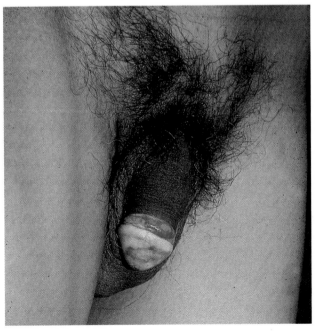

Fig. 92. Zoon's balanitis

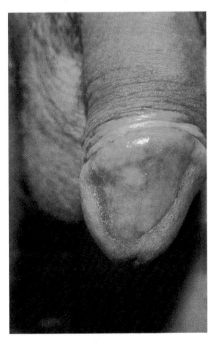

Fig. 93. Fixed drug eruption

Non - Venereal Diseases

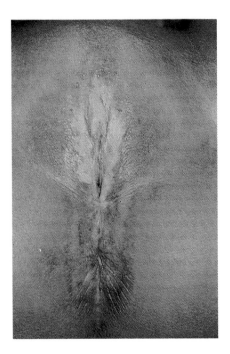

Fig. 94. Lichen sclerosus et atrophicus

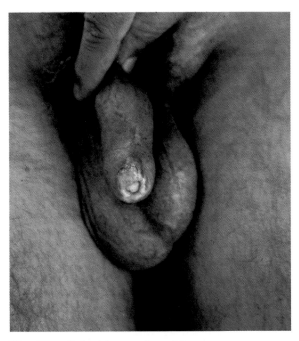

Fig. 95.   Balanitis xerotica obliterans.

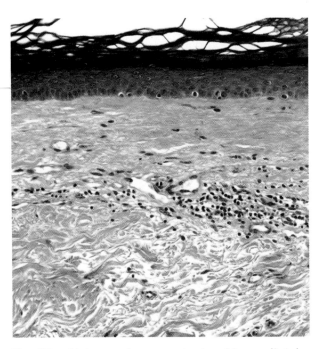

Fig. 96.   Lichen sclerosus et atrophicans (late) -
Sclerosis of papillary dermis with atrophy of
the overlying epidermis

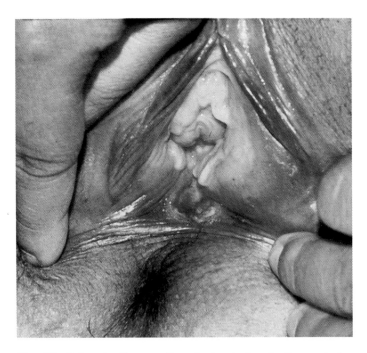

Fig. 97. Behcet's disease - Punched out ulcer in the posterior
commisure

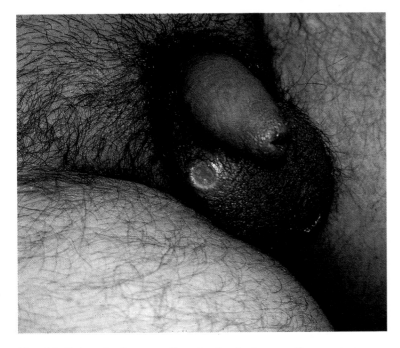

Fig. 98. Behcet's disease - Punched out ulcer on the scrotum

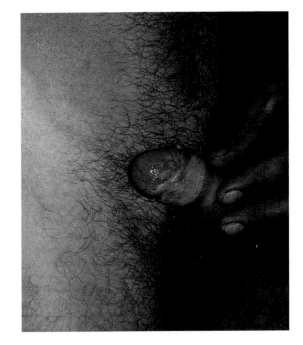

Fig. 99.   Erythroplasia of Queyrat

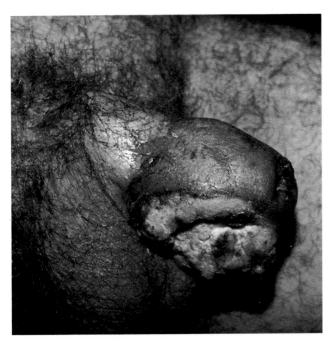

Fig. 100. Buschke Lowenstein tumour

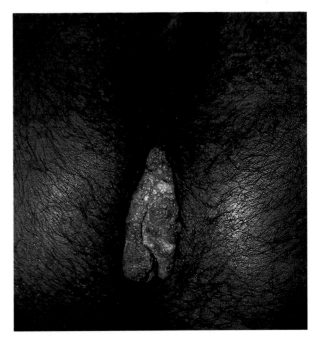

Fig. 101. Buschke Lowenstein tumour

P XXVI

Pre-Malignant and Malignant Lesions

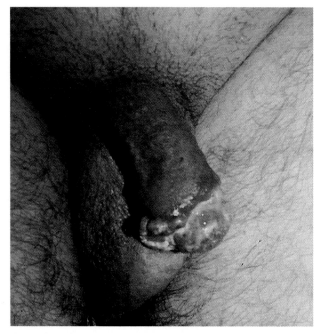

Fig. 102. Squamous cell carcinoma of penis

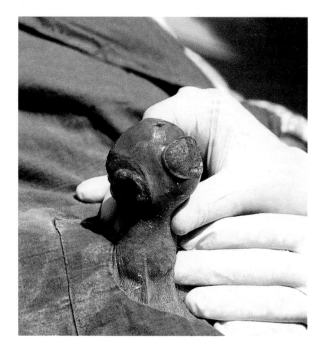

Fig. 103. Squamous cell carcinoma of penis

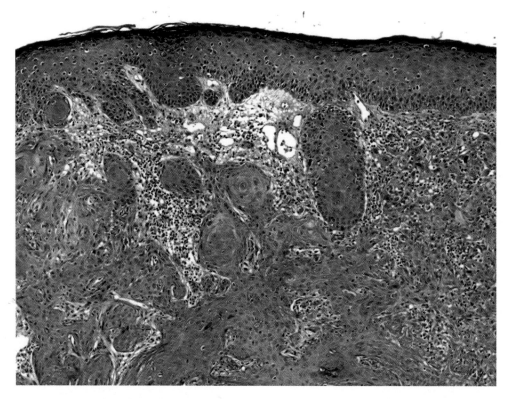

Fig. 104. Squamous cell carcinoma of penis - Photomicrograph of nodules of atypical keratinocytes in the dermis

PART XII
Appendices

Appendix I
History Taking and Proforma in STD

Name	Son/Daughter/Husband/Wife of	Age: Sex: M/F
Address	Occupation/Income	Education level
Referred by self/from Other Departments	Marital status Single/Married/Widow/Widower	I.D. No Date

Complaints with duration
 	
  Genital ulcer   Skin rash
 	
  Genital discharge   Others

Treatment taken for the complaints				
Form	Route	Dose	Duration	Any local application

Recent exposure with dates

If married, ask for marital/ extramarital/premarital contacts	Regarding each exposure, ask for when, where the exposure occurred	With whom (CSW/known/unknown person) Whether protected or unprotected

History of homosexuality

History of vaginal discharge and treatment taken for it	In case of female, menstrual and obstetric history should be elicited

Presenting Complaints

Presenting complaints can be broadly divided into two components

- Complaints related to the genitalia & related areas
- Complaints related to their sexual activity

    (a) Erosion or ulcer in the genitalia and related areas

(b) Discharge—urethral or vaginal
(c) Problems related to the act of micturition-dysuria, dribbling of urine, increased frequency of micturition
(d) Swelling in the inguinal region-lymphadenopathy
(e) Skin and mucous membrane lesions
(f) Growth in the genitalia-genital warts, molluscum contagiosum, malignant tumour
(g) Bone and joint-arthralgia, arthritis

(h) Scrotal swelling-epididymitis, epididymo orchitis,elephantoid changes of the scrotum

(i) Elephantoid changes of the female genitalia

II. Complaints Related to their Sexual Activity

Disinclination towards sexual intercourse

(a) Impotency, Frigidity
(b) Loss of libido
(c) Premature ejaculation
(d) Dysparaeunia
(e) Infertility
(f) Venerophobia/HIV phobia

History Taking

The important points are

(a) History of marital status of the patient

    (i)   Whether married or unmarried (single).

    (ii) If married the number of legal spouses as well as any other regular sex partners.

    (iii) Even in the unmarried, history of having a regular sex partner is to be elicited (this history is important since partner treatment is essential in the control of STD)

(b) History of presenting complaint with duration

(c) History of treatment taken for the present complaint, under which the following is to be elicited, namely

    (i)   Nature of medicine

    (ii) Route of administration (topical, parenteral, oral)

    (iii) Duration of treatment

(d) History of sexual contact (exposure) is to be elicited, namely

    (i)   Nature of contact -marital or extramarital

    (ii) Genito genital, orogenital, anogenital

    (iii) Date of contact (for calculation of incubation period)

    (iv) Whether the patient has used any protective mechanism like condom

(e) History of previous STD and the treatment taken for the same-This is important because the lesion for which the patient has come may be due to the past contact. There are certain STD like syphilis which has got various stages like primary, secondary and late and the primary and secondary lesions have got the tendency to heal on its own with or without proper diagnosis and medication and pass on to later stage. The other example being genital herpes, which has got a tendency to recur without a fresh exposure.

Appendix II
Treatment Guidelines of STD: WHO/ CDC/NACO

WHO (2001)
www.who.int

CDC (2002)
www.cdc.gov

NACO (1996)

Gonococcal infection

Uncomplicated anogenital infection
Recommended regimens
Ciprofloxacin 500 mg orally, as a
single dose
or
Azithromycin, 2 g orally, as a single dose
or
Ceftriaxone, 125 mg by intramuscular
injection, as a single dose
or
Cefixime, 400 mg orally, as a single dose
or
Spectinomycin 2 g by intramuscular
injection, as a single dose

Alternative regimens
Kanamycin 2 g by intramuscular
injection as a single dose
or
Trimethoprim (80mg)/sulfamethoxazole
(400 mg), 10 tablets orally, as a single
dose daily for 3 days

Uncomplicated gonococcal infections
of the cervix, urethra and rectum
Recommended regimens
Cefixime 400 mg orally in a single dose,
or
Ceftriaxone 125 mg IM in a single dose,
or
Ciprofloxacin 500 mg orally in a single
dose
or
Ofloxacin 400 mg orally in a single dose
or
Levofloxacin 250 mg orally in a single
dose

Plus,
If Chlamydial infection is
not ruled out
Azithromycin 1 g orally in a single dose
or
Doxycycline 100 mg orally twice a day
for 7 days.
Alternative regimen
Spectinomycin 2 g in a single IM dose
Single dose cephalosporin regimens include
ceftizoxime (500 mg, administered IM),
Cefoxitin (2 g, administered IM with
probenecid 1 g orally), and cefotaxime
(500 mg, administered IM)
Single dose quinolone regimens include
gatifloxacin 400 mg orally, norfloxacin
800 mg orally, and lomefloxacin
400 mg orally
Uncomplicated gonococcal infection
of the pharynx
Recommended regimen
Ceftriaxone 125 mg IM single dose or
Ciprofloxacin 500 mg orally single dose
              Plus
If Chlamydial infection is not ruled out

Uncomplicated gonococcal infection
Recommended regimens
Cefixime 400 mg orally as a single
dose
or
Azithromycin 2 g orally as a
single dose
or
Ceftriaxone 250 mg intramuscular
(IM) as a single injection
Rectal and pharyngeal gonococcal
infection
Ceftriaxone 500 mg/1 gm IM as
in single dose

WHO (2001) www.who.int	CDC (2002) www.cdc.gov	NACO (1996)
	Azithromycin 1 g orally single dose or Doxycycline 100 mg orally twice daily for 7 days	
Disseminated infection Recommended regimens Ceftriaxone 1g by intramuscular or intravenous injection, once daily for 7 days (alternative third-generation cephalosporins may be required where ceftriaxone is not available but more frequent administrations will be needed) or Spectinomycin 2 g by intramuscular injection, twice daily for 7 days. There are some data to suggest that therapy for 3 days is adequate	**Disseminated gonococcal infection Recommended regimens** Ceftriaxone 1 g IM or IV every 24 hours. **Alternative regimens** Cefotaxime 1 g IV every 8 hours or Ceftizoxime 1 g IV every 8 hours or Ciprofloxacin 400 mg IV every 12 hours or Ofloxacin 400 mg IV every 12 hours or Levofloxacin 250 mg IV daily or Spectinomycin 2 g IM every 12 hours. All of the preceding regimens should be continued for 24–48 hours after improvement begins, at which time therapy may be switched to one of the following regimens to complete at least 1 week of antimicrobial therapy. Cefixime 400 mg orally twice daily or Ciprofloxacin 500 mg orally twice daily or Ofloxacin 400 mg orally twice daily or Levofloxacin 500 mg orally once daily	**Complicated and disseminated gonococcal infection Recommended regimens** Ceftriaxone 1 g IM or IV once daily for 7 days Cefixime 400 mg twice daily orally for 7 days
Adult gonococcal conjunctivitis Recommended regimen Ceftriaxone 125 mg by intramuscular injection as a single dose or Spectinomycin 2 g by intramuscular injection as a single dose or Ciprofloxacin 500 mg orally, as a single dose **Alternative regimen** Kanamycin 2 g by intramuscular injection as a single dose	**Gonococcal conjunctivitis Recommended regimens** Ceftriaxone 1 g IM as a single dose	**Gonococcal conjunctivitis Recommended regimens** Ceftriaxone 500 mg IM as a single dose or Kanamycin 2 g IM as a single dose
Neonatal gonococcal conjunctivitis Recommended regimen Ceftriaxone 50 mg/kg by intramuscular injection as a single dose, to a maximum of 125 mg **Alternative regimen** Kanamycin 25 mg/kg by intramuscular injection as a single dose to a maximum of 75mg or	**Ophthalmia neonatorum Recommended regimens** Ceftriaxone 25-50 mg/kg IV or IM in a single dose, not to exceed 125 mg	**Neonates with gonococcal ophthalmia neonatorum and those born to mothers with gonococcal infections Recommended regimens** Ceftriaxone 50 mg/kg IM as a single dose to a maximum of 125 mg or Kanamycin 25 mg/kg IM as a single dose to a maximum of 75 mg

WHO (2001) www.who.int	CDC (2002) www.cdc.gov	NACO (1996)

Spectinomycin 25 mg/kg by intramuscular injection as a single dose to a maximum of 75 mg

Pregnancy

Ciprofloxacin is contraindicated in pregnancy

In Pregnancy

Gonococcal infections in pregnancy is treated with recommended or alternate cephalosporins, women who cannot tolerate cephalosporin should be administered a single dose spectinomycin 2 gm IM. Quinolones and tetracyclines are contraindicated

Gonococcal infection in pregnancy

Ceftriaxone 250 mg intramuscular (IM) as a single injection
or
Cefixime 400mg orally as a single dose
or
Azithromycin 2 g orally as a single dose (but azithromycin has not been adequately evaluated during pregnancy)

Nongonococcal urethritis

Management of patients who have NGU
Recommended regimens
Azithromycin 1 g orally in a single dose
or
Doxycycline 100 mg orally twice a day for 7 days
Alternative regimens
Erythromycin base 500 mg orally 4 times a day for 7 days
or
Erythromycin ethylsuccinate 800 mg orally four times a day for 7 days
or
Ofloxacin 300mg twice a day for 7 days
or
Levofloxacin 500mg once daily for 7 days

Non gonococcal urethritis (NGU) or cervicitis
Uncomplicated non-gonococal infections
Recommended regimen
Azithromycin 1 g orally in a single dose
or
Doxycycline 100 mg orally twice daily for 7 days
or
Erythromycin base/erythromycin stearate, 500 mg orally 4 times daily for 7 days
Regimen in pregnancy
Erythromycin base/stearate 500 mg orally four times a day for 7 days; Erythromycin should not be taken on empty stomach
or
Amoxycillin 500 mg orally three times a day for 7 days on empty stomach or Azithromycin 1 g orally as a single dose on empty stomach (but azithromycin has not been adequately evaluated during pregnancy)
Neonatal non-gonococcal conjunctivitis
Recommended regimen
Erythromycin syrup 50 mg/kg per day orally in four divided doses for 2 weeks
Infantile pneumonia
Recommended regimen
Erythromycin syrup 50 mg/kg per day orally four divided doses for 3 weeks

Chlamydia trachomatis infections

Chlamydia trachomatis infection (other than lymphogranuloma venereum)
Recommended regimens

Chlamydia infection in adolescents and adults
Recommended regimens

WHO (2001) www.who.int	CDC (2002) www.cdc.gov	NACO (1996)

Doxycycline 100 mg orally, twice daily for 7 days
or
Azithromycin 1 g orally, in a single dose

Alternative regimens
Amoxycillin 500 mg orally, three times a day for 7 days
or
Erythromycin 500 mg orally, four times a day for 7 days
or
Ofloxacin 300 mg orally, twice a day for 7 day
or
Tetracycline 500 mg orally, four times a day for 7 days

Chlamydial infection in pregnancy
Recommended regimen
Erythromycin 500 mg orally four times a day for 7 days
or
Amoxycillin 500 mg orally three times a day for 7 days

Neonatal chlamydial conjunctivitis
Recommended regimen
Erythromycin syrup 50 mg/kg/day orally in four divided doses for 14 days

Alternative regimen
Trimethoprin 40 mg with sulfamethoxazole 200 mg orally, twice daily for 14 days

Azithromycin 1 g orally in a single dose
or
Doxycycline 100 mg orally twice a day for 7 days.

Alternative regimens
Erythromycin base 500 mg orally four times a day for 7 days
or
Erythromycin ethylsuccinate 800 mg orally four times a day for 7 days
or
Ofloxacin 300 mg orally twice a day for 7 days
or
Levofloxacin 500 mg orally for 7 days

In Pregnancy
Recommended regimens
Erythromycin base 500 mg orally four times a day for 7 days
or
Amoxicillin 500mg orally three times daily for 7 days

Alternative regimens
Erythromycin base 250 mg orally four times a day for 14 days
or
Erythromycin ethylsuccinate 800 mg orally four times a day for 7 days
or
Erythromycin ethylsuccinate 400 mg orally four times a day for 14 days
or
Azithromycin 1 g orally, single dose

Syphilis

Early syphilis
Recommended regimens
Benzathine benzylpenicillin 2.4 million IU, by intramuscular injection, at a single session (because of the volume involved, this dose is usually given as two injections at separate sites).

Alternative regimens
Procaine benzylpenicillin 1.2 million IU daily, by intramuscular injection, for 10 consecutive days

Alternative regimen for penicillin-allergic·non-pregnant patients.
Doxycycline 100 mg orally, twice daily for 15 days
or
Tetracycline 500mg orally, 4 times daily for 15 days

Primary and Secondary syphilis
Recommended regimen for adults
Benzathine penicillin G 2.4 million units IM in a single dose

Recommended regimens for children
Benzathine penicillin G 50,000 units/kg/ IM upto the adult dose of 2.4 million units in a single dose

Early syphilis
Recommended regimens
Benzathine benzylpenicillin, 2.4 million IU deep IM in a single session (two equally divided doses in each buttock) after doing intradermal sensitivity test for penicillin
or
Procaine benzylpenicillin, 1.2 million IU (3 vials, each having combination of 1 lakh units of benzyl penicillin G sodium + 3 lakh units of procaine benzylpenicillin), IM once daily for 10 days after doing intradermal sensitivity test for penicillin

Alternative regimen
Doxycycline 100 mg orally twice a day for 15 days
or
Erythromycin base/stearate, 500 mg

WHO (2001)	CDC (2002)	NACO (1996)
www.who.int	www.cdc.gov	

<table>
<tr>
<td valign="top" width="33%">

</td>
<td valign="top" width="33%">

</td>
<td valign="top" width="33%">

orally 4 times a day for 15 days
or
Tetracycline HCl, 500 mg orally 4
times a day for 15 days

</td>
</tr>
<tr>
<td valign="top">

Late latent syphilis
Recommended regimen
Benzathine benzylpenicillin, 2.4 million
IU by intramuscular injection, once
weekly for 3 consecutive weeks
Alternative regimen
Procaine benzylpenicillin, 1.2 million
IU, by intramuscular injection, once
daily for 20 consecutive days
Alternative regimen for pencillin-allergic
non-pregnant patients
Doxycycline, 100mg orally, twice
daily for 30 days
or
Tetracycline, 500mg orally, 4 times
daily for 30 days.

</td>
<td valign="top">

Latent syphilis
Recommended regimens for Adults
Early Latent Syphilis
Benzathine penicillin G 2.4 million units
IM in a single dose.
Late latent syphilis or latent syphilis
of unknown duration
Benzathine penicillin G 7.2 million units
total, administered as three doses of 2.4
million units IM each at 1-week intervals.
Recommended regimens for Children
Early Latent Syphilis
Benzathine penicillin G 50,000 units/kg
IM, up to the adult dose of 2.4 million
units in a single dose.
Late latent syphilis or latent syphilis
of unknown duration
Benzathine penicillin G 50,000 units/kg
IM, up to the adult dose of 2.4 million
units, administered as three doses at
1-week intervals (total 150,000
units/kg up to the adult total dose
of 7.2 million units).

</td>
<td valign="top">

Late Latent (asymptomatic) and late
benign syphilis of more than 2 years
duration or of indeterminate
duration
Recommended regimens
Benzathine benzylpenicillin 2.4 million
IU deep (vide supra) IM weekly for 3
consecutive weeks, after doing
intradermal sensitivity test for penicillin
or
Procaine benzylpenicillin 1.2 million
IU, by intramuscular injection, once
daily for 20 consecutive days after
doing intradermal sensitivity test for
penicillin
Alternative regimen
Doxycycline 100mg orally,
twice daily for 30 days
or
Tetracycline HCl, 500 mg orally,
4 times daily for 30 days.
or
Erythromycin base/stearate,
500 mg orally four times a day
for 30 days

</td>
</tr>
<tr>
<td valign="top">

</td>
<td valign="top">

Tertiary syphilis
Recommended regimen
Benzathine penicillin G 7.2 million
units total, administered as three doses
of 2.4 million units IM each at
1-week intervals

</td>
<td valign="top">

Cardiovascular syphilis
Recommended regimens
Procaine benzylpenicillin, 1.2 million
IU (3 vials, each having a combination
of 1 lakh units of benzylpenicillin G
sodium + 3 lakh units of procaine
benzylpenicillin) IM, daily for 20
consecutive days, after doing
intradermal sensitivity test for
penicillin
Alternative regimen for penicillin-
allergic, non pregnant patients
Doxycycline 100 mg orally twice
daily for 30 days
Tetracycline HCl, 500 mg orally four
times daily for 30 days
Erythromycin base/stearate, 500 mg
orally four times a day for 30 days

</td>
</tr>
<tr>
<td valign="top">

Neurosyphilis
Recommended regimens
Aqueous benzylpenicillin, 12-24
million IU by intravenous injection,
administered daily in doses of 2-4
million IU every 4 hourly for 14 days

</td>
<td valign="top">

Neurosyphilis
Recommended regimens
Aqueous crystalline penicillin G 18–24
million units per day, administered as
3–4 million units IV every 4 hours or
continuous infusion, for 10–14 days.

</td>
<td valign="top">

Neurosyphilis
Recommended regimens
Aqueous benzylpenicillin, 12-24
million IU by intravenous injection,
administered daily in doses of 2-4
million IU every 4 hourly for 14 days

</td>
</tr>
</table>

WHO (2001)	CDC (2002)	NACO (1996)
www.who.int	www.cdc.gov	

Alternative regimens

Procaine benzylpenicillin, 1.2 million IU by intramuscular injection, once daily, and probenecid, 500 mg orally, 4 times daily, both for 10-14 days

Alternative regimens for pencillin allergic non-pregnant patients

Doxycycline 200 mg orally, twice daily for 30 days

or

Tetracycline 500 mg orally, 4 times daily for 30 days

Alternative regimens

Procaine penicillin 2.4 million units IM once daily

Plus Probenecid 500 mg orally four times a day, both for 10–14 days.

after doing intradermal sensitivity test for penicillin

or

Procaine benzylpenicillin, 1.2 million IU by intramuscular injection, once daily + probenecid, 500 mg orally, 4 times daily for 14 days

Alternative regimens

Doxycycline, 100 mg orally, twice daily for 30 days

or

Tetracycline HCl, 500 mg orally, 4 times daily for 30 days

or

Erythromycin base/stearate, 500 mg orally 4 times a day for 30 days

Syphilis in pregnancy
Recommended regimens

Pregnant patients at all stages of pregnancy, who are not allergic to penicillin, should be treated with penicillin according to the dosage schedules recommended for the treatment of non-pregnant patients at a similar stage of the disease.

Alternative regimens for penicillin allergic pregnant patients
Early syphilis

Erythromycin 500mg orally, 4 times daily for 15 days

Late syphillis

Erythromycin 500 mg orally, 4 times daily for 30 days

Syphilis during pregnancy
Recommended regimen

Treatment during pregnancy should consist of the penicillin regimen appropriate for the stage of syphilis

Pencillin allergy:

Patients should be given penicillin after desensitization.

Syphilis in pregnancy
Recommended regimens

Pregnant women who are not hypersensitive to penicillin should be treated with benzathine benzylpenicillin in the same dosage as recommended for non-pregnant patients at the same stage of disease

or

Penicillin hypersensitive pregnant women should be treated with erythromycin base/stearate in the dosage and duration as recommended for non-pregnant patients at the same stage of the disease

Congenital syphilis
Recommended regimens
a. Early congenital syphilis (upto 2 years of age)
And Infants with abnormal cerebrospinal fluid:

Aqueous benzylpenicillin 100 000-150 000 IU/kg day administered as 50 000 IU/kg/dose IV every 12 hours, during the first 7 days of life and every 8 hours thereafter for a total of 10 days

or

Procaine benzylpenicillin 50000 IU/kg by intramuscular injection, as a single daily dose for 10 days.

Congenital Syphilis of 2 or more years duration

Aqueous benzylpenicillin 200000-300000 IU/kg/day by IV or IM injection, a dministered as 50,000 IU/kg every 4-6 hours for 10-14 days

Congenital syphilis

Infants with proven or highly probable congenital syphilis

Recommended regimens

Aqueous crystalline penicillin G 100,000 –150,000 units/kg/day, administered as 50,000 units/kg/dose IV every 12 hours during the first 7 days of life and every 8 hours thereafter for a total of 10 days

or

Procaine penicillin G 50,000 units/kg/dose IM in a single daily dose for 10 days.

More details in chapter on congenital syphilis

Congenital syphilis
Recommended regimens

Aqueous benzylpenicillin 100 000-150 000 IU/kg.day IV in two divided doses daily for 10 days

or

Procaine benzylpenicillin 50000 IU/kg IM in a single daily dose for 10 days

Alternative regimens for penicillin alllergy

Erythromycin base/stearate 7.5-12.5 mg/kg/day orally 4 times a day for 30 days

Late congenital syphilis (More than 2 years duration)

Procaine benzyl penicillin 50,000 IU/kg/day IM for 14 days after doing intradermal sensitivity test for penicillin

or

WHO (2001) www.who.int	CDC (2002) www.cdc.gov	NACO (1996)

Alternate Regimen
Erythromycin 7.5-12.5 mg/kg orally, four times daily for 30 days.

Aqueous benzylpenicillin 2 to 3 lakh units/kg/day IV in divided doses for 14 days
or
Erythromycin base/ stearate 7.5-12.5 mg/kg/day orally 4 times a day for 30 days

Chancroid

Recommended regimen
Ciprofloxacin 500 mg orally, twice daily for 3 days
or
Erythromycin base 500 mg orally, 4 times daily for 7 days
or
Azithromycin 1g orally, as a single dose
Alternative regimen
Ceftriaxone 250 mg by intramuscular injection, as a single dose

Recommended regimens
Azithromycin 1 g orally in a single dose
or
Ceftriaxone 250 mg intramuscularly (IM) in a single dose
or
Ciprofloxacin 500 mg orally twice a day for 3 days
or
Erythromycin base 500 mg orally three times a day for 7 days

Recommended regimens
Azithromycin 1 g orally as a single dose
or
Ceftriaxone 250 mg intramuscularly (IM) as a single dose,
or
Ciprofloxacin 500 mg orally twice a day for 3 days

Genital herpes infections

First clinical episode
Recommended regimen
Acyclovir 200 mg orally, 5 times daily for 7 days
or
Acyclovir 400 mg orally, 3 times daily for 7 days
or
Famciclovir 250 mg, 3 times daily for 7 days
or
Valaciclovir 1g, 2 times daily for 7 days
Recurrent infections
Recommended regimen
Acyclovir 200 mg orally, 5 times daily for 5 days
or
Acyclovir 400 mg 3 times daily for 5 days
or
Acyclovir 800 mg orally twice daily for 5 days
or
Famciclovir 125 mg orally twice daily for 5 days
or
Valacyclovir 500 mg orally twice daily for 5 days
or
Valacyclovir 1000 mg orally once daily for 5 days

First clinical episode of Genital herpes
Recommended regimens
Acyclovir 400 mg orally three times a day for 7–10 days
or
Acyclovir 200 mg orally five times a day for 7–10 days
or
Famciclovir 250 mg orally three times a day for 7–10 days
or
Valacyclovir 1 g orally twice a day for 7–10 days
Recurrent episodes of HSV disease
Recommended regimen
Acyclovir 400 mg orally three times a day for 5 days
or
Acyclovir 200 mg orally five times a day for 5 days
or
Acyclovir 800 mg orally twice a day for 5 days
or
Famciclovir 125 mg orally twice a day for 5 days
or
Valacyclovir 500 mg orally twice a day for 3–5 days
or
Valacyclovir 1.0 g orally once a day

First clinical episode
Recommended regimen
Acyclovir 200 mg orally, 5 times daily for 7 days
or
Acyclovir 400 mg orally, 3 times daily for 7 days
Recurrent infections
Recommended regimen
Acyclovir 200 mg orally,5 times daily for 5 days
or
Acyclovir 400 mg 3 times daily for 5 days
Suppressive therapy
Recommended regimen
Acyclovir 400 mg orally, 2 times daily, continuously atleast for one year; recurrence rate should then be re-assessed after the stoppage of acyclovir
Severe herpes genitalis infections
Acyclovir 5-10 mg/kg IV every 8 hours for 5 to 7 days
Treatment for neonates
Acyclovir 10 mg /kg IV three times a day for 14 day
Herpes and HIV co-infections
Acylovir 400 mg orally five times daily until complete clinical healing of lesions

WHO (2001) www.who.int	CDC (2002) www.cdc.gov	NACO (1996)

Suppressive therapy
Recommended regimen
Acyclovir 400 mg orally, 2 times daily, continuously
or
Famciclovir 250 mg orally twice daily
or
Valacyclovir 500 mg orally once daily
or
Valacyclovir 1000 mg orally once daily
Severe Disease
Acyclovir 5-10 mg/kg IV every 8 hours, 5-7 days or until clinical resolution is attained
Treatment for neonates
Acyclovir 10 mg/kg intravenously three times a day for 10-21 days.
Herpes and HIV co-infection
Acyclovir 400 mg orally 3-5 times daily until clinical resolution is attained.

for 5 days
Suppressive therapy for recurrent genital herpes
Recommended regimen
Acyclovir 400 mg orally twice a day
or
Famciclovir 250 mg orally twice a day
or
Valacyclovir 500 mg orally once a day
or
Valacyclovir 1.0 gram orally once a day
Severe disease
Acyclovir 5-10 mg/kg/body weight IV every 8 hours for 2-7 days or until clinical improvement is observed

or
Acyclovir 5-10 mg/kg IV every 8 hours until complete clinical resolution.

Lymphogranuloma venereum

Recommended regimens
Doxycycline 100 mg orally, twice daily for 14 days
or
Erythromycin 500 mg orally, 4 times daily for 14 days
Alternative regimens
Tetracycline 500 mg orally, 4 times daily for 14 days

Recommended regimen
Doxycycline 100 mg orally twice a day for 21 days
Alternative regimen
Erythromycin base 500 mg orally four times a day for 21 days

Recommended regimens
Doxycycline 100 mg orally twice a day for 2 weeks/tetracycline HCl, 500 mg orally 4 times a day for 2 weeks
or
Erythromycin base/stearate 500 mg orally four times a day for 2 weeks

Recommended regimen
Azithromycin 1 g orally on first day, then 500 mg orally once a day
or
Doxycycline 100 mg orally, twice daily
Alternative regimen
Erythromycin 500 mg orally, 4 times daily
or
Tetracycline, 500 mg orally, 4 times daily
or
Trimethoprim (80 mg)/sulfamethoxazole (400 mg), 2 tablets orally, twice daily for a minimum of 14 days

Granuloma inguinale (Donovanosis)

Recommended regimens
Doxycycline 100 mg orally twice a day for at least 3 weeks
or
Trimethoprim-sulfamethoxazole one double-strength
(160 mg/800 mg) tablet orally twice a day for at least 3 weeks.
Alternative regimens
Ciprofloxacin 750 mg orally twice a day for at least 3 weeks,
or
Erythromycin base 500 mg orally four times a day for at least 3 weeks,
or
Azithromycin 1 g orally once per week for at least 3 weeks.

Recommended regimens
Doxycycline 100 mg orally twice a day for 14 days/tetracycline HCl 500 mg orally 4 times a day for 14 days
or
Erythromycin base/stearate, 500 mg orally 4 times a day for 14 days
or
Azithromycin 500 mg orally twice a day for 14 days

Bacterial vaginosis

Recommended regimen
Metronidazole 400 or 500 mg orally,

Recommended regimens
Metronidazole 500 mg orally twice

Recommended regimen
Metronidazole 400 orally twice daily

WHO (2001) www.who.int	CDC (2002) www.cdc.gov	NACO (1996)
twice daily for 7 days **Alternative regimens** Metronidazole 2 g orally, as a single dose or Clindamycin vaginal cream 2%, 5 g at bedtime intravaginally for 7 days or Metronidazole gel 0.75%, 5g twice daily intravaginally for 5 days or Clindamycin, 300 mg orally twice daily for 7 days	a day for 7 days or Metronidazole gel 0.75% one full applicator (5 g) intravaginally, once a day for 5 days or Clindamycin cream 2% one full applicator (5 g) intravaginally at bedtime for 7 days **Alternative regimens** Metronidazole 2 g orally in a single dose or Clindamycin 300 mg orally twice a day for 7 days or Clindamycin ovules 100 g intravaginally once at bed time for 3 days	for 7 days/metronidazole 2 g orally as a single dose or Tinidazole 2gm orally as a single dose
Bacterial vaginosis in pregnancy **Recommended regimen** Metronidazole 200 or 250 mg orally three times daily for 7 days **Alternative regimen** Metronidazole 2 g orally, as a single dose or Clindamycin 300 mg orally twice daily for 7 days or Metronidazole gel 0.75%, 5 g twice daily intravaginally for 7 days Metronidazole is contraindicated during first trimester.	**Bacterial vaginosis in pregnancy** **Recommended regimens** Metronidazole 250 mg orally three times a day for 7 days or Clindamycin 300mg orally twice a day for 7 days	**Bacterial vaginosis in pregnancy** Metronidazole is contraindicated during the first trimester of pregnancy, but may be used, if necessary, during the second and third trimesters
Trichomonas vaginalis **vaginal infection** **Recommended regimen** Metronidazole 2 g orally, in a single dose or Tinidazole 2 g orally, in a single dose **Alternative regimen** Metronidazole 400 or 500 mg orally, twice daily for 7 days or Tinidazole, 500 mg orally, twice daily for 5 days *Trichomonas vaginalis* **urethritis** **Recommended regimen** Metronidazole 400 or 500 mg orally, twice daily for 7 days or Tinidazole 500 mg, orally twice daily for 5 days	*Trichomonas vaginalis* **infection** **Recommended regimen** Metronidazole 2 g orally in a single dose **Alternative regimen** Metronidazole 500 mg twice a day for 7 days	**Recommended regimen** Metronidazole 2 g orally, in a single dose/metronidazole, 400 mg orally twice daily for 7 days or Tinidazole 2 g orally, in a single dose **In pregnancy** Metronidazole and tinidazole are contraindicated in first trimister, may be used in second and third trimesters. Metronidazlole 400 mg orally twice daily for 7 days. **Neonatal infections** Metronidazole/tinidazole, 5 mg/kg orally 3 times for 7 days.

WHO (2001) www.who.int	CDC (2002) www.cdc.gov	NACO (1996)

Candidiasis

WHO (2001)	CDC (2002)	NACO (1996)
Vulvovaginal candidiasis **Recommended regimen** Miconazole or clotrimazole 200 mg intravaginally, daily for 3 days or Clotrimazole 500 mg intravaginally, as a single dose or Fluconazole 150 mg orally, as a single dose **Alternative regimen** Nystatin 100 000 IU intravaginally, daily for 14 days **Balanoposthitis** Topical application of a nystatin or clotrimazole lotion or cream twice daily for 7 days **Vulvovaginal candidiasis in pregnancy** Only topical azoles (miconazole, clotrimazole, butoconazole, terconazole) should be used to treat pregnant women.	**Uncomplicated Vulvovaginal candidiasis** **Recommended regimens** **Intravaginal Agents:** Butoconazole 2% cream 5 g intravaginally for 3 days or Butoconazole 2% cream 5 g (Butaconazole1 sustained Release), single intravaginal application or Clotrimazole 1% cream 5 g intravaginally for 7–14 days or Clotrimazole 100 mg vaginal tablet for 7 days or Clotrimazole 100 mg vaginal tablet, two tablets for 3 days or Clotrimazole 500 mg vaginal tablet, one tablet in a single application or Miconazole 2% cream 5 g intravaginally for 7 days or Miconazole 100 mg vaginal suppository, one suppository for 7 days or Miconazole 200 mg vaginal suppository, one suppository for 3 days or Nystatin 100,000-unit vaginal tablet, one tablet for 14 days or Ticonazole 6.5% ointment 5 g intravaginally in a single application or Terconazole 0.4% cream 5 g intravaginally for 7 days or Terconazole 0.8% cream 5 g intravaginally for 3 days or Terconazole 80 mg vaginal suppository, one suppository for 3 days **Oral Agent:** Fluconazole 150 mg oral tablet, one tablet in single dose	**Vulvovaginal candidiasis** **Recommended regimen** Miconazole or clotrimazole, 100 mg intravaginally, daily for 6 days or Clotrimazole 500 mg intravaginally, as a single dose or Fluconazole, 150 mg orally, as a single dose **Candidial balanoposthitis** Clotrimazole (1%) cream or Miconazole (2%) cream may be applied locally till complete healing **Vulvovaginal candidiasis in pregnancy** Only topical imidazole (miconazole clotrimazole etc) should be used

Appendix III
Syndromic Approach to Treatment of STD (NACO)

Urethral Discharge

Examine male patients complaining of urethral discharge and/or dysuria for evidence of discharge. If no discharge is seen, massage along the ventral aspect of penis toward the meatus, look for discharge. The common causes of urethral discharge are *N. gonorrohoeae* and/or *C. trachomatis*.

Treatment

Treat for both gonococcal and chlamydial infections.

Recommended Regimen

Azithromycin 2 G orally single dose, under supervision (to treat both gonococcal and chlamydial infections)

Alternate Regimens

Option 1

Cefixime 400 mg orally, single dose, under supervision (to treat gonococcal infection)
Plus
Doxycycline★ 100 mg orally, 2 times daily for 7 days (to treat chlamydial infection)

Option 2

Inj. Ceftriaxone 250 mg IM. single dose (to treat gonococcal infection)
Plus
Doxycycline★ 100 mg orally, 2 times daily for 7 days (to treat chlamydial infection)

★*In individuals allergic/intolerant to doxycycline,*
Erythromycin 500 mg orally, 4 times daily for 7 days.)

Genital Ulcer

The most common STD presenting with genital ulcer (s) are syphilis, chancroid and genital herpes. Treat adequately to cover both syphilis and chancroid or genital herpes depending on history and examination.

Treatment

Ask all patients to wash genital area with soap and water.

> If vesicles are seen or/and history of recurrences present

Treat for genital herpes
First episode: Acyclovir 200 mg orally 5 times daily for 7 days
Recurrent episodes: Acyclovir, 400 mg orally, 3 times daily for 5 days
Note: There is no known cure of herpes but the course of the symptoms can be modified by acyclovir.

> If vesicles are not seen and no history of recurrences Present

Treat for both syphilis and chancroid.

Recommended Regimen

Inj. benzathine penicillin,★ 2.4 million units IM, in 2 equally divided doses. Give one injection in each buttock, after testing for sensitivity for penicillin (to treat syphilis)
Plus
Azithromycin 1G, single dose, orally under supervision (to treat chancroid)

Alternate Regimen

Option 1

Inj. benzathine penicillin,* 2.4 million units IM, in 2 equally divided doses. Give one injection in each buttock, after testing for sensitivity for penicillin (to treat syphilis)
Plus
Inj. ceftriaxone, 250 mg, single dose IM (to treat chancroid)

Option 2. (Do not use in pregnant women)

Inj. benzathine penicillin,* 2.4 million units, IM in 2 equally divided doses. Give one injection in each buttock, after testing for sensitivity for penicillin (to treat syphilis)
Plus
Ciprofloxacin 500 mg two times a day orally for 3 days)

*In individuals allergic/intolerant to penicillin
Doxycycline 100 mg, 2 times daily, for 15 days but
In pregnant women allergic/intolerant to penicillin
Erythromycin base/stearate 500 mg, 4 times daily for 15 days. Ask these women to bring the new born baby for treatment within 7 days of birth

Vaginal Discharge (Without Speculum)

Vaginal discharge is commonly due to vaginitis and/or cervicitis. Cervicitis is caused by *N. gonorrhoeae* and *C. trachomatis* while *Trichomonas vaginalis, Candida albicans,* and bacterial vaginosis cause vaginitis. However, clinical differentiation between the two conditions is difficult. Recent studies suggest that an assessment of the woman's risk status may help in making a diagnosis of cervicitis. If risk assesment is negative, treat for vaginitis. Where it is not possible to differentiate and/or the risk assessment is positive, treat the patients for both cervicitis and vaginitis.

Treatment

Cervicitis

Recommended Regimen

Azithromycin, 2 G orally, single dose, under supervision (to treat both gonococcal and chlamydial infections).

Alternate Regimen

Option 1

Cefixime 400 mg, orally, single dose, under supervision (to treat gonococcal infection)
Plus
Doxycycline* 100 mg orally, 2 times daily for 7 days (to treat chlamydial infection).

Option 2

Inj. Ceftriaxone 250 mg IM, single dose (to treat gonococcal infection)
Plus
Doxycycline* 100 mg orally, 2 times daily for 7 days (to treat chlamydial infections).

*In individuals allergic/intolerant to doxycycline and in all pregnant woman
Give erythromycin base/stearate, 500 mg orally, 4 times daily, for 7 days instead of doxycycline.

Vaginitis

Recommended Regimen

Metronidazole* 2 G orally, single dose, under supervision (to treat trichomoniasis and bacterial vaginosis).
Plus
Fluconazole 150 mg orally, single dose.

Alternate Regimen

Metronidazole 400 mg orally 2 times a day, for 7 days. (to treat trichomoniasis and bacterial vaginosis)
Plus
Clotrimazole pessary, 500 mg intravaginally, once (to treat candidiasis).

*Do not give during the first trimester of pregnancy, however, in symptomatic pregnant women give 100 mg clotrimazole vaginal pessary once daily for 6 days.
*In first trimester of pregnancy donot give metronidazole

Vaginal Discharge (With Speculum)

Vaginal discharge is commonly due to vaginitis and/or cervicitis. Cervicitis is caused by *N. gonorrhoeae* and *C.*

trachomatis while *Trichomonas vaginalis, Candida albicans,* and bacterial vaginosis cause vaginitis. However, clinical differentiation between the two conditions is difficult. Recent studies suggest that an assessment of the woman's risk status may help in making a diagnosis of cervicitis. If risk assesment is negative treat for vaginitis. Where it is not possible to differentiate and/or the risk assessment is positive, treat the patients for both cervicitis and vaginitis.

Treatment

Cervicitis

Recommended Regimen

Azithromycin 2 G orally, single dose, under supervision (to treat both gonococcal and chlamydial infections).

Alternate Regimen

Option 1

Cefixime 400 mg, orally, single dose, under supervision (to treat gonococcal infection)
Plus
Doxycycline★ 100 mg orally, 2 times daily for 7 days (to treat chlamydial infection).

Option 2

Inj. Ceftriaxone 250 mg IM, single dose (to treat gonococcal infection)
Plus
Doxycycline★ 100 mg orally, 2 times daily for 7 days (to treat chlamydial infections).

★In individuals allergic/intolerant to doxycycline and in all pregnant woman
Give erythromycin base/stearate, 500 mg orally, 4 times daily, for 7 days instead of doxycycline.

Vaginitis

Recommended Regimen

Metronidazole★ 2 G orally, single dose, under supervision (to treat trichomoniasis and bacterial vaginosis).
Plus
Fluconazole 150 mg orally, single dose.

Alternate Regime

Metronidazole 400 mg orally 2 times a day, for 7 days. (to treat trichomoniasis and bacterial vaginosis)
Plus
Clotrimazole pessary, 500 mg intravaginally, once (to treat candidiasis).

★Do not give during the first trimester of pregnancy, however, in symptomatic pregnant women give 100 mg clotrimazole vaginal pessary once daily for 6 days.
★In first trimester of pregnancy donot give metronidazole

Scrotal Swelling

A serious complication of gonococcal and chlamydial urethritis is epididymo orchitis. The scrotum becomes swollen, warm and painful. If quick and effective therapy is not given, destruction and scarring of the testicular tissues may occur, causing sub-fertility. Other causes of sub-fertility are mumps virus infection and filariasis

Treatment

Treat for both gonococcal and chlamydial infections.

Recommended Regimen

Azithromycin 2G orally, single dose under supervision (to treat both gonococcal and chlamydial infections)

Alternative Regimen

Option 1

Cefixime 400 mg orally, single dose under supervision (to treat gonococcal infection)
Plus
Doxycycline★ 100 mg orally 2 times daily for 14 days (to treat chlamydial infection)

Option 2

Inj. Ceftriaxone 250 mg IM, single dose (to treat gonococcal infection)
Plus
Doxycycline★ 100 mg orally, 2 times daily, for 14 days (to treat chlamydial infection)

*In individuals allergic/intolerant to doxycycline
Erythromycin 500 mg, 4 times daily orally, for 14 days.

Supportive Therapy

To reduce pain advice bed rest, scrotal elevation with a scrotal support (T-bandage) and analgesics.

Lower Abdominal Pain in Females

Lower abdominal pain is often the presenting feature of women with pelvic inflammatory disease (PID). PID is defined as an infection of the female genital tract above the cervix and therefore means endometritis, salpingitis, tubo-ovarian abscess and peritonitis. PID occurs as a result of ascending infection from the cervix and is caused by *N gonorrhoeae, C. trachomatis* and anaerobic bacteria. Occasionally, PID may be caused by *Mycoplasma hominis.* Infertility due to tubal occlusion and ectopic pregnancy are serious complications of PID.

Treatment

Treat patient for gonococcal and chlamydial infection as well as for anaerobic bacteria.

Recommended Regimen

Azithromycin 2 G orally, single dose under supervision (to treat both gonococcal and chlamydial infections).
Plus
Metronidazole 400 mg orally, 2 times daily, for 14 days (to treat anaerobic bacteria).

Alternate Regimen

Option 1

Cefixime 400 mg orally single dose under supervision (to treat gonococcal infection),
Plus
Doxycycline* 100 mg orally, 2 times daily, for 14 days (to treat chlamydial infection),
Plus
Metronidazole 400 mg orally, 2 times daily, for 14 days (to treat anaerobic bacteria).

Option 2

Inj. ceftriaxone 250 mg IM, single dose (to treat gonococcal infection),
Plus
Doxycycline* 100 mg orally, 2 times daily , for 14 days (to treat chlamydial infections),
Plus
Metronidazole 400 mg orally, 2 times daily, for 14 days (to treat anaerobic bacteria)

*In individuals allergic/intolerant to doxycycline and in all pregnant woman
Erythromycin base/stearate, 500 mg orally, 4 times daily, for 14 days instead of doxycycline.

Caution: PID can be a serious condition. Treating doctor must refer the patient to the hospital if she does not respond to treatment within 3 days and sooner if the condition worsens.

Inguinal Bubo

This is a painful swelling of the lymph node in the inguinal region. It can also result from any kind of acute infection of the skin on the pubic area, genitals, buttocks, anus, thighs, legs feet and toes. A bubo may occur in chancroid or lymphogranuloma venereum (LGV).

Treatment

Recommended Regimen

Doxycycline 100 mg orally, 2 times a day for 21 days.

Alternative Regimen

Option 1

Tetracycline 500 mg orally, 4 times a day for 21 days.

Option 2 (Pregnant and Lactating Females)

Erythromycin base/stearate 500 mg orally, 4 times a day for 21 days.
If bubo becomes fluctuant, aspirate pus with a wide bore needle and syringe. Make entry into bubo through

normal healthy skin from a non-dependent area. Never incise and drain.

Ophthalmia Neonatorum

Ophthalmia neonatorum is a condition, where the baby develops purulent conjunctivitis in one or both eyes within four weeks of birth. It is a medical emergency and unless treatment is initiated within 24 hours there could be permanent damage to the eyes resulting in blindness. The discharge from the eyes may be caused by *N. gonorrhoeae*, *C. trachomatis* and less frequently by other bacteria.

Treatment

Clean the eyes with distilled water or saline.

Recommended Regimen

Inj. ceftriaxone 50 mg/kg body weight, IM single dose, up to maximum of 125 mg (to treat gonococcal infection),
Plus
Erythromycin syrup 50 mg/kg body weight orally, daily in 4 divided doses for 14 days (to treat chlamydial infection)

Alternate Regimen

Kanamycin 25 mg/kg body weight IM single dose, up to a maximum of 75 mg (to treat gonococcal infection),
Plus
Erythromycin syrup 50 mg/kg body weight orally, daily in 4 divided doses for 14 days (to treat chlamydial infection)

Appendix IV
Treatment of Opportunistic Infections in HIV/AIDS

(Maniar JK, Mumbai)

Pathogen or Disease	Treatment	Alternative
Candida	**Thrush** • Clotrimazole troches 10 mg 5x/day × 14 days • Nystatin 500,000/mL units susp. 5 mL gargled or 200,000 units pastilles to suck 4–5/day × 14 days	• Fluconazole 50–100 mg PO/day × 14 days • Itraconazole 100 mg/day liquid solution to gargle
Cryptococcosis Meningitis	• Amphotericin B 0.7–1.0mg/kg/day + 5–FC (flucytosine) 25 mg/kg PO qid × 14 days, then fluconazole 400 mg/day × 8 wks., then 200 mg/day • CSF pressure: OP >250 mm H_2O–drain until $1/2$ initial pressure or < 200; repeat daily until <200 mm H_2O	• Fluconazole 400–800 mg/day PO + 5–FC 25 mg/kg PO qid × 6 to 10 wks., then fluconazole 200 mg/day • *AmBisome* 4 mg/kg/day IV + 5-FC 25 mg PO qid × 10 days, then fluconazole 400 mg/day × 8 wks., then 200 mg/day • Refractory cases: Intrathecal Amphotericin B • Alternative for maintenance: Itraconazole 200 mg/day or Amphotericin B 0.6–1 mg/kg IV 1–2×/wk.
Histoplasmosis	• Amphotericin B 0.7–1.0 mg/kg/day × 3 to 14 days, Itraconazole 200 mg PO bid	• Amphotericin B induction, then maintenance with Fluconazole 800 mg/day PO or Amphotericin B 1 mg/kg/wk. IV
Aspergillosis (invasive)	• Amphotericin B 0.7–1.4 mg/kg/day IV *or* • Lipid formulations: *Abelcet* 5 mg/kg/day, *Amphotec* 4–6 mg/kg/day or • *AmBisome* 5 mg/kg/day IV	• *AmBisome* 3 mg/kg/day IV • Itraconazole 200 mg PO tid × 3 days then 400 mg/day • Caspofungin 70 mg IV/day, then 50 mg IV/day
Cytomegalovirus	**Gastrointestinal** • Ganciclovir 5 mg/kg IV bid × 2 to 3 wks., then either ganciclovir	• Cidofovir: see CMV retinitis (below)

(Contd.)

Pathogen or Disease	Treatment	Alternative
	IV 5 mg/kg/day or valganciclovir 900 mg PO with meals bid × 3 wks then 900 mg PO/day – • Foscarnet IV 90 mg/kg q12h × 3 wks., then IV 90 mg/kg/day	
Cytomegalovirus	**Retinitis** • Intraocular ganciclovir device + oral valganciclovir 900 mg PO bid with meal × 3 wks. then 900 mg/day • Ganciclovir 5 mg/kg IV q12h × 14 to 21 days, then 5 mg/kg IV, 5 to 7 days/wk. • Foscarnet 90 mg/kg IV q12h × 14 to 21 days, then IV 90–120 mg/kg/day	• Cidofovir 5 mg/kg/wk. IV × 2, then 5 mg/kg every 2 wks.; each dose with probenecid 2 gm PO 3 hrs. before each dose and 1 gm at 2 & 8 hrs. after. • Fomivirsen 330 μg intravitreal injection days 1 & 15, then monthly + valganciclovir.
Herpes simplex	**Initial: mild and moderately ill** • Acyclovir 400 mg PO tid or famciclovir 250 mg PO tid or valacyclovir 1 gm PO bid, all 7 to 10 days **Severe or refractory** • Acyclovir 15–30 mg/kg/day IV × >7 days • Valacyclovir 1 gm PO bid • Acyclovir resistance; Foscarnet 60 mg/kg IV q2h ×3	• Foscarnet 60 mg/kg q12h × 3 wks. • Cidofovir 5 mg/kg IV q 2 wks. + probenecid • Topical trifluridine (1% ophthalmic solution) q8h • Topical cidofovir 3% gel q8h
Varicella zoster (VZV)	**Dermatomal** • Valacyclovir 1 gm PO tid 7 days × • Famciclovir 500 mg PO tid 7 days	• Acyclovir 800 mg PO 5 ×/day 7 days • Acyclovir 30 mg/kg/day IV • Foscarnet 60 mg/kg/day IV q12 (acyclovir resistant)
	Disseminated, visceral or ophthalmic Nerve • Acyclovir 30–36 mg/kg/day IV >7 days	• Foscarnet 60 mg/kg/day IV (acyclovir resistant)
Cryptosporidiosis	• Paromomycin 500 mg PO tid with food × 14 to 28 days or • Paromomycin 1 gm PO bid with food + azithromycin 600 mg PO/day × 4 wks., then paraomomycin alone × > 8 wks. • HAART, antiperistaltic (*Lomotil, Loperamide, paregoric*), food supplements	• Atovaquone 750 mg bid with food
Isosporiasis	• TMP-SMX 2 DS PO bid 2 DS tid × 3 wks.	• Pyrimethamine 50–75 mg/day PO + folinic acid

(Contd.)

Pathogen or Disease	Treatment	Alternative
	maintenance TMP-SMX 1–2 DS/day PO	5–10 mg/day × 1 mo. + maintenance pyrimethamine 25 mg + folinic acid 5 mg/day
Microsporidiosis	• Albendazole 400-800mg bid × 3 wks • Metronidazole 500 mg PO tid • HAART, nutritional supplements, antiperistaltic agents (*Lomotil, Imodium, paregoric, etc.*)	• Atovaquone 750 mg PO bid with meals • Thalidomide 100 mg PO day
***P. carinii* pneumonia (PCP)**	• TMP-SMX 15 mg/kg/day –75 mg/kg/day PO or IV × 21 days + pO$_2$ <70 mm Hg or A-a gradient >35 mm Hg: prednisone 40 mg bid × 5 days then 40 mg/day × days, then 20 mg/day to completion of Rx.	• TMP 15 mg/kg/day PO + dapsone 100 mg/day × 21 days • Pentamidine 4 mg/kg/day IV × 21 days • Clindamycin 600 mg IV q8h or 300-450 mg PO q6h + primaquine 15–30 mg base/day × 21 days • Atovaquone 750 mg PO bid with meal × 21 days
Progressive multifocal leucoencephalopalthy	• HAART	• Interferon alpha 3 MU/day IV
Salmonella	• Ciprofloxacin 500 mg PO/400 mg IV bid × >14 days • TMP-SMX 1 DS bid × 5 to 7 days × >14 days • Ceftriaxone 2 gm/day IV × >14 days	
Staph aureus	• Oxacillin/Nafcillin, Cefazolin, Cephalexin, dicloxacillin	• Clindamycin, fluoroquinolone, TMP-SMX
Strep pneumoniae	• Cefotaxime 2 gm IV q6h • Ceftriaxone 2 gm/day IV • Amoxicillin 750 mg PO tid • Fluoroquinolone: Levofloxacin 500 mg PO/IV qd; gatifloxacin 400 mg PO/IV qd; moxifloxacin 400 mg PO/day	• Macrolide (azithromycin, clarithromycin, erythromycin) • Vancomycin
Toxoplasmosis	• Pyrimethamine 100 mg, then 50–100 mg/day PO + folinic acid 10 mg/day (+ sulfadiazine 4-8 gm/day × >6 wks), then maintenance pyrimethamine 25–50 mg/day PO + folinic acid 10–50 mg/day PO + sulhadiazine 5–1 gm PO qid	• Pyrimethamine + folinic acid + clindamycin 900–1200 mg IV q6h or PO 300–450 mg q6h • Pyrimethamine + folinic acid azithromycin 1200 mg/day PO or clarithromycin 1 gm PO bid or atovaquone 750 mg PO qid with food • Maintenance doses: Clindamycin 300–450 mg PO qid, atovaquone 750 mg 2–3×/day, azithromycin 600 mg/day clarithromycin 500 mg bid

Treatment of miscellaneous conditions

Condition	Treatment
Peripheral neuropathy	• d/c d4T, dd1, and/or ddc • Nortriptyline 10 mg, increase by 10 mg/day q 5 days to max. 75 mg/day • Gabapentin 300–1000 mg Po tid • Ibuprofen 600–800 mg tid • Topical capsaicin ointments or lidocaine 20% to 30% ointment • Lamotrigine 25 mg PO/day increased to 300 mg/day over 6 wks. • Phenytoin 200–400/day or carbamazepine 200–400 mg PO bid
HIV-associated dementia	• HAART • Selegiline 5 mg bid or 10 mg
Idiopathic thrombocytopenia	**Asymptomatic** • HAART • Discontinue any contributing drugs **Symptomatic** • HAART • Prednisone 30–60 mg/day with rapid taper to 5–10 mg/day • IVIG 400 mg/kg, days 1, 2, & 14, then q 2 to 3 wks.
Anaemia	**HIV:** HAART **Address Cause:** Marrow infiltrating tumour (lymphoma, KS); infection (TB, parvovirus B19, fungi, esp. Histoplasma), drugs (AZT, amphotericin, ganciclovir, pyrimethamine, dapsone, ribavirin, interferon), anaemia of chronic disease; deficiency state (Fe, folic acid, B12), HIV inhibition of precursors.
Kaposi's sarcoma	**HAART** **Local therapy** • Topical liquid nitrogen • Intra-lesional vinblastine, (0.010–0.002 mg/lesion q 2 wks. x 3) • Radiation or laser **Systemic:** Widespread skin involvement with >25 lesions; failure of local Rx, and/or symptomatic visceral organ involvement. • Liposomal daunorubicin (*DaunoXome*) • *Taxol* (100–500 mg/M 2) • *Adriamycin,* bleomycin + either vincristine or vinblastine • Vincristine/vinblastine • Bleomycin/vinca alkaloids
Non-Hodgkin's lymphoma (NHL)	• EPOCH: Etoposide, vincristine, and doxorubicin + cyclophosphamide + prednisone • Various combinations of methotrexate, bleomycin, doxorubicin, cyclophosphamide, adriamycin, vincristine, corticosteroids ± cranial radiation • CHOP & BACOD + GM–CSF
CNS lymphoma	• Cranial radiation + high dose corticosteroids ± chemotherapy
Dermatophytic fungi	• Topical miconazole or clotrimazole • Refractory: Ketoconazole 200 mg PO/day × 1 to 3 mos. or itraconazole 100 mg/day × 1 to 3 mos. • Nails: Terbinafine 250 mg PO/day × 6 wks. (fingernails) or 12 wks. (toenails) or itraconazole 200 mg PO bid 1 wk/mo × 2 (fingernails) or × 3 to 4 mos (toenails).
Eosinophilic folliculitis	• Astemizole 10 mg/day + topical steroids • Ultraviolet light • Antihistamine (first generation-sedating antihistamines)

Condition	Treatment
Molluscum contagiosum	• HAART, cryotherapy, electrosurgery, curettage, topical cantharidin, or cidofovir
Scabies	• Permethrin cream 5% × 12 hrs.; Repeat 3 to 7 days later (must apply to all skin surfaces); • Topical lindane: Apply to all surfaces except face • Ivermectin 200 mcg/kg × 1
Seborrhea	• Steroid cream (hydrocortisone 1%) ± precipitated sulfur (desonide cream) or topical ketoconazole bid • Scalp-shampoo with selenium sulfide, zinc pyrithione, salicylic acid, coal tar applied daily or ketoconazole shampoo
Staph. folliculitis	• Cephalexin or dicloxacillin 500 mg PO qid × 7 to 21 days
Aphthous ulcers	**Standard** • Topical fluocinonide 0.05% ointment mixed 1:1 with orabase to facilitate application • Mouth washes with dexamethasone (0.5 mg/mL), *Dyclone* (10%), *Benadryl* or viscous lidocaine (2%) (Mile's solution) • Prednisone 40 mg/day PO × 1 to 2 wks., then taper (severe cases) or *Decadron* 0.5 mg/5 mL elixir rinse 1–3×/day **Refractory** • Thalidomide 200 mg PO day × 4 to 6 wks., then 100 mg 2×/wk. • Colchicine 1.5 mg/day
Oral hairy leukoplakia (OHL)	• Usually not treated • Acyclovir 800 mg PO 5×/day × 2 to 3 wks., then 1.2–2 gm/day (famciclovir, valacyclovir, valganciclovir, foscarnet and ganciclovir should be effective) • Tretinoin (*Retin* A) 0.025–0.05% solution applied 2–3×/day
Esophagitis	• **Candida:** Fluconazole, • **CMV:** Ganciclovir, • **HSV:** IV Acyclovir, • **Aphthous:** Prednisone 40 mg/day × 2 wks. then taper slowly or thalidomide 200 mg/day
Diarrhoea Microbial agent specific	**Cryptosporidiosis:** Paromomycin + atovaquone. **Isospora:** TMP-SMX. **Microsporidia:** Albendazole (septata intestinalis only). **Salmonella:** Ciprofloxacin 500 mg PO bid × >14 days; TMP- SMX 1. DS bid × >14 days; cefotaxime 4–8 g/day IV **Shigella:** TMP-SMX 1 DS bid × 3 days; ciprofloxacin 500 mg PO bid × 3 days **E. coli** (Traveler's diarrhoea): ciprofloxacin 500 mg PO bid × 3 days or TMP-SMX 1 DS tid × 3 days **E. histolytica:** Metronidazole 750 mg IV or PO × 5 to 10 days + paromomycin 500 mg PO tid × 7 days **Giardia:** Metronidazole 250–750 mg PO tid × 7 to 10 days
Symptomatic treatment	• Diet modification: Avoid caffeine, fat and milk and/or milk products • Diphenoxylate/atropine (*Lomotil*), loperamide, paregoric (Antiperistaltic agents are contraindicated with *C. difficile* or *E. coli* 0157)
Hepatitis	**HCV** • Indications to treat: Biopsy evidence of bridging fibrosis or moderate inflammation and necrosis + no contraindication to drugs (depression, etc) + patient acceptance + stable HIV • Peginterferon: 180 mcg/wk. (Roche) or 1.5 mcg/kg/wk. (Schering), each with ribavirin 10.6 mg/kg/day × 48 wks. **HBV** • 3 TC 150 mg bid (with concurrent HIV treatment) or 100 mg PO/day or Interferon 30–35 mil U/wk. × 4 mos; famciclovir and adefovir also active.

Appendix V
Prophylaxis of Opportunistic Infections in HIV/AIDS

Prophylaxis to Prevent First Episode of Opportunistic Disease in Adults and Adolescents Infected with Human Immunodeficiency Virus Preventive Regimens (CDC-Guidelines)

Strongly Recommended as Standard of Care

Pathogen	Indication	First choice	Alternative
Pneumocystis carinii	CD4+ count <200/μL or oropharyngeal candidiasis	Trimethoprim-sulfamethoxazole (TMP-SMZ), 1 DS po qd (AI) TMP-SMZ, 1 SS po qd (AI)	Dapsone, 50 mg po bid *or* 100 mg po qd (BI); dapsone, 50 mg po qd *plus* pyrimethamine, 50 mg po qw *plus* leucovorin 25 mg po qw (BI); dapsone 200 mg po plus pyrimethamine, 75 mg po plus leucovorin, 25 mg po qw (BI); aerosolized pentamidine, 300 mg q.month via Respirgard II^TM nebulizer (BI); atovaquone, 1500 mg po qd (BI); TMP-SMZ, 1 DS po tiw (BI)
Mycobacterium tuberculosis Isoniazid-sensitive	TST reaction ≥5 mm or prior positive TST result without treatment or contact with case of active tuberculosis regardless of TST result (BIII)	Isoniazid, 300 mg po *plus* pyridoxine, 50 mg po qd x 9 mo (AII) or isoniazid, 900 mg po *plus* pyridoxine, 100 mg po biw x 9 mo (BII)	Rifampin, 600 mg po qd (BIII) x 4 mo or rifabuin 300 mg po qd (CIII) x 4 mo Pyrazinamide, 15-20 mg/kg po qd x 2 mo *plus* either rifampin, 600 mg po qd (BI) x 2 mo or rifabutin, 300 mg po qd (CIII) x 2 mo
Isoniazid-resistant	Same as above; high probability of exposure to isoniazid-resistant tuberculosis	Rifampin 600 mg po (AIII) or rifabutin, 300 mg po (BIII) pd x 4 mo	Pyrazinamide 15-20 mg/kg po pd plus either rifampin, 600 mg po (BI) or rifabutin, 300 mg po (CIII) qd x 2 mo
Multidrug-(isoniazid and rifampin) resistant	Same as above; high probability of exposure to multidrug-resistant tuberculosis	Choice of drugs requires consultation with public health authorities. Depends on susceptibility of isolate from source patient	——

Pathogen	Indication	First choice	Alternative
Toxoplasma gondii	IgG antibody to Toxoplasma and CD4+ count <100/μL	TMP-SMZ, 1 DS po qd (AII)	TMP-SMZ, 1 SS po qd (BIII): dapsone, 50 mg po qd *plus* pyrimethamine, 50 mg po qw *plus* leucovorin, 25 mg po qw BI); dapsone, (200 mg po plus pyrimethamine, 75 mg po *plus* leucovorin, 25 mg po q w (BI); atovaquone, 1500 mg po qd with or without pyrimethamine, 25 mg po qd plus leucovorin, 10 mg po qd (CIII)
Mycobacterium avium complex	CD4+ count <50/μL	Azithromycin 1,200 mg po qw, (AI) or clarithromycin 500 mg po bid (AI)	Rifabutin, 300 mg po, qd (BI): azithromycin, 1,200 mg po qw *plus* rifabutin, 300 mg po qd (CI)
Varicella zoster virus(VZV)	Significant exposure to chickenpox or shingles for patients who have no history of either condition or, if available, negative antibody to VZV	Varicella zoster Immune globulin (VZIG), 5 vials (1.25 mL each) im, administered ≤96 h after exposure, ideally within 48 h (AIII)	

II. Generally Recommended

Pathogen	Indication	First choice	Alternative
Streptococcus pneumoniae	CD4+ count ≥ 200/μL	23 valent poly saccharide vaccine, 0.5 mL im [BII]	None
Hepatitis B virus	All susceptible (anti-HBc-negative)	Hepatitis B vaccine 3 doses (BII)	None
Influenza virus	All patients (annually, before influenza season)	Inactivated trivalent influenza virus vaccine: one annual dose(0.5 mL) im (BIII)	Oseltamivir, 75 mg po qd (influenza A or B) rimantadine, 100 mg po bid (CIII), or amantadine, 100 mg po bid (CIII) influenza A only)
Hepatitis A virus	All susceptible (anti-HAV-negative patients at increased risk for HAV infection (e.g., illicit drug users, men who have sex with men, haemophiliacs) or with chronic liver disease, including chronic hepatitis B or hepatitis C	Hepatitis A vaccine two doses (BIII)	None

III. Evidence for Efficacy doubtful, but Not Routinely Indicated

Pathogen	Indication	First choice	Alternative
Bacteria	Neutropenia	Granulocyte- Colony stimulating Factor (G-CSF), 5-10 μg/kg sc qd x 2-4 w or granulocyte-macrophage colony-stimulating factor (GM-CSF), 250 μg/m^2 sc iv x 2-4 w (CII)	None

Pathogen	Indication	First choice	Alternative
Cryptococcus neoformans	CD4+ count <50/μL	Fluconazole 100-200 mg po qd (CI)	Itraconazole capsule, 200 mg po qd (CIII)
Histoplasma capsulatum	CD4+ count <100/μL, endemic geographic area	Itraconazole capsule 200 mg po qd(CI)	None
Cytomegalovirus (CMV)	CD4+ count <50/μL and CMV antibody positivity (CI)	Oral ganciclovir 1g po tid	None

Prophylaxis to Prevent Recurrence of Opportunistic Disease in Adults (after chemotherapy for acute disease) in Adults and Adolescents Infected with Human Immunodeficiency Virus Preventive Regimens

Recommended as Standard of Care

Pathogen	Indication	First choice	Alternatives
Pneumocystis. carinii	Prior *P. carinii* pneumonia	Trimethoprim sulfamethoxazole (TMP-SMZ) 1 DS PO qd (AI); TMP-SMZ 1 SS po qd (AI)	Dapsone 50 mg po bid or 100 mg po qd (BI); dapsone 50 mg po qd *plus* pyrimethamine 50 mg po qw *plus* leucovorin 25 mg po qw (BI); dapsone 200 mg po *plus* pyrimethamine, 75 mg po plus leucovorin, 25 mg po qw (BI); aerosolized pentamidine, 300 mg qm via Respirgard II™ nebulizer (BI); atovaquone 1500 mg po qd (BI); TMP-SMZ, 1 DS po tiw (CI)
Toxoplasma gondii	Prior toxoplasmic encephalitis	Sulfadiazine 500-1,000 mg po qid. plus pyrimethamine, 25-50 mg po qd plus leucovorin 10-25 mg po qd (AI)	Clindamycin, 300-450 mg po q 6-8 h plus pyrimethamine, 25-50 mg po qd plus, leucovorin 10-25 mg po qd (BI); atovaquone 750 mg po q 6-12 h with or without pyrimethamine 25 mg po qd plus leucovorin, 10 mg po, qd (CIII)
Mycobacterium avium complex	Documented disseminated disease	Clarithromycin 500 mg po bid (AI) *plus* ethambutol, 15 mg/kg po qd(AII); with or without rifabutin, 300 mg po qd (CI)	Azithromycin 500 mg po qd (AII) *plus* ethambutol, 15 mg/kg po qd (AII); with or without rifabutin 300 mg po qd (CI)
Cytomegalovirus	Prior end-organ disease	Ganciclovir 5-6 mg/kg/day iv 5-7 days/wk or 1,000 mg po tid (AI) or foscarnet, po 90-120 mg/kg iv qd AI) or (for retinitis) ganciclovir sustained-release implant	Cidofovir 5 mg/kg iv qow with probenecid 2 grams 3 hours before the dose followed by 1 gram po 2 hours after the dose and 1 gram po 8 hours after the dose,(total of 4 grams) (AI).

Pathogen	Indication	First choice	Alternative
		q 6-9 months *plus* ganciclovir, 1.0-1.5 g tid (AI)	Fomivirsen 1 vial (330 μg) injected into the vitreous, then repeated every 2-4 wks (AI); valganciclovir 900 mg po qd (BI)
Cryptococcus neoformans	Documented disease	Fluconazole, 200 mg po qd (AI)	Amphotericin B 0.6-1.0 mg/kg iv qw-tiw (AI); itraconazole, 200 mg capsule po qd (BI)
Histoplasma capsulatum	Documented disease	Itraconazole capsule200 mg po bid (AI)	Amphotericin B 1.0 mg/kg iv qw (AI)
Coccidioides immitis	Documented disease	Fluconazole, 400 mg po qd (AII)	Amphotericin B, 1.0 mg/kg iv qw (AI); itraconazole, 200 mg capsule po bid (AII)
Salmonella species,	Bacteremia	Ciprofloxacin, 500 mg po bid for several months(BII)	Antibiotic chemoprophylaxis with another active agent (CIII)

II. Recommended only if subsequent episodes are frequent or severe

Pathogen	Indication	First choice	Alternative
Herpes simplex virus	Frequent/severe recurrences	Acyclovir, 200 mg po tid or 400 mg po bid (AI) Famciclovir 250 mg po bid (AI)	Valacyclovir, 500 mg po bid (CIII)
Candida (oropharyngeal or vaginal)	Frequent/severe recurrences	Fluconazole 100-200 mg, po qd (CI)	Itraconazole solution 200 mg po qd (CI);
Candida (esophageal)	Frequent/severe recurrences	Fluconazole 100-200 mg po qd (BI)	Itraconazole solution, 200 mg po qd (BI);

Prophylaxis to Prevent First Episode of Opportunistic Disease in Infants and Children Infected with Human Immunodeficiency Virus

Strongly Recommended as Standard of Care

Pathogen	Indication	First Choice	Alternatives
Pneumocystis carinii	HIV-infected or HIV-indeterminate, infants aged 1-12 mo;	Trimethoprim- sulfamethoxazole (TMP-SMZ), 150/750 mg/m 2 /d in 2 divided doses po tiw on consecutive days (AII)	Dapsone (children aged >1 mo), 2mg/kg(max 100 mg) po qd or 4 mg/kg (max 200 mg) po qw (CII);
	HIV-infected children aged 1-5 yr with CD4+ count <500/μL or CD4+ percentage <15%;	Acceptable alternative dosage schedules: (AII)	Aerosolized pentamidine (children aged >5 yr), 300 mg qm via Respirgard nebulizer™ (CIII);
	HIV-infected children II aged 6-12 yr with CD4+percentage <15%	•Single dose po on tiw consecutive days •2 divided doses po qd 2 divided doses qd or po tiw on alternate days	Atovaquone (children aged 1-3 mo; and >24 mo, 30mg/kg po qd; children aged4-24 mo, 45 mg/kg po qd(CII)
Mycobacterium	TST reaction, >5mm *or* prior	Isoniazid 10-15 mg/kg max	Rifampin, 10-20

Pathogen	Indication	First choice	Alternative
tuberculosis Isoniazid-sensitive	positive TST result without treatment; or contact with any case of active tuberculosis regardless of TST result	300 mg) po qd x 9 mo (AII) or 20-30 mg/kg (max900) mg po biw x 9 months (BII)	mg/kg (max 600 mg) po qd x 4-6 mo (BIII)
Isoniazid-resistant	Same as above; high probability of exposure to isoniazid-resistant tuberculosis	Rifampin, 10-20 mg/kg (max 600 mg) po qd x 4-6 mo (BIII)	Uncertain
Multidrug-(isoniazid and rifampin) resistant	Same as above; high probability of exposure to multi-drug resistant tuberculosis	Choice of drugs requires consultation with public helath authorities and depends on susceptibility of isolate from source patient	
Mycobacterium avium complex	For children aged>6 yrs, CD4+ count<50/μL; aged 2-6 yrs CD4+ count <75/μL; aged 1-2 yrs, CD4+ count <500/μL; aged <1 yr, CD4+ count <750/μL	Clarithromycin7.5 mg/kg(max 500 mg) po bid (AII), or azithromycin,20 mg/kg (max 1,200 mg) po qw (AII)	Azithromycin, 5 mg/kg 2 (max 250 mg) po qd (AII); children aged ≥6 yrs rifabutin, (max 300 mg po qd (BI)
Varicella zoster virus	Significant exposure to varicellaor shingles with no history of chickenpox or shingles	Varicella zoster i mmune globulin (VZIG), 1 vial (1.25 mL)/10 kg (max 5 vials) im, administered <96 hrs after exposure, ideally within 48 hrs (AII)	None

Generally Recommended

Pathogen	Indication	First choice	Alternative
Toxoplasma gondii	IgG antibody to *Toxoplasma* and severe immunosuppression	TMP-SMZ150/750 mg/m^2/d in 2 divided doses po qd (BIII)	Dapsone (children aged >1 mo), 2mg/kg or 15 mg/m^2 (max 25 mg) po qd *plus* pyrimethamine, 1 mg/kg po qd *plus* leucovorin, 5 mg po every 3 days (BIII) Atovaquone, (aged 1-3 mo and >24 mo, 30 mg/kg po qd; aged 14-24 mo 45 mg/kg po qd) (CIII)
Varicella zoster virus	HIV-infected children who are asymptomatic and not immunosuppressed	Varicella zoster vaccine (see vaccine- preventable pathogens section of this table) (BII)	None
Influenza virus	All patients (annually before influenza season)	Inactivated split trivalent influenza vaccine (see vaccine Preventable section of this table) (BIII)	Oseltamivir (during outbreaks of influenza-A or B) for children ≥ 13 years, 75 mg po qd (CIII); rimantadine or amantadine (during outbreaks of influenza A); aged 1-9 yr, 5 mg/kg in 2 divided doses (max 150 mg/day) po qd; aged ≥10 yr, use adult doses (CIII).

Pathogen	Indication	First choice	Alternative
III. Not Recommended for Most Children; Indicated for Use Only in Unusual Circumstances			
Invasive bacterial infection	Hypogamma globulinemia (i.e., IgG) <400 mg/dL)	IVIG (400mg/kg every 2-4 weeks) (AI)	None
Cryptococcus neoformans	Severe immunosuppression	Fluconazole, 3-6 mg/kg po qd (CII)	Itraconazole, 2-5 mg/kg po every 12-24 h (CII)
Histoplasma capsulatum	Severe immunosuppression endemic geographic area	Itraconazole, 2-5 mg/kg po every 12-24 h (CIII)	None

Prophylaxis to Prevent Recurrence of Opportunistic Disease (after chemotherapy for acute disease) in HIV-infected Infants and Children Preventive Regimens

Recommended for life as standard of care			
Pneumocystis carinii	Prior *P. carinii* pneumonia	TMP-SMZ, 150/750 mg/m²/d in 2 divided doses po tiw on consecutive days (AII) Acceptable alternative schedules for same dosage: (AII) Single dose po tiw on consecutive days; 2 divided doses po qd; 2 divided doses po tiw on alternate days	Daposne (children aged≥1 mo), 2mg/kg (max 100 mg) po qd or 4 mg/kg (max 200 mg) po qw (CII); aerosolized pentamidine (children aged≥5yrs), 300 mg qm via Respirgard II™ nebulizer (CIII); atovaquone (aged 1-3 months and>24 mo., 30 mg/kg po qd aged 4-24 mo., **45 mg/kg po qd**) (CII)
Toxoplasma gondii	Prior toxoplasmic encephalitis	Sulfadiazine, 85-120 mg/kg/d in 2-4 divided doses po qd, *plus* pyrimethamine 1 mg/kg or 15 mg/m² (max 25 mg) po qd *plus* leucovorin, 5 mg po every 3 days (AI)	Clindamycin, 20-30 mg/kg/d in 4 divided doses po qd plus pyrimethamine, 1 mg/kg po qd *plus* leucovorin, 5 mg po. every 3 days (BI)
Mycobacterium avium	Prior disease	Clarithromycin, 7.5 mg/kg (max 500 mg) po bid (AII) *plus* ethambutol 15 mg/kg (max 900 mg) po qd (AII); with or without rifabutin, 5 mg/kg (max 300 mg) po qd (CII)	Azithromycin, 5 mg/kg (max 250 mg) po qd (AII, *Plus* ethambutol, 15 mg/kg (max 900 mg) po qd (AII); with or without rifabutin, 5 mg/kg (max 300 mg) po qd (CII)
Cryptococcus neoformans	Documented disease	Fluconazole, 3-6 mg/kg po qd (AII)	Amphotericin B, 0.5-1.0 mg/kg iv 1-3x/week (AI);

Recommended for life as standard of care

			Itraconazole, 2-5 mg/kg po every 12-24h (BII).
Histoplasma capsulatum	Documented disease	Itraconazole, 2-5 mg/kg po every 12-48 h (AIII)	Amphotericin B, 1.0 mg/kg iv qw (AIII)
Coccidioides immitis	Documented disease	Fluconazole, 6 mg/kg po qd (AIII)	Amphotericin B, 1.0 mg/kg iv qw (AIII); Itraconazole, 2-5 mg/kg po every 12-48 h (AIII)
Cytomegalovirus	Prior end-organ disease	Ganciclovir, 5 mg/kg iv qd or foscarnet, 90-120 mg/kg iv qd (AI)	(For retinitis) Ganciclovir sustained-release *Plus* ganciclovir, 30 mg/kg po tid (BIII)
Salmonella species (non-typhi)	Bacteremia	TMP-SMZ, 150/750 mg/m^2 in 2 divided doses po qd for several months (CIII)	Antibiotic chemoprophylaxis with another active agent (CIII)

Recommended only if subsequent episodes are frequent or severe.

Invasive bacterial Infections	>2 infections in 1-year period	TMP-SMZ, 150/750 mg/m^2, in 2 divided doses po qd (BI); or IVIG, 400 mg/kg every 2-4 wks. (BI)	Antibiotic chemoprophylaxis with another active agent (BIII)
Herpes simplex virus	Frequent/severe recurrences	Acyclovir, 80 mg/kg/d in 3-4 divided doses po qd (AII)	
Candida (oropharyngeal)	Frequent/severe recurrences	Fluconazole, 3-6 mg/kg po qd (CIII)	
Candida (esophageal),	Frequent/severe recurrences	Fluconazole, 3-6 mg/kg po qd (BIII)	Itraconazole solution 5 mg/kg po qd (CIII);

System used to rate the strength of recommendations and quality of supporting evidence

Rating	Strength of the Recommendation
A	Both strong evidence for efficacy and substantial clinical benefit support recommendation for use. **Should always be offered**.
B	Moderate evidence for efficacy — or strong evidence for efficacy but only limited clinical benefit — supports recommendation for use. **Should generally be offered**.
C	Evidence for efficacy is insufficient to support a recommendation for or against use. Or evidence for efficacy might not outweigh adverse consequences (e.g., drug toxicity, drug interactions) or cost of the chemoprophylaxis or alternative approaches. **Optional.**
D	Moderate evidence for lack of efficacy or for adverse outcome supports a recommendation against use. **Should generally not be offered**.
E	Good evidence for lack of efficacy or for adverse outcome supports a recommendation against use. **Should never be offered**.

Recommended for life as standard of care

Quality of evidence supporting the recommendation

I   Evidence from at least one properly randomized, controlled trial.

II   Evidence from at least one well-designed clinical trial without randomization, from cohort or case-controlled analytic studies (preferably from more than one centre), or from multiple time-series studies. Or dramatic results from uncontrolled experiments.

III   Evidence from opinions of respected authorities based on clinical experience, descriptive studies, or reports of expert committees.

Appendix VI
Postexposure Prophylaxis (PEP)

Fig. 1.   Determining the Need for HIV PostexposureProphylaxis (PEP) after an Occupational Exposure★

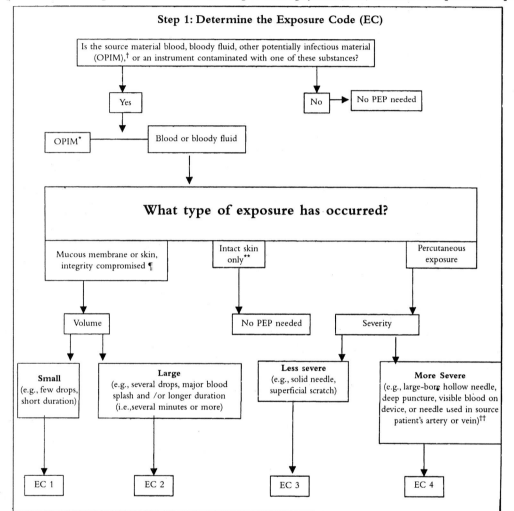

★ this algorithm is inteded to guide initial decisions about PEP and should be used in conjunction with other guidance provided in this report.

† Semen or vaginal secretions; cerebrospinal, synovial, pleural, peritoneal, pericardial, or amniotic fluids; or tissue.

- Exposures to OPIM must be evaluated on a case-by-case basis. In general, these body substances are considered a lowrisk for transmission in health-care settings. Any unprotected contact to concentrated HIV in a research laboratory or production facility is considered an occupational exposure that requires clinical evaluation to determine the need for PEP.

¶ Skin integrity is considered compromised if there is evidence of chapped skin, dermatitis, abrasion, or open wound.

★★ Contact with intact skin is not normally considered a risk for HIV transmission. However, if the exposure was to blood, and the circumstance suggests a higher volume exposure (e.g., an extensive area of skin was exposed or there was prolonged contact with blood), the risk for HIV transmission should be considered.

†† The combination of these severity factors (e.g., large-bore hollowneedle and deep puncture) contribute to an elevated risk for transmission if the source person is HIV-positive.

Fig 1. Determining the Need for HIV Postexposure Prophylaxis (PEP) after an Occupational Exposure★ — *Continued*

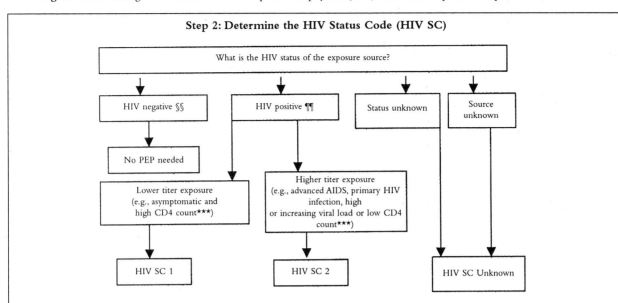

Step 2: Determine the HIV Status Code (HIV SC)

§§ A source is considered negative for HIV infection if there is laboratory documentation of a negative HIV antibody, HIV polymerase chain reaction (PCR), or HIV p24 antigen test result from a specimen collected at or near the time of exposure and there is no clinical evidence of recent retroviral-like illness.

¶¶ A source is considered infected with HIV (HIV positive) if there has been a positive laboratory result for HIV antibody, HIV PCR, or HIV p24 antigen or physician-diagnosed AIDS.

★★★ Examples are used as surrogates to estimate the HIV titer in an exposure source for purposes of considering PEP regimens and do not reflect all clinical situations that may be observed. Although a high HIV titer (HIV SC 2) in an exposure source has been associated with an increased risk for transmission, the possibility of transmission from a source with a low HIV titer also must be considered.

STEP 3: Determine the PEP Recommendation

EC HIV SC PEP recommendation

EC	HIV SC	
1	1	**PEP may not be warranted.** Exposure type does not pose a known risk for HIV transmission. Whether the risk for drug toxicity outweighs the benefit of PEP should be decided by the exposed HCW and treating clinician.
1	2	**Consider basic regimen.** ††† Exposure type poses a negligible risk for HIV transmission. A high HIV titer in the source may justify consideration of PEP. Whether the risk for drug toxicity outweighs the benefit of PEP should be decided by the exposed HCW and treating clinician.
2	1	**Recommend basic regimen.** Most HIV exposures are in this category; no increased risk for HIV transmission has been observed but use of PEP is appropriate.
2	2	**Recommend expanded regimen.** §§§ Exposure type represents an increased HIV transmission risk.
3	1 or 2	**Recommend expanded regimen.** Exposure type represents an increased HIV transmission risk.
Unknown		If the source or, in the case of an unknown source, the setting where the exposure occurred suggests a possible risk for HIV exposure and the EC is 2 or 3, consider PEP basic regimen.

††† Basic regimen is four weeks of zidovudine, 600 mg per day in two or three divided doses, and lamivudine, 150 mg twice daily.

§§§ Expanded regimen is the basic regimen plus either indinavir, 800 mg every 8 hours, or nelfinavir, 750 mg three times a day.

Table 1.   Basic and Expanded Postexposure Prophylaxis Regimens

Regimen category	Application	Drug regimen
Basic	Occupational HIV exposures for which there is a recognized transmission risk (Figure 1).	4 weeks (28 days) of both zidovudine 600 mg every day in divided doses (i.e., 300 mg twice a day, 200 mg three times a day, or 100 mg every 4 hours) and lamivudine 150 mg twice a day.
Expanded	Occupational HIV exposures that pose an increased risk for transmission (e.g., larger volume of blood and/or higher virus titer in blood) (Figure 1).	Basic regimen plus either indinavir 800 mg every 8 hours or nelfinavir 750 mg three times a day.★

★Indinavir should be taken on an empty stomach (i.e., without food or with a light meal) and with increased fluid consumption (i.e., drinking six 8 oz glasses of water throughout the day); nelfinavir should be taken with meals.

Index

Bold number indicates start of the chapter that contains main discussion of the topic